To my husband, Hu Odom, with loving appreciation
for his patience, support, and encouragement.

—*Evie Thomson*

Essentials of Dental Radiography

for Dental Assistants and Hygienists

EIGHTH EDITION

Orlen N. Johnson, BS, DDS, MS
College of Dentistry
University of Nebraska Medical Center
Lincoln, Nebraska

Evelyn M. Thomson, BSDH, MS
Gene W. Hirschfeld School of Dental Hygiene
Old Dominion University
Norfolk, Virginia

PEARSON
Prentice Hall

Upper Saddle River, New Jersey 07458

Library of Congress Cataloging-in-Publication Data

Johnson, Orlen N.
Essentials of dental radiography for dental assistants and hygienists / Orlen N. Johnson, Evelyn M. Thomson.— 8th ed.
p. ; cm.
Includes bibliographical references and index.
ISBN 0-13-171008-7
1. Teeth—Radiography. 2. Dental assistants. I. Thomson, Evelyn M. II. Title.
[DNLM: 1. Radiography, Dental. 2. Dental Assistants. 3. Dental Hygienists. WN 230 J68e 2007]
RK309.D44 2007
617.6'07572—dc22

2006008912

Notice:
The authors and the publisher of this volume have taken care that the information and technical recommendations contained herein are based on research and expert consultation, and are accurate and compatible with the standards generally accepted at the time of publication. Nevertheless, as new information becomes available, changes in clinical and technical practices become necessary. The reader is advised to carefully consult manufacturers' instructions and information material for all supplies and equipment before use, and to consult with a healthcare professional as necessary. This advice is especially important when using new supplies or equipment for clinical purposes. The authors and publisher disclaim all responsibility for any liability, loss, injury, or damage incurred as a consequence, directly or indirectly, of the use and application of any of the contents of this volume.

Publisher: Julie Levin Alexander
Assistant to Publisher: Regina Bruno
Executive Editor: Mark Cohen
Associate Editor: Melissa Kerian
Editorial Assistant: Nicole Ragonese
Media Editor: John J. Jordan
Director of Production and Manufacturing: Bruce Johnson
Managing Production Editor: Patrick Walsh
Production Liaison: Christina Zingone
Production Editor: Jessica Balch, Pine Tree Composition
Manufacturing Manager: Ilene Sanford
Manufacturing Buyer: Pat Brown
Design Director: Cheryl Asherman
Design Coordinator: Christopher Weigand
Cover Designer: Gary Sella
Director of Marketing: Karen Allman
Senior Marketing Manager: Harper Coles
Manager of Media Production: Amy Peltier
Media Project Manager: Stephen Hartner
Composition: Pine Tree Composition, Inc.
Printer/Binder: Courier Westford
Cover Printer: Phoenix Color Corporation

Pearson Education Ltd., *London*
Pearson Education Australia Pty. Limited,
Pearson Education Singapore, Pte. Ltd.
Pearson Education North Asia Ltd., *Hong Kong*
Pearson Education Canada, Ltd., *Toronto*
Pearson Education—Japan, *Tokyo*
Pearson Educación de Mexico, S.A. de C.V.
*Sydney*Pearson Education Malaysia, Pte. Ltd.
Pearson Education, Upper Saddle River, New Jersey

PEARSON
Prentice Hall

10 9 8 7 6 5 4 3 2 1
ISBN 0-13-171008-7

CONTENTS

PREFACE

More than any other subject taught to oral healthcare professionals, dental radiography requires an understanding of theoretical concepts and a mastery of the skills needed to apply these concepts. *Essentials of Dental Radiography for Dental Assistants and Hygienists* provides the student with a clear link between theory and practice. Straightforward and well balanced, *Essentials of Dental Radiography for Dental Assistants and Hygienists* provides in-depth, comprehensive information that is appropriate for an introductory course in dental radiography, without overwhelming the student with non-essential information. It is comprehensive to prepare students for board and licensing examinations and, at the same time, practical, with practice points, procedure boxes, and suggested lab activities that prepare students to apply theory to clinical practice and patient management.

True to its title, *Essentials of Dental Radiography for Dental Assistants and Hygienists* clearly demonstrates its ability to explain concepts that both dental assistants and dental hygienists must know. The examples and case studies used throughout the book include situations that pertain to the roles of both dental assistants and dental hygienists as members of the oral healthcare team.

Essentials of Dental Radiography for Dental Assistants and Hygienists is student-friendly, beginning each chapter with learning objectives from both the knowledge and the application levels. Each objective is tested by study questions presented at the end of the chapter, allowing the student to assess learning outcomes. The objectives and study questions are written in the same order that the material appears in the chapter, guiding the student through assimilation of the chapter content. Key words are listed at the beginning of each chapter and bolded within the text with their definitions, and realistic rationales for learning the material are presented in each chapter introduction. The chapter outline provides a ready reference to locate the topics covered. Meaningful case studies relate directly to radiological applications presented in the chapter and challenge students to apply the knowledge learned in the reading to real-life situations through decision-making activities.

The twenty-eight chapters of the eighth edition have been organized into nine topic sections.

- History and Radiation Basics
- Biological Effects of Radiation and Radiation Protection
- Dental X-ray Film and Processing Techniques
- Dental Radiographer Fundamentals
- Intraoral Techniques
- Radiographic Errors and Quality Assurance
- Mounting and Viewing Dental Radiographs
- Patient Management and Supplemental Techniques
- Extraoral Techniques

Educators can easily utilize the chapters and topic sections in any order and have the option to tailor what material is covered in their courses. The sequencing of material for presentation in this text begins with the basics of radiation physics, biological effects, and protection to give the student the necessary background to operate safely, followed by a description of the radiographic equipment, film, and film processing to help the student understand how radiation is utilized for diagnostic purposes. Prior to learning radiographic techniques, the student will study the fundamentals of infection control, legal and ethical responsibilities, and patient relations. The student will then be prepared to begin to develop the intraoral technique skills necessary to produce diagnostic quality periapical, bitewing, and occlusal radiographs; and learn to mount, evaluate, and interpret the images. Following the interpretation chapters, the student will now possess the basic skills of intraoral radiography and is ready to grasp supplemental techniques and alterations of these basic skills by studying management of special patients. This is also a logical time to discuss digital radiography since this topic fits in with variations on the basics. After all intraoral study is complete, the book ends with extraoral and panoramic techniques.

Educators who have used former editions of this text will recognize immediately that a thorough revision has taken place. These changes represent your request for an up-to-date book that speaks to both dental assisting and dental hygiene students, provides comprehensive information without overwhelming the student with non-essential details and is student-centered. Outstanding features and specific improvements in this edition include the following:

- Updated information on "F" speed film; the new periodontal diseases classification system; the new guidelines from the ADA on selecting patients for radiographs; and the latest research on low dose radiation exposure and low birth weight outcomes.
- Two new chapters: *Recognizing Deviations from Normal Radiographic Anatomy* (chapter 20) and *Supplemental Radiographic Techniques* (chapter 25)
- All chapters were critically evaluated to remove dated material, condense duplicate material, and to improve the presentation of the topics by reorganizing the material covered in each chapter. While the number of chapters (28) remains the same, many chapters now contain more logically ordered content.
- The addition of procedure boxes, which highlight and simplify critical steps of radiographic procedures to prepare students for laboratory application of theory and serve as student outlines, laboratory practice exercises, or as a handy reference when providing radiographic services in a clinical setting.
- The addition of practice points, which call student attention to possible use of theory in real-life situations, providing a "mental break" from studying theory by illustrating how that theory is applied.
- The addition of meaningful case studies to each chapter.
- Suggested activities are included for possible lab exercises, research outside of class time, essay writing, and investigation using the Internet.
- Over 400 new or revised board examination-type study questions have been written. Each question relates back to the objectives at the beginning of the chapter, allowing the student to assess their understanding of the material presented.
- More than 150 new photographs, radiographs, diagrams, and tables have been added or improved.

The focus of the 8th edition of *Essentials of Dental Radiography for Dental Assistants and Hygienists* is on the individual responsibility of the oral radiographer and conveys to the reader the importance of understanding what ionizing radiation is and what it is not; protecting oneself, the patient, and the oral healthcare team from unnecessary radiation exposure; practicing within the scope of the law and ethically treating all patients; producing diagnostic quality radiographs and appropriately correcting errors that diminish radiographic quality; knowing when and how to apply supplemental techniques; and assisting in the interpretation of radiographs for the benefit of the patient.

Whereas *Essentials of Dental Radiography for Dental Assistants and Hygienists* is written primarily for dental assisting and dental hygiene students, practicing dental assistants, dental hygienists, and dentists may find this book to be a helpful reference; particularly when preparing for a re-licensing examination in another jurisdiction. Additionally, *Essentials of Dental Radiography for Dental Assistants and Hygienists* may be a valuable study guide for on-the-job-trained (OJT) oral healthcare professionals who may be seeking radiation safety certification credentials.

ACKNOWLEDGMENTS

A sincere thank you to Dr. Orlen Johnson, for his confidence in selecting me as his co-author for the 8th edition of *Essentials of Dental Radiography for Dental Assistants and Hygienists*. I am truly honored. Thank you also to Mark Cohen, Executive Editor, and Melissa Kerian, Associate Editor, at Prentice Hall and to Jessica Balch, Production Editor, at Pine Tree Composition for their guidance and patience. The quality of this edition is the direct result of the assistance and support of the students, faculty, and staff at the Gene W. Hirschfeld School of Dental Hygiene at Old Dominion University. I would like to express my appreciation to senior dental hygiene students Jennifer Thomas and Ann Poindexter for their assistance with the photographs.

Evelyn Thomson

REVIEWERS

Patricia Boudreau, RDH, MSEd
Program Director, Dental Hygiene
College of Lake County
Grayslake, Illinois

Barbara Bush, RDH, MSEd
Associate Professor, Allied Health
Western Kentucky University
Bowling Green, Kentucky

Barbara J. Crowley, CDA, MEd
Former Department Chair (Retired), Dental Hygiene and Dental Assisting
Pima County Community College
Tucson, Arizona

Sharon K. Dickinson, CDA, CDPMA, RDA, AAS
Program Director, Dental Assisting
El Paso Community College
El Paso, Texas

Tracey Green, BS, CDA
Instructor, Dental Assisting
Massasoit Community College
Canton, Massachusetts

Rita Hallock, RDH, MEd
Assistant Professor, Dental Hygiene
Brevard Community College
Cocoa, Florida

Kristyn Hawkins, RDH
Clinical Lecturer, Dental Education
Indiana University South Bend
South Bend, Indiana

Terri L. Heintz, CDA, RDA
Instructor, Dental Assisting
Des Moines Area Community College
Ankeny, Iowa

Catherine Holl
Instructor, Dental Assisting
San Diego Mesa College
San Diego, California

Linda White Kamp, CDA, BS
Program Head, Dental Assisting
Rowan-Cabarrus Community College
Salisbury, North Carolina

Barbara MacMillan, RDH, CDA, MS
Assistant Professor, Dental Education
Indiana University South Bend
South Bend, Indiana

Betty J. Reynard, RDH, EdD
Program Coordinator, Dental Hygiene
Lamar Institute of Technology
Beaumont, Texas

Pamela J. Sandy, RDH, BS, MA
Professor, Dental Hygiene
Valencia Community College
Orlando, Florida

Donna Solovan-Gleason, RDH, PhD
Program Director, Dental Hygiene
Hillsborough Community College
Tampa, Florida

Shaun Tate, MAEd
Chairperson, Allied Dental Program
Asheville-Buncombe Technical Community College
Asheville, North Carolina

Pam Wood, CDA, RDH, MEd, CAGS
Associate Professor, Dental Hygiene
Community College of Rhode Island
Lincoln, Rhode Island

PART I • HISTORY AND RADIATION BASICS

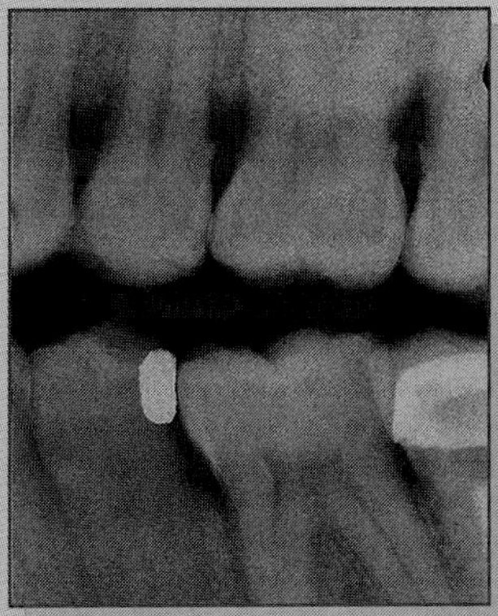

1

History of Dental Radiography

■ OBJECTIVES

Following successful completion of this chapter, you should be able to:

1. Define the key words.
2. State when x-rays were discovered and by whom.
3. Trace the history of radiography, noting the prominent contributors.
4. List two historical developments that made dental x-ray machines safer.
5. Explain how rectangular PIDs reduce patient radiation exposure.
6. Identify the two techniques used to expose dental radiographs.
7. List at least five uses of dental radiographs.
8. Become aware of other imaging modalities available for use in the detection and evaluation of oral conditions.

■ KEY WORDS

Bisecting technique
Computed tomography (CT)
Cone
Digital imaging
Dosage
Magnetic resonance imaging (MRI)
Oral radiography
Panoramic radiography
Paralleling technique
Position indicating device (PID)
Radiograph
Radiography
Radiology
Roentgen ray
Roentgenograph
Tomography
X-ray
X-ray film

CHAPTER OUTLINE

Introduction

Technological advancements continue to impact the way we deliver oral health care. While new methods for diagnosing disease and treatment planning comprehensive care are being introduced, dental radiographs, the images produced by x-rays, remain the basis for many diagnostic procedures and play an essential role in oral health care. **Radiography** is the making of radiographs by exposing and processing x-ray film. The purpose of dental radiography is to provide the oral health care team with radiographs of the best possible diagnostic quality. The goal of dental radiography is to obtain the highest quality radiographs while maintaining the lowest possible radiation exposure risk for the patient.

Dental assistants and dental hygienists meet an important need through their ability to produce diagnostic quality radiographs. The basis for development of the skills needed to expose, process, mount and evaluate radiographic images is a thorough understanding of radiology concepts. All individuals working with radiographic equipment should be educated and trained in the theory of x-ray production. The concepts and theories regarding x-ray production that emerged during the early days of x-radiation discovery are responsible for the quality health care available today. The purpose of this chapter is to present a historical perspective that recognizes the contributions of the early pioneers who supplied us with the fundamentals upon which we practice today and advance toward the future.

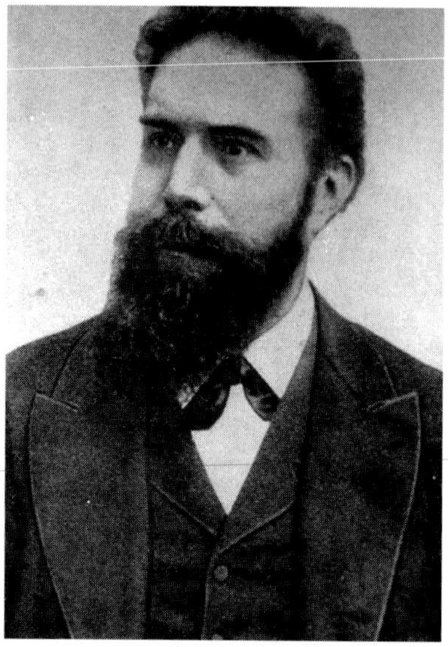

FIGURE 1–1 **Wilhelm Conrad Roentgen (1845–1923).** (Reprinted with permission from Radiology Centennial, Inc., Copyright 1993)

Discovery of the X-ray

Oral **radiology** is the study of x-rays and the techniques used to produce radiographs. We begin that study with the history of dental radiography and the discovery of the x-ray. The x-ray revolutionized the methods of practicing medicine and dentistry by making it possible to visualize internal body structures non-invasively. Professor Wilhelm Conrad Roentgen's (pronounced "rent'gun") (Figure 1–1) experiment in Bavaria (Germany) on November 8, 1895, produced a tremendous advance in science. Professor Roentgen's curiosity was aroused during an experiment with a vacuum tube called a Crookes tube (named after William Crookes, an English chemist). He observed that a fluorescent screen near the tube began to glow when the tube was activated by passing an electric current through it. Examining this strange phenomenon further, he noticed that shadows could be cast on the screen by interposing objects between it and the tube. Further experimentation showed that such shadow images could be permanently recorded on photographic film (Figure 1–2). For his work, Dr. Roentgen was awarded the first Nobel Prize for physics, in 1901.

In the beginning, Roentgen was uncertain of the nature of this invisible ray that he had discovered. When he later reported his finding at a scientific meeting he spoke of it as an **x-ray** because the symbol *x* represented the unknown. After his findings were reported and published, fellow scientists honored him by calling the invisible ray the **roentgen ray** and the image produced on photosensitive film a **roentgenograph.** Because a photographic negative and an x-ray film have basic similarity and the x-ray closely resembles the radio wave, the prefix *radio-* and the suffix *-graph* have been combined into **radiograph.** The latter term is used by oral health care professionals because it is more descriptive than x-ray and easier to pronounce than roentgenograph.

Early Pioneers

A few weeks after Professor Roentgen announced his discovery, Dr. Otto Walkhoff, a German physicist, was the first to expose a prototype of a dental radiograph. This was accomplished by covering a small, glass photographic plate with black paper to protect it from light, and then wrapping it in a sheath of thin rubber to prevent moisture damage during the 25 minutes that he held the film in his mouth. A similar exposure can now be made in 1/10 second. The resulting radiograph was experimental and had little diagnostic value because it was impossible to prevent film movement, but it did prove that the x-ray would have a role in dentistry. The length of the exposure made the experiment a dangerous one for Dr. Walkhoff; the dangers of overexposure to radiation were not known at that time.

We will probably never know who made the first dental radiograph in the United States. It was either Dr. William Herbert Rollins, a Boston dentist and physician, Dr. William James Morton, a New York physician, or Dr. C. Edmund Kells, a New Orleans dentist. Dr. Rollins was one of the first to alert the profession to the need for radiation hygiene and protection and is considered by many to be the first advocate for the science of radiation protection. Unfortunately, his advice was not taken seriously by many of his fellow practitioners for a long time.

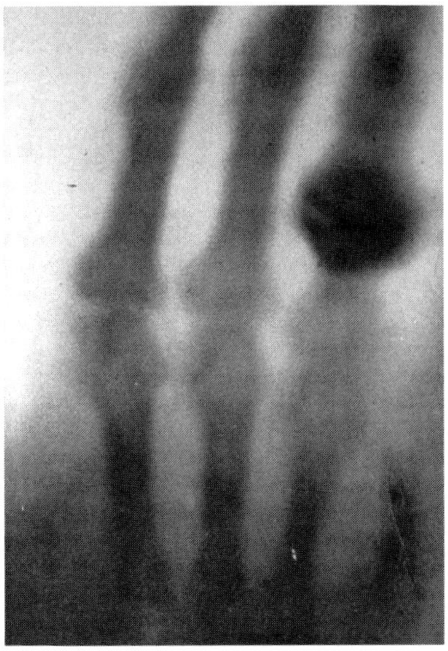

FIGURE 1-2 This famous radiograph, purported to be Mrs. Bertha Roentgen's hand, was taken on December 22, 1895. (Reprinted with permission from Radiology Centennial, Inc., Copyright 1993)

Dr. Morton is known to have taken radiographs very early, on skulls. He gave a lecture on April 24, 1896, before the New York Odontological Society calling attention to the possible usefulness of roentgen rays in dental practice. One of Dr. Morton's radiographs revealed an impacted tooth, which was otherwise undetectable.

Most people claim Dr. Kells took the first dental radiograph on a living subject in the United States. He was the first to put the radiograph to practical use in dentistry. Dr. Kells made numerous presentations to organized dental groups and was instrumental in convincing many dentists that they should use **oral radiography** as a diagnostic tool. At that time, it was customary to send the patient to a hospital or physician's office on those rare occasions when dental radiographs were prescribed.

Two other dental x-ray pioneers should be mentioned, William David Coolidge and Howard Riley Raper. The most significant advancement in radiology came in 1913 when Dr. Coolidge, working for the General Electric Company, introduced the hot cathode tube. The x-ray output of the Coolidge tube could be predetermined and accurately controlled. Professor Raper, Indiana Dental College, wrote the first dental radiology textbook, *Elementary and Dental Radiology*, and introduced bitewing radiographs in 1925.

Because x-rays are invisible, the pioneers in the field of radiography were not aware that continued exposure produced accumulations of radiation effects in the body and, therefore, could be dangerous to both patient and radiographer. When radiography was in its infancy, it was common practice for the dentist or dental assistant to help the patient hold the film in place while making the exposure. These oral health care professionals were exposed to unnecessary radiation. Frequent repetition of this practice endangered their health and occasionally led to permanent injury or death. Fortunately, although the hazards of prolonged exposure to radiation are not completely understood, scientists have learned how to reduce them drastically by proper use of fast film, safer x-ray machines, and strict adherence to safety protocol.

Practice Point

Never hold the film packet in the patient's oral cavity during the exposure. If the patient can not tolerate film packet placement or hold still throughout the exposure, the patient's parent or guardian may have to be utilized to assist or an extraoral radiograph may have to be substituted. The parent or guardian should be protected with lead, or lead equivalent barriers such as an apron or gloves when they will be in the path of the beam.

Today, when almost half of the radiation-producing equipment used in the United States is in dental offices, it is worth noting that initially few hospitals and only the most progressive physicians and dentists possessed x-ray equipment. This limited use of dental radiography can be attributed to the fact that the early equipment was primitive and sometimes dangerous. Also, x-rays were used for entertainment purposes by charlatans at fairgrounds so people often associated them with quackery. Resistance to change, ignorance, apathy, and fear delayed the widespread acceptance of radiography in dentistry for years.

Table 1–1 lists the early dental radiology pioneers.

Dental X-ray Machines

Dental x-ray machines manufactured before 1920 were an electrical hazard to oral health care professionals because of the open, uninsulated high-voltage supply wires. In 1919, William David Coolidge and General Electric introduced the Victor CDX shockproof dental x-ray machine. The x-ray tube and high-voltage transformer were placed in an oil-filled compartment that acted as a radiation shield and electrical insulator. Modern x-ray machines use this same basic construction. Variable, high-kilovoltage machines were introduced in the middle 1950s, allowing increased target–film distances to be used, which in turn increased the use of the paralleling technique.

Within the last 30 years, major progress has been made in restricting the size of the x-ray beam. One such development is the replacement of the pointed **cone** through which x-rays pass from the tube head toward the patient by open cylinders. When the pointed cones were first used, it was not realized that the x-rays were scattered through contact with the material of the cones. Because cones were used for so many years, many still refer to the open cylinders or rectangular tubes as cones.

TABLE 1-1 **Early Dental Radiology Pioneers**

Name	Event	Year
W. C. Roentgen	Discovered x-rays	1895
C. E. Kells	May have taken first dental radiograph in U.S.	1896
W. J. Morton	May have taken first dental radiograph in U.S.	1896
W. H. Rollins	May have taken first dental radiograph in U.S.	1896
	Published "X Light Kills," warning of x-ray dangers	1901
O. Walkhoff	First to make a dental radiograph	1896
W. A. Price	Suggested basics for both bisecting and paralleling techniques	1904
A. Cieszynski	Applied "rule of isometry" to bisecting technique	1907
W. D. Coolidge	Introduced the hot cathode tube	1913
H. R. Raper	Wrote first dental x-ray textbook	1913
	Introduced bitewing radiographs	1924
F. W. McCormack	Developed paralleling technique	1920
G. M. Fitzgerald	Designed a "long-cone" to use with the paralleling technique	1947

The term **position indicating device (PID)** is more descriptive of its function of directing the x-rays, rather than of its shape. A further improvement has been the introduction of rectangular lead-lined PIDs. These limit the size of the x-ray beam that strikes the patient to the actual size of the dental film (Figure 1–3).

Panoramic radiography became popular in the 1960s with the introduction of the panoramic x-ray machine. Panoramic units are capable of exposing the entire dentition and surrounding structures on a single film. Today, many oral health care practices have a panoramic x-ray machine.

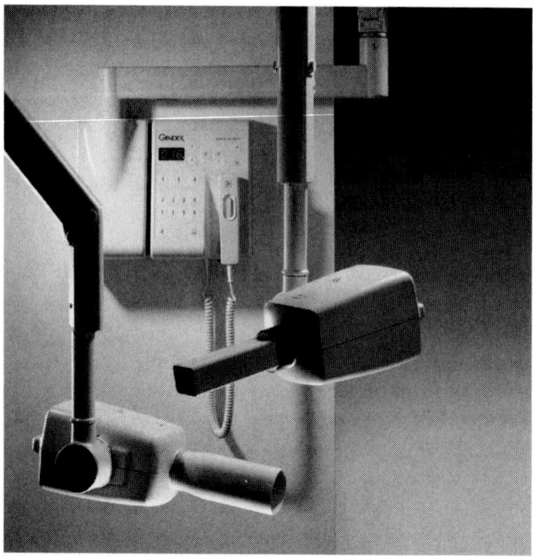

FIGURE 1–3 **Comparison of circular and rectangular PIDs.** (Image courtesy of Gendex Dental Corporation)

Dental X-ray Film

Early dental **x-ray film** packets consisted of glass photographic plates wrapped in black paper and rubber. In 1913, the Eastman Kodak Company marketed the first hand-wrapped, moisture-proof dental x-ray film packet. It wasn't until 1919 that the first machine-wrapped dental x-ray film packet became commercially available (from Kodak).

Early film had emulsion on only one side and required long exposure times. Today, both sides of the dental x-ray film are coated with emulsion and require only about 1/16th the amount of exposure required 50 years ago.

The film base has also greatly improved. Early base material was cellulose nitrate, which was highly flammable. In the 1920s, cellulose acetate replaced the nitrate base and was used until the early 1960s, when polyester (Dacron) was introduced. With the introduction of automatic film processors, it was necessary to have a thinner base that did not warp.

Dental X-ray Techniques

Two basic techniques are employed in intraoral radiography. The first and earliest technique is called the **bisecting technique.** The second and newer technique is referred to as the **paralleling technique.** The paralleling method is the technique of choice and is taught in all dental assisting, dental hygiene, and dental schools.

In 1904, Dr. Weston A. Price suggested the basics of both the bisecting and paralleling techniques. As others were working on the same problems and were unaware of Price's contributions, the credit for developing the techniques went to others.

In 1907, A. Cieszynski, a Polish engineer, applied the *rule of isometry* to dental radiology and is given credit for suggesting the bisecting technique. The bisecting technique was the only method used for many years.

The search for a less complicated technique that would produce better radiographs more consistently resulted in the development of the paralleling technique by Dr. Franklin McCormack in 1920. Dr. G. M. Fitzgerald, Dr. McCormack's son-in-law, designed a long "cone" PID and made the paralleling technique more practical in 1947.

Advancements in the Use of Dental Radiography

Today, few oral health care practices are without x-ray units; many have a unit in each operatory and supplement these with a panoramic-type x-ray machine. It is difficult to imagine how a modern oral health care practice would be able to provide quality care for patients without radiography (Figure 1–4). While no diagnosis can be based solely on radiographic evidence without a visual and physical examination, many conditions might go undetected if not for radiographic examinations (Table 1–2).

Radiography, aided by the introduction of transistors and computers, is benefited by the incorporation of minicomputer technology that permits significant radiation reduction in modern x-ray units. The introduction of a computed approach with instant images (both radiographic and photographic) has the potential greatly to improve the quality of dental care. This recent and exciting advancement in dental radiography is called **digital imaging** (Chapter 26). Digital imaging systems used in dentistry replace film with an alternative sensor. Image sensors now are comparable to film in dimensions of the exposed field of view and approach film in overall radiographic quality. Their advantages include a reduction in radiation **dosage,** and there is no need for the purchase of film and processing chemistry, or the disposal of spent chemicals hazardous to the environment.

Other imaging modalities routinely used in medicine often aid in the diagnosis and treatment planning of oral conditions.

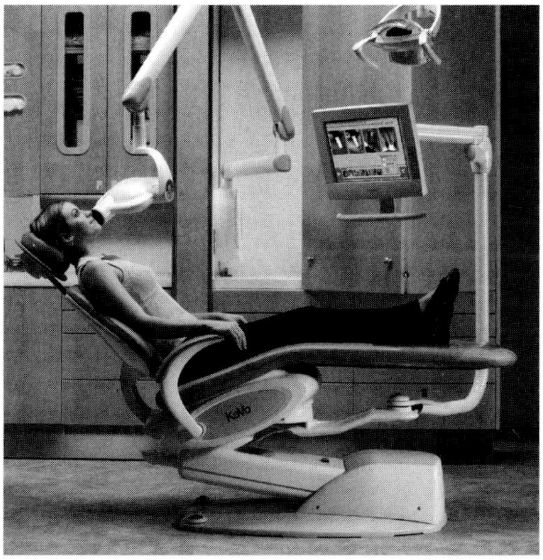

FIGURE 1–4 **Radiography in a modern oral health care practice.** (Image courtesy of Gendex Dental Corporation)

TABLE 1–2 **Uses of Dental Radiographs**

- To detect, confirm, and classify dental diseases and lesions
- To detect and evaluate trauma
- To evaluate growth and development
- To detect missing and supernumerary (extra) teeth
- To document the dental condition of a patient
- To educate the patient about their dental health

While not commonly performed in dental practices, the dental assistant and the dental hygienist should be aware of these procedures and be familiar with how these diagnostic techniques compare to oral radiography. Dental patients may be referred for such images, and copies of these images may be sent to the dental practice for interpretation and consultation. Imaging techniques such as tomography, computed tomography, and magnetic resonance imaging are just three types of imaging modalities occasionally used to aid in the diagnosis of oral conditions.

Tomography is a method of radiography by which a single selected plane is radiographed, with the outlines of structures in other planes eliminated. This principle is used in most panoramic-type x-ray machines and in evaluating the temporomandibular joint (TMJ) and dental implants.

Computed tomography (CT) scanning has been used since the early 1970s. CT images require the use of radiation, but are computer-generated and need no film or film–screen combinations. Originally called CAT scans, CTs are used in dentistry for diagnosing lesions—especially within the salivary glands—and for planning implant cases.

Magnetic resonance imaging (MRI) is a technique for obtaining cross-sectional pictures of the human body without exposing the patient to x-rays. The patient is placed within a large MRI machine that generates a static magnetic field. The nuclei of certain atoms within the body react to the magnetic field, and a picture is obtained. Non-ionizing radiofrequency energy is used to produce the images instead of x-rays. In dentistry, MRIs are used to visualize soft tissue components of the temporomandibular joint and to view pathologic conditions.

The discovery of x-radiation revolutionized the practice of preventive oral health care. Future technological advances undoubtedly will improve both the diagnostic use and the safety of radiography in the years ahead.

REVIEW—Chapter Summary

Professor Wilhelm Conrad Roentgen's discovery of the x-ray on November 8, 1895 revolutionized the methods of practicing medicine and dentistry by making it possible to visualize internal body structures non-invasively. The usefulness of the x-ray as a diagnostic tool was recognized almost immediately and many dental radiology pioneers contributed to its advancement. The use of radiographs in medical and dental diagnostic procedures is now essential.

Important roles for the dental assistant and the dental hygienist include exposing, processing, mounting, and evaluating dental radiographs. It is of vital importance that the person taking the x-ray exposure understands how x-rays are produced, controlled, and used to achieve the best diagnostic results.

Improved equipment, advanced techniques, and educated personnel make it possible to obtain radiographs with high diagnostic value and minimal risk of unnecessary radiation to patient or operator.

RECALL—Study Questions

For questions 1–5, match each term with its definition.

a. Radiograph
b. Radiography
c. Radiology
d. Roentgen ray
e. X-ray

________ 1. The study of x-radiation.
________ 2. Image or picture produced by x-rays.
________ 3. An older term given to x-radiation in honor of its discoverer.
________ 4. The original term Roentgen applied to the invisible ray he discovered.
________ 5. The making of radiographs by exposing and processing x-ray film.

6. Who discovered the x-ray?
   a. C. Edmund Kells
   b. William Rollins
   c. Franklin McCormack
   d. Wilhelm Conrad Roentgen
7. When were x-rays discovered?
   a. 1695
   b. 1795
   c. 1895
   d. 1995
8. Who is believed to have exposed the prototype of the first dental x-ray film?
   a. A. Cieszynski
   b. Otto Walkhoff
   c. Wilhelm Conrad Roentgen
   d. C. Edmund Kells
9. Who is considered by many to be the first advocate for the science of radiation protection?
   a. Weston Price
   b. William Morton
   c. William Herbert Rollins
   d. Franklin McCormack
10. Dental x-ray machines replaced the original pointed "cone" with an open-cylinder PID to reduce the size of the x-ray beam *and* to reduce the radiation dose to the patient.
    a. The first part of the statement is true but the second part of the statement is false.
    b. The first part of the statement is false but the second part of the statement is true.
    c. Both parts of the statement are true.
    d. Both parts of the statement are false.
11. Who is given credit for suggesting the bisecting technique?
    a. A. Cieszynski
    b. William Rollins
    c. G. M. Fitzgerald
    d. Otto Walkhoff
12. Who is given credit for developing the paralleling technique?
    a. W. D. Coolidge
    b. H. R. Raper
    c. William Morton
    d. Franklin McCormack
13. List five uses of dental radiographs.
    a. ____________________
    b. ____________________
    c. ____________________
    d. ____________________
    e. ____________________
14. Which imaging modality does not require the use of ionizing radiation?
    a. Magnetic resonance imaging
    b. Computed tomography
    c. Digital imaging
    d. Tomography

REFLECT—Case Study

Your patient today tells you that she recently watched a television documentary on the dangers of excess radiation exposure. Based on your reading in this chapter, develop a brief conversation between you and this patient explaining how historical developments have increased dental radiation safety, in order to put the patient at ease.

RELATE—Laboratory Application

Perform an inventory of the x-ray machine used in your facility. Using the historical lessons learned in this chapter, identify the parts of the x-ray machine, type of film or digital sensor used, and the safety protocol and posted exposure factors in place. Specifically list the following:

a. Unit manufacturer
   Using the Internet, research the manufacturer's Web site to determine the company origin. How old is the company? Are they a descendant of an original manufacturer? Who developed the design for the x-ray unit produced today? Do they offer different unit designs? What is the reason your facility chose this model?
b. Shape and length of the PID
   Does the machine you are observing reduce radiation exposure? Why or why not? Why was the PID you are observing chosen over other shapes and lengths?
c. Names of the dials on the control panel.
   How does this differ from the dental x-ray machines used in dental practices in the early 1900s? What exposure factors are inherent to the unit, and what factors may be

varied by the radiographer? What are the advantages and disadvantages to using an x-ray machine where the exposure settings are fixed? Variable?

d. What are the recommended exposure settings for various types of radiographs? How do these differ from the settings used by the early pioneers?

e. Describe the film or digital sensor used to produce a radiographic image.

   What is the film size, speed, and how is it packaged? Does the film or sensor used in your facility allow you to produce a quality radiograph using the least amount of radiation? What is the rationale for using this film type in your facility?

f. Are the safety protocols regarding unit operation known to all operators? How is this made evident? List the safety protocols in place in your facility.

BIBLIOGRAPHY

Eastman Kodak. *Radiation Safety in Dental Radiography.* Rochester, NY: Eastman Kodak, 1998.

Langland, O. E., Langlais, R. P., Preece, J. W. *Principles of Dental Imaging,* 2nd ed. Philadelphia: Williams & Wilkins, 2002.

White, S. C., Pharoah, M. J. *Oral Radiology. Principles and Interpretation,* 5th ed. St. Louis: Elsevier, 2004.

2

Characteristics and Measurement of Radiation

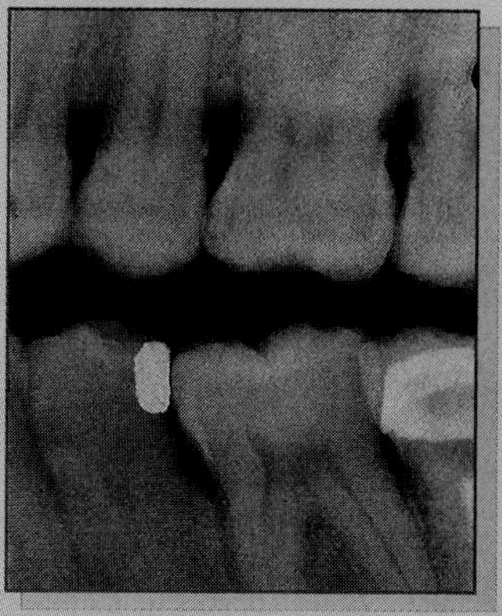

CHAPTER OUTLINE

■ OBJECTIVES

Following successful completion of this chapter, you should be able to:

1. Define the key words.
2. Draw and label a typical atom.
3. Describe the process of ionization.
4. Differentiate between radiation and radioactivity.
5. Discuss the difference between particulate radiation and electromagnetic radiation and give two examples of each.
6. Explain the relationship between wavelength and frequency.
7. Explain the inverse relationship between wavelength and penetrating power of x-rays.
8. List the properties of x-rays.
9. List and describe the two processes by which kinetic energy is converted to electromagnetic energy.
10. List and describe the four possible interactions of dental x-rays with matter.
11. Define the terms used to measure x-radiation.
12. Match the traditional terms of x-radiation measurement to the corresponding Système Internationale (SI) units.
13. Identify three sources of naturally occurring background radiation.

■ KEY WORDS

Absorbed dose
Absorption
Alpha particle
Angstrom (Å)
Atom
Atomic number
Atomic weight
Background radiation
Beta particle
Binding energy
Characteristic radiation
Coherent scattering
Compton effect (scattering)
Coulombs per kilogram (C/kg)
Decay
Dose
Dose equivalent
Electromagnetic radiation

Electromagnetic spectrum	Neutron
Electron	Photoelectric effect
Element	Photon
Energy	Proton
Energy levels	Rad
Exposure	Radiation
Frequency	Radioactivity
Gamma rays	Radiolucent
General/bremsstrahlung radiation	Radiopaque
Gray (Gy)	Rem
Hard radiation	Roentgen (R)
Ion	Secondary radiation
Ion pair	Sievert (Sv)
Ionizing radiation	Soft radiation
Ionization	Système Internationale
Isotope	Velocity
Kinetic energy	Wavelength
Molecule	Weighting factor

Introduction

The word "radiation" is attention-grabbing. When news headlines incorporate words such as *radiation*, *radioactivity*, and *exposure*, the reader pays attention to what follows. Patients often link dental x-rays with other types of radiation exposures they read about or see on TV. Patients assume that oral health care professionals who are responsible for taking dental x-rays are knowledgeable regarding all types of ionizing radiation exposures and can adequately answer their questions. While the study of quantum physics is beyond the scope of this book, it is important that dental assistants and dental hygienists understand what dental radiation is, what it can do, and what it cannot do. In this chapter we will explore the characteristics of x-radiation and look at where dental x-rays fit in relation to other types and sources of radiations.

Prior to studying the production of x-rays, the radiographer should have a base knowledge of atomic structure. The scientist understands the world to consist of matter and energy. Matter is defined as anything that occupies space and has mass. Thus all things that we see and recognize are forms of matter. Energy is defined as the ability to do work and overcome resistance. Heat, light, electricity, and x-radiation are forms of energy. Matter and energy are closely related. Energy is produced whenever the state of matter is altered by natural or artificial means. The difference between water, steam, and ice is the amount of energy associated with the molecules. Such an energy exchange is produced within the x-ray machine and will be discussed later.

Atomic Structure

To understand radiation, we must understand atomic structure. Currently we know of 105 basic **elements** occurring either singly or in combination in natural forms. Each element is made up of atoms. An **atom** is the smallest particle of an element that still retains the properties of the element. If any given atom is split, the resulting components no longer retain the properties of the element. Atoms are generally combined with other atoms to form molecules. A **molecule** is the smallest particle of a substance that retains the properties of that substance. A simple molecule such as sodium chloride (table salt) contains only two atoms, whereas a complex molecule like DNA (deoxyribonucleic acid) may contain hundreds of atoms.

Atoms are extremely minute and are composed of three basic building blocks: electrons, protons, and neutrons.

- **Electrons** have a negative charge and are constantly in motion orbiting the nucleus.
- **Protons** have a postitive charge. The number of protons in the nucleus of an element determines its **atomic number.**
- **Neutrons** have no charge.

The atom's arrangement in some ways resembles the solar system (Figure 2–1). The atom has a nucleus as its center or sun, and the electrons revolve around it like planets. The protons and neutrons form the central core or nucleus of the atom. The electrons orbit around the nucleus in paths called shells or energy levels. Normally, the atom is electrically neutral, having equal numbers of protons in its nucleus and electrons in orbit.

The nucleus of all atoms except hydrogen contains at least one proton and one neutron (hydrogen in its simplest form has only a proton). Some atoms contain a very high number of each. The electrons and the nucleus normally remain in the same position relative to one another. To accommodate the electrons revolving about the nucleus, the larger atoms have several concentric orbits at various distances from the nucleus. These are referred to as electron shells, which some chemists now call

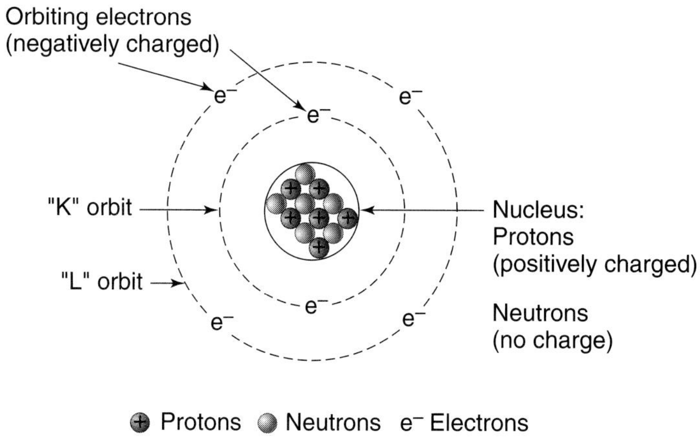

FIGURE 2-1 **Diagram of carbon atom.** In the neutral atom, the number of positively charged protons in the nucleus is equal to the number of negatively charged orbiting electrons. The innermost orbit or energy level is the K shell, the next is the L shell, and so on.

energy levels. The innermost level is referred to as the K shell, the next as the L shell, and so on, up to 7 shells (Figure 2–1).

Electrons are maintained in their orbits by the positive attraction of the protons known as **binding energy.** The binding energy of an electron is strongest in the intermost K shell and becomes weaker in the outer shells.

Ionization

Atoms that have gained or lost electrons are electrically unstable and are called ions. An **ion** is defined as a charged particle. The formation of ions is easier to understand if we review the normal structural arrangement of the atom. The atom normally has the same number of protons (positive charges) in the nucleus as it has electrons (negative charges) in the orbital levels. When one of these electrons is removed from its orbital level in a neutral atom, the remainder of the atom loses its electrical neutrality.

An atom from which an electron has been removed has more protons than electrons, is positively charged, and is called a positive ion. The negatively charged electron that has been separated from the atom is a negative ion. The positively charged atom ion and the negatively charged electron ion are called an **ion pair. Ionization** is the formation of ion pairs. When an atom is struck by an x-ray photon, an electron may be dislodged and an ion pair created (Figure 2–2). As high-energy electrons travel on, they push out (like charges repel) electrons from the orbits of other atoms, creating additional ion pairs. These unstable ions attempt to regain electrical stability by combining with another oppositely charged ion.

Ionizing Radiation

Radiation is defined as the emission and movement of **energy** through space in the form of electromagnetic radiation (x- and **gamma rays**) or particulate radiation (**alpha** and **beta particles**). Any radiation that produces ions is called **ionizing radiation.** Only a portion of the radiation portrayed on the electromagnetic spectrum, the x-rays and the gamma and cosmic rays, are of the ionizing type. In dental radiography, our concern is limited to the changes that may occur in the cellular structures of the tissues as the ions are produced by the passage of x-rays through the cells. The mechanics of biologic tissue damage is explained in Chapter 5.

Radioactivity

Radioactivity is defined as the process whereby certain unstable elements undergo spontaneous disintegration (decay) in an effort to attain a stable nuclear state. Unstable **isotopes** are radioactive and attempt to regain stability through the release of energy, by a process known as **decay.** Dental x-rays do not involve the use of radioactivity.

Scientists have learned to produce several types of radiations that are identical to natural radiations. Ultraviolet waves are produced artificially for sun lamps or fluorescent lights and for numerous other uses. Another recent man-made radiation is the laser beam, whose potential impact on oral health is still being explored.

Electromagnetic Radiation

Electromagnetic radiation is the movement of wave-like energy through space as a combination of electric and magnetic fields. Electromagnetic radiations are arranged in an orderly fashion according to their energies in what is called the **electromagnetic spectrum** (Figure 2–3). The electromagnetic spectrum consists of an orderly arrangement of all known radiant energies. X-radiation is a part of the electromagnetic spectrum, which also includes cosmic rays, gamma rays, ultraviolet rays, visible light, infrared, television,

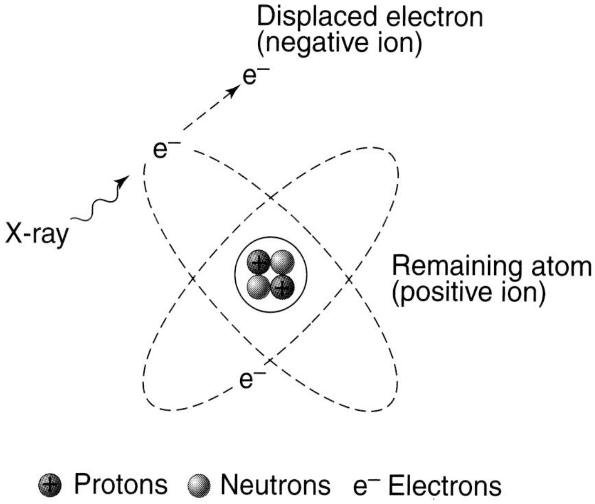

FIGURE 2-2 Ionization is the formation of ion pairs. When an atom is struck by an x-ray, an electron may be dislodged and an ion pair results.

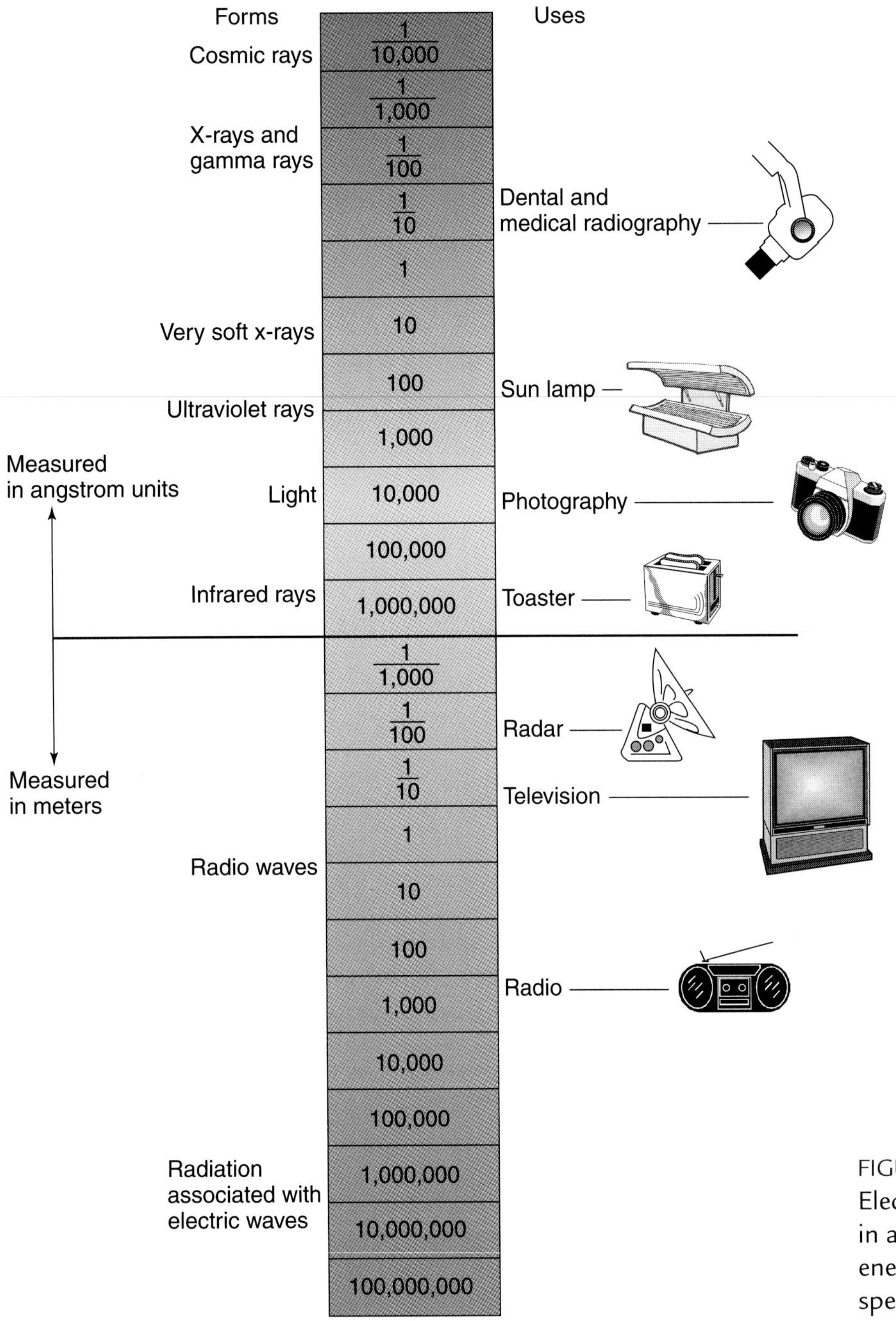

FIGURE 2–3 **The electromagnetic spectrum.** Electromagnetic radiations are arranged in an orderly fashion according to their energies in what is called the electromagnetic spectrum.

radar, microwave, and radio waves. All energies of the electromagnetic spectrum share the following properties:

- Travel at the speed of light
- Have no electrical charge
- Have no mass or weight
- Pass through space as particles and in a wave-like motion
- Give off an electrical field at right angles to their path of travel and a magnetic field at right angles to the electric field
- Have energies that are measurable and different

Electromagnetic radiations display two seemingly contradictory properties. They are believed to move through space as both a particle and a wave. Particle or quantum theory assumes the electromagnetic radiations are particles, or quanta. These particles are called photons. **Photons** are bundles of energy that travel through space at the speed of light. The wave theory assumes that electromagnetic radiation is propagated in the form of waves similar to waves resulting from a disturbance in water. Electromagnetic waves exhibit the properties of wavelength, frequency, and velocity.

- **Wavelength** is the distance between two similar points on two successive waves, as illustrated in Figure 2–4. The symbol for wavelength is the Greek letter lambda (λ). Wavelength may be measured in the metric system or in **angstrom (Å)** units (1 Å is about 1/250,000,000 in. or 1/100,000,000

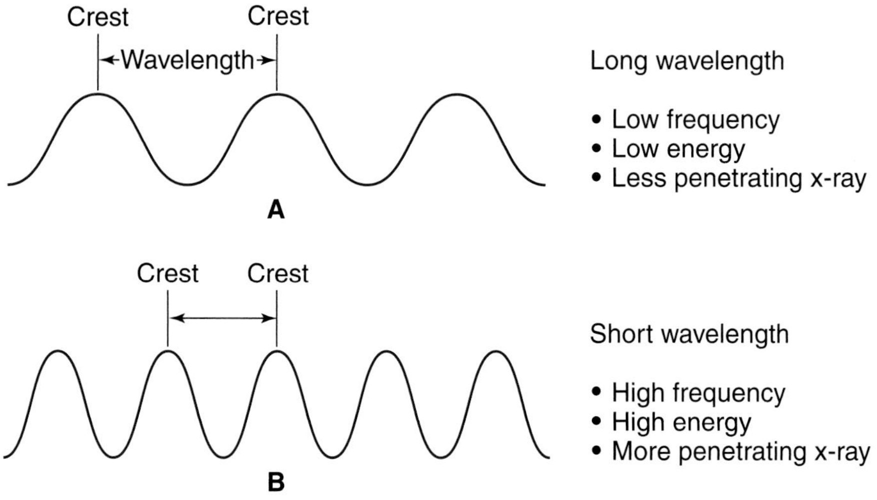

FIGURE 2–4 **Differences in wavelengths and frequencies.** Only the shortest wavelengths with extremely high frequency and energy are used to expose film in dental radiography. Wavelength is determined by the distances between the crests. Observe that this distance is much shorter in (**B**) than in (**A**). The photons that comprise the dental x-ray beam are estimated to have over 250 million such crests per inch. Frequency is the number of crests of a wavelength passing a given point per second.

cm). The shorter the wavelength, the more penetrating the radiation.

- **Frequency** is a measure of the number of waves that pass a given point per unit of time. The symbol for frequency is the Greek letter nu (ν). The special unit of frequency is the hertz (Hz). One hertz equals 1 cycle per second. The higher the frequency, the more penetrating the radiation.
- Wavelength and frequency are inversely related. When the wavelength is long, the frequency is low, resulting in low-energy, less penetrating x-rays (Figure 2–4). And when the wavelength is short, the frequency is high, resulting in high-energy, more penetrating x-rays.
- **Velocity** refers to the speed of the wave. In a vacuum, all electromagnetic radiations travel at the speed of light (186,000 miles/sec or 3×10^8 m/sec).

No clear-cut separation exists between the various radiations represented on the electromagnetic spectrum; consequently, overlapping of the wavelengths is common. Each form of radiation has a range of wavelengths. This accounts for some of the longer infrared waves being measured in meters, while the shorter infrared waves are measured in angstrom units. It therefore follows that all x-radiations are not the same wavelength. The longest of these are the Grenz rays, also called **soft radiation,** that have only limited penetrating power and are unsuitable for exposing dental radiographs. The wavelengths used in diagnostic dental radiography range from about 0.1 to 0.5 Å and are classified as **hard radiation,** a term meaning radiation with great penetrating power. Still shorter wavelengths are produced by super-voltage machines when greater penetration is required, as in some forms of medical therapy and industrial radiography.

Properties of X-rays

X-rays are believed to consist of minute bundles (or quanta) of pure electromagnetic energy called photons. These have no mass or weight, are invisible, and cannot be sensed. Because they travel at the speed of light (186,000 miles/sec or 3×10^8 meters/sec), these x-ray photons are often referred to as "bullets of energy." X-rays have the following properties. They

- Are invisible
- Travel in straight lines
- Travel at speed of light
- Have no mass or weight
- Have no charge
- Interact with matter causing ionization
- Can penetrate opaque tissues and structures
- Can affect photographic film emulsion (causing a latent image)
- Can affect biological tissue

X-ray photons have the ability to pass through gases, liquids, and solids. The ability to penetrate materials or tissues depends on the wavelength of the x-ray and the thickness and density of the object. The composition of the object or the tissues determines whether the x-rays will penetrate and pass through it or whether they will be absorbed in it. Materials that are extremely dense and have a high **atomic weight** will absorb more x-rays than thin materials with low atomic numbers. This partially explains why dense structures such as bone and enamel appear **radiopaque** (white or light gray) on the radiograph, whereas the less dense pulp chamber, muscles, and skin appear **radiolucent** (dark gray or black).

Production of X-rays

X-rays are generated inside an x-ray tube located in the tube head of a dental x-ray machine (Chapter 3). X-rays are produced whenever high-speed electrons are abruptly stopped or slowed down. Bodies in motion are believed to have **kinetic energy** (from the Greek word *kineticos*, "pertaining to motion"). In a dental x-ray tube, the kinetic energy of electrons is converted to electromagnetic energy by the formation of general or *bremsstrahlung* radiation (German for "braking") and characteristic radiation.

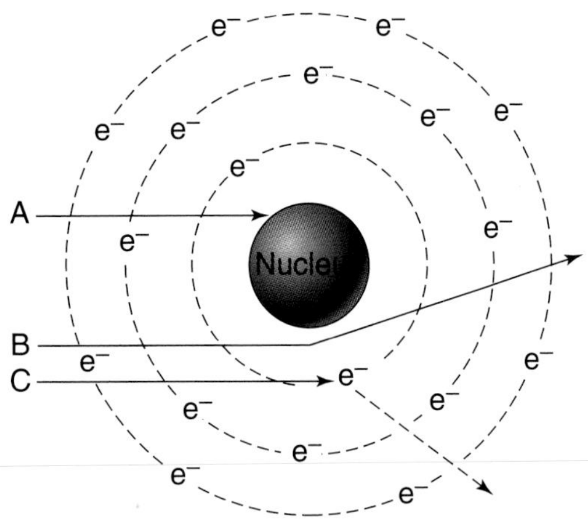

FIGURE 2-5 **General/bremsstrahlung and characteristic radiation.** High-speed electron (**A**) collides with the nucleus and all of its kinetic energy is converted into a single x-ray. High-speed electron (**B**) is slowed down and bent off its course by the positive pull of the nucleus. The kinetic energy lost is converted into an x-ray. The impact from both A and B electrons produce general radiation. Characteristic radiation is produced when high-speed electron (**C**) hits and dislodges a K shell (orbiting) electron. Another electron in an outer shell quickly fills the void and an x-ray is emitted. Characteristic radiation only occurs above 70 kVp with a tungsten target.

- **General/bremsstrahlung radiation** is produced when high-speed electrons are stopped or slowed down by the tungsten atoms of the dental x-ray tube. Referring to Figure 2–5, observe that the impact from both (A) and (B) electrons produce general/bremsstrahlung. When a high-speed electron collides with the nucleus of an atom in the target metal, as in (A), all of its kinetic energy is transferred into a single x-ray photon. In (B), a high-speed electron is slowed down and bent off its course by the positive pull of the nucleus. The kinetic energy lost is converted into an x-ray. The majority of x-rays produced by dental x-ray machines are formed by general/bremsstrahlung radiation.
- **Characteristic radiation** is produced when a bombarding electron from the tube filament collides with an orbiting K electron of the tungsten target as shown in Figure 2–5 (C). The K-shell electron is dislodged from the atom. Another electron in an outer shell quickly fills the void, and an x-ray is emitted. The x-rays produced in this manner are called characteristic x-rays. Characteristic radiation can only be produced when the x-ray machine is operated at or above 70 kilovolts (kVp) because a minimum force of 69 kVp is required to dislodge a K electron from a tungsten atom. Characteristic radiation is of minor importance because it accounts for only a very small part of the x-rays produced in a dental x-ray machine.

Interaction of X-rays with Matter

A beam of x-rays passing through matter is weakened and gradually disappears. Such a disappearance is referred to as **absorption** of x-rays. When so defined, absorption does not imply an occurrence such as a sponge soaking up water, but refers to the process of transferring the energy of the x-rays to the atoms of the material through which the x-ray beam passes. The basic method of absorption is ionization.

When a beam of x-rays pass through matter, four possibilities exist:

1. No interaction. The x-ray can pass through an atom unchanged and no interaction occurs (Figure 2–6). In dental radiography about 9 percent of the x-rays pass through the patient's tissues without interaction.
2. **Coherent scattering** (unmodified scattering, also known as Thompson scattering). When a low-energy x-ray passes near an atom's outer electron, it may be scattered without loss of energy (Figure 2–6). The incoming x-ray interacts with the electron by causing the electron to vibrate at the same frequency as the incoming x-ray. The incoming x-ray ceases to exist. The vibrating electron radiates another x-ray of the same frequency and energy as the original incoming x-ray. The new x-ray is scattered in a different direction than the original x-ray. Essentially, the x-ray is scattered unchanged. Coherent scattering accounts for about 8 percent of the interactions of matter with the dental x-ray beam.
3. **Photoelectric effect.** The photoelectric effect is an all-or-nothing energy loss. The x-ray imparts all of its energy to an orbital electron of some atom. This dental x-ray, since

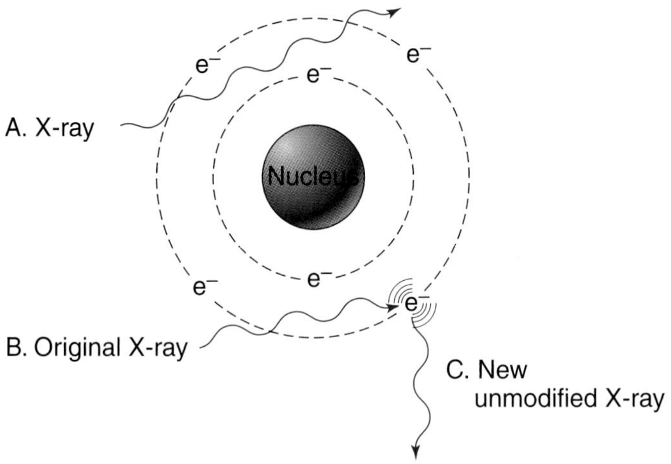

FIGURE 2-6 **X-rays interacting with atom.** X-ray (**A**) can pass through an atom unchanged and no interaction occurs. Incoming x-ray (**B**) interacts with the electron by causing the electron to vibrate at the same frequency as the incoming x-ray. The incoming x-ray ceases to exist. The vibrating electron radiates new x-ray (**C**) with the same frequency and energy as the original incoming x-ray. The new x-ray is scattered in a different direction than the original x-ray.

it consisted only of energy in the first place, simply vanishes. The electromagnetic energy of the x-ray is imparted to the electron in the form of kinetic energy of motion and causes the electron to fly from its orbit with considerable speed. Thus, an ion pair is created (Figure 2–7). Remember, the basic method of the interaction of x-rays with matter is the formation of ion pairs. The high-speed electron (called a photoelectron) knocks other electrons from the orbits of other atoms (forming secondary ion pairs) until all of its energy is used up. The positive ion atom combines with a free electron and the absorbing material is restored to its original condition. In dental radiography, the photoelectric effect interaction takes place during dental x-radiation production about 30 percent of the time.

4. **Compton effect.** The Compton effect (often called Compton scattering) is similar to the photoelectric effect in that the dental x-ray interacts with an orbital electron and ejects it. But in the case of Compton interaction, only a part of the dental x-ray energy is transferred to the electron and a new, weaker x-ray is formed and scattered in some new direction (Figure 2–8). This **secondary radiation** may even travel in a direction opposite to that of the original x-rays. The new x-ray may undergo another Compton scattering or it may be absorbed by a photoelectric effect interaction. The positive ion atom combines with a free electron and the absorbing material is restored to its original condition. Thus, it is important to remember that the Compton effect causes x-rays to be scattered in all directions.

A question often asked is, "Do x-rays make the material they pass through radioactive?" The answer is no. Dental x-rays have no effect on the nucleus of the atoms they interact with. Therefore, equipment, walls, and patients do not become radioactive after exposure to x-rays.

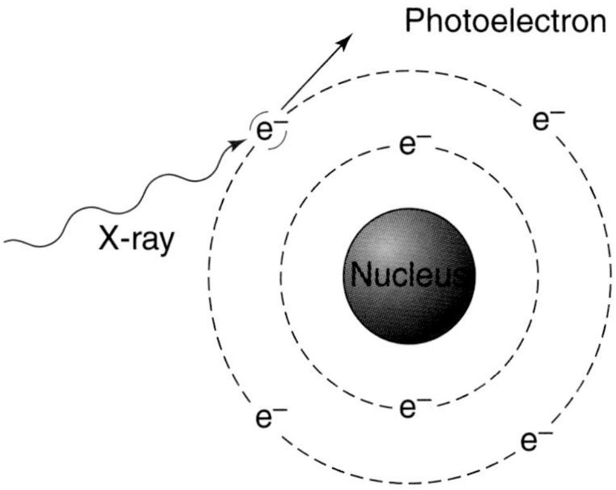

FIGURE 2–7 **Photoelectric effect.** The incoming x-ray gives up all of its energy to an orbital electron of the atom. The x-ray is absorbed and simply vanishes. The electromagnetic energy of the x-ray is imparted to the electron in the form of kinetic energy of motion and causes the electron to fly from its orbit. Thus, an ion pair is created. The high-speed electron (called a photoelectron) knocks other electrons from the orbits of other atoms forming secondary ion pairs.

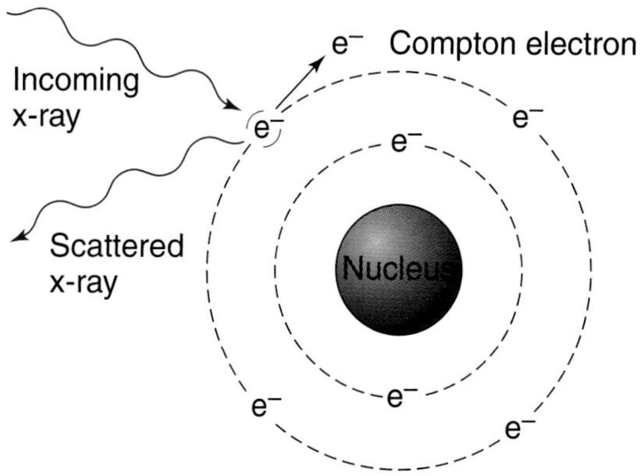

FIGURE 2–8 **Compton scattering.** Compton scattering is similar to the photoelectric effect in that the incoming x-ray interacts with an orbital electron and ejects it. But in the case of Compton interaction, only a part of the x-ray energy is transferred to the electron and a new, weaker x-ray is formed and scattered in some new direction. The new x-ray may undergo another Compton scattering or it may be absorbed by a photoelectric effect interaction.

Practice Point

"How long should you wait after exposure before entering the room where the radiation was?"

X-rays travel at the speed of light and cease to exist within a fraction of a second. This question is similar to asking, "How long will it take for the room to get dark after turning off the light switch?"

Units of Radiation

The terms used to measure x-radiation are based on the ability of the x-ray to deposit its energy in air, soft tissues, bone, or other substances. The International Commission on Radiation Units and Measurements (ICRU) has established standards that clearly define radiation units and radiation quantities. At the present time, two sets of terms are used for units of radiation (Table 2–1). The older system, referred to as the traditional

TABLE 2–1 **Radiation Measurement Terminology**

Quantity	Système International (SI) Unit	Traditional Unit
Exposure	coulombs per kilogram (C/kg)	roentgen (R)
Absorbed dose	gray (Gy)	rad
Dose equivalent	sievert (Sv)	rem

units, is being phased out. Gaining greater acceptance is the metric equivalent known as the Système Internationale (SI). The traditional units are:

1. Roentgen (R)
2. Rad (radiation absorbed dose)
3. Rem (radiation equivalent in man)

The **Système Internationale (SI)** units are:

1. Coulombs per kilogram (C/kg)
2. Gray (Gy)
3. Sievert (Sv)

The American Dental Association requires the use of SI terminology on national board examinations. In this book, we will use the new SI units first, followed by the traditional units.

A "quantity" may be thought of as a description of a physical concept such as time, distance, or weight. The measure of the quantity is a "unit" such as minutes, miles (kilometers), or pounds (kilograms).

For practical x-ray protection measurement, three quantities are used. They are:

1. Exposure
2. Absorbed dose
3. Dose equivalent

Exposure

Exposure can be defined as the measurement of ionization in air produced by x- or gamma rays. The units for measuring exposure are **coulombs per kilogram (C/kg)** and the **roentgen (R)**. A coulomb is a unit of electrical charge. Therefore, the unit C/kg measures electrical charges (ion pairs) in a kilogram of air.

- **Roentgen (R):** One roentgen is the amount of x- or gamma rays that will produce 2.08×10^9 (about 2 billion) ion pairs in 1 cc of air at standard conditions of pressure and temperature (Figure 2–9).

To avoid confusion with the name of the person for whom a unit may be named, the word is capitalized when referring to the person (Roentgen) but when referring to the unit, the word is written in lowercase (roentgen). The abbreviation for the unit is, however, capitalized (R). The roentgen only applies to x- or gamma radiation and only measures ion pairs in air. It does not measure the radiation absorbed by tissues or other materials. Therefore, it is not a measurement of **dose.** An exposure does not become a dose until the radiation is absorbed in the tissues.

Absorbed Dose

Absorbed dose is defined as the amount of energy deposited in any form of matter (such as teeth, soft tissues, treatment chair, air, and so on), by any type of radiation (alpha or beta particles, gamma or x-rays). The units for measuring the absorbed dose are the **gray (Gy)** and the **rad** (radiation absorbed dose).

- **Gray (Gy):** A unit for measuring absorbed dose that is replacing the rad. One gray equals 1 joule (J) (a unit of energy) per kilogram of tissue. One gray equals 100 rads.
- **Rad** (radiation absorbed dose): A special unit of absorbed dose equal to 0.01 J/kg of tissue. For x-rays absorbed in the soft tissues, the rad is approximately numerically equivalent to the roentgen.

Dose Equivalent

Dose equivalent is a term used for radiation protection purposes to compare the biological effects of the various types of radiation. Dose equivalent is defined as the product of the absorbed dose times a biological-effect qualifying or **weighting factor.** Because the weighting factor for x-rays is 1, the absorbed dose and the dose equivalent are equal. The units for measuring the dose equivalent are the **sievert (Sv)** and the **rem** (roentgen equivalent man).

- **Sievert (Sv):** A unit used to measure the dose equivalent. One sievert equals 1 Gy times a biological-effect weighting

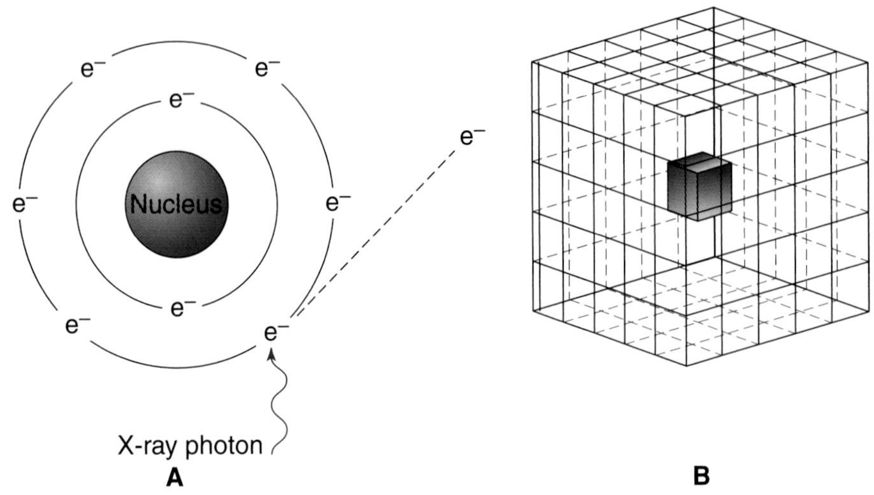

FIGURE 2-9 **Schematic representation.** (**A**) Ionization of an oxygen atom. (**B**) One roentgen is the amount of radiation that will produce about 2 billion oxygen ion pairs in 1 cubic cm of air surrounded by an infinite amount of air.

factor. Because the weighting factor for x- and gamma radiation equals 1, the number of sieverts is identical to the absorbed dose in grays for these radiations. One sievert equals 100 rems.

- **Rem** (roentgen equivalent [in] man): A unit used to measure the dose equivalent. One rem equals one rad times a biological-effect weighting factor. Because the weighting factor for x- and gamma radiation equals 1, the number of rems is identical to the absorbed dose in rads for these radiations. One rem equals 0.01 sievert.

In dental radiology, grays and sieverts are equal, while roentgens, rads, and rems are considered to be numerically equal; however, it should be pointed out that only x-rays and gamma rays are measured in coulombs per kilogram or roentgens. Grays or rads and sieverts or rems are used to measure all radiations: gamma and x-rays, alpha and beta particles, neutrons, and high-energy protons.

A simplified comparison of the terms explains the coulomb per kilogram or roentgen as a measurement of x-ray exposure in air; the gray or rad represents the amount of energy the tissues absorb; and the sievert or rem represents the relative biological effect of radiation absorbed in the body tissues.

Because these units of measurement are fairly large, smaller multiples of these units are commonly used in dental radiology. For example, the word *milli* means "one-thousandth of" and we express a smaller dose of a gray as a milligray (mGy).

Background Radiation

Dental x-rays are artificially produced, and along with medical x-rays account for approximately 11 percent of the total radiation exposure to the population. However, it is important that we not overlook the fact that the greatest exposure to ionizing radiations to the population is from naturally occurring, background sources of radiation (Figure 2–10). **Background radiation** is defined as ionizing radiation that is always present in our environment. The human race has always been subjected to exposure from natural background radiations originating from the following sources:

- Cosmic radiations from outer space
- Terrestrial radiations from the earth and its environments
- Background radiations from naturally occurring radionuclides (unstable atoms that emit radiations) that are deposited in our bodies by inhalation and ingestion

The average natural background radiation levels for the United States population is estimated to be about 3 mSv (millisievert) or 300 mrem (millirem) per year. The exact amount varies

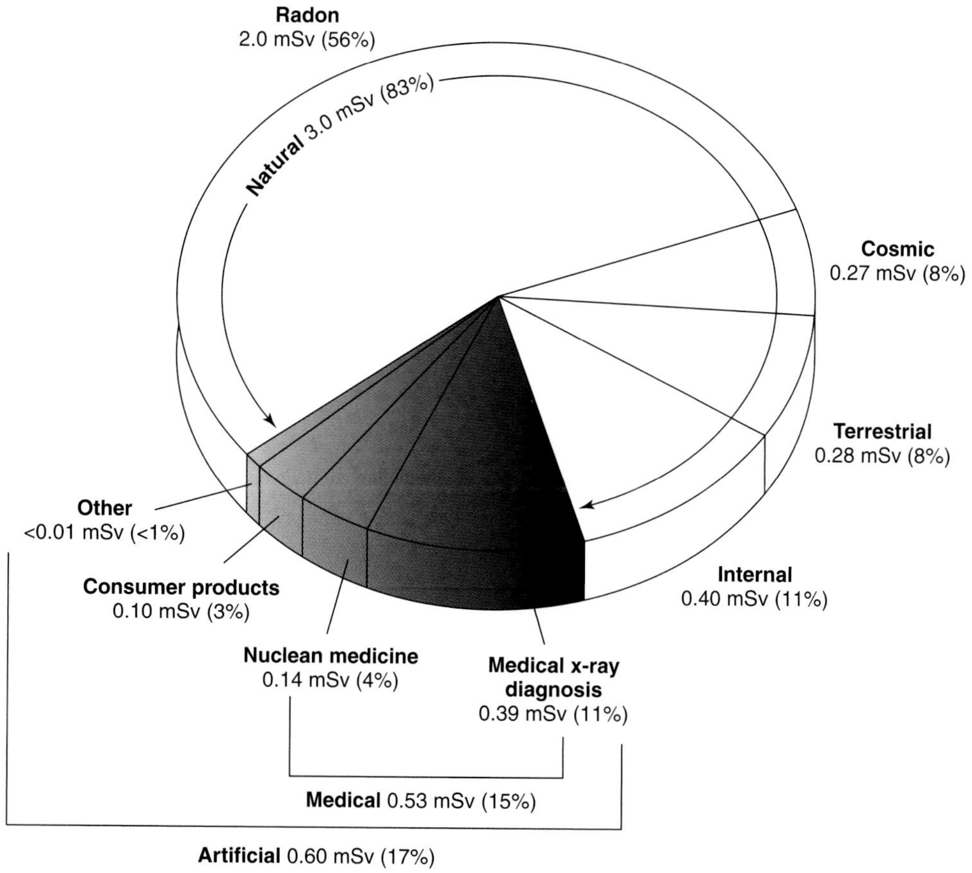

FIGURE 2–10 **Annual dose equivalent of ionizing radiations.** This chart illustrates the approximate percentage of exposure of the U.S. population to background and artificial radiations. (Reprinted from S. C. White and M. J. Pharoah, *Oral Radiology Principles and Interpretation,* 5th edition, p. 49, copyright 2004, with permission from Elsevier.)

according to locality, the amount of radioactive material present, and the intensity of the cosmic rays—this intensity varies according to altitude and latitude. For example, persons living on the Colorado plateau receive an increased dose of background radiation because of the increased cosmic radiation at the higher altitude and more terrestrial radiation from soils enriched in naturally occurring uranium that raise the levels of terrestrial radionuclides located there.

REVIEW—Chapter Summary

The three basic building blocks of an atom are protons, neutrons, and electrons. Protons and neutrons make up the central nucleus, which is orbited by the electrons. The number of protons determines the chemical element.

Ionization is the formation of charged particles called ions. A positive ion and a negative ion are called an ion pair. Ionizing radiation is defined as any radiation that produces ions.

Electromagnetic radiation is the movement of wave-like energy through space. Electromagnetic waves exhibit the properties of wavelength, frequency, and velocity. Short-wavelength x-rays, called hard radiation, are very penetrating. Long-wavelength x-rays, called soft radiation, have limited penetrating power. The electromagnetic spectrum consists of an orderly arrangement of all known radiant energies.

X-rays are invisible, travel in straight lines at the speed of light, interact with matter causing ionization, affect photographic film, and affect living tissue. X-rays are produced whenever high-speed electrons are abruptly stopped or slowed down. They may pass through a patient with no interaction, or they may be absorbed by the photoelectric effect or scattered by either Compton scattering or coherent scattering.

For practical x-ray measurement three quantities are used. They are exposure, absorbed dose and dose equivalent. The units for measuring exposure are coulombs per kilogram (C/kg) and the roentgen (R). The units for measuring the absorbed dose are the gray (Gy) and the rad (radiation absorbed dose). The units for measuring the dose equivalent are the sievert (Sv) and the rem (roentgen equivalent man).

The ever-present background radiation consists of cosmic radiation, terrestrial radiations, and naturally occurring radionuclides that are deposited in our bodies by inhalation and ingestion.

RECALL—Study Questions

1. What term describes the smallest particle of an element that retains the properties of that element?
   a. Atom
   b. Molecule
   c. Photon
   d. Isotope
2. Draw and label a typical atom.
3. Which of these subatomic particles carries a negative electric charge?
   a. Proton
   b. Neutron
   c. Nucleus
   d. Electron
4. Radiant energy sufficient to remove an electron from its orbital level of an atom is called
   a. Atomic.
   b. Electronic.
   c. Ionizing.
   d. Ultrasonic.
5. What term describes the process by which unstable atoms undergo decay in an effort to obtain nuclear stability?
   a. Absorption
   b. Radioactivity
   c. Radiolucent
   d. Ionization
6. *Electromagnetic radiation* is a combination of electric and magnetic energy emitted in the form of rays or waves, while *particulate radiation* consists of bits of matter traveling at high speeds.
   a. The first part of the statement is correct, but the second part of the statement is incorrect.
   b. The first part of the statement is incorrect, but the second part of the statement is correct.
   c. Both parts of the statement are correct.
   d. Both parts of the statement are incorrect.
7. What is the distance between two similar points on two successive waves called?
   a. Wavelength
   b. Frequency
   c. Velocity
   d. Energy level
8. Which x-ray wavelength has the most penetrating power?
   a. 0.1 Å
   b. 0.5 Å
   c. 0.8 Å
   d. 1.0 Å
9. Which of these electromagnetic radiations has the shortest wavelength?
   a. Radar
   b. Ultraviolet rays
   c. Infrared rays
   d. X-rays
10. Which of these forms of radiation has the greatest penetrating power?
    a. Visible light
    b. X-rays
    c. Sunlamp
    d. Radio waves
11. Which of these forms of radiation is least capable of causing ionization of body tissue cells?
    a. Cosmic rays
    b. Gamma rays
    c. X-rays
    d. Infrared light

12. List five properties of x-rays.
    a. ____________________
    b. ____________________
    c. ____________________
    d. ____________________
    e. ____________________
13. Radiation produced when high-speed electrons are stopped or slowed down by the tungsten atoms of the dental x-ray tube is called:
    a. General/bremsstrahlung
    b. Characteristic
    c. Coherent
    d. Compton
14. What term best describes the process of transferring the energy of the x-rays to the atoms of the material through which the x-ray beam passes?
    a. Compton scattering
    b. Photoelectric effect
    c. Absorption
    d. Bremsstrahlung
15. Which of these terms is the unit used to measure radiation exposure?
    a. Angstrom (Å)
    b. Gray (rad)
    c. Sievert (rem)
    d. Coulombs per kilogram (roentgen)
16. The Système Internationale (SI) unit that is replacing the rem is:
    a. Gray
    b. Sievert
    c. Rad
    d. Coulomb/kilogram
17. List the three sources of background radiation.
    a. ____________________
    b. ____________________
    c. ____________________
18. What is the average amount of background radiation to an individual in the United States?
    a. 1 mSv (100 millirem) per year
    b. 2 mSv (200 millirem) per year
    c. 3 mSv (300 millirem) per year
    d. 4 mSv (400 millirem) per year

REFLECT—Case Study

While taking a full mouth series of dental radiographs on your patient, he begins to consider the number of radiographs which are made in this operatory on a daily basis. He begins to ask you questions such as, "How long do you have to wait after each exposure before you can re-enter the room?" and "Are the walls and equipment in this room becoming radioactive from all the exposures taken in here?" Prepare a conversation with this patient addressing these two questions based on what you learned in this chapter on radiation physics.

RELATE—Laboratory Application

Research recent media (magazine or journal articles, newspaper reports, or the Web) for stories on radiation exposure. Select an article for review and critique the article for clarity and readibility. Summarize how many different types of radiation are mentioned in the article. What units of radiation measurement does the author use? Does the article use these terms in a manner that is appropriate for what is being measured? Consider the type of radiation described in this article. Is it naturally occuring/background radiation or a radiation generated by an artificial or man-made source? How many key words from this chapter can you find in the article? Anticipate what questions your patient may have for you after reading this article.

BIBLIOGRAPHY

Bushberg, J. T., Seibert, J. A., Leidholdt, E. M. Jr., & Boone, J. M. *The Essential Physics of Medical Imaging,* 2nd ed. Baltimore, MD: Lippincott Williams & Wilkins, 2001.

Langland, O. E., Sippy, F. H., & Langlais, R. P. *Textbook of Dental Radiology,* 2nd ed. Springfield, IL: Charles C. Thomas, 1984.

United States Nuclear Regulatory Commission, Office of Public Affairs. *Fact Sheet.* Washington, DC, 2003.

White, S. C., & Pharoah, M. J. *Oral Radiology. Principles and Interpretation,* 5th ed. St. Louis: Elsevier, 2004.

3

The Dental X-ray Machine: Components and Functions

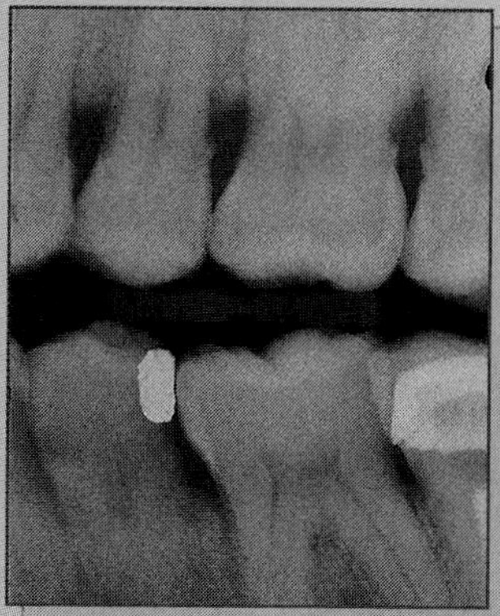

CHAPTER OUTLINE

■ OBJECTIVES

Following successful completion of this chapter, you should be able to:

1. Define the key words.
2. Identify the three major components of a dental x-ray machine.
3. Identify and explain the function of the five controls on most dental x-ray machines.
4. State the three conditions necessary for the production of x-rays.
5. Draw and label a dental x-ray tube.
6. Trace the flow of electricity through the three transformers, describing the function and location of each.
7. Trace the production of x-rays from the time the exposure button is activated until x-rays are released from the tube.
8. Demonstrate, in sequence, steps in operating the dental x-ray machine.

■ KEY WORDS

Alternating current (AC)
Amperage
Ampere (A)
Anode
Autotransformer
Cathode
Central ray
Collimator
Control panel
"Dead-man" switch
Direct current (DC)
Electric current
Electrical circuits
Electrode
Electron cloud
Exposure button
Extension arm
Filament
Filter
Focal spot
Focusing cup
Impulse
Incandescence
Intensity
Kilovolt (kV)
Kilovolt peak (kVp)
Line switch
Milliampere (mA)
Polychromatic
Port
Primary beam
Quality
Quantity
Radiator

Step-down transformer
Step-up transformer
Target
Thermionic emission
Timer
Transformer
Tube head
Tungsten
Useful beam
Volt (V)
Voltage
Voltmeter
X-ray tube
Yoke

Introduction

At the time of exposure, the radiographer who activates the exposure button is responsible for the radiation dose incurred by the patient. The role of exposing dental radiographs is an important one for the dental assistant and dental hygienist, making it essential that these professionals possess an understanding of how the x-ray machine works to produce ionizing radiation. To operate dental x-ray equipment safely and competently, the radiographer needs to develop a base knowledge of the components of the dental x-ray machine and possess an understanding of how these components work together to produce ionizing radiation. The purpose of this chapter is to discuss the conventional dental x-ray machine, its components and functions.

Evolution of the Dental X-ray Machine

Improvements in early x-ray generating machines began to occur after the dangers of radiation exposure became evident. The Coolidge hot cathode vacuum tube, invented by Dr. W. D. Coolidge in 1913, improved the previous erratic radiation output of earlier machines. Then during the mid-1950s, variable kilovoltage machines were introduced that allow for different penetrating abilities of the x-beam. In 1966, the recessed PID was introduced (Figure 3–1). On x-ray machines of conventional design, the x-ray tube is located in the front section of the tube head; on those employing a recessed design, the x-ray tube is located in the back of the tubehead. This configuration allows for a sharper image. (The role a longer x-ray tube-to-

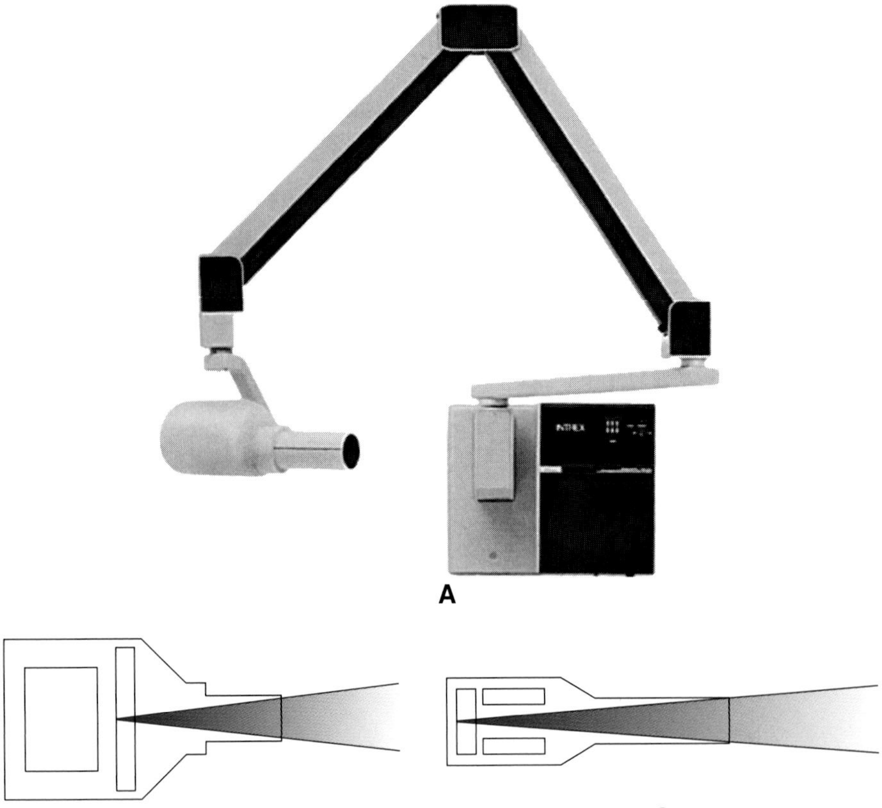

FIGURE 3–1 **Comparison of conventional and recessed tube position within the tube head.** (**A**) Intrex recessed tube x-ray machine. (**B**) Conventional position with tube in front of transformer. Because x-ray source is in front, the beam pattern quickly flares out. (**C**) With a recessed tube a relatively more parallel x-ray beam is produced. This will produce a sharper radiographic image. (Courtesy of S. S. White Dental Products International)

object distance plays in producing sharp images is discussed in Chapter 4.)

In 1974, the federal government began regulating the manufacture and installation of all dental x-ray machines. There are also state and local governing agencies that set guidelines on the safe installation and use of dental x-ray equipment. New technology employing miniaturized solid-state transformers and rare-earth materials for filtration of the x-ray beam has also contributed to the development of a modern dental x-ray machine that is safe, compact, easy to position, and simple to operate.

Dental X-ray Machine Components

While dental x-ray machines vary in size and appearance, they have similar structural components (Figure 3–2). The typical dental x-ray machine consists of three parts:

1. The **control panel,** which contains the regulating devices.
2. The **extension arm** or bracket, which enables the tube head to be positioned.
3. The **tube head,** which contains the x-ray tube from which x-rays are generated.

Control Panel

The **electric current** enters the control panel either through a cord plugged into a grounded outlet in the wall or through a direct connection to a power line in the wall. The control panel may be integrated with the extension arm and tube head (Figure 3–3) or it may be remote from the unit, mounted on a shelf or wall (Figure 3–4). One control panel may serve two or more tube heads (Figure 3–5). Dental x-ray machines are available with variable controls allowing for manual adjustment of the milliamperage and the kilovoltage of the incoming electricity (Figure 3–5); or these controls may be preset by the manufacturer. If the milliamperage and the kilovoltage are pre-set by the manufacturer, the control panel will indicate at what variables these units are pre-set. Five major controls may be operated or will be pre-set on dental x-ray machines: (1) the line switch to the electrical outlet, (2) the milliampere selector, (3) the kilovoltage selector, (4) the timer, and (5) the exposure button. The function of each of these is discussed here.

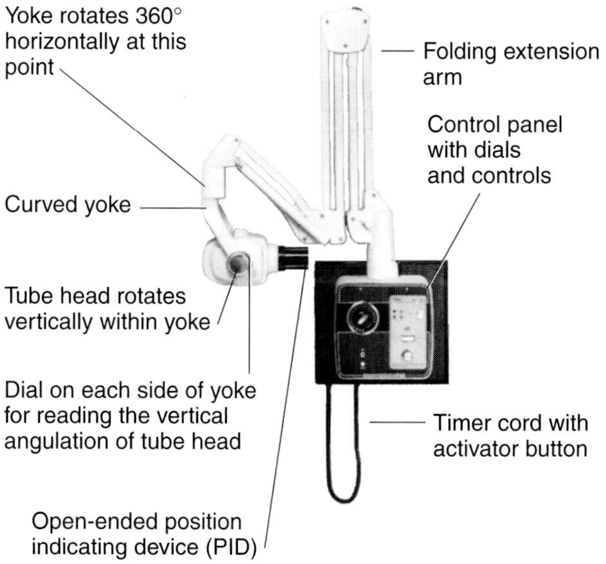

FIGURE 3–2 **Typical wall-mounted dental x-ray machine.** (Courtesy of Ritter-Midwest Division of Sybron Corporation)

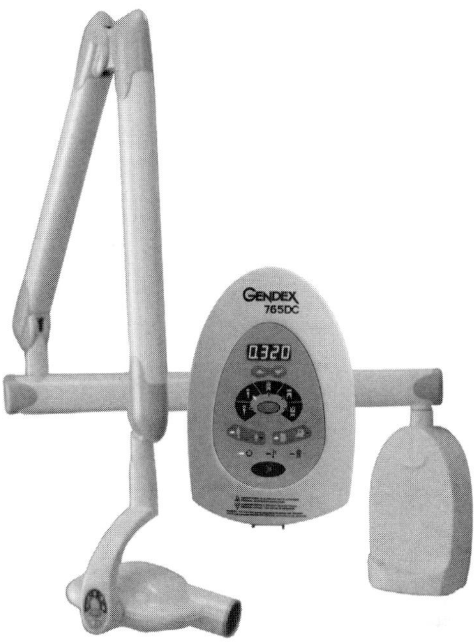

FIGURE 3–3 **Control panel integrated with tube head support.** (Image courtesy of Gendex Dental Corporation)

Line Switch

The **line switch** on the control panel of the dental x-ray machine may be a toggle switch that can be flicked on or off with light finger pressure, or it may be an ON/OFF push button. It is generally located on the side or face of the cabinet or control panel. In the ON position, this switch energizes the circuits in the control panel but not the low- or high-voltage circuits. An indicator light turns on indicating the machine is operational. In the OFF position, the transformers are totally disconnected from the supply of electric current.

Milliampere (mA) Selector

The **milliampere** selector measures the amount of current passing through the wires of the circuit. The milliampere selector may be a knob or push button or key pad (Figure 3–5). On a preset x-ray machine, it is connected directly to the ON/OFF switch. On some machines, a needle on the control panel dial indicates that current is available for operation. The **amperage** selected determines the available number of free electrons at the cathode filament and, therefore, the amount of x-rays produced.

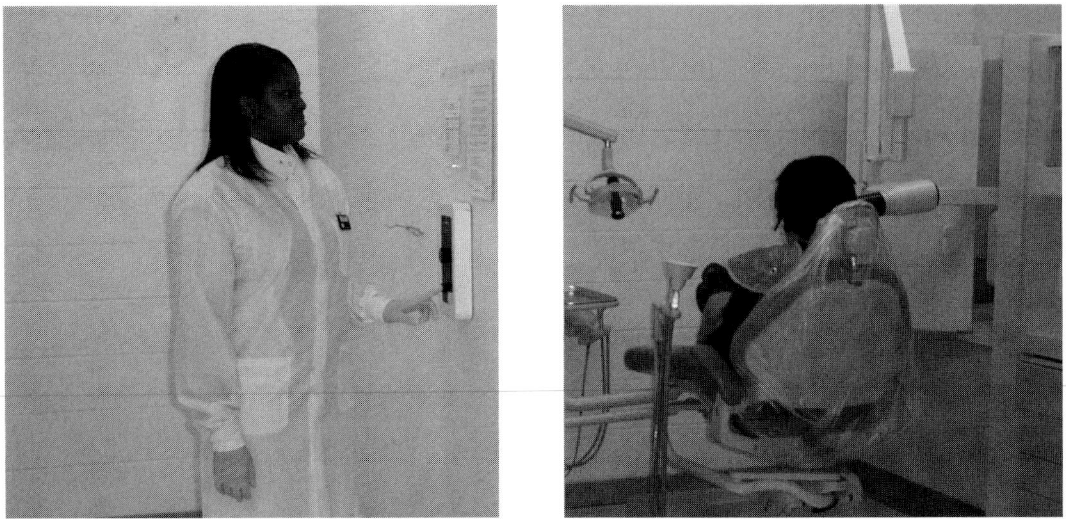

FIGURE 3–4 **Control panel mounted in protected area.**

Kilovolt Peak (kVp) Selector

The **voltmeter** measures the difference in potential or voltage across the x-ray tube. A **kilovolt peak (kVp)** selector (Figure 3–5) in the form of push buttons, knobs, key pads or dials enables the operator to change the peak kilovoltage. The kVp selected determines the speed of electrons traveling toward the target on the anode and therefore, the penetrating ability of the x-rays produced.

Timer

The timer is set by turning the selector knob, depressing the marked push button, or touching a keypad. The **timer** (Figure 3–5) serves to regulate the duration of the interval that the current will pass through the x-ray tube. X-ray machines equipped with a vacuum-type electronic timer are accurate up to 1/60-second intervals. Time settings of less than a second may be indicated in fractions and in **impulses** (there are 60 impulses in a second). For example, a 1/10-second exposure lasts 6 impulses, 1/5 second for 12 impulses, and so forth. New x-ray machines with electronic digital timers are accurate to 1/100-second intervals and work well with digital radiography systems. The **time** selected determines the duration of the exposure.

Exposure Button

Depressing the **exposure button** or key pad or switch activates the x-ray production process. The exposure button may be located on the handle of the timer cord (Figure 3–6), the control panel, or at a remote location in a protected area (Figure 3–7). If the exposure button is located on the end of the timer cord, the cord must be sufficiently long to enable the operator to step into an area of protection from radiation, usually at least 6 ft (1.83 m) from the source of the x-ray beam. Because the possibility exists that the operator may not utilize the full length of the timer cord to be safely protected from the x-rays generated, an exposure switch permanently mounted to the control panel or other protected area is preferred. In fact, many state regulations now require that the exposure button be permanently mounted in a protected area. Older x-ray machines equipped with exposure buttons on timer cords must be modified to attach the exposure button to an unmovable, permanent mount to meet this requirement.

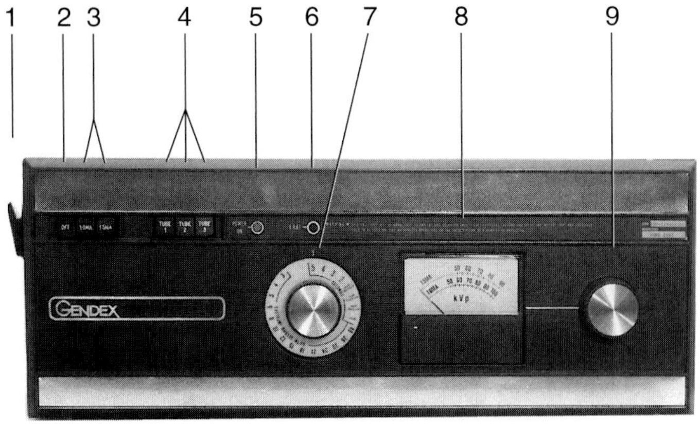

FIGURE 3–5 **Control panel of Gendex dental x-ray machine.** (**1**) Exposure button holder, (**2**) main ON/OFF switch, (**3**) mA control, (**4**) x-ray tube selector, (**5**) power ON light, (**6**) x-ray emission light, (**7**) timer control, (**8**) kVp meter, (**9**) kVp control. This master control unit accommodates three remote tube heads. This unit permits variable kVp and mA selection for settings of 50 kVp to 90 kVp at 15 mA, and 50 kVp to 100 kVp at 10 mA.

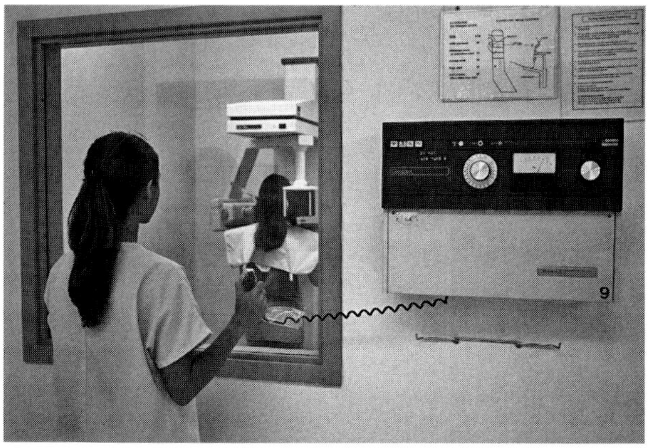

FIGURE 3-6 **Exposure button on the handle of the timer cord.** Operator is exposing a panoramic radiograph from behind a lead-lined glass window.

All dental x-ray machines are required to be equipped with a **"dead-man"** exposure **switch** that automatically terminates the exposure when the finger ceases to press on the timer button. This makes it necessary to maintain firm pressure on the button during the entire exposure. Failure to do so results in the formation of an insufficient number of x-rays to properly expose the film. When the exposure button is activated the operator will hear an audible beep (required by law) that indicates x-rays are being generated. Additionally, exposure buttons installed directly on the control panel allow the operator to observe an light indicating that x-rays are being generated.

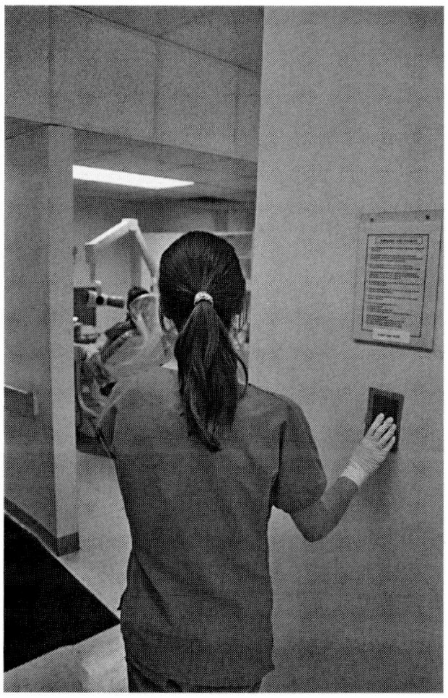

FIGURE 3-7 **Exposure button in remote location.** This location allows the radiographer to stand in a position at least 6 ft (1.83 m) from the head of the patient at an angle of 90 degrees to 135 degrees out of the primary beam. (See Chapter 6.)

The manufacturing trend is toward simpler and automated controls. In addition to pre-set milliamperage and kilovoltage, most new dental x-ray machines have an electrical timer that automatically resets itself and does not have to be altered unless a change in the exposure time is desired.

Extension Arm

The folding **extension arm** is a support from which the tube housing is suspended (Figure 3–2). The extension arm allows for moving and positioning the tube head. The extension arm is hollow to permit the passage of electrical wires from the control panel to the tube head from one or both sides at a point where the tube head attaches to the yoke. The tube head is attached to the extension arm by means of a **yoke** that can revolve 360 degrees horizontally where it is connected. In addition, the tube head can be rotated vertically within the yoke. All sections of the extension arm and yoke are heavily insulated to protect the patient and the operator from electrical shock.

Practice Point

After use, the extension arm bracket should be folded into a neutral, closed position. The tube head is finely counterbalanced in its suspension from the extension arm. This balance can be disturbed if the tube head is left suspended for prolonged time periods with the extension arm stretched out. This may lead to instability and tube head drifting.

Tube Head (Tube Housing)

The **tube head** (sometimes called tube housing) (Figure 3–8) is a tightly sealed heavy metal (usually cast aluminum), lead-lined housing that contains the dental x-ray tube, insulating oil, and step-up and step-down transformers. The metal housing performs several important functions:

1. It protects the x-ray tube from accidental damage.
2. It increases the safety of the x-ray machine by grounding its high-voltage components (the x-ray tube and the transformers) to prevent shock.
3. It prevents overheating of the x-ray tube by providing a space filled with oil, gas, or air to absorb the heat created during the production of x-rays.
4. Its lead liner absorbs any x-rays produced except the primary beam that exits through the port in the direction of the position indicating device (PID).

Electricity

Since electricity is needed to produce dental x-rays, an understanding of basic electrical concepts is necessary. Electricity has been defined as electrons in motion. An electric current is a move-

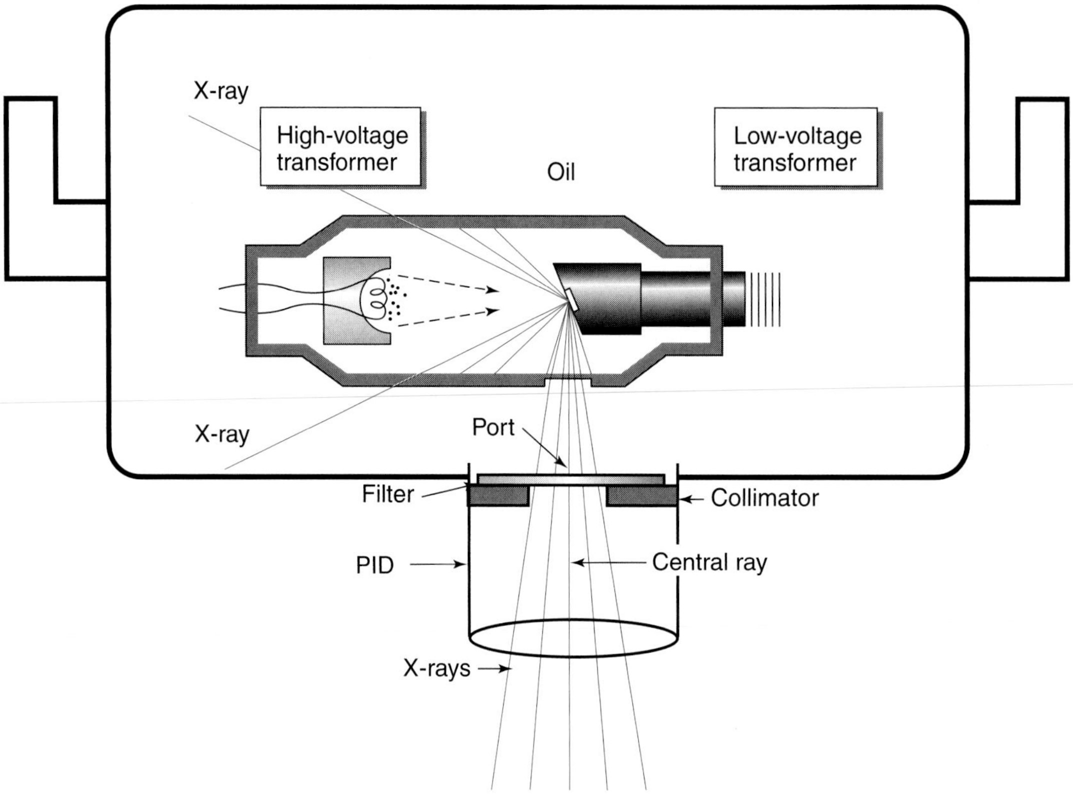

FIGURE 3-8 **Dental x-ray tube head, containing dental x-ray tube, transformers, and oil.** When an electric current is applied to the high-voltage circuit (between the cathode and the anode), each electron is propelled from the cathode to the target on the anode, producing heat and x-rays. X-rays are emitted in all directions. Most of the x-rays travel toward the port because of the 20-degree angle of the anode target. These x-rays make up the primary x-ray beam and exit the tube head via the port. The central ray is the x-ray in the center of the primary beam.

ment of electrons through a conducting medium (such as copper wire). Electric current can flow in either direction along a wire or conductor. It can flow steadily in one direction (direct current) or flow in pulses and change directions (alternating current).

Direct Current

Direct current (DC), flows continuously in one direction. The unidirectional current is similar to that used in flashlight batteries. Direct current dental x-ray machines are well suited for use with digital imaging (see Chapter 26).

Alternating Current

The ordinary household current used in the United States is a 110-V, 60-cycle **alternating current (AC)**, which changes its direction of flow 60 times per second (Figure 3–9). Thus the alternating current has two phases—one positive and the other negative—and alternates between these phases. Most dental x-ray machines operate on 110- or 220-V alternating current.

The electrical terms *amperage*, the measurement of the number of electrons moving through a wire conductor and *voltage*, the measurement of electrical force that causes electrons to flow through a conductor, will be used to describe x-rays generated as well.

Amperage

Amperage measures the number of electrons that move through a conductor. The **ampere (A)** is the unit of quantity of electric current. An increase in amperage results in an increase in the number of electrons that are available to travel from the cathode to anode when the tube is activated. This results in a production of more x-rays. Only a small current is required to operate the x-ray machine; therefore, the term **milliampere (mA)**, denoting 1/1,000 of an ampere, is used. The majority of dental x-ray machines operate in ranges from 7 to 15 mA. On some x-ray units, the milliamperage can be varied by the operator; on others, it is pre-set by the manufacturer.

Voltage

Voltage or **volt (V)** is the electrical pressure (sometimes called potential difference) between two electrical charges. In radiography the voltage determines the speed of the electrons when

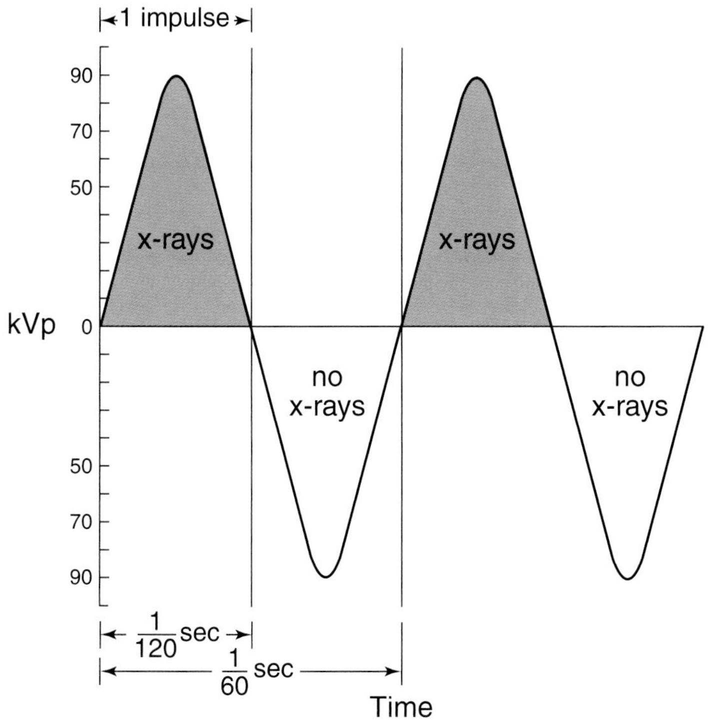

FIGURE 3–9 **Sine wave of 60-cycle alternating current operating at 90,000 V (90 kVp).** Ordinary household electric current is called 60-cycle alternating current because the current changes its direction of flow 60 times a second. During the time that the x-ray tube is producing x-rays, the cathode and the anode each change from negative to positive 60 times per second. The crest of the wave represents the maximum voltage when the current is moving in one direction, while the trough of the wave represents the maximum voltage when the current is moving in the other direction. The total cycle takes place in 1/60 sec. This alternation in current direction occurs every 1/120 sec (twice during each full cycle) on x-ray machines of conventional design. It produces the x-rays in a series of bursts, or impulses, rather than in a continuous flow.

traveling from cathode to anode. This speed of the electrons, in turn, determines the energy (penetrating power) of the x-rays produced. When the voltage is increased, the electrons travel faster and produce the hardest type of radiation.

Because dental x-ray equipment operates at very high voltages, it is customary to express voltage in terms of **kilovolts.** A kilovolt equals 1,000 V and is abbreviated **kV.** The voltage varies during an exposure, producing a **polychromatic** beam (x-rays of many different energies) containing high-energy rays and also containing soft rays that have barely enough energy to escape from the tube. The highest voltage to which the current in the tube rises during an exposure is called the **kilovolt peak (kVp).** Thus if the x-ray machine controls are set at 75 kVp (75,000 V), the maximum x-ray energy that can be produced during this exposure is 75 kVp. Dental x-ray machines currently manufactured operate within a range of 65 kVp to 100 kVp.

The X-ray Tube

X-rays are produced when a stream of high-speed electrons are stopped or slowed down. Therefore, three conditions must exist for x-rays to be produced:

1. A source of free electrons
2. High voltage to impart speed to the electrons
3. A target that is capable of stopping the electrons

The x-ray tube and the circuits within the machine are designed to create these conditions. The **x-ray tube,** located inside the tube head, is a glass bulb from which the air has been pumped out to create a vacuum (Figure 3–10). An **anode** (the positive electrode) and a **cathode** (the negative electrode) are sealed within the tube, and the two protruding arms of the electrodes permit the passage of the current through the tube (Figure 3–11).

Electrons are created at the filament wire of the cathode. This process, known as **thermionic emission,** occurs whenever a wire is heated to **incandescence** (glowing red with heat). A familiar example of this phenomenon is the tungsten electric light bulb. The radiographer, by adjusting the milliamperage, can accurately control the thermionic emission. The vacuum offers a minimum resistance to the stream of electrons flowing across the space between the cathode and anode. In most dental x-ray tubes, the space between the electrodes is less than 1 in. (25.4 mm). The cathode and the anode are connected to

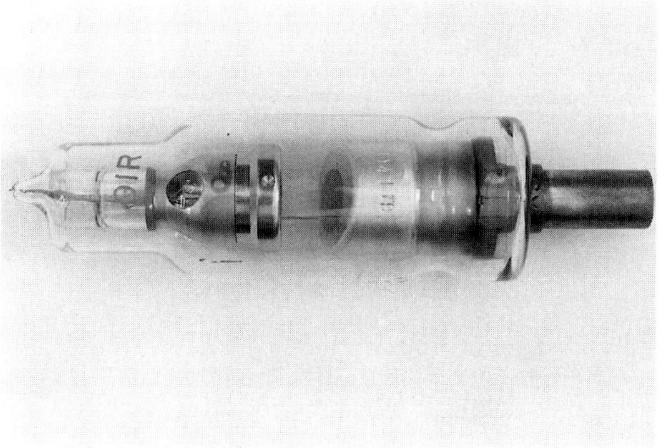

FIGURE 3–10 **Photograph of a dental x-ray tube.**

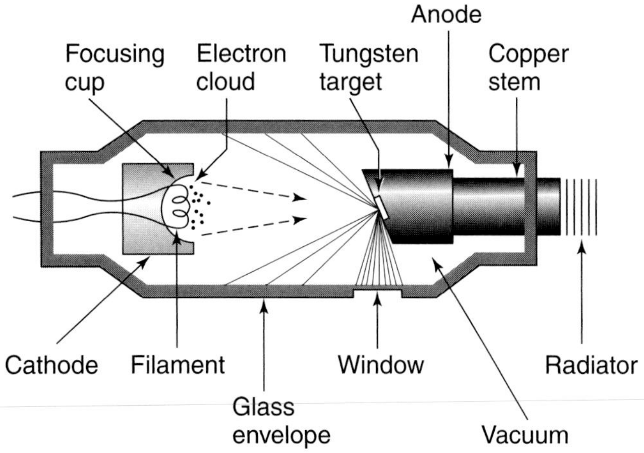

FIGURE 3-11 **Drawing of a typical dental x-ray tube.**

the outside of the tube by massive copper wires, which permit a high-voltage current to flow across the tube when the x-ray machine is in operation.

Cathode

The purpose of the cathode is to supply electrons necessary to produce x-rays. The cathode, or negative electrode, consists of a thin, spiral filament of **tungsten** wire. This **filament** wire, when heated to incandescence (red hot and glowing), produces the electrons (Figure 3–12). Tungsten's high atomic number makes it possible to liberate electrons, through thermionic emission, from their orbital shells when the metal is heated. The wire filament is recessed into a molybdenum **focusing cup,** which directs the electrons toward the target on the anode (Figure 3–13).

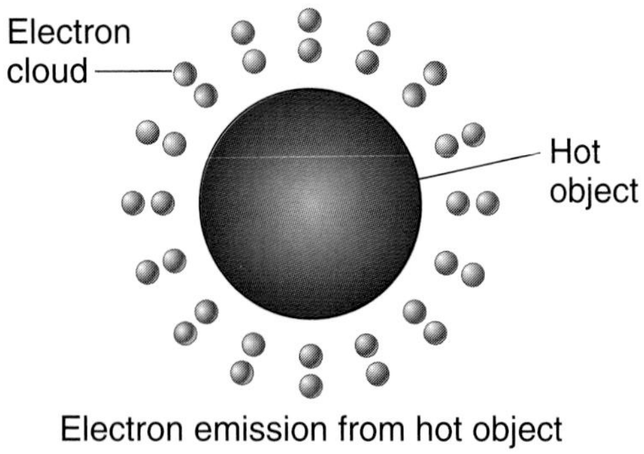

FIGURE 3-12 **Cross section of a filament wire.** The filament wire in the cathode is heated to incandescence. The attached electrons are literally boiled out of the wire and become available as a source of free electrons, thus fulfilling the first requirement for x-ray production. The milliamperage selected by the operator will determine the number of electrons available to be accelerated across to the target of the anode.

Anode

The purpose of the anode is to stop the high-velocity electrons, converting their kinetic energy into x-rays (electromagnetic energy). The anode, or positive **electrode,** consists of a copper bar with a tungsten plate imbedded in the end that faces the focusing cup of the cathode. On dental x-ray machines, this tungsten plate, called the **target,** is set into the copper at an angle of 20 degrees to the cathode. The angle assures that most of the x-rays (the primary beam) are produced in one direction.

When the tube is in operation, a cloud of electrons first forms around the filament wire of the cathode as the tube warms. Later, when the high-voltage current is applied, these electrons are attracted and electrically charged to propel toward a rectangular area on the surface of the target known as the focal spot.

Focal Spot

The **focal spot** is a small rectangular area on the target of the anode to which the focusing cup directs the electron beam. X-rays originate at the focal spot. Its size is controlled by the manufacturer. A small focal spot not only improves the sharpness on the radiograph but concentrates the electrons and creates enormous heat. The smaller the focal spot, the sharper the radiographic image.

Electrical Circuits

An **electrical circuit** is a path of electrical current. There are two electrical circuits used in producing dental x-rays.

1. A filament circuit provides low voltage (3–8 V) to the filament of the x-ray tube to provide the source of electrons needed for the production of x-rays.
2. A high-voltage circuit provides the high voltage (65–100 kV) necessary to accelerate the electrons from the cathode filament to the anode target.

Transformers

A **transformer** is an electromagnetic device for changing the alternating current coming into the machine. Transformers are required to decrease (step down) or increase (step up) the ordinary 110-V current that enters the x-ray machine (Figure 3–14).

Step-down Transformer

A **step-down** (low-voltage) **transformer** decreases the voltage from the wall outlet to approximately 5 V, just enough to heat the filament and form an electron cloud.

Step-up Transformer

A **step-up** (high-voltage) **transformer** increases the voltage as required by the technique the radiographer is using. The high-voltage current, 65–100 kVp, begins to flow through the cathode–anode circuit when the exposure button on the line

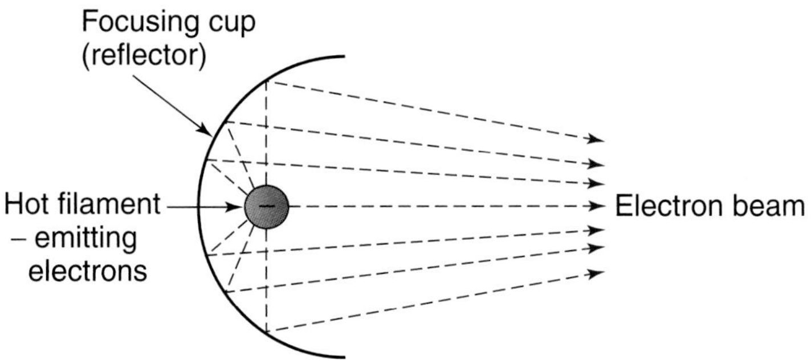

FIGURE 3–13 **Formation of electron beam by focusing cup.** A reflector, or focusing cup, within the cathode structure into which the filament is placed, focuses the electron beam in a similar manner as light is focused by a flashlight reflector. When the high-voltage circuit is activated, the free electrons are accelerated toward the focal spot on the anode target.

switch is depressed. The step-up and step-down transformers are located in the tube head.

Autotransformer

An **autotransformer** is a voltage compensator that corrects minor fluctuations in the current flowing through the wires. The output of the autotransformer is regulated by the kVp selector dial on the control panel. The kVp dial selects the desired voltage and applies it across the primary of the high voltage transformer.

The autotransformer is located in the control panel. By turning a knob on the control panel, the operator causes a selector switch to slide over a series of tabs that regulate the voltage by either decreasing or increasing it. This action is comparable to fine tuning on a radio.

Many transformers used in conventional x-ray machines are heavy and bulky. The trend is toward using lighter weight and miniaturized solid-state components. This has the added advantage of reducing the size and the weight of the tube head, thus making it easier for the operator to position it.

Principles of X-ray Tube Operation

A summation of the fundamentals of x-ray generation is in order prior to examining the radiation output of the x-ray machine. Before x-ray production can begin, the machine must be turned on and the necessary settings made on the control panel. The process of x-ray production is initiated by firmly pressing the exposure button. This permits the current to enter the filament circuit of the x-ray machine. A step-down transformer reduces the voltage before it enters the filament circuit and heats the filament of the cathode to incandescence, separating electrons from their atoms. The degree to which the filament is heated depends on the milliamperage that is selected: The higher the mA, the more electrons in the **electron cloud.** These electrons are now in a state of excitation as they hover around the filament wire recessed in the focusing cup. After a time delay of less than 1/2 second, the line current enters the cathode–anode high-voltage circuit. A step-up transformer then increases the voltage to impart sufficient force to propel the free electrons to the focal spot on the target at the anode. These high-velocity electrons are stopped by the tungsten atoms in the target resulting in the production of general radiation (bremsstrahlung) and characteristic radiation. This kinetic energy (the high-velocity electrons) is converted into 99 percent heat and 1 percent x-rays (Chapter 2).

The metal tungsten (symbol W and atomic number 74; also known as wolfram) is ideally suited for use in the filament and target because it can withstand extremely high temperatures (melting point 3370°C). Because it is subjected to such extreme heat and has low thermal conductivity, the tungsten plate is imbedded in a core of copper. Copper is highly conductive and carries the heat off to the **radiator,** which is just outside the tube (refer to the tube diagram in Figure 3–11). In an oil-cooled tube, the large mass of copper conducts the heat out of the tube into a radiator that transfers the heat to the oil surrounding the tube. In an air-cooled tube, the heat is transferred through the copper and the radiator into the air inside the tube head.

The x-rays produced by the energy exchange within the tube are emitted in all directions within the tube housing. Many of

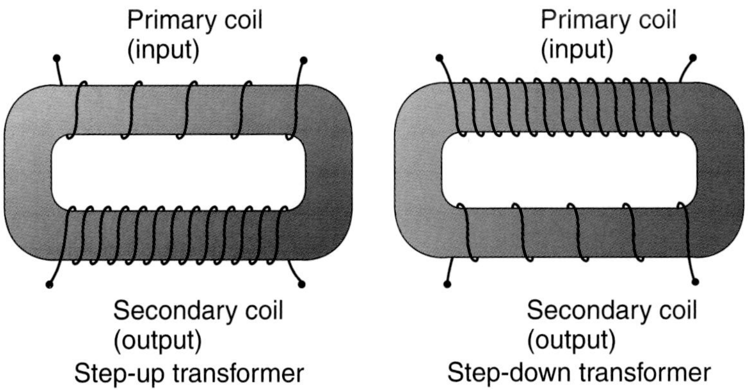

FIGURE 3–14 **Simplified diagram of the step-up and step-down transformers.**

these x-rays are absorbed by the glass tube, oil, air, wires, transformers, and the tube head lining. A window (a thin area in the glass envelope) is located at a point where the emission of x-rays is most intense. In turn, this window is aligned with an opening in the tube housing called the **port** that is covered by a permanent seal of glass, beryllium, or aluminum.

If the tube head is properly sealed, the port is the only place through which the x-rays can escape the tube head (Figure 3–8). These x-rays make up the primary beam. The PID (position indicating device) fits over the port and can be moved to aim the primary beam of x-rays in the desired direction. Upon completion of the predetermined exposure, the high-voltage current is automatically shut off, and x-ray production stops.

The X-ray Beam

X-rays are produced in 360-degree direction at the focal spot of the target. However, because of the angle of the anode, a high concentration of x-rays travels toward the port of the tube head. Only a beam of radiation the size of the port seal is allowed to exit the tube head. The other x-rays are stopped (absorbed) by the contents and walls of the tube head. After the beam exits through the port, the lead **collimator** (explained in Chapter 6) further restricts the x-ray beam to the desired size.

The x-ray beam is cone-shaped because x-rays travel in diverging straight lines as they radiate from the focal spot. This beam of x-rays is called the **primary beam** or the **useful beam.** The primary beam is the original useful beam of x-rays that originates at the focal spot and emerges through the port of the tube head. The **central ray** is the x-ray in the center of the primary beam.

The x-ray beam formed at the focal spot is **polychromatic,** consisting of x-rays of various wavelengths. Only x-rays with sufficient energy to penetrate oral structures are useful for diagnostic radiology. X-rays of low penetrating power (long wavelength) add to the patient dose but not to the information on the film. To remove the soft x-rays, a thin sheet of aluminum called a **filter** is placed in the path of the x-ray beam. Filtration is explained in detail in Chapter 6.

The **intensity** of the x-ray beam refers to the quantity and quality of the x-rays. **Quantity** refers to the number of x-rays in the beam. **Quality** refers to the energy or penetrating ability of the x-ray beam (see Chapter 4). **Intensity** is defined as the product of the number of x-rays (quantity) and the energy of the x-rays (quality) per unit of area per unit of time. Intensity of the x-ray beam is affected by milliamperage (mA), kilovoltage (kVp), exposure time, and distance.

Operation of the Dental X-ray Machine

The operation of each dental x-ray machine is explained fully in the operating manual provided by the manufacturer. All persons operating an x-ray machine should study the manual until they are thoroughly familiar with the operational capability and maintenance requirements of the machine. To achieve consistent results, the radiographer should follow a systematic and orderly procedure (Procedure Box 3–1). Additionally, whenever x-ray exposures are made on patients, it is assumed here and in all subsequent instructions that:

- The radiographer is competent and can follow radiation safety protocol. (Some states require anyone placing and

PROCEDURE 3–1

OPERATION OF THE DENTAL X-RAY MACHINE

1. Turn power on. A light on the control panel will indicate that the machine is ready to operate.
2. Unless preset by unit manufacturer, select mA and kVp best suited for the exposure to be made.
3. Set timer for the desired exposure time.
4. Place film packet into the film-holding device and position in the patient's oral cavity.
5. Utilizing the extension arm and yoke, adjust the tube head by aligning the PID so that the central beam of radiation is directed toward the center of the film at the appropriate horizontal and vertical angulations.
6. Establish appropriate location from the tube head.
7. Depress exposure button and hold it down firmly until the exposure is completed. The audible signal and x-ray exposure indicator light will activate for the duration of the exposure.
8. Remove the film packet from the patient's oral cavity after the exposure.
9. When the procedure is complete, fold the tube head support extension arm into the closed, neutral position.
10. Turn off the power to the x-ray machine.

exposing dental radiographs to successfully complete a training course in radiation safety and protection.)

- The radiographer performs all radiographic procedures in accordance with federal, state, and local regulations and recommendations.
- Infection control is maintained throughout the procedure (see Chapter 9).
- The procedure has been explained and the patient has given consent.
- The patient has received verbal instructions and is able to cooperate with the procedure.
- Film-holding devices are utilized for all intraoral radiographs.

Practice Point

For maximum effectiveness in exposing dental radiographs, prepare the patient and the x-ray equipment and set the controls on the x-ray unit prior to positioning the film packet in the oral cavity. Following an orderly sequence in positioning the film packets reduces the likelihood of errors and retakes.

REVIEW—Chapter Summary

All x-ray machines, regardless of size and voltage range, operate similarly and have the same components (control panel, extension arm, and tube head) and electrical parts (x-ray tube, low- and high-voltage circuits, and a timing device).

The control panel may be integrated with the x-ray machine tube head support or it may be remote from the unit, mounted on a shelf or wall. There are five major controls that may be operated or will be pre-set on most dental x-ray machines: (1) the line switch to the electrical outlet, (2) the milliampere selector, (3) the kilovoltage selector, (4) the timer, and (5) the exposure button.

A folding extension arm is a support from which the tube housing is suspended. The tube head is a tightly sealed heavy metal housing that contains the dental x-ray tube, insulating oil, and step-up and step-down transformers.

Three conditions must exist to produce x-rays: (1) a source of free electrons, (2) high voltage to accelerate them, and (3) a target to stop them. The dental x-ray tube creates these conditions. X-rays are produced only when the unit is turned on and a firm pressure is maintained on the exposure button.

Electric current flows into the x-ray machine and proceeds either through the step-down transformer or the step-up transformer. The step-down transformer reduces the electric current from the wall outlet to heat up the filament inside the focusing cup of the cathode (negative) side of the tube. Thermionic emission results in freed electrons available to make x-rays. The step-up transformer increases the electric current to impart kinetic energy to the freed electrons to cause them to propel across the tube to strike the target (on the focal spot) at the anode (positive) side of the tube.

The degree to which the filament is heated and, hence, the quantity of electrons made available depends on the millamperage setting. Quantity refers to the number of x-rays in the beam. The higher the mA, the more electrons available. The penetrating ability or quality of the resultant x-rays is determined by the kilovoltage setting. The higher the kVp, the more penetrating the x-rays.

The beam of radiation that exits the port seal of the tube head is the primary or useful beam. The polychromatic beam must be filtered to allow only x-rays with sufficient energy to reach the oral structures.

The radiographer must be familiar with the operation of the machine and the patient must understand the procedure and provide consent. To achieve consistent results, the radiographer should follow a systematic and orderly procedure.

RECALL—Study Questions

1. All of the following may be located on the control panel *except* one. Which one is this *exception?*
   a. mA selector
   b. kVp selector
   c. Focusing cup
   d. Line switch
2. How many impulses are equivalent to 1/4 second?
   a. 6
   b. 15
   c. 24
   d. 40
3. Fill in the blanks.
   a. 30 impulses = _____ second.
   b. 45 impulses = _____ second.
   c. 1/3 second = _____ impulses.
   d. 3/10 second = _____ impulses.
4. Which of the following activates the x-ray production process?
   a. Exposure button
   b. Milliamperage
   c. Voltmeter
   d. Timer selector
5. The x-ray machine component that allows the operator to position the tube head is called the:
   a. Timer cord.
   b. Control panel.
   c. Dead-man switch.
   d. Extension arm.
6. To get the biggest increase in the quantity of electrons available, increase the:
   a. mA (milliamperage).
   b. kVp (kilovoltage).
   c. PID (position indicating device).
   d. DC (direct current).
7. Which term describes the electrical pressure (difference in potential) between two electrical charges?
   a. Amperage
   b. Voltage
   c. Ionization
   d. Incandescence

8. List the three conditions that must exist for x-rays to be produced.
   a. ______________________
   b. ______________________
   c. ______________________
9. Draw and label a typical dental x-ray tube.
10. The process of heating the cathode wire filament until red hot and electrons boil off is called:
    a. Autotransformation.
    b. Self-rectification.
    c. Thermionic emission.
    d. Kilovoltage peak.
11. What metal is used for the filament in the x-ray tube?
    a. Lead
    b. Copper
    c. Tungsten
    d. Molybdenum
12. What metal is used for the target in the x-ray tube?
    a. Copper
    b. Tungsten
    c. Aluminum
    d. Molybdenum
13. Which of these must be charged negatively during the time that the x-ray tube is operating in order to produce x-rays?
    a. Radiator
    b. Target
    c. Anode
    d. Cathode
14. Which of these terms describes an electromagnetic device within the x-ray tube head for changing the voltage of alternating current?
    a. Transformer
    b. Collimator
    c. Radiator
    d. Rectifier
15. Which part of the x-ray tube is heated when the electric current is allowed to flow through the low-voltage circuit?
    a. Target
    b. Filament
    c. Focal spot
    d. Tube housing
16. What percent of the kinetic energy inside the x-ray tube is converted into x-rays?
    a. 1%
    b. 50%
    c. 75%
    d. 99%
17. Which term describes the opening in the tube housing that allows the primary beam to escape?
    a. Yoke
    b. Filament
    c. Port
    d. Focusing cup
18. Which term best describes an x-ray beam that is composed of a variety of wavelengths?
    a. Collimated
    b. Short-scale
    c. Filtered
    d. Polychromatic
19. Which of the following removes the low-energy, long-wavelength energy from the beam?
    a. Transformer
    b. Collimator
    c. Filter
    d. Radiator

REFLECT—Case Study

To help you understand the practical use of altering exposure variables on a dental x-ray machine, consider the following patients with these characteristics:

1. A 9-year-old female, height 4′ 8″ and weight 85 pounds, who has been assessed for bitewing radiographs to determine the evidence of caries.
2. A 21-year-old male college football player, height 6′ 1″, 280 pounds, who has been assessed for periapical radiographs of suspected impacted third molars.
3. A 58-year-old female, diagnosed with Bell's palsy with slight head and neck tremors, who has been assessed for a full mouth series for the evaluation of periodontal disease.

Would you select an increased or decreased amount of radiation to produce diagnostic quality radiographic images for each of these patients?

Which of these three exposure variables—milliamperage, kilovoltage, or time—control(s) the amount of radiation produced?

Which exposure variable would be the *best* choice to alter to increase or decrease the amount of radiation produced for each of these patients?

Would you select an increased or decreased penetrating ability of the x-ray beam to produce diagnostic quality radiographic images for each of these patients?

Which of the three exposure variables—milliamperage, kilovoltage, or time—control(s) the penetrating ability of the x-ray beam?

Which exposure variable would be the *best* choice to alter to increase or decrease the penetrating ability of the x-ray beam?

Suppose that you wanted to decrease the amount of time of the exposure, as may be needed when patient movement is anticipated, (as in the case of patient 3) but still wanted to produce enough radiation to achieve a diagnostic quality radiographic image. Which variable—milliamperage or kilovoltage—would you adjust? Would you increase or decrease this variable?

Think of other characteristics patients may present with that would require you to adjust these x-ray machine variables. Keep in mind that increasing one factor may necessitate decreasing an opposing factor. Discuss the rationale for your choices.

RELATE—Laboratory Application

Obtain an inanimate object of varying densities that can be exposed at different exposure variables and compare the results. For example expose a seashell placed on a size #2 intraoral film at the following exposure settings: 7 mA, 70 kVp, 10 impulses. Expose subsequent films varying one or more of the exposure settings. Using a view box, analyze the resultant radiographic images. Identify which settings produced darker or lighter images, and which settings produced low or high contrast images. (See Chapter 4 for definitions of radiographic density and contrast.)

BIBLIOGRAPHY

Bushberg, J. T., Seibert, J. A., Leidholdt, E. M. Jr., & Boone, J. M. *The Essential Physics of Medical Imaging,* 2nd ed. Baltimore, MD: Lippincott Williams & Wilkins, 2001.

Eastman Kodak. *Successful Intraoral Radiography.* Rochester, NY: Eastman Kodak, 1998.

White, S. C., & Pharoah, M. J. *Oral Radiology: Principles and Interpretation,* 5th ed. St. Louis: Elsevier, 2004.

4

Producing Quality Radiographs

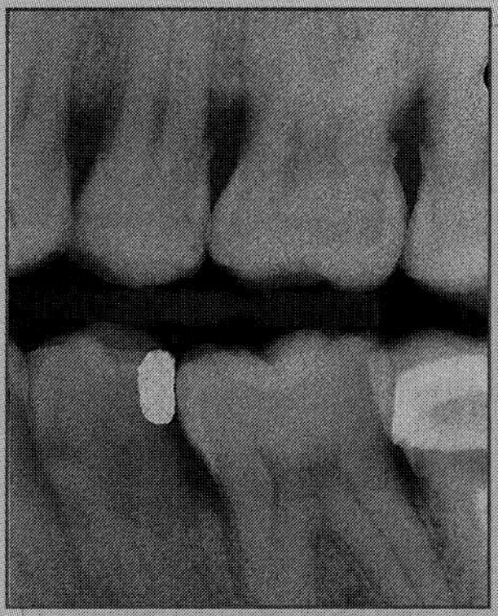

CHAPTER OUTLINE

■ OBJECTIVES

Following successful completion of this chapter, you should be able to:

1. Define the key words.
2. Evaluate a radiographic image identifying the basic requirements of acceptability.
3. Differentiate between radiolucent and radiopaque areas on a dental radiograph.
4. Define radiographic density and contrast.
5. List the rules for casting a shadow image.
6. Differentiate between subject contrast and film contrast.
7. List the factors that influence magnification and distortion.
8. List the geometric factors that affect image sharpness.
9. Summarize the factors affecting the radiographic image.
10. Describe how mA, kVp, and exposure time affect film density.
11. Discuss how kVp affects the image contrast.
12. Explain target–surface, object–film, and target–film distances.
13. Demonstrate the practical use of the inverse square law.

■ KEY WORDS

Contrast
Crystal
Definition
Density
Distortion
Exposure chart
Exposure factors
Exposure time
Extraoral radiography
Film contrast
Focal spot
Geometric factors
Grid
Intensifying screen
Intraoral radiography
Inverse square law
Kilovoltage peak (kVp)
Long-scale contrast
Magnification
Milliampere (mA)
Milliampere/second (mAs)
Motion
Object–film distance
Penumbra
Position indicating device (PID)
Radiographic contrast
Radiolucent
Radiopaque
Sharpness
Short-scale contrast
Subject contrast
Target–film distance
Target–object distance
Target–surface distance

Introduction

Each patient presents with a unique set of characteristics for which a customized approach to exposure settings is needed. The dental radiographer has an ethical responsibility to produce the highest diagnostic quality radiographs for patients who agreed to be exposed to ionizing radiation. To consistently produce diagnostic quality radiographs at the lowest possible radiation dose, the dental radiographer needs to understand the inter-relationships of the components of the dental x-ray machine.

There are three basic requirements for an acceptable diagnostic radiograph (Figure 4–1).

1. All parts of the structures radiographed must be shown on the film as close to their natural shapes and sizes as the patient's oral anatomy will permit. Distortion and superimposition of structures should be at a minimum.
2. The area examined must be shown completely, with enough surrounding tissue to distinguish between the structures shown.
3. The film should be free of errors and of proper density, contrast, and definition.

The quality of a radiograph depends upon both the physical factors and the subjective opinion of the individual who reads it. The purpose of this chapter is to describe the physical attributes of a quality radiographic image and to study the factors that affect these attributes.

Terminology

The following terms should be used when describing radiographic images: radiolucent, radiopaque, density, contrast, and sharpness.

When a dental radiograph is viewed on a light source the image appears black and white, with various shades of gray in between. The terms used to describe the black and white areas are radiolucent and radiopaque, respectively.

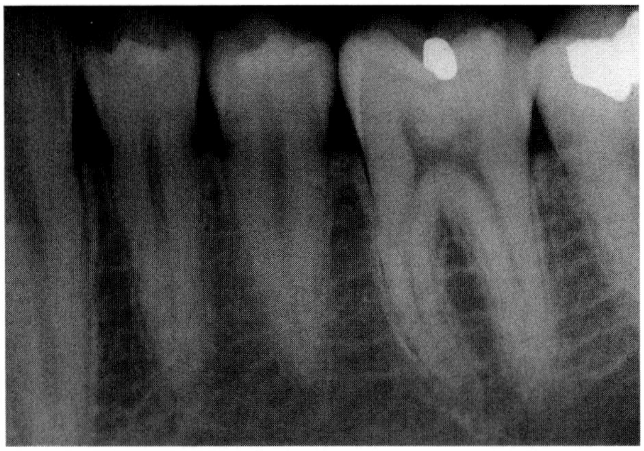

FIGURE 4–1 **An acceptable diagnostic radiograph.**

Radiolucent

Radiolucent refers to that portion of the image that is dark or black (Figure 4–1). Structures that appear radiolucent permit the passage of x-rays with little or no resistance. Soft tissues and air spaces are examples of structures that appear radiolucent on a radiograph.

Radiopaque

Radiopaque refers to that portion of the image that is light or white (Figure 4–1). Structures that appear radiopaque are dense and absorb or resist the passage of x-rays. Enamel, dentin, and bone are examples of structures that appear radiopaque on the radiograph.

Radiolucent and radiopaque are relative terms. For instance, even though both enamel and dentin are radiopaque, dentin is more radiolucent (appears darker) than enamel.

Three visual image characteristics that directly influence the quality of the radiographic image are density, contrast, and sharpness.

Density

Density, also known as film blackening, is the amount of light transmitted through the film (Figure 4–2). If a great deal of light is transmitted through the film, the radiograph is said to have little density. If the radiograph is very dense (black), little light will be transmitted through the film. The blackness in a dental radiograph results when x-rays strike sensitive crystals in the film emulsion and subsequent processing causes the crystals to turn black. Thus the degree of darkening of the radiograph is increased when the milliamperage or the exposure time is increased and more x-rays are produced to reach the film emulsion.

Radiographs need just the right amount of density to be viewed properly. If the density is too light or too dark, the images of the teeth and supporting tissues cannot be visually separated from each other. The ideal radiograph has the proper amount of density for the interpreter to view black areas (radiolucent), white areas (radiopaque), and the gray areas.

Contrast

Contrast refers to how sharply dark and light areas are differentiated (Figure 4–3). A film with good contrast will contain black, white, and many shades of gray. A radiograph that shows just a few

A

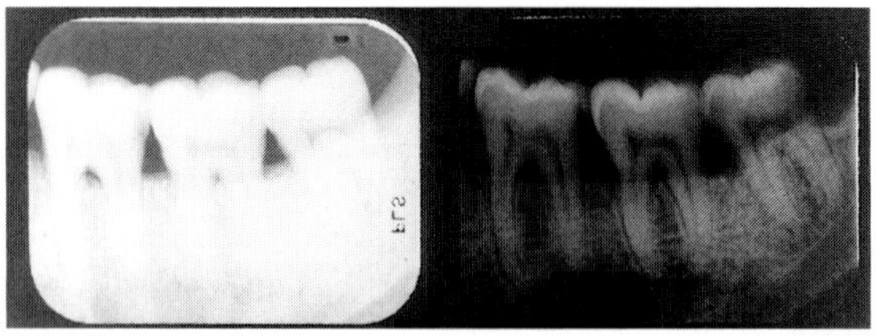

B

FIGURE 4–2 **Radiographic density.** Radiograph (**A**) is underexposed and appears too light (less dense). Radiograph (**B**) is overexposed and appears too dark (more dense).

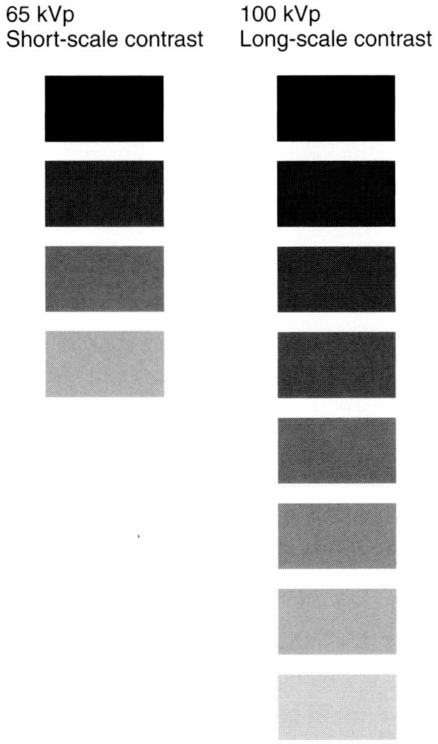

FIGURE 4–3 Penetrometer tests demonstrate radiographically that a longer contrast scale results from the use of 100 kilovolt exposures. Dental radiographs exposed at 100 kVp have long-scale contrast. Radiographs exposed at 65 kVp have short-scale contrast. (Courtesy of General Electric Company, Medical Systems Division)

shades is said to have short-scale contrast, while one that shows many variations in shade is said to possess long-scale contrast.

The term **short-scale contrast** (Figure 4–4) describes a radiograph in which the density differences between adjacent areas are large. The contrast is high because there are fewer shades of gray and more black against white. The gray tones indicate the differences in absorption of the x-ray photons by the various tissues of the oral cavity or the head and neck region. The radiograph is radiolucent (dark) where the tissues are soft or thin and radiopaque (white) where the tissues are hard or thick. Such radiographs result when low (65–75) kVp is applied. Short-scale contrast radiographs are purported to make dental caries easier to recognize; however, fine detail, such as that regarding the periodontium, may be difficult to distinguish on short-scale images.

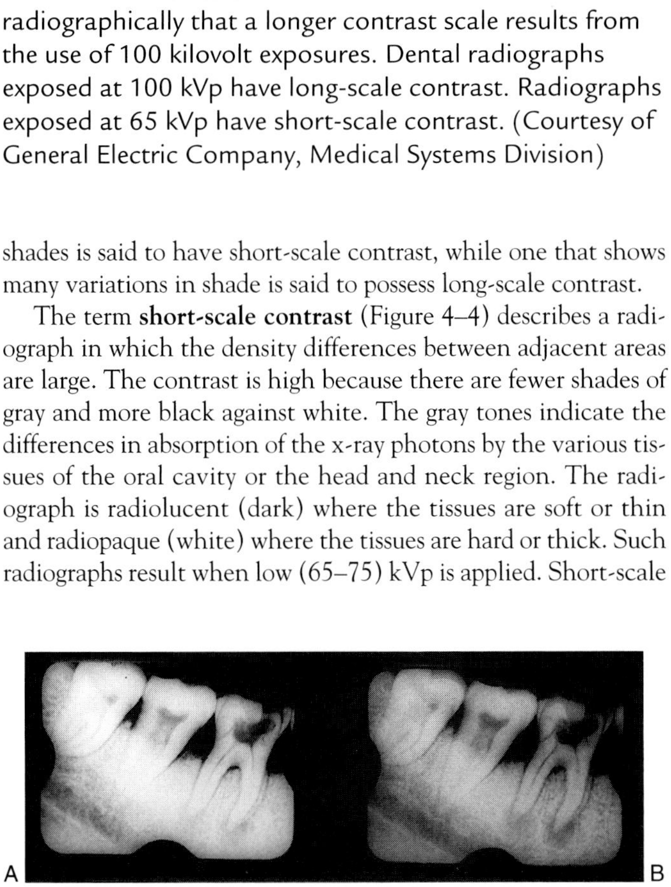

FIGURE 4–4 **Radiographic contrast.** Radiograph (**A**) exposed at 60 kVp, has high contrast. Radiograph (**B**) exposed at 90 kVp, has low contrast.

The term **long-scale contrast** (Figure 4–4) describes a radiograph in which the density differences between adjacent areas are small. The contrast is low and very gradual because there are many shades of gray. Such radiographs result when high (85–100) kVp is applied. More detailed information can be obtained from such radiographs, provided that a view box with variable light control is used. The ideal kVp to use is strictly a matter of individual preference.

Practice Point

In the past it was thought that high-kVp techniques resulted in a lower radiation dose to the patient. That is not necessarily so. High-kVp techniques do result in lower *exposures* to the patient, but not lower *doses* (see Chapter 2 for an explanation of the difference between exposure and dose). Compared to high-kVp techniques, low-kVp techniques result in a higher entrance dose but a lower exit dose to the patient's head and neck region. This is because the x-rays are less penetrating. High-kVp techniques result in a lower entrance dose but a higher exit dose because the x-rays are more penetrating. The total dose to the patient is essentially the same with either kVp technique. While the dose is distributed through the patient's anatomical structures differently, from a radiological health aspect, the dose is the same.

Sharpness

Sharpness/definition is a geometric factor that refers to the detail and clarity of the outline of the structures shown on the radiograph. Unsharpness is generally caused by movement of the patient, film, or the tube head during exposure.

Shadow Casting

A radiograph is a two-dimensional image of three-dimensional objects. Therefore, it is necessary to apply the rules for creating a shadow image to produce a quality radiographic image. The following rules for casting a shadow image will help to reproduce the size and shape of the objects radiographed accurately.

Rules for Casting a Shadow Image

1. Small focal spot: to reduce the size of the **penumbra** (partial shadow around the objects of interest) resulting in a sharper image and slightly less magnification.
2. Long target-object distance: to reduce the penumbra and magnification.

3. Short object-film distance: to reduce penumbra and magnification.
4. Parallel relationship between object and film: to prevent distortion of the image.
5. Perpendicular relationship between the central ray of the x-ray beam and the object and film: to prevent distortion of the image.

Because x-rays belong to the same electromagnetic spectrum as light (see Chapter 2), these two energies share many of the same characteristics. Therefore, when considering the application of shadow cast rules it is helpful to compare the shadows cast by light with the shadows that x-rays will cast of the structures of the oral cavity. For example, if you were outside during the morning hours when the sun was low on the horizon, the sun's rays would be directed at your body at a low angle, casting a shadow that was elongated, or longer than your actual height. If you were outside at midday, when the sun was directly overhead, the sun's rays would be directed at your body at a steep angle, casting a shadow that was foreshortened, or shorter than your actual height. At some time during the day, the sun's light would be cast at the precise angle to your body that your shadow on the ground would be at the same length as your actual height. Directing a flashlight at an object, such as the child's game of producing hand puppet shadows, is another example of shadow casting. Depending on the direction of the flashlight beam alignment and the distance the light must travel to reach the object, accurate or distorted shadow images result.

Shadow cast rules are often referred to as the **geometric factors** that contribute to the quality of the radiographic image. Geometric factors are those factors that relate to the relationships of angles, lines, points, or surfaces. Each of the shadow cast rules will be discussed in detail as to its role in producing quality radiographic images.

Factors Affecting the Radiographic Image

The dental radiographer must have a working knowledge of the factors that affect the radiographic image. The detail and visibility of a radiograph depends upon two independent factors—radiographic contrast and sharpness/definition (Table 4–1).

Radiographic Contrast

Radiographic contrast can be defined as the visible difference between densities on a radiograph. The radiographic contrast depends upon two separate factors: (1) subject contrast, the result of differences in absorption of the x-ray by the tissues under examination; and (2) film contrast, a characteristic of the film and processing.

Subject Contrast

The three factors that affect the **subject contrast** are the subject (patient), kilovoltage, and scattered radiation.

a. **Subject (patient).** The subject contrast is the result of differences in absorption of the x-rays by the tissues under examination. The subject to be radiographed must have contrast. A radiograph of a 1-in. sheet of plastic would show no contrast since the plastic is of uniform thickness and composition. Patients have contrast because human tissues vary in size, thickness, and density.
b. **Kilovoltage peak (kVp).** There is an inverse relationship between kVp and contrast (Figure 4–4). In relative terms, higher kilovoltages produce lower subject contrast. The blacks are grayer, the whites are grayer, and there are many steps (or shades) of gray in between. Lower kilovoltages produce higher subject contrast. The blacks are blacker, the whites are whiter, and there are fewer steps (or shades) of gray in between.
c. **Scattered radiation.** In Chapter 2 we learned that Compton scattering occurs whenever x-rays interact with matter such as the tissues of the patient's head. These scattered x-rays add a uniform exposure to the radiograph, thereby decreasing the contrast. For **intraoral radiography** (inside the mouth), a collimator (lead diaphragm) is used to keep the beam size as small as possible to help reduce scatter radiation. For **extraoral radiography** (outside the mouth), grids are sometimes used to absorb scattered x-rays. A **grid** is a mechanical device composed of thin strips of lead alternating with a radiolucent material (plastic). The grid is placed between the patient and the film in order to absorb scattered x-rays (see Figure 27–8).

TABLE 4–1 **Summary of Factors That Affect the Radiographic Image**

Detail—Visibility			
Radiographic Contrast		Sharpness / Definition	
Subject Contrast	Film Contrast	Geometric Factors	Crystal Size
Subject	Film type	Focal spot size	Crystal size
kVp	Exposure	Target–film distance	
Scattered radiation	Processing	Object–film distance	
		Motion	
		Screen thickness	
		Screen–film contact	

Film Contrast

Film contrast is the inherent contrast built into the film by the manufacturer. Film contrast is affected by: film type, exposure, and processing.

a. **Film type.** Each film has its own built-in contrast. Film contrast is determined by the film manufacturer.
b. **Exposure.** An underexposed or an overexposed film will result in poor contrast and reduce viewing quality of the radiograph. The radiographer must always use the proper exposure settings to produce quality radiographic images.
c. **Processing.** Maximum film contrast can only be obtained through meticulous film processing procedures (Chapter 8). If improper development time or temperature is used, the radiograph will not have the ideal contrast the manufacturer built into it.

Sharpness / Definition

Sharpness, also known as **definition,** refers to the clarity of the outline of the structures on the image of a radiograph. Sharpness is the result of two separate things: geometric factors and crystal size (see Table 4–2).

Geometric Factors

The **geometric factors** that contribute to the radiographic image are the first three shadow cast rules—focal spot size, target–film distance, object–film distance—and three additional geometric factors—motion, screen thickness, and screen–film contact.

a. **Focal spot size.** As explained in Chapter 3, the **focal spot** is the small area on the target where bombarding electrons are converted into x-rays. The smaller the focal spot area, the sharper the image appears (Figure 4–5). A large focal spot creates more penumbra (partial shadows) and therefore loss of image sharpness (Figure 4–6). Ideally, the focal spot should be a point source; then no penumbra would be present. However, a single point source would create extreme heat and burn out the x-ray tube. Focal spot size is determined by the manufacturer of the x-ray machine. To

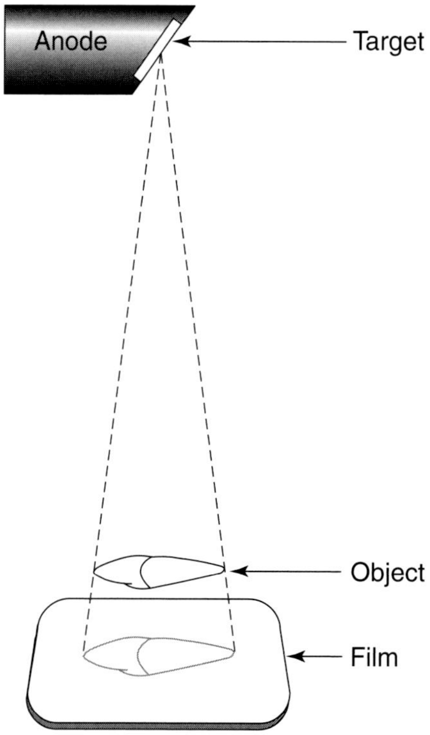

FIGURE 4–5 Using a small focal spot on the target, a long target–film distance, and a short object–film distance will result in a sharp image.

TABLE 4–2 **Factors Influencing Sharpness**

Factors	Modify	Sharpness
Focal spot size	Small focal spot	Increase sharpness
	Large focal spot	Decrease sharpness
Target–film distance	Long target–film distance	Increase sharpness
	Short target–film distance	Decrease sharpness
Object–film distance	Short object–film distance	Increase sharpness
	Long object–film distance	Decrease sharpness
Motion	No movement	Sharp image
	Movement	Fuzzy image
Screen thickness	Thin screen	Increase sharpness
	Thick screen	Decrease sharpness
Screen–film contact	Close contact	Increase sharpness
	Poor contact	Decrease sharpness
Film crystal size	Small crystals	Increase sharpness
	Large crystals	Decrease sharpness

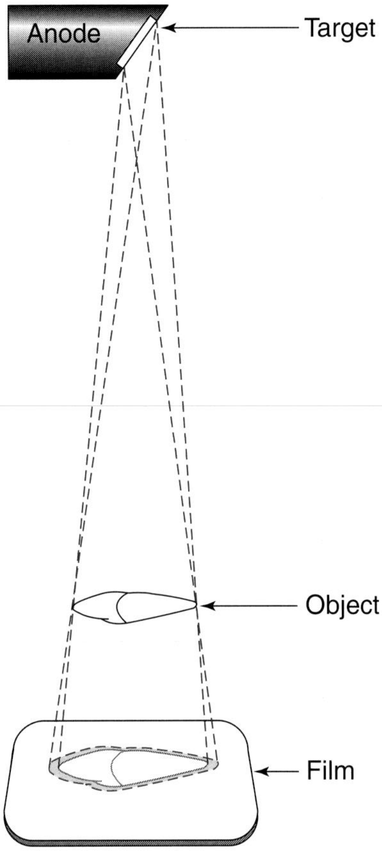

FIGURE 4-6 Large focal spot on the target and long object-film distance results in more penumbra and therefore loss of image sharpness.

ensure that the focal spot remains small, the tube head must remain perfectly still during the exposure. Even slight vibration of the tube head increases the size of the focal spot (Figure 4–7).

Practice Point

The tube head must remain perfectly still during exposure. Even slight vibration of the tube head increases the size of the focal spot, which in turn produces an unsharp image.

b. **Target–film distance.** The **target–film distance** is the distance between the source of x-ray production (which is at the target on the anode inside the tube head) and the film. PIDs are used to establish the target–film distance. PIDs are classified as being short or long and come in standard lengths of 8 inches (20.5 cm), 12 inches (30 cm), and 16 inches (41cm) for intraoral projections. The shorter the target–film distance, the more divergent the x-ray beam (Figure 4–8). A long target–film distance has x-rays in the center of the beam that are nearly parallel. Therefore, the image on the radiograph will be sharper. Also a longer target–film distance will result in less image magnification (explained later in this chapter).

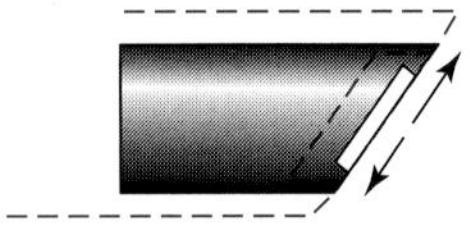

FIGURE 4-7 **Movement of the tube head.** Motion, even slight, of the tube head will effectively create a larger surface area of the focal spot, resulting in penumbra.

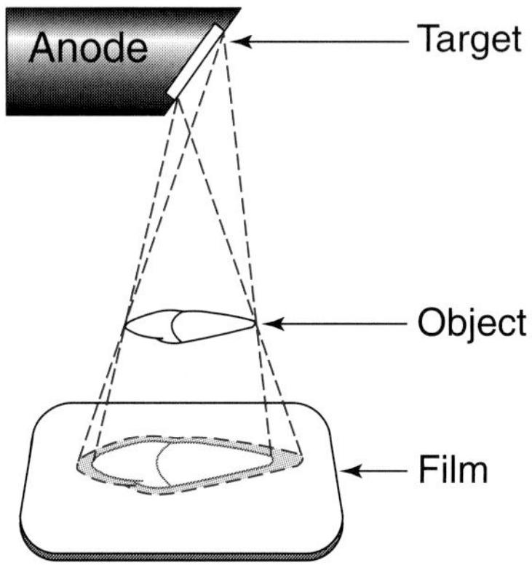

FIGURE 4-8 Large focal spot on the target and short target-film distance results in more penumbra and therefore loss of image sharpness.

c. **Object–film distance.** The **object–film distance** is the distance between the object being radiographed (the teeth) and the dental x-ray film. The film should always be placed as close to the teeth as possible. The closer the proximity of the film to the teeth, the sharper the image and the less magnification (image enlargement). The image will become fuzzy (more penumbra) and magnified, as the object–film distance is increased (Figure 4–6).

d. **Motion.** Movement of the patient and/or the film in addition to the tube head results in a loss of image sharpness (Figure 4–9).

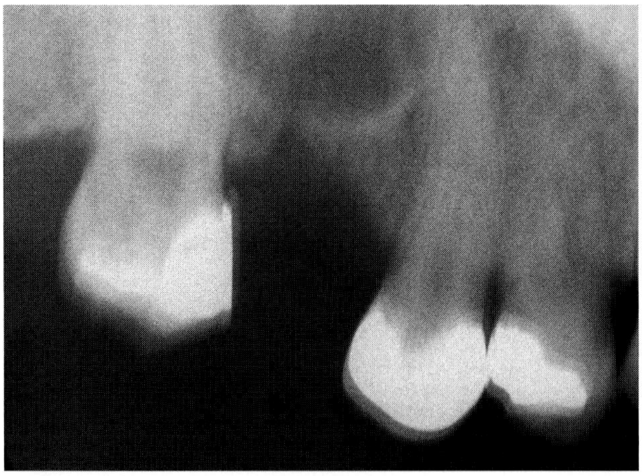

FIGURE 4-9 Blurry, unsharp image caused by movement of the patient, the film, or the tube head.

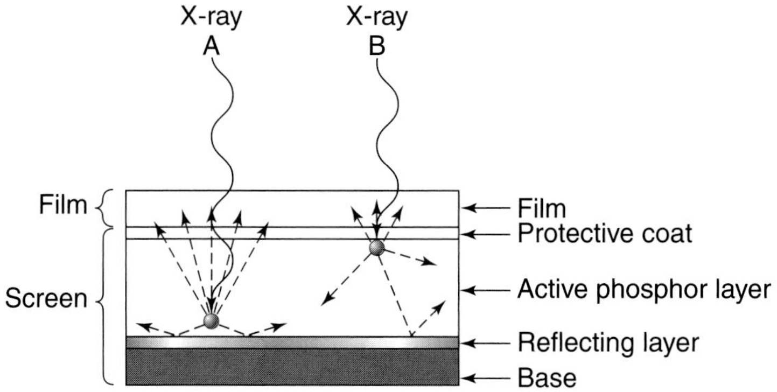

FIGURE 4–10 **Screen thickness.** X-ray A strikes a crystal far from the film and the divergent light exposes a wide area of the film resulting in unsharpness. X-ray B strikes a crystal close to the film, resulting in less divergence of the light that exposes the film and therefore a sharper image. The thicker the screen, the less sharp the image.

e. **Screen thickness. Intensifying screens** (often referred to as screens), used in extraoral radiography, are made of crystals that emit light when struck by x-rays. The light, in turn, exposes the film and helps to produce the image. Intensifying screens require less radiation to produce a radiographic image than direct exposure film, resulting in less radiation exposure to the patient. However, the use of intensifying screens decreases the sharpness of the radiographic image (Figure 4–10). The thicker the screen, the less radiation required to expose the film; however, these thicker screens produce a less sharp radiographic image. Generally, the radiographer should use the highest speed screen and film combination, determined by the thickness of the phosphor layer, that is consistent with good diagnostic results. Intensifying screens are explained in detail in Chapter 27.

f. **Screen–film contact.** The film should be in close physical contact with the intensifying screen. Poor screen–film contact results in the wider spread of light and fuzziness (penumbra) of the image. Intensifying screens should be examined periodically for proper screen–film contact. Additionally, only one film should be placed in contact with the screen. Attempting to make a duplicate image by placing two films into one cassette is not acceptable practice unless using a film made especially for this purpose.

Crystal Size of Intraoral Film

Sharpness is influenced by the size of the **crystals** within the emulsion of the film. Similar to the crystal size of the intensifying screens, the smaller the size of the crystals within the film emulsion, the sharper the radiographic image.

X-ray film emulsion contains crystals that are struck by x-rays when exposed and in turn produce the radiographic image. Sharpness of the radiographic image is relative to the size of the crystals. High-speed film requiring less radiation for exposure uses larger crystals that produce less image sharpness. Blurriness occurs because larger crystals do not produce object outlines as well as small crystals. However, this loss of sharpness is tolerated because of the reduction in patient exposure. Image definition (sharpness of details) is more distinct when crystals are small, but small crystal size contributes to a slow speed film, requiring the patient to receive a larger dose of radiation. Dental x-ray film is explained in detail in Chapter 7.

Magnification/Enlargement

Magnification or enlargement is the increase in size of the image on the radiograph compared to the actual size of the object. In Chapter 3, we learned that x-rays travel in diverging straight lines as they radiate from the focal spot of the target. Because of these diverging x-rays, there is some magnification present in every radiograph.

Magnification is mostly influenced by the **target–object distance** and the object–film distance. The target–object distance is determined by the length of the PID. When a long PID is used, the x-rays in the center of the beam are more parallel, resulting in less image magnification (Figure 4–11). The object–film distance should be kept to a minimum. Always place the film as

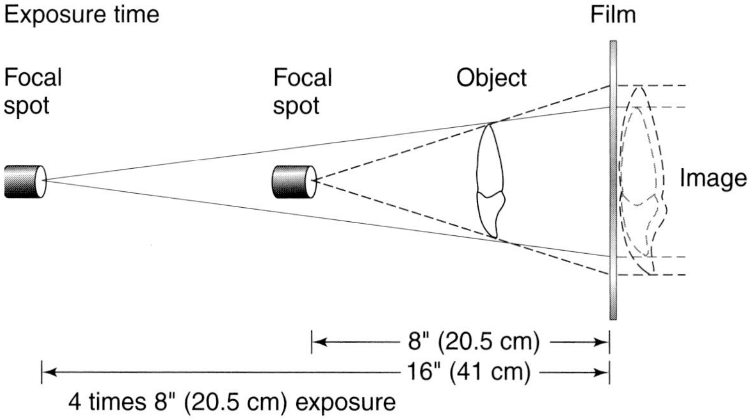

FIGURE 4–11 **Magnification.** Comparison of 8-in. (20.5-cm) and 16-in. (41-cm) target–film distance. The image is magnified (enlarged) when the target–film distance is shortened and the object (tooth)–film distance is held constant. Ideally, the distance from the target to the object should be as long as possible and the object (tooth)–film distance should be as short as possible. When using the 16-in. (41-cm) target–film distance, the exposure time must be lengthened to four times that required at an 8-in. (20.5-cm) target–film distance. (Courtesy of Dentsply Rinn)

close to the teeth as possible, while maintaining a parallel relationship between the long axis of the teeth and the film plane, to decrease magnification.

Increasing the target–object distance and decreasing the object–film distance will minimize image magnification. Note that these two shadow cast rules for reducing magnification also increase image sharpness.

Distortion

Distortion is the result of unequal magnification of different parts of the same object. Distortion results when the film is not parallel to the object (Figure 4–12) and/or when the central ray of the x-ray beam is not perpendicular to the object and film plane (Figure 4–13). To minimize image distortion, the two shadow cast rules for film packet and x-ray beam positioning must be followed. Rule 4 and Rule 5 state that the film plane must be positioned parallel to the long axis of the tooth and the central ray of the x-ray beam must be aligned perpendicular to both the film and the tooth.

Effects of Varying the Exposure Factors

Two visual characteristics of the radiographic image, density and contrast, have a tremendous influence on the diagnostic quality of the radiograph. Here we will see what effect the x-ray machine exposure factors settings have on the density and contrast.

The milliamperage, the exposure time, and the kilovoltage are known as the **exposure,** control, or radiation **factors.** Whenever one of the exposure factors is altered, one or a combination of the other factors must be altered proportionally to maintain radiographic density (Table 4–3). For example, exposure time will need to be decreased when milliamperage or kilovoltage is increased to maintain optimal film density. Distance, or PID length, is an additional variable factor that is explained later in this chapter.

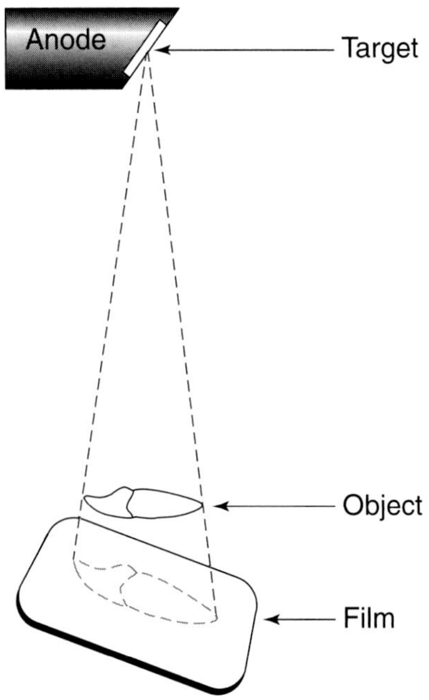

FIGURE 4–12 **Object and film are not parallel, resulting in distortion.**

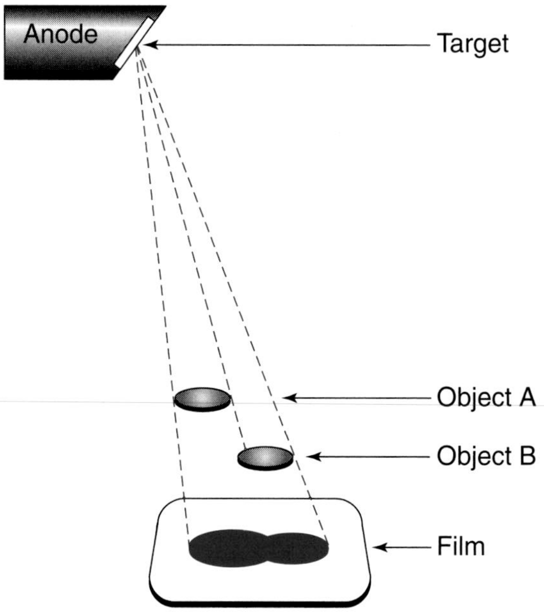

FIGURE 4–13 Central ray of x-ray beam is not perpendicular to the objects and film, resulting in distortion and overlapping of object A and object B. Note object A is magnified larger than object B because object A is a greater distance from the film than object B.

Variations in Milliamperage (mA)

The amount of electric current used in the x-ray machine is expressed in **milliamperes (mA).** The mA selected by the operator, or pre-set by the unit manufacturer, determines the quantity or number of x-rays that are generated within the tube. The density of the radiograph is affected whenever the milliamperage

TABLE 4–3 **Effect of Varying Exposure Factors on Film Density**

Exposure Adjustment[a]	Film Density
Increase mA	Darker
Decrease mA	Lighter
Increase time	Darker
Decrease time	Lighter
Increase kVp	Darker[b]
Decrease kVp	Lighter[b]

[a]When any exposure factor is increased, or decreased, one or more of the other exposure factors must be adjusted to maintain optimum film density.
[b]Varying kVp primarily affects the film contrast, but it will also (secondarily) affect the film density. Increase kVp for less contrast and decrease kVp for more contrast.

is changed. Increasing the mA increases (darkens) the density of the radiograph, whereas decreasing the mA decreases (lightens) the density of the radiograph.

Variations in Exposure Time

Exposure time is the interval that the x-ray machine is fully activated and x-rays are produced. The principal effect of changes in exposure time is on the density of the radiograph. Increasing the exposure time darkens the radiograph, while decreasing exposure time lightens it. Opinions differ on optimum density and contrast because visual perception varies from person to person; some practitioners may prefer lighter radiographs, while others may prefer darker radiographs. Of the three controls, exposure time is easiest to change. In fact, many x-ray machines today have pre-set fixed milliamperage and kilovoltage, so that time is the only exposure factor that can be changed by the operator.

Milliampere/seconds (mAs)

Since both milliamperage and exposure time are used to regulate the number of x-rays generated and have the same effect on radiographic density, they are often combined into a common factor called **milliampere/seconds (mAs).** Combining the milliamperage with the exposure time is an effective way to determine the total radiation generated.

A simple formula for determining this total is: mA multiplied by the exposure time (in seconds or impulses) equals mAs.

$$\text{mA} \times \text{s} = \text{mAs}$$

PROBLEM. Consider a practical problem using this formula. Assume the following exposure factors are in use: 10 mA, 0.6 sec, 90 kVp, and 16-in. (41-cm) target–film distance. If the mA is increased to 15, but the kVp and target–film distance remain constant, what should the new exposure time be to maintain image density?

SOLUTION. The only exposure factor that was changed is the mA, which was increased from 10 mA to 15 mA. We need to compensate for the increase in mA by decreasing the exposure time.

$$\text{mA} \times \text{s} = \text{mAs}$$

$$10\ \text{mA} \times 0.6\ \text{sec.} = 6\ \text{mAs}$$

$$15\ \text{mA} \times ?\ \text{sec.} = 6\ \text{mAs}$$

$$?\ \text{sec.} = \frac{6\ \text{mAs}}{15\ \text{mAs}}$$

$$?\ \text{sec.} = 0.4\ \text{sec}$$

ANSWER. The new exposure time is 0.4 sec.

When the mA is increased, the exposure time must be decreased to produce identical radiographic image density between the first and second radiographs. A practical use for applying this formula would be when patient movement is anticipated—in this case, increasing the amount of radiation produced, so that the duration of exposure could be shortened.

Variations in Kilovoltage (kVp)

The quality of the radiation (wavelength or energy of the x-ray photons) generated by the x-ray machine is determined by the kilovoltage peak (kVp). The more the kVp is increased, the shorter the wavelength and the higher the energy and penetrating power of the x-rays produced. Kilovoltage is the only exposure factor that directly influences the contrast of a dental radiograph. However, increasing the kVp will also increase the number (quantity) of x-rays produced. Therefore, the number of x-rays that enter the emulsion coating of the x-ray film also increases, resulting in increased density of the radiograph. As the kVp of the x-ray beam is increased for the purpose of producing a lower contrast image, the density of the radiograph is held constant by reducing the milliampere-seconds (mAs) or exposure time. Since the exposure time is usually the easiest exposure factor to change, the following rule applies: When increasing the kVp by 15, for example from 70 kVp to 85 kVp, decrease the exposure time by dividing by 2, when decreasing the kVp by 15, increase the exposure time by multiplying by 2. Thus one exposure factor balances the other to produce a radiographic image of acceptable density.

Effects of Variations in Distances

The operator must take into account several distances to produce the ideal diagnostic quality image:

- The distance between the x-ray source (at the focal spot on the target) and the surface of the patient's skin
- The distance between the object to be x-rayed (usually the teeth) and the film
- The distance between the x-ray source and the recording plane of the film

Various terms are used in dental literature to describe these distances. The terms target–surface (skin), anode–surface, focus–surface, tube–surface, and source–surface are synonymous, as are target–film, anode–film, focus–film, and source–film. In this text, the terms target–surface distance, object–film distance, target–object distance, and target–film distance are used (Figure 4–14).

Target–Surface Distance

Generally, whenever the film is positioned intraorally, the length of the **target–surface distance** depends on the length of the position indicating device used. All intraoral techniques require the open end of the PID be positioned to almost touch the patient's skin to standardize the distance used and the image density.

Object–Film Distance

The object–film distance depends largely on the method that is employed to hold the film in position next to the teeth. When the bisecting technique is used (see Chapter 12), the film is

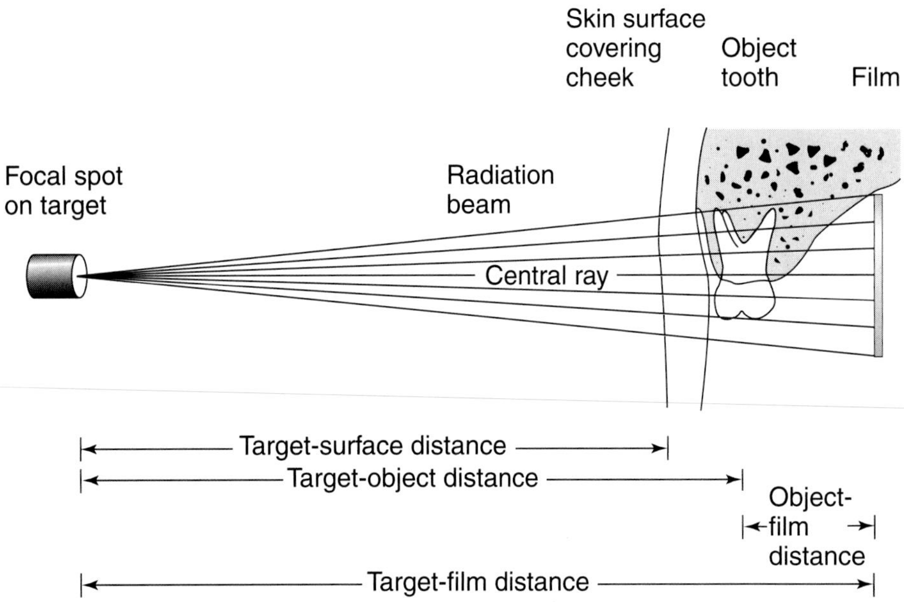

FIGURE 4-14 **Distances.** Relationship among target, skin surface, object (tooth), and x-ray film distance.

pressed against the palatal or lingual tissues as close as the oral anatomy will permit. This results in the object–film distance being shorter in the area of the crown where the tooth and film touch than in the area of the root, where the thickness of the bone and gingiva may cause a divergence between the long axis of the tooth and the film (Figure 4–15). The least divergence occurs in the mandibular molar areas. The greatest divergence is in the maxillary anterior areas, where the palatal structures may curve sharply.

With the paralleling technique, most film holders are designed so that the film is held parallel to the average long axis of the tooth being radiographed. This necessitates positioning the film sufficiently into the lingual area of the oral cavity, away from the teeth to avoid impinging on the supporting bone and gingival structures. This technique results in object–film distances that are often more than 1 in. (25 mm). The paralleling technique compensates for this increased object–film distance by recommending an increase in the target–film distance (use a longer PID) to help offset the distortion, explained next.

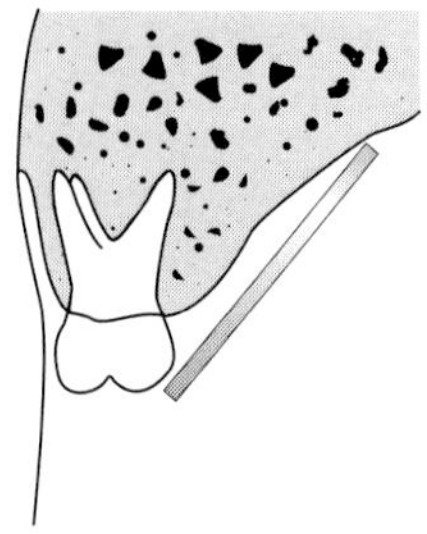

FIGURE 4-15 **Object–film distance.** This film packet placement places the crown of the tooth closer to the film than the root.

Target–Film Distance

The target–film distance is the sum of the target–object and the object–film distance (Figure 4–14). The quality of the radiographic image improves whenever the target–film distance is increased. Magnification is reduced, and sharpness of detail (definition) is increased. Increasing the target-film distance reduces the fuzzy outline (penumbra) that is seen around the radiographic images. Hence, positioning the film far enough from the teeth to enable it to be held parallel and using a long 16-in. (41-cm) PID will increase the quality of the image definition. These techniques are described in detail in Chapter 12.

The location of the x-ray tube within the tube housing can affect the target–film distance. In the conventional dental x-ray machine, the target (located on the anode within the tube) is situated in the tube head in front of the transformers. The attached PID length can be visibly determined. When the tube is recessed within the tube head, located behind the transformers enough space is gained within the tube head so that a long target–film distance is achieved even though a short PID is in place (see Figure 3–1).

Inverse Square Law

The x-ray photons, traveling in straight lines, spread out (diverge) as they radiate away from the source (target). It follows that the intensity of the beam is reduced as this occurs (Figure 4–16). How much the beam intensity decreases is based on the **inverse square law,** which states that the intensity of radiation varies inversely as the square of the distance from its source.

The inverse square law may be written as:

$$\frac{I_1}{I_2} = \frac{(D_2)^2}{(D_1)^2}$$

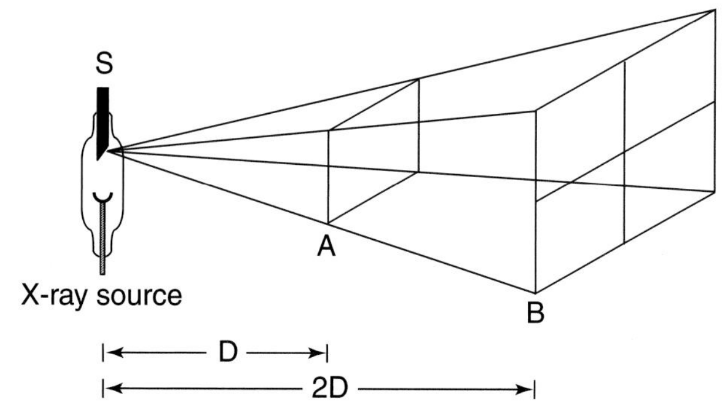

FIGURE 4–16 **Inverse square law.** Relationship of distance (D) to the area covered by x-rays emitted from the x-ray tube. X-rays emerging from the tube travel in straight lines and diverge from each other. The areas covered by the x-rays at any two points are proportional to each other as the square of the distances measured from the source of radiation. (Reproduced with permission from Wuehrmann AH, Manson-Hing LR. ***Dental Radiology,*** 5th ed. St. Louis: C. V. Mosby, 1981)

where: I_1 is the original intensity.
I_2 is the new intensity.
D_1 is the original distance.
D_2 is the new distance.

The inverse square law is applied when considering the distance between the source of radiation and the film, as in the length of the PID and when considering the distance between the source of radiation and the operator, as in where the operator stands to maintain radiation protection during exposure. The distance between the source of radiation and the film will have an affect on the image quality. When changing the PID length, a corresponding change must occur in the exposure time to maintain film density. When changing the distance an operator stands from the source of radiation, it is important to understand how the intensity of the radiation decreases by the square of the distance increased.

Consider the following problem where distance is considered as a means of operator protection.

PROBLEM. A dental radiographer stands 3 feet (0.9 m) from the source of radiation where the measured intensity is 100 milliroentgens (mR) per minute. The radiographer then moves to a new location 6 ft (1.8 m) from the source of radiation. What is the radiation intensity at the new location?

SOLUTION.

$$I_1 = 100 \text{ mR/min}$$

$$D_1 = 3 \text{ ft}$$

$$D_2 = 6 \text{ ft}$$

Find I_2.

$$\frac{100}{I_1} = \frac{6^2}{3^2}$$

$$\frac{100}{I_2} = \frac{2^2}{1^2}$$

$$\frac{100}{I_2} = \frac{4}{1}$$

$$\left(\frac{1}{4}\right)\frac{100}{I_2} = \frac{4}{1}\left(\frac{1}{4}\right)$$

$$I_2 = 25 \text{ mR per minute}$$

ANSWER. The intensity at the new location is 25 mR/min.

In this case, the radiographer's new location is a safer place to stand during exposure, since this new location at 6 ft away from the source of radiation receives only one-fourth the exposure of the old location at 3 ft away for the source of radiation.

Consider the following problem where distance is considered when changing the length of the PID.

PROBLEM. A quality dental radiograph is obtained using an 8-in. (20.5 cm) PID and an exposure time of 3 impulses. The 8-in. (20.5 cm) PID is removed from the tube head and replaced with a 16-in. (41 cm) PID. What should the new exposure time be to maintain image density of radiographs exposed at this new target–film distance?

We know that the radiation intensity at a distance of the 16 inches (41 cm) will be less than the intensity at the old distance of 8 inches (20.5 cm). Applying the inverse square law formula we would see that the intensity of the radiation will have decreased by the square of the distance, producing a radiographic image that would be less dense (lighter) than the original radiograph produced using an 8-in. (20.5 cm) PID. To produce a radiograph of equal density using a 16-in. (41 cm) PID, use the following modification of the inverse square law formula to determine the new exposure setting:

$$\frac{I_1}{I_2} = \frac{(D_1)^2}{(D_2)^2}$$

where:
I_1 is the original exposure time (in impulses).
I_2 is the new exposure time (in impulses).
D_1 is the original distance.
D_2 is the new distance.

SOLUTION.

$$I_1 = 3 \text{ impulses}$$

$$D_1 = 8 \text{ inches}$$

$$D_2 = 16 \text{ inches}$$

Find I_2.

$$\frac{3}{I_2} = \frac{8^2}{16^2}$$

$$\frac{3}{I_2} = \frac{1^2}{2^2}$$

$$\frac{3}{I_2} = \frac{1}{4}$$

$$\frac{(4)3}{I_2} = \frac{1(4)}{4}$$

$$I_2 = 12 \text{ impulses}$$

ANSWER. The impulse setting required to maintain film density at the new 16-in. (41 cm) source-to-film distance is 12 impulses.

Since the x-rays emerging from the tube travel in straight lines and diverge from one another, it follows that the intensity of the beam is reduced unless a corresponding increase is made in one or a combination of the target–film distance exposure factors. Such changes in exposure factors are essential to maintaining optimum film density. Usually time is the easiest exposure factor to change. This formula is useful for obtaining the appropriate exposure time when only the target–film distance is altered.

Exposure Charts

Operators may memorize exposure factors needed for a particular technique; however, safety protocol dictates that **exposure charts,** available commercially or custom made by the practice, be posted at the x-ray unit control panel for easy reference. In fact, in some locations regulations require that exposure charts be posted. These charts show at a glance how much exposure time is required for a film of any given speed when used with all possible combinations of exposure time, milliamperage, and peak kilovoltage.

Some dental x-ray machine manufacturers have incorporated the commonly used film speeds and other exposure factors into the dial of the control panel. With these units, the operator only has to set the pointer to the desired combination for a film of a given speed and the unit automatically sets the required exposure factors.

REVIEW—Chapter Summary

An acceptable diagnostic radiograph must show the areas of interest—the designated teeth and surrounding bone structures—completely and with minimum distortion and maximum sharpness. When evaluating a radiographic image, the oral health care professional should utilize appropriate scientific terminology such as density, contrast, sharpness, magnification and distortion. The term radiolucent refers to the dark or black portion of the image, while radiopaque refers to the light or white portion of the image. High contrast images, those with black and white and few shades of gray, are called short-scale, while low contrast images, those with grayer whites and grayer blacks with many shades of gray, are called long-scale.

The dental radiographer must have a working knowledge of the factors that affect the radiographic image. The detail and visibility of a radiograph depends upon two factors—radiographic contrast and sharpness/definition. Radiographic contrast is composed of both subject contrast and film contrast. Sharpness is determined by geometric factors and crystal size of the film emulsion.

To create a sharp image, the radiographer must follow the rules for casting a shadow image: small focal spot, long target–film distance, short object–film distance, parallel relationship between object and film, and perpendicular relationship between central ray of the x-ray beam and the object and film. Image magnification and loss of sharpness is further reduced by limiting movement of the tube head and PID, the patient, and the film during exposure.

While not all dental x-ray units allow the operator to manually alter all exposure factors, when available, the radiographer should take advantage of the ability to vary the exposure factors to produce radiographs that have the desired image qualities. When altering one exposure factor, a corresponding change must be made to another factor to produce identical radiographic image density. When changing the PID length, the inverse square law must be utilized to adjust the exposure time to produce identical radiographic image density.

RECALL—Study Questions

1. List the three criteria for acceptable radiographs.
   a. ______________________
   b. ______________________
   c. ______________________
2. Dense objects absorb the passage of x-rays *and therefore* appear radiolucent on the resultant radiographic image.
   a. The first part of the statement is true but the second part of the statement is false.
   b. The first part of the statement is false but the second part of the statement is true.
   c. Both parts of the statement are true.
   d. Both parts of the statement are false.
3. The degree of darkening of the radiographic image is referred to as:
   a. Contrast
   b. Definition
   c. Density
   d. Penumbra
4. Which of the following describes the radiographic image produced with a kVp exposure setting of 100?
   a. Short scale
   b. Long scale
   c. High contrast
   d. Low density
5. Subject contrast is affected by:
   a. Processing procedures.
   b. Type of film.
   c. Scattered radiation.
   d. Crystal size.

6. What factor has the greatest effect on image sharpness?
   a. Movement
   b. Filtration
   c. Kilovoltage
   d. Amperage
7. As crystals in the film emulsion increase in size, the radiographic image sharpness increases, *and* the amount of radiation needed to expose the film at an acceptable density decreases.
   a. The first part of the statement is correct but the second part of the statement is incorrect.
   b. The first part of the statement is incorrect but the second part of the statement is correct.
   c. Both parts of the statement are correct.
   d. Both parts of the statement are incorrect.
8. What term best describes a fuzzy shadow around the outline of the radiographic image?
   a. Magnification
   b. Distortion
   c. Detail
   d. Penumbra
9. Distortion results when:
   a. Object and film are not parallel.
   b. X-ray beam is perpendicular to the object and film.
   c. Using a short object–film distance.
   d. Using a small focal spot.
10. The dental radiograph will appear less dense (lighter) if one increases the:
    a. mA.
    b. kVp.
    c. Exposure time.
    d. Target–film distance.
11. The exposure factors in an oral health care facility are: 10 mA, 0.9 sec, 70 kVp, and 16-in. (41-cm) target–film distance. The radiographer increases the mA to 15, but leaves the kVp and target–film distance constant. To maintain identical image density, what should the new exposure time be?
    a. 0.3
    b. 0.6
    c. 1.2
    d. 1.8
12. Which of the following is appropriate to increase radiographic contrast while maintaining image density?
    a. Increase the kVp and increase the exposure time.
    b. Increase the kVp and decrease the exposure time.
    c. Decrease the kVp and increase the exposure time.
    d. Decrease the kVp and decrease the exposure time.
13. Based on the inverse square law, what happens to the intensity of the x-ray beam when the target–film distance is doubled?
    a. Intensity is doubled.
    b. Intensity is not affected.
    c. Intensity is one-half as great.
    d. Intensity is one-fourth as great.
14. A radiographer stands 4 ft (1.22 m) from the head of the patient while exposing a dental film. Her personnel monitoring device measures the radiation dose at that position to be 0.04 millisievert (mSv). The radiographer decides to move to a new location 8 ft (2.44 m) from the head of the patient. What is the dose at the new location?
    a. 0.01 mSv
    b. 0.02 mSv
    c. 0.08 mSv
    d. 0.16 mSv
15. A patient presents whose radiographs must be taken utilizing the bisecting technique. The radiographer decides to replace the 16-in. (41 cm) PID with an 8-in. (20.5 cm) PID to better accommodate the bisecting technique. Currently the impulse setting, with the 16-in. (41 cm) PID, is 12. To maintain image density, what will the new impulse setting be with the 8-in. (20.5 cm) PID?
    a. 3
    b. 6
    c. 24
    d. 48

REFLECT—Case Study

You have just been hired to work in a new oral health care facility. Prior to providing patient services, you are being asked to help develop exposure settings and equipment recommendations for the practice. The equipment and film manufacturers' suggestions are as follows:

F Speed Film   8-in. (20.5 cm) PID   85 kVp

	Impulses	
Bitewings	Adult	Child
Posterior	10	8
Anterior	6	4
Periapicals		
Maxillary anterior	8	6
Maxillary premolar	12	8
Maxillary molar	14	10
Mandibular anterior	6	4
Mandibular premolar	8	6
Mandibular molar	10	8

1. You recommend that the facility replace the 8-in. (20.5 cm) PID with a 16-in. (41 cm) PID. Develop a new exposure chart for using the new 16-in. (41 cm) PID.
2. You recommend using a kVp setting of 70 when exposing radiographs for the purpose of detecting caries. Develop a new exposure chart for 70 kVp.
3. You recommend using a kVp setting of 90 when exposing radiographs for the purpose of evaluating supporting bone and periodontal disease. Develop a new exposure chart for 90 kVp.

RELATE—Laboratory Application

For a comprehensive laboratory practice exercise on this topic, see E. M. Thomson, *Exercises in Oral Radiography Techniques: A Laboratory Manual,* 2nd ed. Upper Saddle River, NJ: Prentice Hall, 2007. Chapter 9, "Exposure Variables—Factors Affecting the Radiographic Image."

BIBLIOGRAPHY

Eastman Kodak. *Successful Intraoral Radiography.* Rochester, NY: Eastman Kodak, 1998.

Langland, O. E., Sippy, F. H., & Langlais, R. P. *Textbook of Dental Radiology,* 2nd ed. Springfield, IL: Charles C. Thomas, 1984.

Thomson, E. M. and Tolle, L. A practical guide for using radiographs in the assessment of periodontal disease, Part I. *Practical Hygiene* 3:1, 1994.

White, S. C., & Pharoah, M. J. *Oral Radiology: Principles and Interpretation,* 5th ed. St. Louis: Elsevier, 2004.

Part II • Biological Effects of Radiation and Radiation Protection

5

Effects of Radiation Exposure

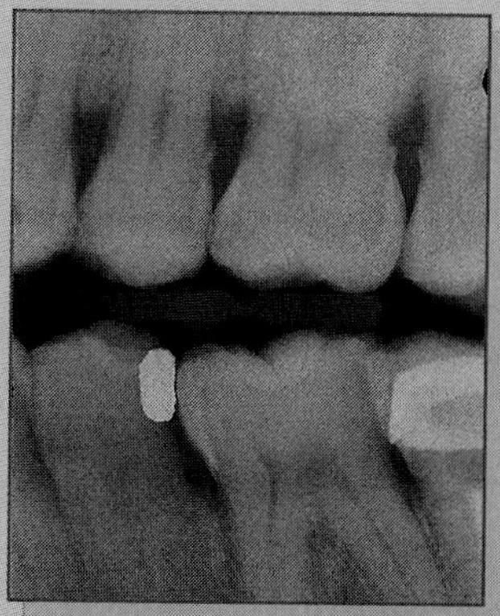

CHAPTER OUTLINE

OBJECTIVES

Following successful completion of this chapter, you should be able to:

1. Define the key words.
2. Explain the difference between the direct theory and the indirect theory of biological damage.
3. Determine the relative radiosensitivity or radioresistance of various kinds of cells in the body.
4. Explain the difference between somatic effect and genetic effect.
5. Explain the difference between a threshold dose–response curve and a non-threshold dose–response curve.
6. Identify the factors that determine radiation injuries.
7. List the sequence of events that may follow exposure to radiation.
8. Explain the difference between deterministic and stochastic effects.
9. List the possible short- and long-term effects of irradiation.
10. Identify critical tissues for dental radiography in the head and neck region.
11. Discuss the risk versus benefit of dental radiographs.
12. Utilize effective dose equivalent to make radiation exposure comparisons.
13. Adopt an ethical responsibility to follow ALARA.

KEY WORDS

Acute
Acute radiation syndrome (ARS)
ALARA (as low as reasonably achievable)
Cumulative effect
Deterministic (non-stochastic) effect
Direct theory
Dose rate
Dose–response curve
Effective dose equivalent
Genetic cells
Genetic effect
Genetic mutations
Indirect theory
Ionization
Irradization
Irreparable injury
Latent period
Law of B and T

Lethal dose (LD)	Recovery period
Microsievert (μSv)	Risk
Non-threshold dose–response curve	Somatic cells
Period of injury	Somatic effect
Radioresistant	Stochastic effect
Radiosensitive	Threshold dose–response curve

Introduction

Patients are often concerned with the safety of dental x-ray procedures. Such concerns are shared by oral health care professionals. The fact that ionizing radiation produces biological damage has been known for many years. The first x-ray burn was reported just a few months following Roentgen's discovery of x-rays in 1895. As early as 1902, the first case of x-ray-induced skin cancer was reported in the literature. Events such as the 1945 bombing of Hiroshima and the 1986 Chernobyl nuclear power plant accident have continued to generate unfavorable attitudes toward ionizing radiation, and concern over the use of x-rays in dentistry and medicine as well. While public concern is warranted, there are also some sensational and unsubstantiated articles appearing in newspapers and magazines, on television, and the Internet. Much of what we know about the effects of radiation exposure comes from data that is extrapolated from high doses and high dose rates. Studies of occupational workers exposed to chronic low levels of radiation have shown no adverse biological effect (U.S. Nuclear Regulatory Commission, http://www.nrc.gov/what-we-do/radiation/affect.html). However, even the radiation experts have not been able to determine whether or not a threshold level exists below which radiation effects would not be a risk. Because even the experts cannot always predict a specific outcome from an amount of radiation exposure, the radiation protection community conservatively assumes that any amount of radiation may pose a risk. The purpose of this chapter is to explain the theories of radiation injury and to identify factors that increase the risk of producing a biological response.

Theories of Biological Effect Mechanisms

As pointed out in Chapter 2, x-rays belong to the ionizing portion of the electromagnetic spectrum. X-rays have the ability to detach and remove electric charges from the complex atoms that make up the molecules of body tissues. This process, known as **ionization,** creates an electrical imbalance within the normally stable cells. Because disturbed cellular atoms or molecules generally attempt to regain electrical stability, they often accept the first available opposite electrical charge. In such cases, the undesirable chemical changes become incompatible with the surrounding body tissues. During ionization, the delicate balance of the cell structure is altered, and the cell may be damaged or destroyed.

There are two generally accepted theories on how radiation damages biological tissues: (1) the direct (or target) theory and (2) the indirect (or poison-water) theory (Figure 5–1).

- **Direct theory:** According to the direct theory, x-ray photons collide with important cell chemicals and break them apart by ionization, causing critical damage to large molecules (Figure 5–2). However, most dental x-ray photons probably pass through the cell with little or no damage. A healthy cell can repair any minor damage that might occur. Moreover, the body contains so many cells that the destruction of a single cell or a small group of cells will have no observable effect.
- **Indirect theory:** Based on the assumption that radiation can cause chemical damage to the cell by ionizing the water within it (Figure 5–3). Since about 80 percent of body weight is water and ionization can dissociate water into hydrogen and hydroxyl radicals, the theory proposes that new chemicals such as hydrogen peroxide could be formed under certain conditions.

These chemicals act as a poison to the body, causing cellular dysfunction. Fortunately, when the water is broken down during irradiation, the ions have a strong tendency to recombine immediately to form water again instead of seeking out new combina-

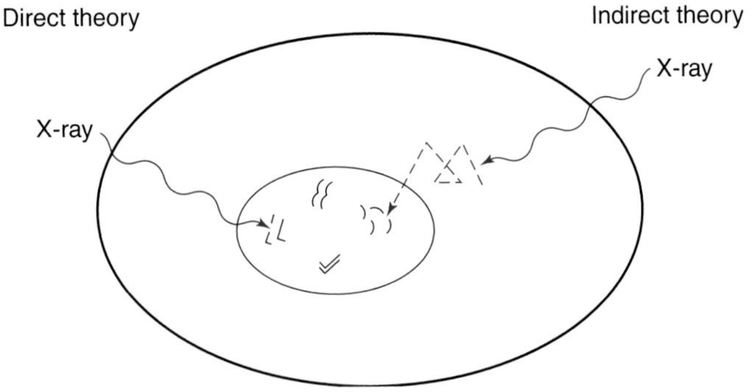

FIGURE 5–1 **Direct theory and indirect theory.** In the direct theory, x-ray photons collide with large molecules and break them apart by ionization. The indirect theory is based on the assumption that radiation can cause chemical damage to the cell by ionizing the water within it.

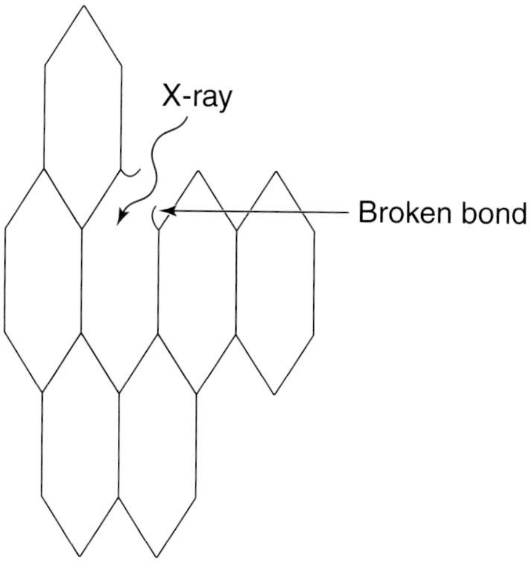

FIGURE 5-2 **Direct theory.** Radiation breaks the bonds connecting atoms in molecules causing ionization, thus producing harmful effects.

tions. This tendency holds cellular damage to a minimum. Under ordinary circumstances, even when a new chemical is formed, other cells that are not affected can take over the functions of the damaged cells until recovery takes place. Only in extreme instances, where massive irradiation has taken place, will entire body tissues be destroyed or death result. However, it should be remembered that cellular destruction is not the only biological effect; the potential exists for the cell to become malignant.

Cell Sensitivity to Radiation Exposure

The terms **radiosensitive** and **radioresistant** are used to describe the degree of susceptibility of various cells and body tissues to radiation. The cell is most susceptible to radiation injury during mitosis (cell division).

All cells are not equally sensitive to radiation. The relative sensitivity of cells to radiation was first described in 1906 by two French scientists, Bergonie and Tribondeau, and is known as the **law of B and T.** The first half of the law of B and T states that actively dividing cells, such as white blood cells, are more sensitive than slowly dividing cells. Embryonic and immature cells are more sensitive than mature cells of the same tissue. The second half of the law of B and T states that the more specialized a cell is, the more radioresistant the cell.

Based on these factors, it is possible to rank various kinds of cells in descending order of radiosensitivity:

High sensitivity

- White blood cells (lymphocytes)
- Red blood cells (erythrocytes)
- Immature reproductive cells
- Epithelial cells
- Endothelial cells
- Connective tissue cells
- Bone cells
- Nerve cells
- Brain cells
- Muscle cells

Low sensitivity

Additionally, a distinction should be made between irradiation of somatic cells and reproductive cells. **Somatic cells** are all of the cells of the body, except the reproductive cells. A **somatic effect** occurs when the biological change or damage occurs in the irradiated individual, but is not passed along to offspring. A **genetic effect** describes the changes in hereditary material that do not manifest in the irradiated individual, but in future generations.

The experts do not fully understand all these effects or their future consequences. Scientists believe that some of these effects are **cumulative,** especially if exposure is too great and the intervals between exposures too frequent for the body cells to repair themselves. Unless the damage is too severe or the subject is in extremely poor health, many body cells (somatic cells) have a recovery rate of almost 75 percent during the first 24 hours; after that, repair continues at the same rate.

In determining whether or not an exposure is potentially harmful, the radiographer should consider the quantity and the duration of the exposure and which body area is to be **irradiated.** Continued exposure over prolonged periods alters the ability of the **genetic cells** (eggs and sperm) to reproduce normally. Current

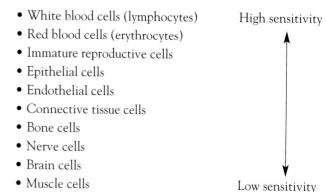

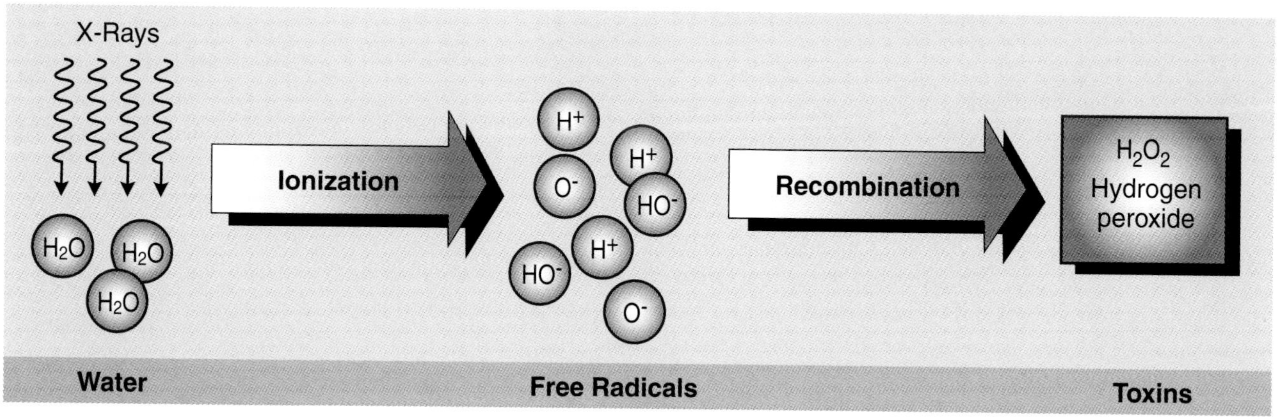

FIGURE 5-3 **Indirect theory.** X-rays ionize water, resulting in the formation of free radicals, which recombine to form toxins.

evidence indicates that chromosome damage is cumulative, increasing in effect by each successive additional radiation exposure, and genetic cells cannot repair themselves. Radiation may alter the genetic material in the reproductive cells so that mutations (abnormalities) may be produced in future generations.

The Dose–Response Curve

Radiation doses, like doses of drugs or other biologically harmful agents, can be plotted with response or damage produced, in an attempt to establish acceptable levels of exposure. In plotting these two variables, a **dose–response curve** is produced. A **threshold dose–response curve** indicates that there is a "threshold" amount of radiation, below which no biological response would be expected; a **non-threshold dose–response curve** indicates that any amount of radiation, no matter how small, has the potential to cause a biological response. These two possibilities are illustrated in Figure 5–4.

Unfortunately, radiobiologists have been unable to determine radiation effects at very low levels of exposure (for example, doses below 100 mSv) and cannot be certain whether or not a threshold dose exists. (To help put 100 mSv into perpective, a full mouth series of 18 F-speed films, at 90 kVp with 16 in. [41 cm] length PID is approximately 30 mSv skin exposure.) Therefore, the radiation protection community takes the conservative approach and considers any amount of ionizing radiation exposure as being non-threshold. This assumption has been made in the establishment of radiation protection guidelines and in radiation control activities. The concept that every dose of radiation produces damage and should be kept to the minimum necessary to meet diagnostic requirements is known as the **ALARA** concept, where ALARA stands for **as low as reasonably achievable.** ALARA is explained in detail in Chapter 6.

Factors That Determine Radiation Injury

Biological responses to low doses of radiation exposure are often too small to be detected. The body's defense mechanisms and ability to repair molecular damage often result in no residual effects. In fact, the following five outcomes are possible: (1) nothing—the cell is unaffected by the exposure; (2) the cell is injured or damaged but repairs itself and functions at pre-exposure levels; (3) the cell dies, but is replaced through normal biological processes; (4) the cell is injured or damaged, repairs itself, but now functions at a reduced level; (5) the cell is injured or damaged, and repairs itself incorrectly or abnormally, resulting in a biophysical change (tumor or malignancy). Determining which of these five outcomes might occur depends on all of the following.

- **Total dose:** The total dose of radiation depends on the type, energy, and duration of the radiation. The greater the dose, the more severe the probable biological effect.
- **Dose rate:** The rate at which the radiation is administered or absorbed is very important in the determination of what effects will occur. Since a considerable degree of recovery occurs from the radiation damage, a given dose will produce less effect if it is divided (thus allowing time for recovery between dose increments) than if it is given in a single exposure. For instance, an exposure of 1 R/week for 100 weeks would result in far less injury than a single exposure of 100 R.
- **Area exposed:** The amount of injury to the individual depends on the area or volume of tissue irradiated. The larger the area exposed, other factors being equal, the greater the injury to the organism. Exposure should be confined to as small an area as practical. Intraoral dental radiographic exposures use a very small (2.75 in. or 7 cm) beam diameter to limit the area of radiation exposure to the area of diagnostic concern, and this area can be further limited by the use of rectangular collimation (see Figure 6–4).
- **Variation in species:** Various species have a wide range of radiosensitivity. Lethal doses for plants and microorganisms are usually hundreds of times higher than those for mammals.
- **Individual sensitivity:** Individuals vary in sensitivity within the same species. The genetic makeup of some individuals may pre-dispose them to ionizing radiation damage. For this reason the **lethal dose (LD)** for each species is expressed

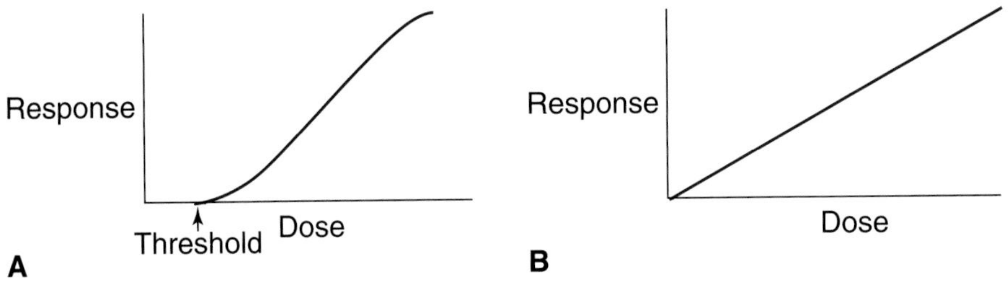

FIGURE 5–4 **Diagram of dose–response curve.** (**A**) A typical "threshold" curve. The point at which the curve intersects the base line (horizontal line) is the threshold dose that is the dose below which there is no response. If an easily observable radiation effect, such as erythema (reddening of the skin) is taken as "response," then this type of curve is applicable. (**B**) A linear "non-threshold" curve, in which the curve intersects the base line at its origin. Here it is assumed that any dose, no matter how small, causes some response.

in statistical terms, usually as the LD 50/30 for that species, or the dose required to kill 50% of the individuals in a large population in a 30-day period. For humans, the LD 50/30 is estimated to be 4.5 grays (Gy) or 450 rads (grays and rads are units of absorbed dose; see Chapter 2).

- **Variation in cell sensitivity:** Within the same individual, a wide variation in susceptibility to radiation damage exists among different types of cells and tissues. As the law of B and T points out, the cells that rapidly divide or have a potential for rapid division are more sensitive to radiation than those that do not divide. Furthermore, primitive or non-specialized cells are more sensitive than those that are highly specialized. Within the same cell families, then, the immature forms, which are generally primitive and rapidly dividing, are more radiosensitive than the older, mature cells, which have specialized function and have ceased to divide.
- **Variation in tissue sensitivity:** Some tissues (organs) of the body are more radiosensitive than others. For instance, blood-forming organs such as the spleen and red bone marrow are more sensitive than the highly specialized heart muscle.
- **Age:** Younger, more rapidly dividing cells are more radiosensitive than older, mature cells so it follows that children may be more susceptible to injury than adults from an equal dose of radiation. Also, in children the distance from the oral cavity to the reproductive and other sensitive organs is less than for adults. Therefore the dental doses to the critical organs may be higher than they would be for an adult. Additionally, an increase in radiation sensitivity is observed again in old age. As the body ages, the cells may begin to lose the ability to repair damage.

Sequence of Events Following Radiation Exposure

The sequence of events following radiation exposure are latent period, period of injury, and recovery period, assuming, of course, that the dose received was non-lethal.

- **Latent period:** Following the initial radiation exposure, and before the first detectable effect occurs, a time lag called the latent period occurs. The latent period may be very short or extremely long, depending on the initial dose. Effects that appear within a matter of minutes, days, or weeks are called short-term effects and those that appear years, decades, and even generations later are called long-term effects. Again, this relates to the types of cells involved and their corresponding rates of mitosis (cell division).
- **Period of injury:** Following the latent period, certain effects can be observed. One of the effects seen most frequently in growing tissues exposed to radiation is the stoppage of mitosis, or cell divisions. This may be temporary or permanent, depending upon the radiation dosage. Other effects include breaking or clumping of chromosomes, abnormal mitosis, and formation of giant cells (multi-nucleated cells associated with cancer.
- **Recovery period:** Following exposure to radiation, some recovery can take place. This is particularly apparent in the case of short-term effects. Nevertheless, there may be a certain amount of damage from which no recovery occurs, and it is this **irreparable injury** that can give rise to later long-term effects (Figure 5–5).

Radiation Effects on Tissues of the Body

Low levels of radiation exposure do not usually produce an observable adverse biological effect. As the dose of radiation increases, and enough cells are destroyed, the affected tissue will begin to exhibit clinical signs of damage. The severity of these clinical manifestations are dependent on the dose and dose rate. For example, erythema (redness of the skin) would not be expected from exposing the skin to sunlight for a few seconds. However, as the time of exposure to sunlight increased, the erythema would be expected to increase proportionally. When the severity of the change is dependent on the dose, the effect is called a **deterministic (non-stochastic) effect.**

When a biological response is based on the probability of occurrence rather then the severity of the change, it is called a **stochastic effect.** The occurrence of cancer is a stochastic effect of radiation exposure. When the dose of radiation is increased, the "probability" of the stochastic effect (cancer) occurring increases, but not its severity.

Short- and Long-term Effects of Radiation

The effects of radiation are classified as either short-term or long-term. Short-term effects of radiation are those seen minutes, days, or months after exposure. When a very large dose of radiation is delivered in a very short period of time, the latent period is short. If the dose of radiation is large enough (generally over 1.0 Gy or 100 rads, whole-body), the resultant signs and symptoms that comprise these short-term effects are collectively known as **acute radiation syndrome (ARS).** ARS symptoms include erythema

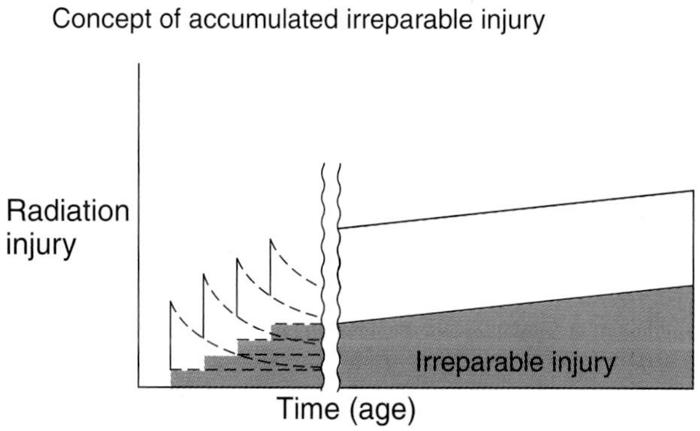

FIGURE 5–5 **Concept of accumulated irreparable injury.** After exposure to radiation cell recovery can take place. However, there may be a certain amount of damage from which no recovery occurs, and it is this irreparable injury that can give rise to later long-term effects.

(redness of the skin), nausea, vomiting, diarrhea, hemorrhage, and hair loss. ARS is not a concern in dentistry, because dental x-ray machines cannot produce the very large exposures necessary to cause it.

Long-term effects of radiation are those that are seen years after the original exposure. The latent period is much longer (years) than that associated with the acute radiation syndrome (hours or days). Delayed radiation effects may result from a previous **acute,** high exposure that the individual has survived or from chronic low-level exposures delivered over many years. From the public health point of view, the possibility of long-term effects on the large number of people receiving low, chronic exposures is cause for greater concern than the short-term radiation effects from acute exposures that involve only a few individuals.

There is no unique disease associated with the long-term effects of radiation. However, there is a statistical increase in the incidence of certain already existing conditions. Because of the low normal incidence of these conditions, one must observe large numbers of exposed persons in order to evaluate this kind of an increase.

The long-term effects observed have been somatic damage, which may result in an increased incidence of cancer, embryological defects, cataracts, life span shortening, and genetic mutations. The first four conditions are somatic effects and only involve the individual exposed. Genetic mutations involve hereditary material and may have an adverse effect for many generations after the original exposure.

- **Cancer:** Anything that is capable of causing cancer is called a *carcinogen*. X-rays, like certain drugs, chemicals, and viruses, have been shown to have carcinogenic effects. Carcinogenic mechanisms are not clearly understood. Moreover, cancer is probably "caused" by the simultaneous interaction of several factors, and the presence of some of these factors without the others may not be sufficient to cause the disease.

  Some explanations for the carcinogenic action of x-rays include the following: x-rays activate viruses already present in cells; x-rays damage chromosomes, and certain diseases (such as leukemia) are associated with chromosomal injury; x-rays cause mutations in somatic cells, which may result in uncontrolled growth of cells; and x-rays ionize water, which results in chemical "free radicals" that may cause cancer.

  Any one or a combination of these theories may explain how cancer is caused. X-radiation is only one of a number of possible carcinogens involved, and the precise mechanism is not yet understood. Much of the evidence that x-radiation is carcinogenic comes from studies of early radiation workers, including dentists, who were exposed to large amounts of radiation (Figures 5–6 and 5–7).
- **Embryological defects:** The immature, undifferentiated, rapidly growing cells of the embryo are highly sensitive to radiation. The first trimester of a pregnancy when the fetus undergoes the period of major organogenesis (formation of organs) is especially critical. High doses of radiation may cause birth abnormalities, stunting of growth, and mental retardation. The dose from a dental x-ray examination is less than 0.0003 to 0.003 milligrays (0.03 to 0.3 millirads), the use of a leaded apron reduces this potential dose to zero.
- **Low birth weight:** Medical (not dental) x-radiation exposure of pregnant females has been associated with an increase in the incidence of full-term pregnancies resulting in below normal birth weight infants. Because the reproductive organs are not located in a critical area, exposure of necessary dental radiographs has not been contraindicated during pregnancy. In 2004 the American Medical Association published research that investigated the effect on pregnancy outcomes of radiation exposure of the pregnant female's hypothalamus and the pituitary and thyroid glands, that suggests that dental radiation exposure may be associated with full-term low birth weight infants. More research

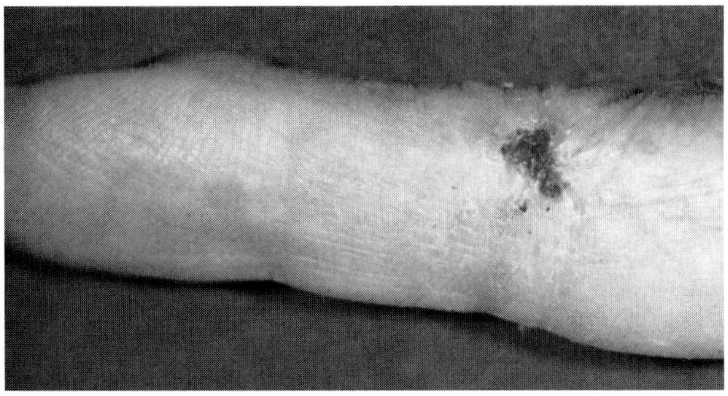

Figure 5–6 **Ulcerated lesion.** Early carcinoma on the finger of a dentist who admitted holding films in the patient's oral cavity during exposure.

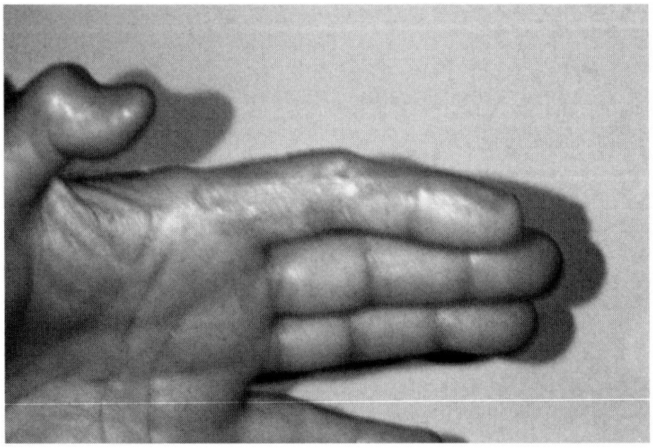

FIGURE 5–7 **Radiation injury on the finger of a dentist caused by holding films in the patient's oral cavity during exposure.** Many of these lesions become squamous cell carcinoma (cancer).

in this area may lead to altered guidelines on the assessment of pregnant females for dental radiographs. Exposing dental radiographs on pregnant females is discussed further in Chapter 24.

- **Cataracts:** When the lens of the eye becomes opaque, it is called a cataract. Various agents, including x-rays, have been known to cause cataracts. It takes at least 2 Gy (200 rads) of x-radiation to cause cataract formation. The dose to the eye from dental radiographic procedures is in the order of milligrays (millirads). Dental x-rays have never been reported to cause cataracts.
- **Life-span shortening:** Life-span shortening effects caused by x-radiation have been demonstrated in animal experiments. The effect seems to be caused by premature aging. However, life span shortening has never been demonstrated in humans.
- **Genetic mutations:** X-radiation is known to sometimes cause changes in the genetic material of cells. These changes are referred to as genetic mutations. The genetic material is the means by which hereditary traits are passed from one generation to another. Drugs, chemicals, and even elevated body temperatures are also capable of causing mutations. Genetic effects are especially important, because there may be no level of radiation that will not produce at least some effect.

  While there have been mutations that have occurred in nature that have helped a species survive, most geneticists agree that the majority of genetic mutations are harmful. Because of their damaging effects, they are gradually eliminated from the population by natural means, since individuals with this damage are less likely to reproduce themselves successfully than are normal individuals. The more severe the condition produced by the mutation, the more rapidly it will be eliminated. As a balance to this natural elimination of harmful mutations, new ones are constantly occurring. Natural background radiation probably accounts for a small proportion of naturally occurring mutations.

  Since the scattered radiation reaching the gonads from dental radiography is less than 0.0001 that of the exposure to the surface of the face, the dental contribution to genetic mutations is extremely small, ranging from 0.0 to about 0.002 milligrays (0.2 millirad) per radiograph. By using a lead apron and thyroid collar, the dose is essentially reduced to zero.

Risk Estimates

A **risk** may be defined as the likelihood of injury or death from some hazard. The primary risk from dental radiography is radiation-induced cancer and possibly, the potential to affect pregnancy outcomes. Otherwise, the facial and oral structures, composed largely of bone, nerve, and muscle tissue, are fairly radioresistant (Table 5–1).

Risk estimates vary, depending upon several factors, such as speed of film, collimation, and the technique used. In dental radiology, the most critical areas in the head and neck are the mandible (red bone marrow), the lens of the eye, the thyroid gland and possibly the hypothalamus-pituitary-thyroid combination. The mandible contains an estimated 15 g of red bone marrow. However, it should be noted that this is only about 1 percent of the total amount of red bone marrow in the adult body. While x-radiation will cause cataracts, the dental radiation exposure to the lens of the eye during some maxillary exposures is well below the dose needed to produce cataracts. The thyroid gland is relatively radiosensitive. Until recently the focus has been on radiation exposure causing cancer of the thyroid gland. A recent study published in the Journal of the American Medical Association (2004) has demonstrated a possible link between radiation exposure to the thyroid gland and/or to the hypothalamus-pituitary-thyroid combination of a pregnant female and low birth weight infants delivered after the full 9-month term.

Until more is documented regarding this phenomenon, the focus is on radiation-induced cancer as the primary risk from dental radiography. The potential risk of a full mouth dental x-ray examination inducing cancer in a patient has been estimated to be 2.5 per 1,000,000 examinations. It should be noted that every day we assume hundreds of risks such as climbing stairs, crossing the street, riding a bicycle, and driving a car. Activities with a fatality risk of 1 in 1,000,000 include riding 300 miles in

TABLE 5–1 Critical Organs and Doses for Dental Radiography

Critical Organ	Effect	Minimum Dose Required to Produce Effect	Dental Dose from an FMS
Eye	cataract	2,000 mSv	0.4 mSv
Hematopoietic	leukemia	50 mSv	8.0 mSv
Skin	cancer	250 mSv	12.6 mSv
Thyroid gland	cancer	65 mSv	0.4 mSv
Gonads	sterility	4,000 to 6,000 mSv	0.005 mSv *(no lead apron)* to 0.0003 mSv *(lead apron)*

TABLE 5-2 **One in One Million Fatality Risk**

Risk	Nature
Smoking 1.4 cigarettes/day	Cancer
Riding 10 miles on a bicycle	Accident
Travel 300 miles by auto	Accident
Travel 1,000 miles by airplane	Accident

an automobile, traveling 1,000 miles in an airplane, or smoking 1.4 cigarettes a day (Table 5–2). People accept these risks every day because we perceive a benefit from them.

- **Risk versus benefit:** Dental radiographs should be taken only when the benefit outweighs the risk of biologic injury to the patient. When dental radiographs are properly prescribed (see Chapter 6), exposed, and processed, the health benefits to the patient far outweigh any risk of injury. There have been no reports of radiation injuries caused by normal dental procedures since safety protocols have been adopted.

Practice Point

Dental radiographs should be prescribed only when necessary. Consider the following case: If a female patient is assessed for bitewing radiographs, and then she reveals that she may be pregnant, would the need for the bitewing radiographs change? Would she still need the radiographs? Or would these once-needed radiographs now be radiographs that can wait? If radiographs can wait, they are not necessary radiographs.

Radiation Exposure Comparisons

Patients often have questions regarding the amount of radiation dental radiographs are adding to their accumlated lifetime exposure. The exact amount of radiation exposure produced when taking dental radiographs varies, depending on many factors, such as film speed, technique used, collimation type (circular or rectangular). Additionally, dental exposures are often quoted as skin surface amounts rather than amounts to the more important bone marrow and other deeper structures. For example, comparing the skin dose of a chest x-ray (which is approximately 0.2 mSv) and a single periapical radiograph (which is approximately 2.5 mSv) does not take into consideration that the chest x-ray delivers its dose to a larger area and to more tissues of the body than the single periapical radiograph.

To aid in making more accurate comparisons between different radiographic exposures, the **effective dose equivalent** is used to compare the risk of the radiation exposure producing a biological response. The effective dose equivalent compensates for the differences in area exposed and the tissues, critical or less critical, that may be in the path of the x-ray beam. Using the example above, the effective dose equivalent for the chest x-ray is approximately 80 μSv, and the effective dose equivalent for the single periapical using F-speed film and a round PID is approximately 1.3 μSv. The effective dose equivalent is expressed using the term **microsievert (μSv,)** meaning 1/1,000,000 of a sievert.

The effective dose equivalent can be used to compare dental radiation exposures with days of natural background exposure. The average effective dose equivalent from naturally occuring background radiation to the population of the United States is approximately 8 μSv per day. A full mouth series of radiographs using F-speed film and a round PID has an effective dose equivalent of approximately 23.4 μSv. Therefore, the full mouth series is equal to approximately 2.9 days of naturally occurring background radiation exposure (Table 5–3).

Much about radiation effects remains to be discovered. Future research may demonstrate that human beings are not as sensitive to radiation damage as we now believe. But until we have such evidence, common sense dictates improving radiographic safety techniques in every way possible.

TABLE 5-3 **Effective Dose Equivalent**[a]

Examination	Effective Dose	Days of Natural Exposure[b]
Single intraoral exposure[c]	1.3 μSv	0.2
Bitewing radiographs[c] (4 films)	5.2 μSv	0.7
Full mouth series[c] (18 films)	23.4 μSv	2.9
Panoramic radiograph	7 μSv	0.9
Chest x-ray	80 μSv	10
Upper GI	2440 μSv	305
Lower GI	4060 μSv	507.5

[a]Modified from White, S. C., & Pharoah, M. *Oral Radiology: Principles and Interpretation,* 5th ed. St. Louis: Elsevier, 2004.
[b]Fractions rounded up.
[c]F-speed, round PID.

Practice Point

Be careful not to tell the patient that a full mouth series is equal to 2.9 days "in the sun." Naturally occurring background radiation includes not only the sun, or cosmic energy, but terrestrial and internal sources of background radiation (see Chapter 2). Additionally, most patients are aware that exposure to the sun's rays is harmful and many take precautions against putting themselves at risk for skin damage. To compare dental x-rays to sun exposure may provoke a response from the patient to avoid dental x-rays as well.

REVIEW—Chapter Summary

Ionizing radiation has the potential to produce biological damage because x-rays can detach subatomic particles from larger molecules and create an electrical imbalance within a normally stable cell. This potential for cellular damage is of concern to everyone—the general public and those who work with radiation.

There are two generally accepted theories on how radiation may cause damage to cellular tissues: (1) the direct or target theory, and (2) the indirect or poison-water theory. Whether cell damage from radiation is physical or chemical, it has been established that minor damage is soon repaired by a healthy body.

The terms radiosensitive and radioresistant are used to describe the degree of susceptibility of various cells and body tissues to radiation. According to the law of B and T, cells that are highly specialized and have a lesser reproductive capacity are considered to be radioresistant, and cells that are undifferenciated and have a greater capacity for reproduction are considered to be radiosensitive.

Genetic and somatic cell reaction to the ionization that occurs during radiation exposure depends on the age, size, and health of the patient, the output of the x-ray machine, the duration of the exposure, the degree of tissue radiosensitivity, and the area of exposure: local or whole-body. In dental radiography, the main concern is that damage to genetic cells may result in altering the chromosomes and creating mutations in future generations.

The dose–response curve is a method used to plot the dosage of radiation administered with the response produced in order to establish responsible levels of radiation exposure. The conservative view that every dose of radiation potentially produces damage and should be kept to a minimum is expressed by the ALARA concept—as low as reasonably achievable.

The factors that determine the amount of radiation injury include total dose, dose rate, area exposed, variation in species, individual sensitivity, variation in cell sensitivity, variation in tissue sensitivity, and age. The lethal dose for each species is expressed in statistical terms—the LD 50/30 for that species. Assuming that the dose received is not lethal, the sequence of events following radiation exposure are (1) a latent period, (2) a period of injury, and (3) a recovery period.

The term deterministic (non-stochastic) is used when referring to a tissue response, such as erythema, whose severity is directly related to the radiation dose. The term stochastic effect is used when referring to a tissue response, such as cancer, that is based on the probability of occurrence rather then the severity of the response.

The effects of radiation exposure may be short- or long-term. Short-term effects often include erythema and general discomfort. Long-term effects may result in an increased incidence of cancer, embryological defects, poor pregnancy outcomes, cataracts, life-span shortening, and genetic mutations.

The potential benefits of dental radiographs outweigh the risk. With proper radiation safety protocol, there is minimal risk of injury caused by necessary dental radiographic procedures.

While the most critical areas in the head and neck are (1) the red bone marrow in the mandible, (2) lens of the eye, and (3) thyroid gland, most facial tissues are fairly radioresistant.

The effective dose equivalent can be used to compare the risks of different radiation exposures and to compare dental radiation exposures with days of natural background exposure. The effective dose equivalent is expressed using the term μSv or microsievert, meaning 1/1,000,000 of a sievert.

RECALL—Study Questions

1. The primary cause of biological damage from radiation is:
   a. Ionization.
   b. Direct effect.
   c. Indirect effect.
   d. Genetic effect.
2. Direct injury from radiation occurs when the x-ray photons:
   a. Ionize water and form toxins.
   b. Pass through the cell.
   c. Strike critical cell molecules.
   d. All of the above.
3. Indirect injury from radiation occurs when the x-ray photons:
   a. Ionize water and form toxins.
   b. Pass through the cell.
   c. Strike critical cell molecules.
   d. All of the above.
4. According to the law of B and T, cells with a high reproductive rate are described as:
   a. Radiopaque.
   b. Radiolucent.
   c. Radioresistant.
   d. Radiosensitive.
5. Which of these cells are most radiosensitive?
   a. Muscle cells
   b. Nerve cells
   c. Red blood cells
   d. Mature bone cells
6. Which of these cells are most radioresistant?
   a. Red blood cells
   b. Muscle cells
   c. Epithelial cells
   d. White blood cells
7. When the effect of a radiation exposure is observed in the offspring of an irradiated person, but not in the irradiated person, this is called the:
   a. Somatic effect.
   b. Genetic effect.
   c. Direct effect.
   d. Indirect effect.

8. A dose–response curve indicating that any amount of radiation, no matter how small, has the potential to cause a biological response is a called:
   a. Stochastic
   b. Non-stochastic
   c. Threshold
   d. Non-threshold
9. ALARA stands for _____ _____ _____ _____ _____.
10. List the five possible biological responses of an irradiated cell.
   a. ____________________
   b. ____________________
   c. ____________________
   d. ____________________
   e. ____________________
11. All of the following are factors that determine radiation injury *except* one. Which one is this *exception?*
   a. Size of the irradiated area
   b. Amount of radiation
   c. Patient gender
   d. Dose rate
12. A lethal dose (LD) of LD 50/30 refers to the amount of radiation:
   a. That would kill 50% of a species within a 30-day period.
   b. That would kill 30% of a species within a 50-day period.
   c. That would ionize 50% of the cells in the body within a 30-minute period.
   d. That would ionize 30% of the cells in the body within a 50-minute period.
13. According to the factors that determine radiation injury, based on age, who is the most radiosensitive?
   a. 6 year old
   b. 16 year old
   c. 26 year old
   d. 46 year old
14. Which of the following is the correct sequence of events following radiation exposure?
   a. Period of injury, latent period, recovery period
   b. Latent period, period of injury, recovery period
   c. Latent period, recovery period, period of injury
   d. Recovery period, latent period, period of injury
15. When a biological response is based on the probability of occurrence rather than the severity of the change, it is called a:
   a. Short-term effect.
   b. Non-stochastic effect.
   c. Deterministic effect.
   d. Stochastic effect.
16. Which of the following is a short-term effect of radiation exposure?
   a. Embryological defects
   b. Cataracts
   c. Acute radiation syndrome
   d. Cancer
17. Full-term, low birth weight is possibly associated with radiation exposure to which of the following?
   a. Thyroid gland
   b. Hypothalamus
   c. Pituitary gland
   d. All of the above
18. During a dental radiograph exposure, approximately how much smaller is the dose of radiation in the gonadal area than at the surface of the face?
   a. 0.10
   b. 0.01
   c. 0.001
   d. 0.0001
19. All of the following are considered critical for dental radiography because they are in the head and neck area *except* one. Which one is this *exception?*
   a. Mandible
   b. Lens of the eye
   c. Brain and spinal cord
   d. Thyroid gland
20. Which of the following units of radiation measurement most accurately compares different radiation exposures?
   a. Dose equivalent
   b. Absorbed dose
   c. Effective absorbed dose
   d. Effective dose equivalent

REFLECT—Case Study

Retaking a radiograph because of a technique or processing error causes an increase in radiation exposure for the patient. Discuss ways a retake radiograph affects the factors that determine radiation injury.

RELATE—Laboratory Application

Calculate your radiation dose. Visit the United States Environmental Protection Agency at www.epa.gov/radiation/students/calculate.html, where you can estimate your average annual radiation dose. Based on the questions posed by this calculator, what conclusions can you draw about (1) the source of radiation exposure; (2) region in which people live; (3) sources of internal radiation exposure; and (4) situations and/or products with the ability to increase your dose of radiation exposure?

BIBLIOGRAPHY

Eastman Kodak. *Radiation Safety in Dental Radiography.* Rochester, NY: Eastman Kodak, 1998.

Hujoel, P. P., Bollen, A., Noonan, C. J., & del Aguila, M. A. Antepartum dental radiography and infant low birth weight. *JAMA* 291(16): 1987–1993, 2004.

National Academy of Sciences, National Research Council. *The Effects on Populations of Exposure to Low Levels of Ionizing Radiation* (BEIR III report). Washington, DC: National Academy Press, 1980.

National Council on Radiation Protection and Measurements. *Implementation of the Principle of as Low as Reasonably Achievable (ALARA) for Medical and Dental Personnel.* Washington, DC: 1991. NCRP report no. 107.

U. S. Nuclear Regulatory Commission. "How Does Radiation Affect the Public?" http://www.nrc.gov/what-we-do/radiation/affect.html.

White, S. C., & Pharoah, M. J. *Oral Radiology: Principles and Interpretation,* 5th ed. St. Louis: Elsevier 2004.

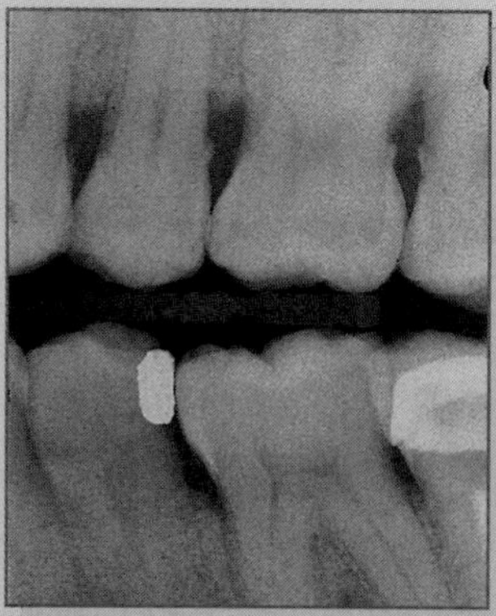

6

Radiation Protection

CHAPTER OUTLINE

■ OBJECTIVES

Following successful completion of this chapter, you should be able to:

1. Define the key words.
2. Adopt the ALARA concept.
3. Summarize the radiation protection methods for the patient.
4. Summarize the radiation protection methods for the operator.
5. Utilize the selection criteria guidelines to explain the need for prescribed radiographs.
6. Explain the roles communication, working knowledge of quality radiographs, and education play in preventing unnecessary radiation exposure.
7. Explain the roles technique and exposure choices play in preventing unnecessary radiation exposure.
8. List the two functions of a collimator.
9. State the federally mandated diameter of the intraoral dental x-ray beam at the patient's skin.
10. Explain the difference between round and rectangular collimation.
11. Explain the function of the filter.
12. State the filtration requirements for an intraoral dental x-ray unit that operates above and below 70 kVp.
13. Compare inherent, added, and total filtration.
14. Explain how PID shape and length contribute to reducing patient radiation exposure.
15. Advocate the use of the lead apron and thyroid collar for every patient for every x-ray exposure.
16. Identify the fastest and slowest speed film currently available for dental radiography use.
17. Explain the role film holders play in reducing patient radiation exposure.
18. Explain the role darkroom protocol and film handling play in reducing patient radiation exposure.
19. Explain the roles time, shielding, and distance play in protecting the operator from unnecessary radiation exposure.
20. Utilize distance and location to take a position the appropriate distance and angle from the x-ray source at the patient's head during an exposure.
21. Describe personnel monitoring devices used to detect radiation.
22. State the maximum permissible dose (MPD) for radiation workers and for the general public.
23. List the organizations responsible for recommending and setting exposure limits.

KEY WORDS

Added filtration	Personnel monitoring
ALARA (as low as reasonably achievable)	Personnel monitoring device
Aluminum equivalent	PID (position indicating device)/BID (beam indicating device)
Area monitoring	Primary beam
Collimation	Primary radiation
Dosimeter (radiation monitoring device)	Protective barrier
Exposure factors	Radiation leakage
Film badge	Radiation workers
Film holder	Re-take radiographs
Filter	Scatter radiation (secondary radiation)
Filtration	Selection criteria
Half-value layer	Structural shielding
Inherent filtration	Thermoluminescent dosimeter (TLD)
Lead apron	Thyroid collar
Lead equivalent	Total filtration
Maximum permissible dose (MPD)	
Monitoring	

Introduction

In Chapter 5 we learned that radiation exposure in sufficient doses may produce harmful biological changes in human beings. Although it is the consensus of radiobiologists that the dose received from a dental x-ray exposure is not likely to be harmful, even the experts do not know what risk a small dose carries. Therefore, it must be assumed that any dose may be capable of potential risk. The patient has agreed to be subjected to the risks of radiation exposure because he/she believes that the oral health care practitioner will follow safety protocols that protect the patient from excess exposure.

In this chapter we discuss radiation safety protocols, including selection criteria used in prescribing dental radiographs and methods to minimize x-ray exposure to both the dental patient and the radiographer.

ALARA

The oral health care team has an ethical responsibility to embrace the **ALARA (as low as reasonably achievable)** concept, recommended by the International Commission on Radiological Protection to minimize radiation risks. The ALARA concept implies that "any radiation dose that can be reduced without major difficulty, great expense, or inconvenience should be reduced or eliminated." ALARA is not simply a phrase, but a culture of professional excellence. ALARA should guide practice principles. In an ideal world, the oral health care team would like to glean the diagnostic benefits of dental radiographs with a zero dose radiation exposure to the patient. In reality, this is not possible; dental radiographs will result in a small but acceptable level of risk. The best way to prevent this risk from increasing is to keep the exposure ALARA.

Protection Measures for the Patient

Professional Judgment

The benefits of radiographs in dentistry outweigh the risks when proper safety procedures are followed. The most important way to assure that the patient receives a reasonably low dose of radiation is to use evidenced-based **selection criteria** when determining which patients need radiographs. Guidelines developed by an expert panel of health care professionals convened by the Public Health Service and adopted by the American Dental Association have been published to assist in deciding when, what type, and how many radiographs should be taken (Table 6–1). These guidelines allow the dentist to base his/her decision regarding x-rays for the patient on expert recommendations. While the dentist prescribes the radiographic exam for the patient based on these guidelines, these recommendations are subject to clinical judgment and may not apply to every patient.

Evidenced-based selection criteria guidelines are applied only after reviewing the patient's health history and completing a clinical examination. The time frames suggested in the guidelines are utilized in the absence of positive historical findings and signs and symptoms presented by the patient. For example, a patient who presents with a toothache would most likely be assessed for a radiographic exam of this symptom even if he/she had radiographs within the suggested time frame for this patient's category. However, a radiographic examination should not wait until a patient presents with pain or other symptom of pathology. The time frames suggested by the selection criteria guidelines are preventive measures that are evidence-based effective. While the dentist utilizes these guidelines to prescribe the radiographic exam for the patient, the dental hygienist may utilize the guidelines during initial examination of the patient to make a preliminary assessment for the recommendation of radiographic need; the dental hygienist and the dental assistant rely on the selection criteria guidelines to assist with explaining radiographic need to the patient. Once the decision to expose radiographs is made, every reasonable effort must be made to minimize exposure to the patient and to the operator and to those who may be in the area of the x-ray machine.

Practice Point

Completing an accurate dental history may reveal that the patient has recently had radiographs taken at a previous oral health care practice. Every effort should be made to have a copy of these radiographs forwarded to your practice to avoid additional radiation exposure for the patient.

Technical Ability of the Operator

- **Communication.** Reduction of radiation exposure begins with communication skills. The patient's cooperation must be secured to perform radiographic examinations accurately and safely. Patient protection during a radiographic procedure should begin with clear, concise instructions. When responsibilities are adequately defined through effective communication, the patient understands what must be done and can more fully cooperate with the radiographer and avoid re-take mistakes.
- **Working knowledge of quality radiographs.** The operator should understand what a quality dental radiograph should image. Based on this knowledge, the operator needs to take every precaution against re-taking radiographs. **Retake radiographs** are necessary when the first exposure results in errors that compromise image quality. When a radiograph is re-taken, the second exposure now unnecessarily doubles the dose and dose rate of radiation for the patient. The best way to avoid re-take radiographs is to develop an understanding of common technique and processing errors (see Chapter 16). Armed with this knowledge, the operator can better avoid those mistakes that increase patient radiation exposure. Re-takes may also be avoided if the area of interest is imaged on an adjacent film.
- **Education.** Continuing education is the corner stone of all health care professions. Rapidly advancing technology is constantly changing the scope of oral health care practice. Many of the methods and procedures learned for the practice of oral health care as little as five years ago may be obsolete in today's world. With these advancements come new and improved ways to provide oral health care for the patient. For example, we may soon see the elimination of the darkroom used in dental radiography with the increasing use of computers in health care and the advancement of digital imaging. New technology continues to contribute to the reduction of dental radiation exposure. The use of digital imaging equipment for radiography can reduce the patient's radiation dose by 50 to 80 percent over film-based radiography. The radiographer who continues to learn about and adopt these new practices will further help decrease radiation exposure for the patient and him/herself.

Technique Standards

- **Intraoral technique choice.** The paralleling technique should be the operator's first choice when exposing periapical radiographs. The paralleling technique yields more accurate and precisely sized radiographic images (see Chapter 12). However, consideration should also be given to which technique, paralleling or bisecting, would yield the best results for the patient. The more efficient and convenient the technique, the less likely there will be retake radiographs. The operator should be skilled at both techniques and should possess the knowledge upon which to base the decision regarding which one to use to avoid unnecessary radiation exposure to the patient.
- **Exposure factors.** Operating the dental x-ray machine includes selecting the appropriate **exposure factors**—kilovoltage (kVp), milliamperage (mA), and time—for the patient and the area to be imaged. The radiographer should possess a working knowledge of appropriate exposure factors to avoid overexposing the patient or the area unnecessarily. Additionally, underexposures that result in re-take radiographs also lead to overexposure of the patient when a re-take radiograph results. A working knowledge of the exposure factors includes the ability to adjust each of the variables—the kilovoltage (kVp), milliamperage (mA), and time—in relationship to each other. In Chapter 4, we learned that an adjustment in one variable usually leads to a necessary counter-adjustment in another variable to maintain exposure control. To assist in radiation safety, exposure charts should be posted near the control panel for easy reference.

Equipment Standards

Using proper equipment is the next step in reducing radiation exposure to the patient. All dental x-ray machines in the U.S. are safe from a radiological health point of view. The Federal Performance Standard for Diagnostic X-Ray Equipment became effective on August 1, 1974. The provisions of the standard require that all x-ray equipment manufactured after that date meet certain radiation safety requirements including collimation, filtration, and PID (a position indicating device)

TABLE 6-1 **Guidelines for Prescribing Dental Radiographs**

	CHILDREN		ADOLESCENT	ADULT	
TYPE OF ENCOUNTER	Primary Dentition *(prior to eruption of first permanent tooth)*	Transitional Dentition *(after eruption of first permanent tooth)*	Permanent Dentition *(prior to eruption of third molars)*	Dentate or Partially Edentulous	Edentulous
New Patient Being evaluated for dental disease and dental development	Individualized radiographic exam consisting of selected periapical/occlusal views and/or posterior bitewings if proximal surfaces cannot be visualized or probed. Patients without evidence of disease and with open proximal contacts may not require a radiographic exam at this time.	Individualized radiographic exam consisting of posterior bitewings with panoramic exam or posterior bitewings and selected periapical images.	Individualized radiographic exam consisting of posterior bitewings with panoramic exam or posterior bitewings and selected periapical images. A full mouth intraoral radiographic exam is preferred when the patient has clinical evidence of generalized dental disease or a history of extensive dental treatment.		Individualized radiographic exam, based on clinical signs and symptoms.
Recall Patient* With clinical caries or at increased risk for caries**	Posterior bitewing exam at 6–12 month intervals if proximal surfaces cannot be examined visually or with a probe.			Posterior bitewing exam at 6–18 month intervals.	Not applicable.
Recall Patient* With no clinical caries and not at risk for caries**	Posterior bitewing exam at 12–24 month intervals if proximal surfaces cannot be examined visually or with a probe.		Posterior bitewing exam at 18–36 month intervals.	Posterior bitewing exam at 24–36 month intervals.	Not applicable.
Recall Patient With periodontal disease	Clinical judgment as to the need for and type of radiographic images for the evaluation of periodontal disease. Imaging may consist of, but is not limited to, selected bitewing and/or periapical images of areas where periodontal disease (other than nonspecific gingivitis) can be identified clinically.				Not applicable.
Patient For monitoring of growth and development	Clinical judgment as to the need for and type of radiographic images for the evaluation and/or monitoring of dentofacial growth and development.		Clinical judgment as to the need for and type of radiographic images for evaluation and/or monitoring of dentofacial growth and development. Panoramic or periapical exam to assess developing third molars.	Not usually indicated.	
Patient With other circumstances including, but not limited to, proposed or existing implants, pathology, restorative/endodontic needs, treated periodontal disease and caries remineralization.	Clinical judgment as to the need for and type of radiographic images for the evaluation and/or monitoring in these circumstances.				

*Clinical situations for which radiographs may be indicated include but are not limited to:

A. Positive historical findings
1. Previous periodontal or endodontic treatment
2. History of pain or trauma
3. Familial history of dental anomalies
4. Postoperative evaluation of healing
5. Remineralization monitoring
6. Presence of implants or evaluation for impact placement

B. Positive clinical signs/symptoms
1. Clinical evidence of periodontal disease
2. Large or deep restorations
3. Deep carious lesions
4. Malposed or clinically impacted teeth
5. Swelling
6. Evidence of dental/facial trauma
7. Mobility of teeth
8. Sinus tract ("fistula")
9. Clinically suspected sinus pathology
10. Growth abnormalities
11. Oral involvement in known or suspected systemic disease
12. Positive neurologic findings in the head and neck
13. Evidence of foreign objects
14. Pain and/or dysfunction of the temporomandibular joint
15. Facial asymmetry
16. Abutment teeth for fixed or removable partial prosthesis
17. Unexplained bleeding
18. Unexplained sensitivity of teeth
19. Unusual eruption, spacing or migration of teeth
20. Unusual tooth morphology, calcification or color
21. Unexplained absence of teeth
22. Clinical erosion

**Factors increasing risk for caries may include but are not limited to:
1. High level of caries experience or demineralization
2. History of recurrent caries
3. High titers of cariogenic bacteria
4. Existing restoration(s) of poor quality
5. Poor oral hygiene
6. Inadequate fluoride exposure
7. Prolonged nursing (bottle or breast)
8. High-sucrose frequency diet
9. Poor family oral health
10. Developmental or acquired enamel defects
11. Developmental or acquired disability
12. Xerostomia
13. Genetic abnormality of teeth
14. Many multisurface restorations
15. Chemo/radiation therapy
16. Eating disorders
17. Drug/alcohol abuse
18. Irregular dental care

Data from U.S. Dept. of Health and Human Services: The Selection of Patients for Dental Radiographic Examinations. *Revised 2004 by the American Dental Association: Council on Dental Benefit Program, Council on Dental Practice, Council on Scientific Affairs.*

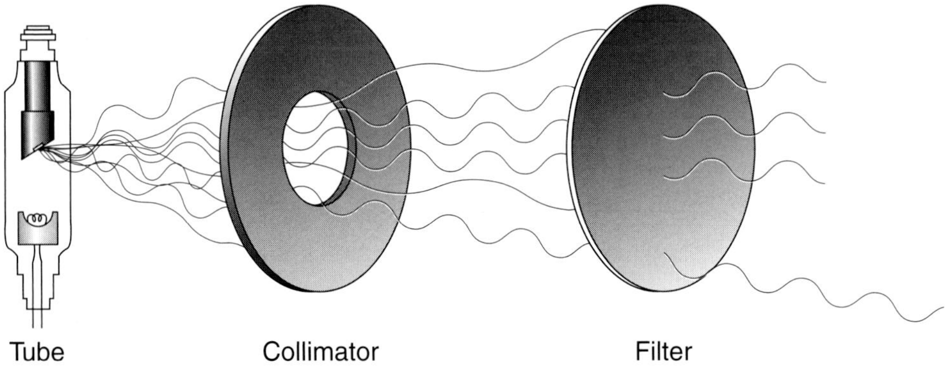

FIGURE 6–1 **Collimator and filter.** The collimator is a lead washer that restricts the size of the x-ray beam. The filter is an aluminum disc that filters (removes) the long wavelength x-rays.

- **Collimation** controls the size and shape of the useful beam. **Collimation** of the beam is accomplished by using a lead diaphragm or washer (Figure 6–1). The function of the collimator is to reduce the size of the x-ray beam and thus the volume of irradiated tissue. The collimator is placed in the path of the **primary beam** as it exits the tube housing at the port (Figure 6–2). Collimators may have either a round or a rectangular opening. Federal regulations require that round opening collimators restrict the x-ray beam to 2.75 in. (7 cm) at the patient end of the PID (Figure 6–3). Rectangular collimators restrict the beam to the approximate size of the film (Figure 6–4), which reduces the area of radiation exposure over a round-collimated beam. Although rectangular collimation reduces patient radiation exposure by up to 70 percent, most dental x-ray machines have round openings. Figure 6–5 shows how much excess radiation the patient receives with the circular collimator when exposing a #2-sized film. Rectangular collimation may also be achieved through the use of external collimators that attach to the PID or film holding device (Figure 6–6 and Figure 6–7).

  Collimation reduces **scatter radiation** (sometimes called **secondary radiation**). Scattered radiation is radiation that has been deflected from its path by impact during its passage through matter. In addition to increasing patient radiation dose, scattered radiation decreases the quality of the radiographic image by fogging the film. Hence two important functions of collimation are:
  - Reduces the radiation dose to the patient by reducing the volume of tissue exposed
  - Reduces scatter radiation that causes poor contrast of the radiograph (see Chapter 4)
- **Filtration** is the absorption of the long wavelength, less penetrating, x-rays of the polychromatic x-ray beam by passage of the beam through a sheet of material called a **filter** (Figure 6–1). A filter is an absorbing material (usually aluminum) placed in the path of the x-ray beam in order to remove a high percentage of the soft x-rays (the longer wavelengths) and reduce patient radiation dose.

  In the dental x-ray machine, these aluminum filter disks vary in thickness. The **half-value layer (HVL)** of an x-ray beam is the thickness (measured in millimeters) of aluminum that will reduce the intensity of the beam by one-half. Measuring the HVL determines the penetrating quality of the x-ray beam. The HVL is more accurate

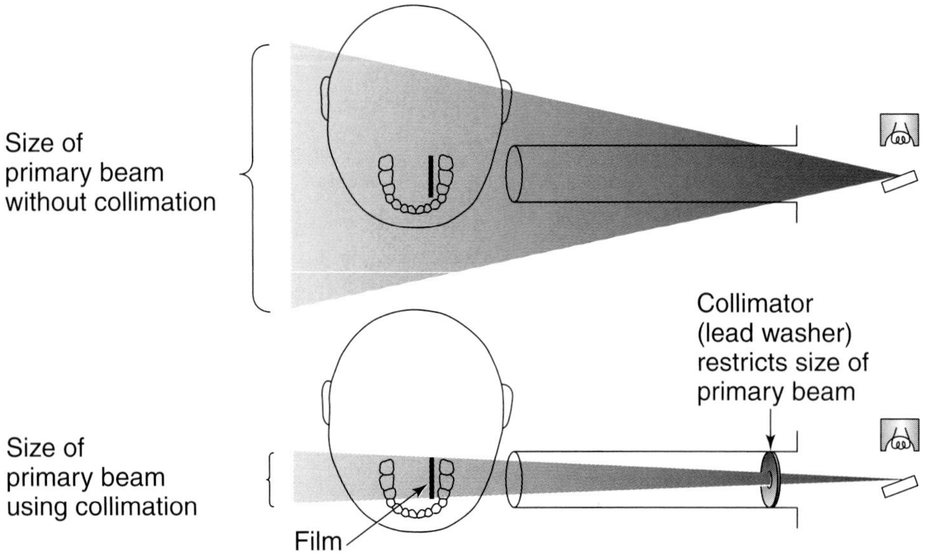

FIGURE 6–2 **Effect of collimation on primary beam.** Lead collimators control the shape and size of the primary beam. The beam is limited to the approximate size of the film.

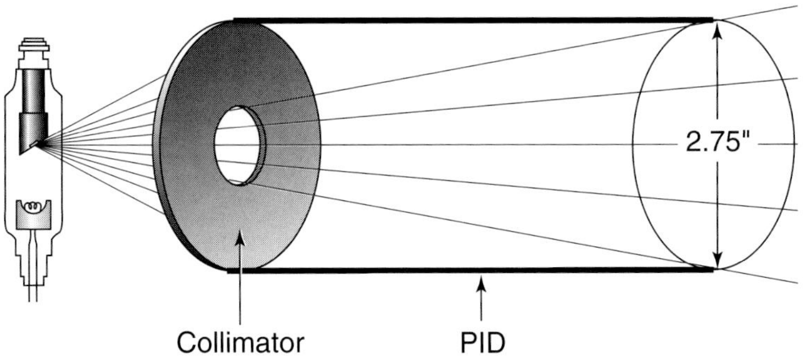

FIGURE 6-3 The collimator restricts the size of the primary beam to 2.75 in. (7 cm) at the end of the PID.

than kilovoltage to describe the x-ray beam quality and penetration. Two similar x-ray machines operating at the same kilovoltage may not produce x-rays of the same quality and penetration. The half-value layer is used by radiological health personnel when determining filtration requirements.

Filters may be sealed into the tube head or inserted into the port where the PID attaches. Pure aluminum or its equivalent will not hinder the passage of high-energy x-rays, but will absorb a high percentage of the low-energy x-rays. The latter do not contribute to the radiographic image. However, they are harmful to the patient because they are absorbed by the skin and increase the patient's dose (Figure 6–8).

Any material the x-ray beam passes through filters the beam. Filtration may be built into the tube head (inherent), or it may be added.

Inherent filtration is the filtration built into the machine by the manufacturer. This includes the glass of the x-ray tube, the insulating oil, and the material that seals the port. All x-ray units have some built-in filtration. Usually the inherent filtration is not sufficient to meet state and federal standards, requiring filtration be added.

Added filtration is the placement of aluminum discs in the path of the x-ray beam between the port seal of the tube head and the PID. When the inherent filtration is not sufficient to meet present safety standards, a disk of aluminum of the appropriate thickness (usually 0.5 mm) can be inserted between the port of the tube head and the PID. Several manufacturers have introduced x-ray units in which the traditional aluminum filter is replaced with samarium, a rare-earth metal.

Total filtration is the sum of the inherent and added filtration expressed in millimeters of **aluminum equivalent.** Beam **filtration** must comply with state and federal laws. Present safety standards require an equivalent of 1.5 mm aluminum for x-ray machines operating in ranges below 70 kVp and a minimum of 2.5 mm aluminum for machines operating at or above 70 kVp.

- The **position indicating device (PID)** (or **beam indicating device BID)** is an extension of the tube housing and is used to direct the primary x-ray beam. The shape and length of the PID has an effect on the radiation dose the patient receives. Modern PIDs may be shaped as round cylinders or rectangular tubes. A rectangular PID reduces patient radiation exposure by up to 70 percent over round, cylinder PIDs (Figures 6–4 and 6–5). The pointed, closed-end plastic cone, originally designed as an aiming device, is no longer used (Figure 6–9). The tip of pointed, closed-end cones was supposed to indicate the central ray and aid in aiming the x-ray beam at the center of the film packet. When pointed cones were first used, it was not realized that many of the x-rays were deflected through contact with the material of the cones, thus producing scatter radiation.

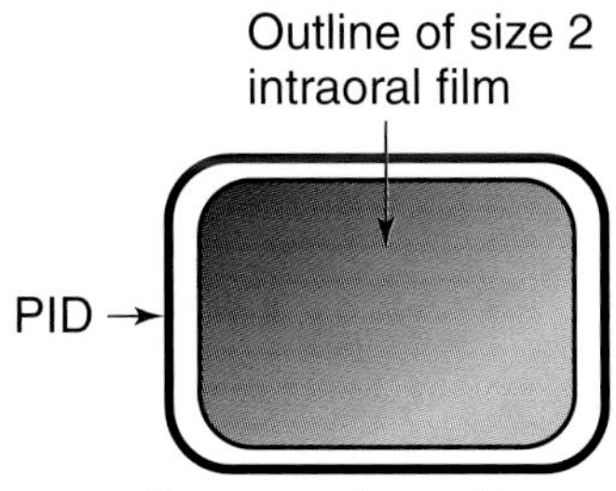

FIGURE 6-4 The rectangular collimator restricts the beam to the approximate size of a #2 film.

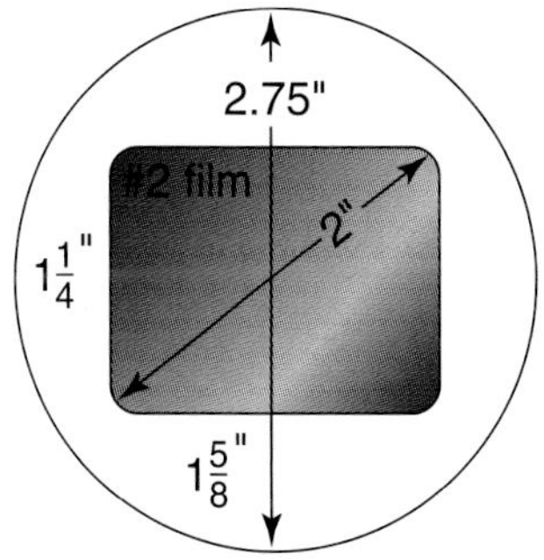

FIGURE 6-5 Circular collimation provides a large enough area of exposure to adequately cover a size #2 intraoral film packet. The patient also receives excess radiation not needed for the exposure of the film.

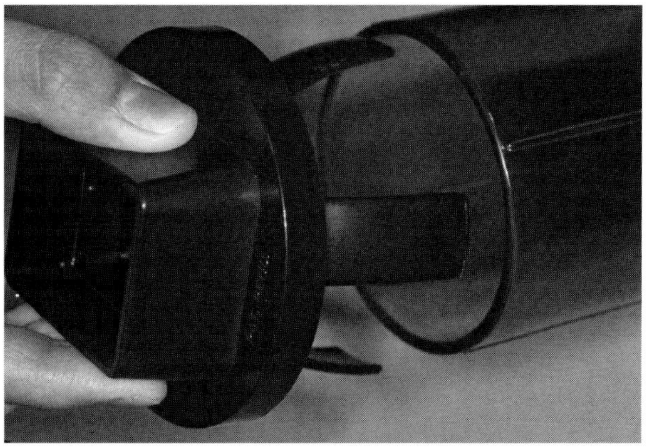

FIGURE 6-6 External collimator that attaches to the PID reduces the area of radiation exposure.

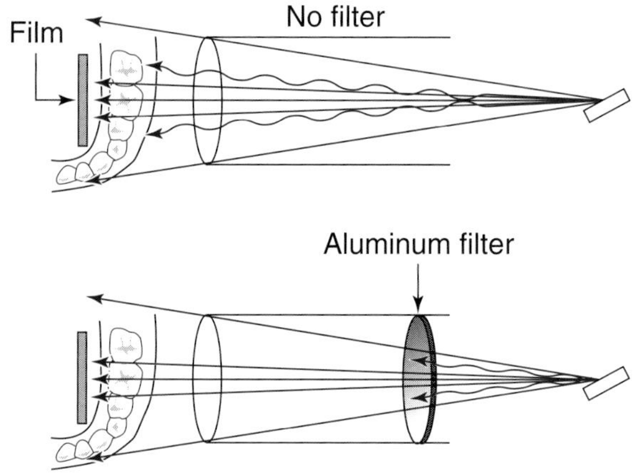

FIGURE 6-8 **Effect of filtration on skin exposure.** Aluminum filters selectively absorb the long wavelength x-rays.

Practice Point

Pointed, closed-end cones are no longer used in dentistry. Because these pointed cones were used for so many years, many still refer to the open cylinders or rectangular tubes as "cones." The term position-indicating device (PID) is more descriptive of its function of directing the x-rays, rather than of its shape.

The length of the PID helps to establish the desired target-surface distance. Both circular and rectangular PIDs are available in various lengths: 8 in. (20.5 cm), 12 in. (30 cm), and 16 in. (41 cm) (Figure 6–10). The longer the PID (12-in. or 16-in. length), the less radiation dose to the patient and the better quality radiographic image (see Figure 4–11). With a longer PID, there is less divergence of the beam, creating a smaller diameter of exposure (Figure 6–11).

It is important to note that the dental x-ray machine may appear to have a short PID when it actually may be long. Some dental x-ray machines feature a recessed PID, where the tube is recessed back in the tubehead behind the transformers, therefore creating a longer target–surface distance (see Figure 3–1).

All intraoral techniques require that the end of the PID be placed as close to the patient's skin as possible, without touching, during the exposure. This is necessary to establish the desired target–surface distance.

- **The lead apron** is a protective barrier against scattered radiation. Made of 0.25-mm lead or **lead-equivalent** materials (Figure 6–12), it should be placed over the patient's

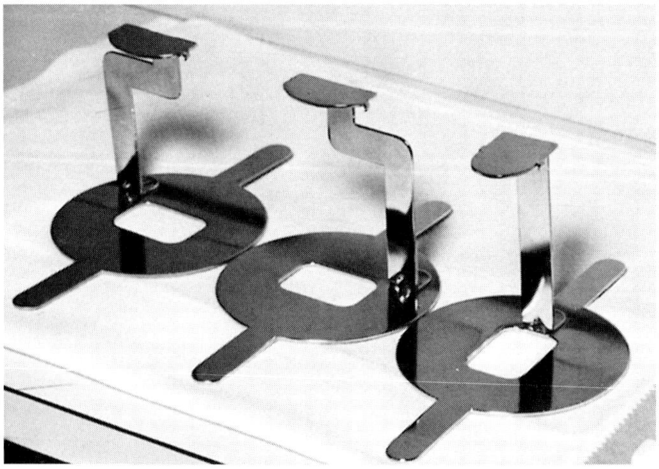

FIGURE 6-7 Set of Precision® instruments featuring metal collimating shield that restricts the x-ray beam to the size of the opening, providing just enough radiation to expose the film properly. (Courtesy of Isaac Masel Company)

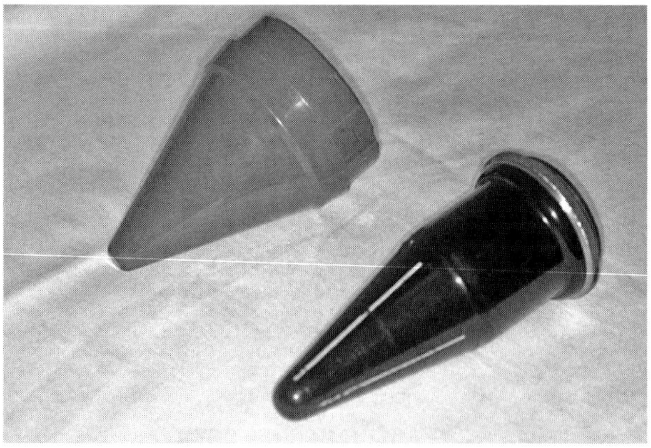

FIGURE 6-9 Plastic closed-ended, pointed "cones" are no longer used.

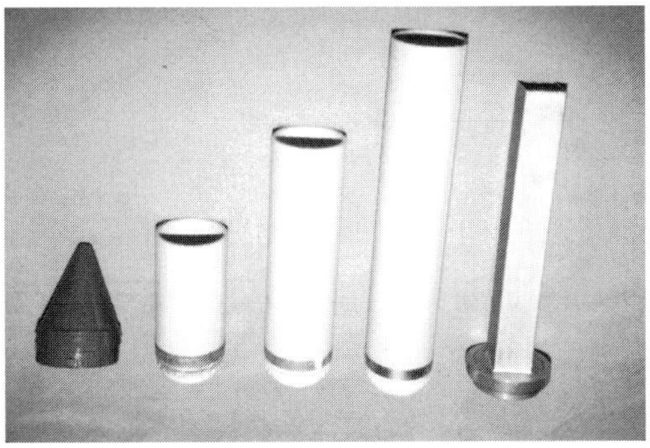

FIGURE 6-10 **PID lengths vary.** Left to right: 8 in. (20.5 cm) pointed, closed-end PID; 8 in. (20.5 cm), 12 in. (30 cm), 16 in. (41 cm) circular PIDs; and 16 in. (41 cm) rectangular PID.

body to protect the reproductive organs and other radiosensitive tissues from scatter radiation. Several states have laws requiring the use of a lead apron over the abdominal area. Even if it is not legally required, the use of a lead or lead-equivalent apron is important, and in keeping with the ALARA concept, should be used on all patients during all intraoral dental x-ray exposures. Lead aprons should be stored flat or hung unbent. Folding the lead apron may cause the lead material to crack. This is most likely to occur when aprons are repeatedly folded in the same place day after day. Cracks in the material allow radiation to penetrate and thus render the apron defective. Lead or lead-equivalent aprons are available with or without an attached thyroid collar.

- **Thyroid collar.** Lead or lead equivalent aprons are available with an attached thyroid collar. The thyroid collar contains 0.25-mm lead or lead-equivalent materials and protects the radiosensitive thyroid gland in the neck region during the exposure of intraoral radiographs. Unattached or detachable thyroid collars are available as a separate piece to supplement lead aprons without a thyroid collar attached (Figure 6–12).

Practice Point

The use of a thyroid collar is contraindicated when exposing panoramic radiographs using rotational panoramic equipment because the collar or upper part of the apron to which it is attached may obscure diagnostic information or interfere with the rotation of the panoramic unit. This is one of the reasons lead aprons are available without thyroid collars.

- **Fast film** requires less radiation for exposure and is essential from the standpoint of exposure reduction. In fact, after rectangular collimation, high-speed film is the single most effective method of reducing radiation to the patient. Currently, intraoral dental x-ray film is available in three speed groups, D, E and F. E-speed film, when compared to D-speed film, is twice as fast and therefore requires only one-half the exposure time. F-speed film will reduce radiation exposure 20 percent compared to E-speed film. The American Dental Association and the American Academy of Oral and Maxillofacial Radiology recommend the use of the fastest speed film currently available.
- **Film-holding devices** that position the film packet intraorally are recommended. The use of a **film holder** eliminates having the patient hold the film in the oral cavity with the fingers (Figure 6–13). Unnecessarily exposing the patient's fingers is not ethical practice in keeping with ALARA. The use of film holders with external aiming devices also assists the operator in aligning the x-ray beam, which may afford the patient additional protection by reducing the number of re-takes that may result from alignment errors (Figure 6–14). These devices also stabilize the film in the mouth and reduce the possibility of movement and film bending that often result when the patient uses a finger to hold the film packet in position. There are also film holders on the market that provide rectangular collimation to further reduce the exposure reaching the patient's tissues (Figure 6–7).

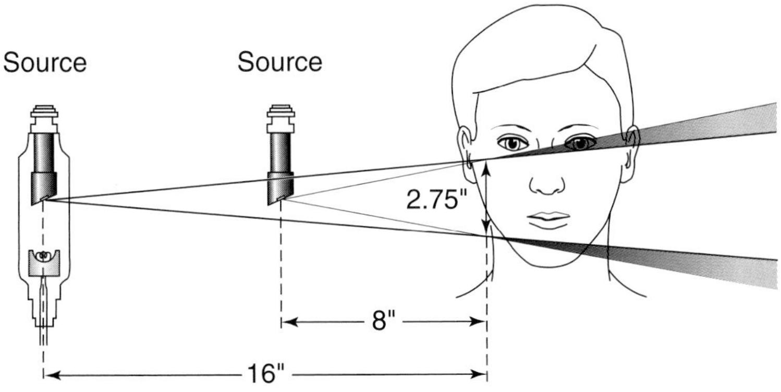

FIGURE 6-11 **Source–film distance.** The longer the source–film distance, the more parallel the rays and the less tissue exposed. Note the beam size at the patient's skin entrance is 2.75 in. (7 cm) for both source–film distances; it is the exit beam size that increases to expose a larger area when using the shorter source–film distance.

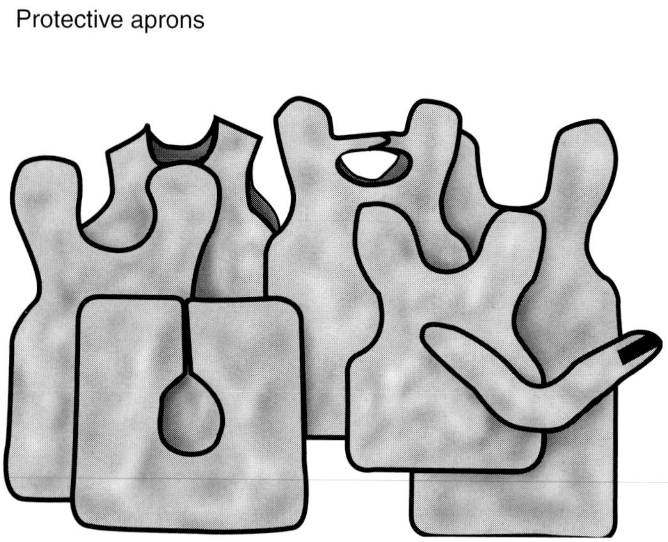

FIGURE 6–12 Lead aprons and thyroid collars are available in a wide range of sizes. Aprons are available with an attached thyroid collar, or the thyroid collar may be separate part. (Courtesy of Dentsply Rinn)

Optimum Film Processing

An often-overlooked step in producing diagnostic radiographs is film processing. Processing errors increase patient radiation exposure by resulting in re-take radiographs. The patient deserves the attention that must be paid to meticulous processing procedures and careful film handling to produce ideal diagnostic quality radiographs. Darkroom procedures should be outlined and followed carefully (see Chapter 8).

Careful attention to chemical replenishment and following the time–temperature method of processing produces radiographs of ideal quality and avoids re-takes. There are ethical considerations to proper processing protocols as well. In the past, it was sometimes observed that an unethical practitioner would call for overexposing (increasing the radiation dose to the patient) and underdeveloping the film in an attempt to save time during certain procedures. Another unethical practice noted in the recent history has been to let processing chemicals go too long between replenishment or solution change. As the processing chemistry weakens, the resultant images appear less dense (lighter). Unethical practitioners would increase the dose of radiation to compensate for the weakening processing solutions. It was the patient who bore the brunt of this practice by enduring the additional radiation burden. Patient protection techniques should be used at all times to keep radiation exposures as low as possible (Table 6–2).

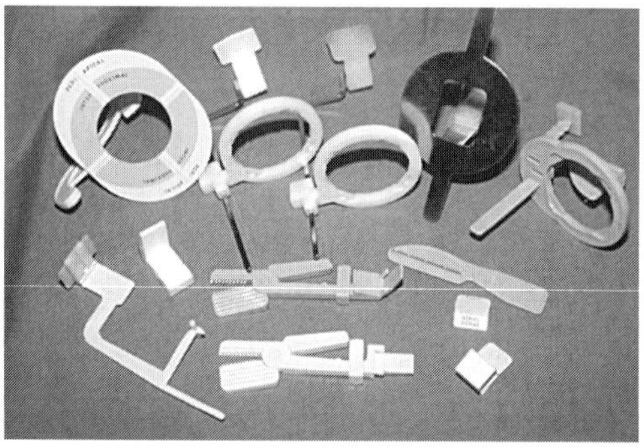

FIGURE 6–13 There are many film holding devices available to fit most situations. The use of a film holder prevents asking patients to put their fingers in the path of the primary beam.

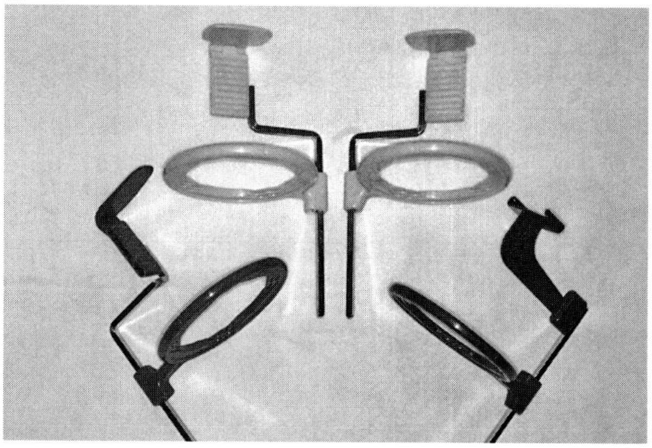

FIGURE 6–14 RINN XCP® film holders manufactured by Dentsply Rinn. Note the external aiming device to assist with determining the correct angulation.

Protection Measures for the Operator

All the radiation protection measures we have discussed to protect the patient also benefit the operator (Table 6–3). Additionally, radiation protection methods for the radiographer include

TABLE 6–2 **Summary of Protection Methods for the Patient**

Evidenced-based prescribing
Communication
Working knowledge of quality radiographs
Education
Intraoral technique selected
Exposure factors posted
Collimation
Filtration
Open-ended, 16-in. (41 cm) rectangular PID
Lead apron with thyroid collar
F-speed film
Film holders
Darkroom protocol
Proper exposure factors

TABLE 6-3 Summary of Methods to Protect the Operator

All patient protection measures
Time
Avoid retakes
Never hold the tube head
Never hold film for the patient
Shielding
Position behind a barrier
Use leaded protective clothing when necessary
Distance
6 ft (1.82 m) at 90° to 135° from the head of the patient.
Radiation monitoring

time, shielding, and distance. The operator should spend a minimal amount of time, protected by shielding, at the greatest distance from the source of radiation to avoid unnecessary exposure.

Time

When careful attention is focused on producing the highest quality radiographs, the need for re-take radiographs is decreased, which in turn decreases the time the radiographer spends near the x-ray machine. Additionally, the dental radiographer should avoid the pitfalls that may lure him/her into the path of the primary beam. For example, a drifting tubehead should never be held during the exposure. **Radiation leakage** from the tubehead can expose the operator to a significant amount of radiation. If the tubehead drifts, it should be serviced to stabilize it.

If a patient must be stabilized during the procedure, as is sometimes the case with a small child, a parent or guardian may have to be asked to assist with the procedure. The parent or guardian should be protected with lead, or lead-equivalent barriers such as an apron or gloves, when they will be in the path of the x-ray beam. The radiographer must never place him/herself in the primary beam.

Film-holding devices should be used to stabilize a film in the patient's oral cavity. If film packet placement with a film holding device is difficult to achieve, as is the case with a patient with a small mouth, low and/or sensitive palatal vault, or an exaggerated gag reflex, the radiographer should experiment with other holders, smaller sized films, or the bisecting technique. The radiographer must not hold the film packet in the patient's mouth. Additionally, another member of the oral health care team must not be allowed to place themselves in the path of the primary beam while the radiographer presses the exposure button.

Shielding

Structural shielding provides the radiographer with additional protection from scattered radiation. Most oral health care practices are located in buildings which have incorporated adequate shielding in walls such as these regularly used construction materials: plaster, cinderblock, 2½ to 3 inches of drywall, 3/16 inch steel, or 1 millimeter of lead. Additionally, lead-lined walls or windows, thick or specially constructed partitions between the rooms, or specially constructed lead screens offer excellent protection for the operator during exposure (see Figure 3–6.) Safe installation of most dental x-ray machines will provide an exposure button permanently mounted behind a **protective barrier,** providing protection for the operator (see Figure 3–4).

Distance

If access to a barrier is not possible, as may be the case in an open-bay designed practice setting, distance plays an important role in safeguarding the radiographer during patient exposures. The operator should always stand as far away as practical—at least 6 ft (1.8 m)—from the head of the patient (the source of scatter radiation) while making the exposure. The intensity of the x-radiation diminishes the farther the x-rays travel (Figure 6–15). A careless operator who stands close to the patient while making an exposure can receive unnecessary scatter radiation.

The safest place for the operator to stand is from 90° to 135° out of the primary beam, behind the bulkiest part of the patient's head (Figure 6–16 and Figure 3–7). The head absorbs most of the **primary radiation** and much of the scatter radiation.

In addition to the operator protection protocol, all persons, whether other oral health care team members or other patients not directly concerned with the x-ray exposure, must also be protected by shielding and/or distance.

Radiation Monitoring

The only way to make sure that x-ray equipment is not emitting too much radiation and that operators are not receiving more than the maximum permissible dose is to use radiation measuring devices to monitor equipment and personnel. In radiography, **monitoring** is defined as periodic or continuing measurement to determine the dose rate in a given area or the dose received by an operator.

Area Monitoring

Area monitoring involves making an on-site survey to measure the output of the dental x-ray unit, to check for possible high-level radiation areas in the operatory, and to determine if any radiation is passing through walls. Special equipment is needed to detect the exact amount of ionizing radiation at any given area. Numerous companies specialize in area monitoring. In some regions, this service may be performed by qualified state personnel.

Personnel Monitoring

Personnel monitoring requires oral health care professionals to wear a radiation monitoring device or **dosimeter** (Figure 6–17). The use of these radiation measuring devices serves to record any radiation dose possibly received by the operator. While **personnel monitoring devices** play a valuable role it should be noted that they are limited in their ability to be precise. Some merely indicate that radiation has been received; others show the amount,

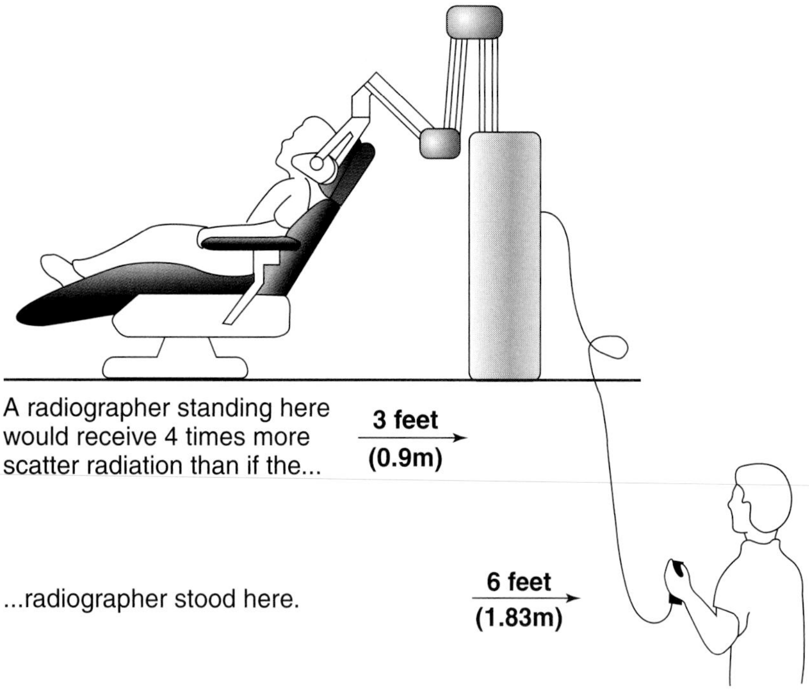

FIGURE 6-15 Distance is an effective means of reducing exposure from scatter radiation.

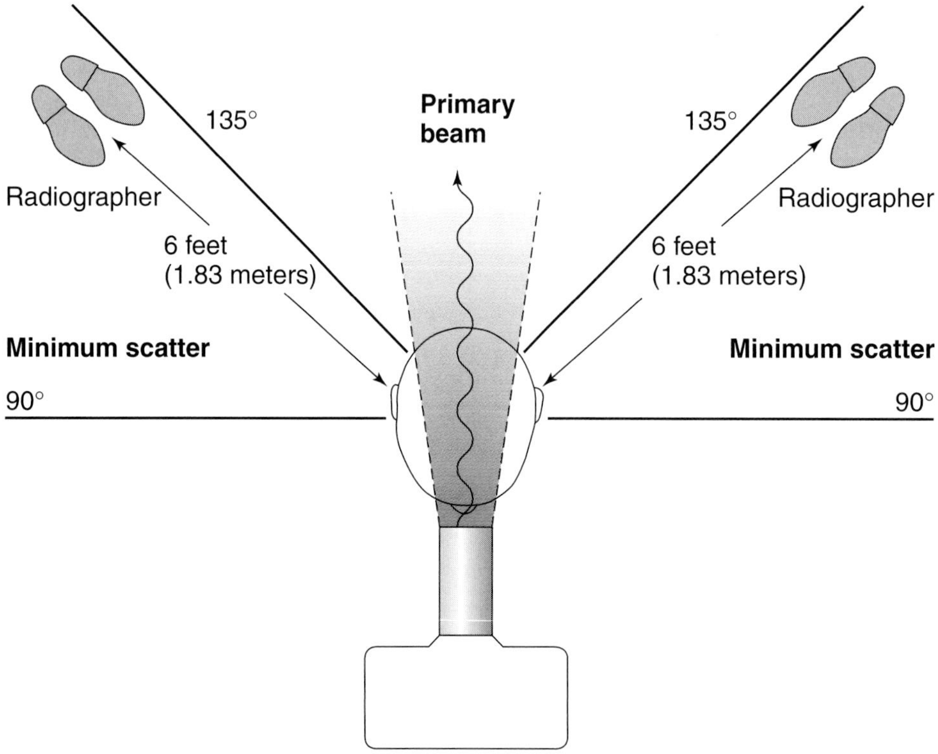

FIGURE 6-16 When structural shielding is not available, the radiographer should stand in a position at least 6 ft (1.83 m) from the head of the patient at an angle of 90° to 135° out of the primary beam.

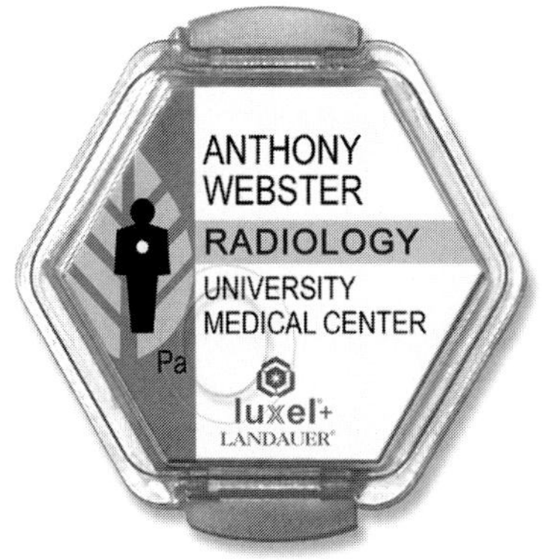

FIGURE 6-17 A TLD badge used for radiation measurement that is worn by the radiographer. (Courtesy of Landauer, Inc.)

and still others measure the amount and type of radiation. The use of computers and advancing technology in this area continue to improve the ability of dosimeters to estimate exposures. However, the personnel monitoring device does not "protect" the wearer from radiation.

The likelihood of dental radiation exposing an oral health care professional who is following ALARA is so small that only a few states consider dental radiation monitoring mandatory. Even so, more and more oral health care professionals are deciding to provide monitoring devices and services for themselves and their employees, even when the service is not mandated by law. As a risk management tool, monitoring radiation exposure—or more likely, the lack of exposure—helps to determine whether or not the operator is maintaining radiation safety protocols; aids in providing the radiographer with peace of mind; and assists in the area of risk management by providing a health record of exposures, or lack of exposures, for personnel.

Types of Personnel Monitoring Devices

For a fee, radiation monitoring companies provide the measuring devices to the oral health care team to use. After use, the devices are returned to the company who evaluates the device and provides the dental practice with a report regarding exposure or lack of exposure. This report compares the operator's exposure reading with the maximum allowable level and the monitoring company updates the subscriber's records to keep the wearer in full compliance with all federal and state safety regulations. The reports from a radiation monitoring service are the most reliable permanent records of accumulated doses of occupational radiation exposure.

- The **film badge** consists of a radiosensitive film loaded in a plastic or metal holder. It has a clip-on attachment for wearing on personal protective clothing, gown, or uniform. Ring or bracelet-type badges are available for other health care professionals, such as radiological technicians, whose hands may be positioned in such a way as to incur a dose of radiation exposure. The film badge is lined with various thicknesses of filters of different materials that make it possible to measure the types of radiation received. Exposure through these filters is determined by "reading" the processed film electronically. The film badge is worn by the operator for one month, after which time the operator removes the film packet from the badge and returns the film packet to the monitoring company for evaluation. A film badge records only the exposure received in the body area in which it is worn.
- The **thermoluminescent dosimeter (TLD)** is also provided in a badge form with a clip-on attachment for wearing on personal protective clothing, gown, or uniform. The thermoluminescent dosimeter (TLD) is worn by the operator for three months, after which time the one-piece constructed TLD is returned to the company for evaluation. The word thermoluminescent is from the Greek word *therme* meaning heat, and the Latin word *lumen*, meaning light and ascent, meaning any giving off of light caused by absorption of radiant energy. The TLD contains crystals, usually lithium fluoride, that absorb energy when exposed to radiation. When the crystals are heated after being exposed to radiation, energy in the form of visible light is given off. The total light emitted is proportional to the amount of radiation (energy) absorbed by the crystals. TLDs are very accurate.

Organizations Responsible for Recommending/Setting Exposure Limits

As early as 1902, studies were undertaken to determine the effect of radiation exposure on the body and to consider setting limits on radiation exposure. The International Commission on Radiological Protection (ICRP) was formed in 1928, and in 1929 the National Council on Radiation Protection and Measurements (NCRP) was created in the United States. The ICRP and the NCRP do not actually set the laws governing the use of ionizing radiation, but their suggestions and recommendations are so highly regarded that most all regulatory bodies use recommendations from these organizations to formulate legislation controlling the use of radiation. The American Dental Association (ADA) and its various committees and affiliated organizations, such as the American Academy of Oral and Maxillofacial Radiology (AAOMR), work closely with all organizations to assure that oral health care patients receive state-of-the-art treatment in radiation safety (Table 6–4).

Maximum Permissible Dose (MPD)

The National Council on Radiation Protection and Measurements (NCRP) developed radiation protection guides referred to as the **maximum permissible dose (MPD)** for the protection of radiation workers and the general public. Maximum permissible dose is defined as the dose equivalent of ionizing radiation that, in the light of present knowledge, is not expected to cause detectable body damage to average persons at any time during

TABLE 6-4 Radiation Protection Organizations

Organization	Web Site
International Commission on Radiological Units and Measurements (ICRU)	www.icru.org
International Commission on Radiological Protection (ICRP)	www.icrp.org
National Council on Radiation Protection and Measurements (NCRP)	www.ncrp.com
U.S. Nuclear Regulatory Commission (NRC)	www.nrc.gov
U.S. Environmental Protection Agency (EPA)	www.epa.gov
U.S. Food and Drug (FDA)	www.fda.gov
U.S. Occupational Safety and Health Administration (OSHA)	www.osha.gov
American Academy of Oral and Maxillofacial Radiology (AAOMR)	www.aaomr.org
American Dental Association (ADA)	www. ada.org

their lifetime. These limits do not apply to medical or dental radiation used for diagnostic or therapeutic purposes. Over the years, the acceptable limits have been constantly revised downward; they are now about 700 times smaller than those originally proposed in 1902, mainly because many aspects of tissue damage from radiation are still not clearly understood.

Maximum limits were set higher for workers than for the public, but the suggested limits of the maximum permissible accumulated dose for both groups were purposely set far lower than it was believed the body could safely accept.

- **Radiation workers.** The maximum permissible dose (MPD) for oral health care professionals is the same as for other radiation workers. According to these guidelines, the whole-body dose may not exceed 50 mSv (5 rem) per year. There is no established weekly limit, but state public health personnel usually use a weekly dose of 1.0 mSv (0.1 rem) when inspecting dental offices.

  The 50 mSv (5 rem) yearly limit for radiation workers has two very important exceptions. It does not apply to persons under 18 years or to any female members of the oral health care team who are known to be pregnant. Persons under 18 years are classified as part of the general public and can accumulate only 5 mSv (0.5 rem) per year. In the case of pregnant women, it is recommended that exposure to the fetus be limited to 5 mSv (0.5 rem), not to be received at a rate greater than 0.5 mSv (0.05 rem) per month.
- **General public.** The general public is permitted 5 mSv (0.5 rem) per year, or one-tenth the dose permitted radiation workers. It should be noted that the MPD has been established for incidental or accidental exposures, and does not include doses from medical and dental diagnostic or therapeutic radiation. Necessary medical and dental diagnostic or therapeutic radiation is not counted in the permissible dose limits. If a patient needs radiographic services, then that patient needs the radiographic services. An oral health care team member who requires medical, dental diagnostic, or therapeutic radiation would become the "patient" and then the general public MPD would apply.

Guides for Maintaining Safe Radiation Levels

Radiation Safety Legislation

The Tenth Amendment gives the states the constitutional authority to regulate health. Because many federal agencies are involved in the development and use of atomic energy, the federal government has preempted the control of radiation. Certain provisions of the Constitution and Public Law 86-373 have enabled the states to assume this pre-empted power and pass laws that spell out radiation safety measures to protect the patient, the operator, or anyone (the general public) near the source of radiation. In fact, even counties and cities have passed ordinances to protect their citizens from radiation hazards. Most states and a few localities require periodic inspection or monitoring of the equipment and its surroundings.

The entry of the federal government into the regulation of x-ray machines began in 1968 with the enactment of the Radiation Control for Health and Safety Act, which standardized the performance of x-ray equipment. Subsequently, the Consumer-Patient Radiation Health and Safety Act of 1981 was passed requiring the various states to develop minimum standards for operators of dental x-ray equipment. Several states responded to this by enacting educational requirements for the certification of individuals who place and expose dental radiographs.

Since the laws concerning radiation control vary from state to state, individuals working with x-rays must be familiar with the regulations governing the use of ionizing radiation in their locale. Regardless of laws, failure to observe safety protocol cannot be justified ethically.

REVIEW—Chapter Summary

Oral health care professionals have an ethical responsibility to adopt the ALARA concept—as low as reasonably achievable—which implies that any dose that can be reduced without major difficulty, great expense or inconvenience, should be reduced or eliminated.

The most important step in keeping the patient's exposure to a minimum is the use of evidenced-based selection criteria to assess patients for radiographic need.

The technical ability of the radiographer will aid in preventing unnecessary radiation exposure to the patient. Technical ability includes communication, working knowledge of quality radiographs, and education. Technique standards, including the choice of paralleling or bisecting technique, and the selection of exposure factors also aid in preventing unnecessary radiation exposure. Equipment standards that play an important role in reducing patient radiation dose include collimation, filtration, and PID length.

Collimation is the control of the size and shape of the useful beam. Federal regulations require that round opening collimators restrict the x-ray beam to 2.75 in. (7 cm) at the patient end of the PID. Rectangular collimation reduces patient radiation dose by 70 percent over round collimation. Collimation reduces scattered radiation that contributes to poor contrast of radiographic images.

Filtration is the absorption of the long wavelength, less penetrating x-rays from the x-ray beam by passage through a sheet of material called a filter. The half-value layer (HVL) of an x-ray beam is the thickness (measured in millimeters) of aluminum that will reduce the intensity of the beam by one-half. Present safety standards require an equivalent of 1.5 mm aluminum filtration for dental x-ray machines operating in ranges below 70 kVp and a minimum of 2.5 mm aluminum for machines operating at or above 70 kVp. Total filtration is the sum of inherent and added filtration.

The position indicating device (PID) is an extension of the tube housing and is used to direct the primary x-ray beam. The length of the PID helps to establish the desired target–surface distance. PIDs have either a round or rectangular shape. Rectangular PIDs reduce patient radiation dose by 70 percent. Standard PID lengths are 8 in. (20.5 cm), 12 in. (30 cm), and 16 in. (41 cm). The longer the PID, the less radiation exposure to the patient.

All patients should be draped with a lead apron and lead thyroid collar in preparation for all intraoral x-ray exposures.

Fast film requires less radiation for exposure. Film speed groups D, E or F are currently available for use in dental radiography. Film speed F reduces patient radiation exposure by 20 percent over film speed E. Film speed E reduces patient radiation exposure by 50 percent over film speed D.

The use of film holders eliminates using the patient's fingers to stabilize the film packet intraorally, avoiding unnecessary radiation exposure of the patient's fingers.

Optimum film processing using time-temperature techniques in an adequately equipped darkroom will help avoid re-takes, which increase patient radiation exposure.

To reduce the chance of operator exposure time spent near the source of radiation should be reduced; structural shielding employed; or the operator should be in a position at least 6 feet away from the source of radiation at an angle of 90–135 degrees.

Film badges and TLDs can be utilized to monitor radiographers for possible radiation exposure. The International Commission on Radiological Protection (ICRP) and the National Council on Radiation Protection and Measurements (NCRP) recommend dose limits. Federal, state, and local agencies set regulations governing exposure. The American Dental Association and the American Academy of Oral and Maxillofacial Radiology work closely with all agencies responsible for radiation safety.

The maximum permissible dose (MPD) is 50 mSv (5 rem) per year for radiation workers and 5 mSv (0.5 rem) for the general public, radiation workers who are pregnant, and children under 18 years of age.

RECALL—Study Questions

1. Who has an ethical responsibility to adopt ALARA?
   a. The dental assistant
   b. The dental hygienist
   c. The dentist
   d. All of the above
2. Based on the selection criteria guidelines, what is the radiographic recommendation for bitewing radiographs on an adult recall patient with no clinical caries and no high-risk factors for caries?
   a. Every 6–12 months
   b. Every 12–18 months
   c. Every 18–24 month
   d. Every 24–36 months
3. Communication, working knowledge of a quality radiographic image, and education all aid in protecting the patient against unnecessary radiation exposure by:
   a. Using lower exposure factors.
   b. Reducing the risk of re-take radiographs.
   c. Collimating and filtering the primary beam.
   d. Creating a longer target–surface distance.
4. Radiation protection from secondary radiation may be increased by the use of an aluminum filter and a lead collimator *because* the filter regulates the size of the tissue area that is exposed and the collimator prevents low energy radiation from reaching the tissue.
   a. Both statement and reason are correct.
   b. Both statement and reason are not correct.
   c. The statement is correct, but the reason is not correct.
   d. The statement is not correct, but the reason is correct.
5. What material is the collimator made of?
   a. Lead
   b. Tungsten
   c. Samarium
   d. Aluminum
6. What is the minimum total filtration that is required by an x-ray machine that can operate in ranges above 70 kVp?
   a. 1.5 mm of aluminum equivalent
   b. 1.5 mm of lead equivalent
   c. 2.5 mm of aluminum equivalent
   d. 2.5 mm of lead equivalent
7. What is the federally mandated size of the diameter of the primary beam at the end of the PID (at the skin of the patient's face)?
   a. 1.75 in. (4.5 cm)
   b. 2.75 in. (7 cm)
   c. 3.75 in. (10 cm)
   d. 4.75 in. (12 cm)
8. Which of the following contributes the most to reducing patient radiation exposure?
   a. 8 in. (20.5 cm) round PID
   b. 12 in. (30 cm) round PID
   c. 16 in. (41 cm) round PID
   d. 16 in. (41 cm) rectangular PID
9. During x-ray exposure, the lead apron and thyroid collar should be placed on:
   a. Children.
   b. Females.
   c. Males.
   d. All patients.
10. Which of the following contributes the most to reducing patient radiation exposure?
    a. D speed film
    b. E speed film
    c. F speed film

11. All of the following aid in reducing patient radiation exposure *except* one. Which one is this *exception?*
    a. Slow speed film
    b. Careful film handling
    c. Darkroom protocol
    d. Film holders
12. The principal hazard to the dental radiographer during x-ray procedures is produced by:
    a. Direct radiation.
    b. Scattered radiation.
    c. Gamma radiation.
    d. Alpha radiation.
13. What is the recommended minimum distance that the operator should stand from the source of the radiation?
    a. 3 ft (0.91 m)
    b. 6 ft (1.83 m)
    c. 9 ft (2.74m)
    d. 12 ft (3.66m)
14. Film badges and TLDs are used to:
    a. Protect the operator from unnecessary radiation exposure.
    b. Reduce the radiation exposure received by the patient.
    c. Monitor radiation exposure the dental radiographer may incur.
    d. Record an on-site survey of the radiation output of the x-ray unit.
15. The annual maximum permissible whole-body dose for oral health care personnel is:
    a. 0.5 mSv.
    b. 5.0 mSv.
    c. 50 mSv.
    d. 500 mSv.
16. The annual maximum permissible whole-body dose for the general public is:
    a. 0.5 mSv.
    b. 5.0 mSv.
    c. 50 mSv.
    d. 500 mSv.

REFLECT—Case Study

Use the selection criteria guidelines to make a preliminary recommendation and/or to explain to the patient why the dentist has prescribed or has not prescribed radiographs. Consider the following three cases:

1. A 17-year-old patient presents with a healthy oral assessment. No active caries were clinically detected. No periodontal pockets were noted. His record indicates that his last radiographs were bitewings taken 6 months ago. Based on the evidence-based selection criteria guidelines, what would be the most likely recommendation for radiographs for this patient?
2. A 25-year-old female recall patient presents for her 6-month check-up. While her homecare is good, Class II (multi-surface) restorations are present on several molars and premolars. Her last radiographs were bitewings taken 3 years ago. Based on the evidenced-based selection criteria guidelines, what would be the most likely recommendation for radiographs for this patient?
3. A 45-year-old male patient, new to your practice, presents with a moderate periodontal condition and evidence of generalized dental disease. He reveals that he has not been "to the dentist" in several years, but is here today to begin to "take care of his teeth." Based on the evidenced-based selection criteria guidelines, what would be the most likely recommendation for radiographs for this patient?

RELATE—Laboratory Application

Using Table 6–2: Summary of Protection Methods for the Patient and Table 6–3: Summary of Methods to Protect the Operator as a guide, perform an inventory of your facility. Make a list of all of the radiation protection methods used at your facility. Compare and contrast these with the safety protocols you learned in this chapter.

Begin with the first patient radiation protection method listed in Table 6–2, evidence-based prescribing. Investigate how the dentist at your facility determines who will need radiographs. What guidelines do the dental hygienist and the dental assistant use to help them in explaining the need for necessary radiographs to the patient? Does your facility use guidelines similar to the evidence-based guidelines you learned about in this chapter? Describe them. Compare and contrast the methods your facility uses to determine radiographic need to the guidelines you learned about in this chapter. Is your facility meeting or exceeeding this safety method for reducing patient radiation dose? If not, what is the rationale for not meeting this standard?

Proceed to the next item on the list in Table 6–2, Communication. Observe the communication between the oral health care professionals at your facility prior to, during, and following patient x-ray exposure. What are some examples of dialogue that contributed to aiding in the protection of patients from unnecessary radiation exposure? Was there any communication that you think could have been added? Again, compare and contrast the communication standards the professionals at your facility use to decrease the likelihood of unnecessary radiation exposure using the guidelines you learned about in this chapter. Is your facility meeting or exceeeding this safety method for reducing patient radiation dose? If not, what is the rationale for not meeting this standard?

Proceed through the list of items in Table 6–1 and Table 6–2. Use observation and interviewing techniques to thoroughly investigate how each of these items is applied at your facility. Based on what you learned in this chapter, determine whether or not your facility is adequately applying all possible methods of reducing radiation expsoure to patients and operators.

BIBLIOGRAPHY

ADA Council on Scientific Affairs. An Update on Radiographic Practices: Information and Recommendations. *J. Am. Dent. Assn.* 2001;132:234–238.

Eastman Kodak: *Radiation Safety in Dental Radiography.* Rochester, NY: Eastman Kodak, 1998.

International Commission on Radiological Protection. *1990 Recommendations of ICRP.* Publication 60. Stockholm: Annuals of the ICRP, 1991;21/1–3.

National Council on Radiation Protection and Measurements. *Implementation of the Principle of As Low as Reasonably Achievable (ALARA) for Medical and Dental Personnel.* Washington, DC: NCRP, 1991. NCRP report no. 107.

National Council on Radiation Protection and Measurements. *Limitation of Exposure to Ionizing Radiation.* Washington, DC: NCRP, 1993. NCRP report no. 116.

National Council on Radiation Protection and Measurements. *Radiation Protection in Dentistry.* Washington, DC: NCRP, 2003. NCRP report no. 145.

Public Health Service, Food and Drug Administration, American Dental Association Council on Dental Benefit Program, Council on Dental Practice, Council on Scientific Affairs. *The Selection of Patients for Dental Radiographic Examinations.* Washington, DC: U.S. Dept. of Health and Human Services, 1987; revised 2004.

Part III • Dental X-ray Film and Processing Techniques

7

Dental X-ray Film

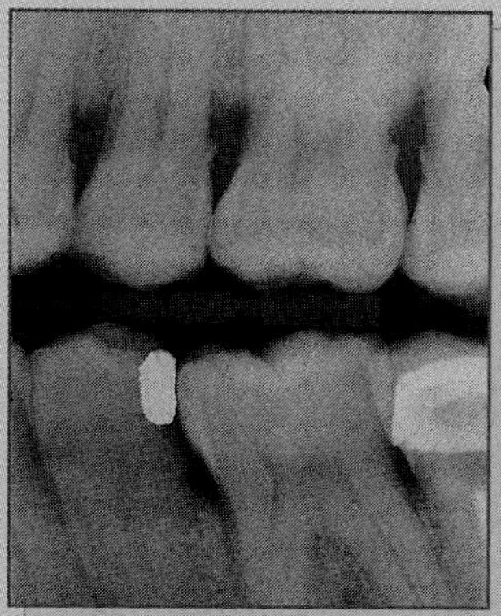

CHAPTER OUTLINE

■ OBJECTIVES

Following successful completion of this chapter, you should be able to:

1. Define the key words.
2. List and describe the four parts of an intraoral film.
3. Describe latent image formation.
4. List and describe the four parts of an intraoral film packet.
5. Differentiate between the tube side and the back side of an intraoral film packet.
6. Identify the intraoral film speeds currently available for dental radiographs.
7. Match the intraoral film size with customary usage.
8. Match the type of intraoral projection with radiographic need.
9. Explain the difference between intraoral film and screen extraoral film.
10. List typical extraoral film sizes.
11. Compare and contrast duplicating film with radiographic film.
12. List the seven conditions that fog stored film.

■ KEY WORDS

Antihalation coating
Bitewing radiograph
Duplicating film
Emulsion
Extraoral film
Film packet
Film speed
Gelatin
Halide
Identification dot
Intensifying screen
Intraoral film
Latent image
Occlusal radiograph
Pedodontic film
Periapical radiograph
Screen film
Silver halide crystals
Solarized emulsion
Tube side

Introduction

Since it is radiation's interaction with film that allows us to utilize x-rays in preventive oral health care, the dental assistant and dental hygienist should possess a working knowledge of how radiographic film records an image. Additionally, determining how film can best be utilized to provide the most diagnostic information while exposing the patient to the least amount of radiation possible is the key to radiation safety. The purpose of this chapter is to explain film composition, introduce film category types, and discuss film protection and storage to aid the dental assistant and dental hygienist in making appropriate decisions regarding film use and handling.

Composition of Dental X-ray Films

The films used in dental radiography are photographic films that have been especially adapted in size, emulsion, film speed, and packaging for dental uses. Figure 7–1 is a schematic cross-sectional drawing of dental x-ray film.

Film Base

The purpose of the film base is to provide support for the fragile emulsion and to provide strength for handling. Films used in dental radiography have a thin, flexible, clear, or blue-tinted polyester base. The blue tint enhances contrast and image quality. The base is covered with a photographic emulsion on both sides.

Adhesive

Each emulsion layer is attached to the base by a thin layer of adhesive.

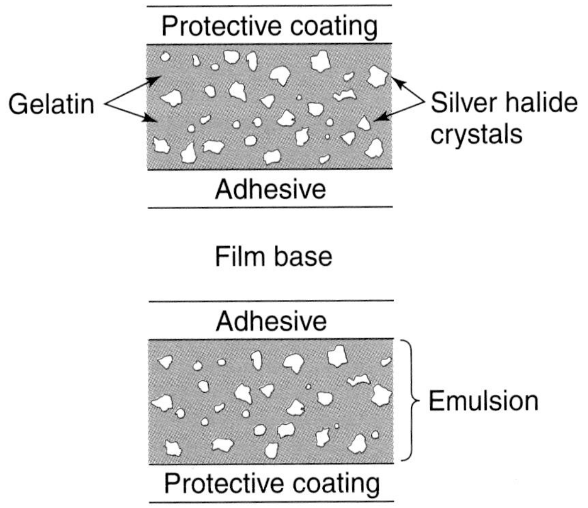

FIGURE 7–1 **Schematic cross-section drawing of dental x-ray film.** The rigid but flexible film base is coated on both sides with an emulsion consisting of silver halide (bromide and iodide) crystals embedded in gelatin. Each emulsion layer is attached to the base by a thin layer of adhesive. The emulsion layers are covered by a supercoating of gelatin to protect the emulsion from scratching and handling.

Emulsion

The **emulsion** is composed of **gelatin** in which crystals of silver **halide** salts are suspended. The function of the gelatin is to keep the silver halide crystals evenly suspended over the base. The gelatin will not dissolve in cold water, but swells, thus exposing the silver halide crystals to the chemicals in the developing solution. The gelatin shrinks as it dries, leaving a smooth surface that becomes the radiograph.

The **silver halide crystals** are compounds of a halogen (either bromine or iodine) with another element. In radiography, as well as in photography, that element is silver. Dental film emulsion is about 90–99 percent silver bromide and 1–10 percent silver iodide. Silver halide crystals are sensitive to radiation. It is the silver halide crystals which, when exposed to x-rays, retain the latent image.

Protective Layer

The supercoating of gelatin to protect the emulsion from scratching and rough handling that covers the emulsion layers is called the protective layer.

Latent Image Formation

During radiation exposure the x-rays strike and ionize some, but not all, of the silver halide crystals, resulting in the formation of a **latent image** (invisible image). Not all of the radiation penetrating the patient's tissue will reach the film emulsion. For example, metal restorations such as an amalgam or crown will absorb the x-ray energy and stop the radiation from reaching the film. It should be noted that there will be varying amounts of radiation reaching the film. Enamel and bone will absorb, or stop, more of the x-rays from reaching the film than the less dense structures such as the dentin or pulp chambers of the teeth. The varying thicknesses of the objects in the path of the beam will allow more or less radiation to pass through and reach the film emulsion. When radiation does reach the emulsion, the silver halide crystals are ionized, or separated into silver and bromide ions that store this energy as a latent image. These energy centers store the invisible image pattern until the processing procedure produces a visual image (see Chapter 8).

During the developing stage of the processing procedure, the exposed silver halide crystals—which have stored a latent image—are changed into black specks of silver, resulting in the black or radiolucent areas observed on a dental radiograph. The amount of black silver specks varies depending on the structures radiographed, and whether or not those structures allowed the x-rays to pass through and reach the film emulsion. While thin structures permit the passage of x-rays, thick, dense structures will not. These dense structures will appear clear/white or radiopaque on the radiograph as a result of the fixer step during film processing (see Chapter 8).

Types of Dental X-ray Film

Depending on where the film is to be used—inside or outside the mouth—the film is classified as intraoral or extraoral.

Intraoral Films

Intraoral films are designed for use inside the oral cavity. The use of an intraoral film outside the oral cavity is contraindicated because of the increased dose of radiation needed to produce an acceptable radiographic density.

Film Packet

The film manufacturer cuts the films to the sizes required in dentistry. Small films suitable for intraoral (inside the mouth) radiography are made into what is called a **film packet.** The terms film packet and film are often used interchangeably. Figure 7–2 shows the front or **tube side** and the back side of an intraoral film packet.

All intraoral film packets are assembled similarly. The film is first surrounded by black, light-protective paper. Next, a thin sheet of lead foil to shield the film from backscatter radiation is placed on the side of the film that will be away from the radiation source. An outer wrapping of moisture-resistant paper or plastic completes the assembly (Figures 7–3 and 7–4).

The film packet consists of:

1. Film
2. Black paper wrapping
3. Lead foil
4. Moisture-resistant outer wrapping

- **Film.** Film packets may contain one or two films. When a packet containing two x-ray films is exposed, duplicate

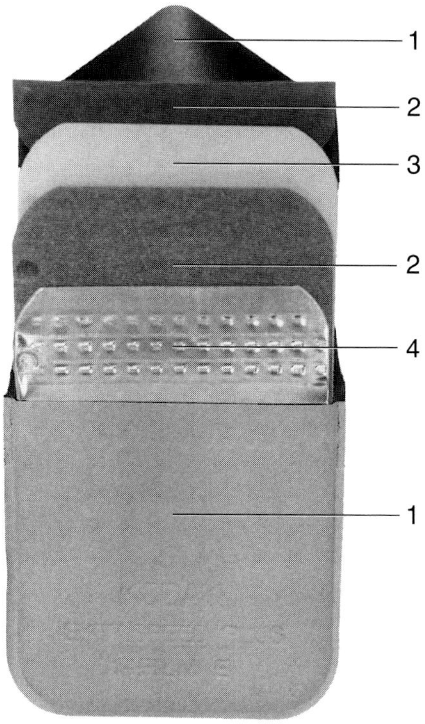

FIGURE 7–3 **Photograph of the back of an open film packet.** (**1**) Moisture-resistant outer wrap. (**2**) Black paper. (**3**) Film. (**4**) Lead foil backing.

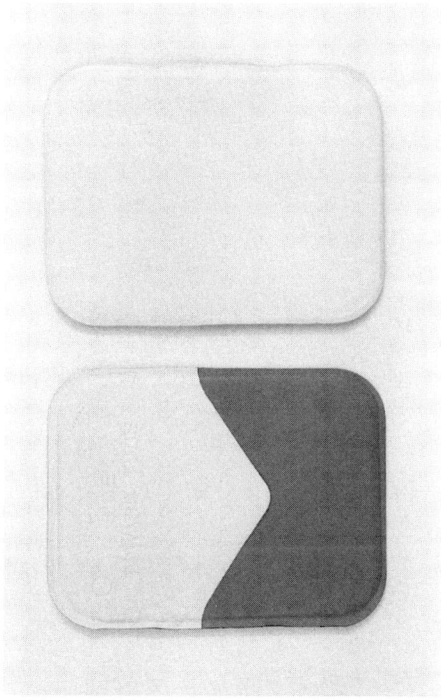

FIGURE 7–2 Intraoral film packets showing the front or tube side (white, unprinted side of the film packet) *(top)* and the back side (color-coded side) of the film packet *(bottom)*.

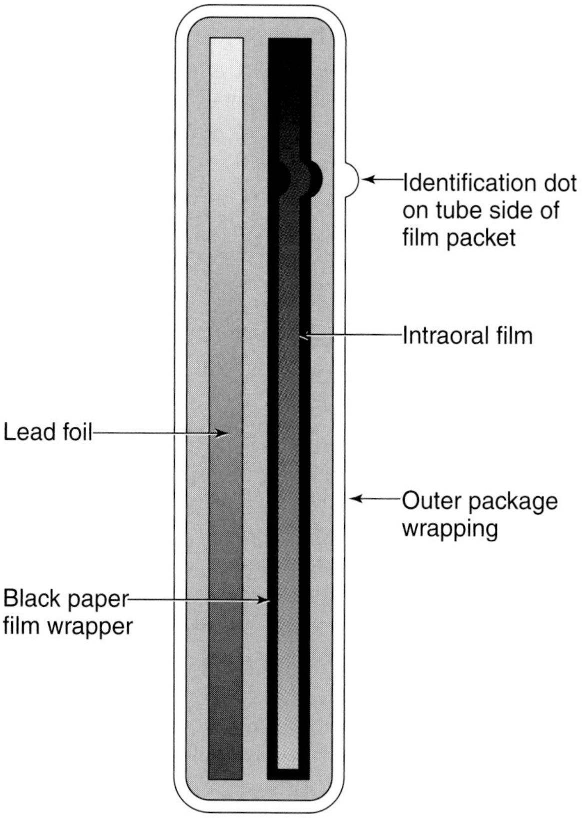

FIGURE 7–4 **Cross-section of a film packet.**

radiographs result, at no greater radiation exposure to the patient. A duplicate radiograph allows the oral health care practice to keep one of the radiographs as a part of the patient's permanent record, while sending the other, identical radiograph out for consultation or referrals with specialists, as evidence for third party payment, for legal evidence, or when a patient is moving to another location, which requires seeking another primary care practitioner.

Practice Point

Several court rulings and a California law concerning the patient's right of access to dental records require the dentist to furnish records (including x-ray films) to the patient on demand. This has increased the use of two-film packets.

A small raised **identification dot** is located in one corner of the film. The raised dot is used to determine film orientation and is used to distinguish the right radiographs from the left radiographs (see Chapter 18).

- **Black paper wrapping** is wrapped around the film. The purpose of the black paper wrapping is to protect the film from light.
- **Lead foil.** A sheet of lead foil is located in the back of the film packet, behind the film. The purpose of the lead foil backing is to absorb scattered radiation. Scattered x-rays strike the film emulsion from the back side of the film (the side away from the tube), fogging or reducing the clarity of the image. The lead foil is embossed with a pattern that becomes visible on the developed x-ray film in the event that the packet is accidentally positioned backwards during the exposure.
- **Moisture-resistant outer wrapping.** The packet covering is an outer wrapping of moisture-resistant paper or soft vinyl plastic. The purpose of the wrapping is to hold the packet contents and to protect the film from light and moisture. Each film packet has two sides, a front side or tube side that faces the tube (radiation source) and a back side away from the source of radiation (Figure 7–2).
  - **Tube Side.** The tube side is a solid white (either paper or plastic) outer moisture-resistant wrapping that is either smooth or slightly pebbly, to prevent slippage. There is a small embossed dot evident near one of the film corners. The embossed dot will be used later to aid in identifying the image as either the patient's right or left side; however, it is important to know which corner it is located on during the film placement step.

    In intraoral radiography, the tube side of the film faces the source of radiation. When placing the film intraorally, the tube side will face the lingual surfaces of the teeth of interest.
  - **Back side.** The back side containing the tab for opening the film packet is white, or may be color coded (Table 7–1). To aid in determining which is the front and back side of the film packet the following information is usually printed on the back side:
    - Manufacturer's name
    - Film speed
    - Number of films in the packet (one or two)
    - Circle or mark indicating the location of the identifying dot
    - The statement "Opposite side toward tube"

Practice Point

During intraoral film packet placement, the embossed dot should be positioned away from the area of interest. Usually, when taking periapical radiographs, the area of interest is the apices of the teeth; therefore, the embossed dot should be positioned toward the occlusal. To assist with positioning the embossed dot out of the way, intraoral film manufacturers have packaged film so that the embossed dot can be observed on the outer moisture-resistant wrapping.

Film Packaging

Intraoral film packets are packaged in cardboard boxes or plastic trays. Depending on the size, intraoral films are usually packaged 25, 50, 130 or 150 to a box, the most popular being the 130- or 150-film packages. A layer of lead foil surrounds the films inside the container to protect them from damage by stray radiation while being stored.

Film Emulsion Speeds (Sensitivity)

Speed refers to the amount of radiation required to produce a radiograph of acceptable density. The faster the **film speed,** the less radiation required to produce an acceptable density radiograph. Factors that determine film speed are:

- **Size of silver halide crystal.** The larger the crystal, the faster the film speed.
- **Thickness of emulsion.** Emulsion is coated on both sides of the film base to increase film speed. The thicker the emulsion, the faster the film speed.

TABLE 7–1 **Kodak Film Packet Color Codes**

	One-film packet	Two-film packet
Ultra-speed (D)	Green	Gray
Insight (F)	Lavender	Tan

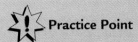

- **Special radiosensitive dyes.** Manufacturers add special dyes that help to increase the film speed.

While the thickness of the emulsion and the addition of radiosensitive dyes aid in increasing film speed (film sensitivity), the most important factor in increasing film speed is the size of the silver halide crystals in the emulsion. The larger the crystals, the faster the film speed, resulting in less radiation exposure to produce an acceptable image. However, image sharpness is more distinct when the crystals are small. The larger crystals used in high-speed (fast) film result in a certain amount of graininess that reduces the sharpness of the radiographic image. It has been determined that this slight loss of image sharpness does not interfere with diagnosis and is tolerated because of the reduction in patient radiation exposure.

Speed Groups

Trademark names like *Ultra*-speed or *Insight* tell little or nothing about the actual film speed. The American National Standards Institute (ANSI) groups film speed using letters of the alphabet, speed group A for the slowest through F for the fastest. At the present time, F-speed is the fastest film available and film speeds slower than D are no longer used. In addition to labeling the film packages, film speed is printed on the back side of each individual film packet.

Currently only D-speed, E-speed, and F-speed films are available. Kodak introduced their F-speed film in 2000 and subsequently stopped manufacturing E-speed film in late 2001. Both the American Dental Association and the American Association of Oral and Maxillofacial Radiology recommend using the fastest speed film currently available to aid in reducing unnecessary radiation to patients. Although F-speed film requires less radiation to produce an acceptable image, some practitioners have not stopped using the slower D-speed film. Faster speed films contain a larger crystal size that contributes to a decrease in image resolution. Some practitioners who are accustomed to viewing D-speed images resist the change. However, it should be noted that changes in the visual acuity of today's films have improved the image of the faster speed films. Additionally, it should be noted that studies of film speed comparisons have failed to indicate that faster speed films are less diagnostic. The use of high-speed film has made it possible to reduce patient exposure to radiation to a fraction of the time formerly deemed necessary. Fast speed film has contributed more to radiation safety than any other factor except rectangular collimation.

Film Size

There are five sizes of intraoral film: #0, #1, #2, #3, and #4. The larger the number, the larger the size of the film (Figure 7–5).

- **Size 0.** The #0 films are especially designed for small children and thus are often called pedo (from the Greek word *paidos*, child) or **pedodontic films.**
- **Size 1.** The #1 films may also be used for children. In adults, the use of the narrow #1 film is normally limited to exposing radiographs of the anterior teeth. Although it shows only two or three teeth, this film is ideal for areas where the oral cavity is narrow and curves a great deal.
- **Size 2.** The wider #2 film is generally referred to as the standard film, or PA for periapical film. This film size is used in at least 75 percent of all intraoral radiography. The #2 films are commonly used on both larger children, especially those with a mixed dentition, and adults.
- **Size 3.** The extra-long #3 film is also called the long bitewing film. These films usually come with a pre-attached bite tab.
- **Size 4.** The #4 films are the largest of the intraoral films. Size 4 films are generally referred to as occlusal films.

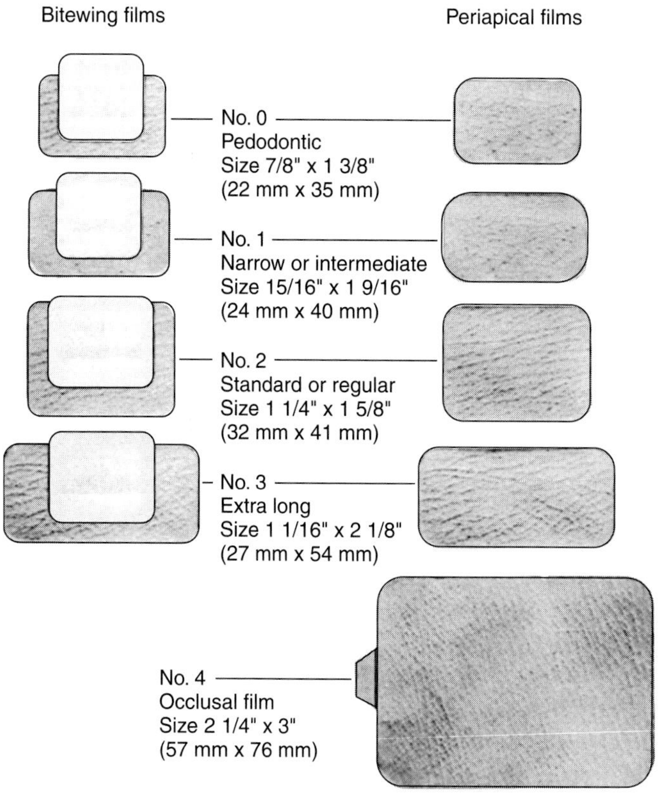

FIGURE 7–5 **Intraoral film.** With the exception of the large occlusal film, all intraoral film sizes are available both with and without an attached bite tab for use in taking bitewing projections. (Courtesy of Dentsply Rinn)

Types of Projections

There are three types of intraoral film projections: bitewing, periapical, and occlusal.

- **Bitewing radiographs** (Figure 7–6) are used to examine the crowns of the teeth, especially the surfaces of the teeth that touch each other. Additionally, bitewings radiographs image a portion of the alveolar bone crests. Bitewing radiographs image the coronal portions of both the maxillary (upper) and mandibular (lower) teeth and crestal bone on the same film. Bitewing radiographs are particularly valuable when determining the extent of proximal caries.

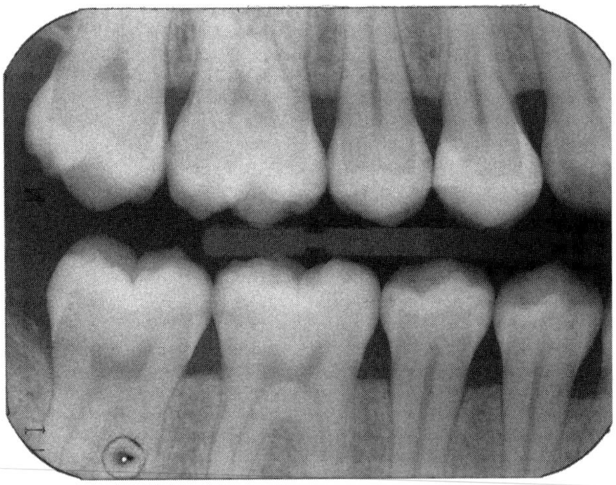

FIGURE 7-6 **Bitewing radiograph.**

Vertical bitewing radiographs (see Chapter 14) provide additional information regarding the supporting periodontia. Both vertical and horizontal bitewing radiographs may be exposed using film sizes #0, #1, or #2. Film size #3 is especially designed to expose horizontal bitewing radiographs. Bitewing film sizes, especially the size #3 film packet, may be purchased with an attached flap or tab on which the patient must bite to hold the film packet in place between the occlusal surfaces of the maxillary and mandibular teeth.

- **Periapical radiographs** (Figure 7–7) (from the Greek word *peri*, for around and the Latin word *apex* for the root tip) are used to make a detailed examination of the entire tooth, from crown to root tip or apex. Additionally, periapical radiographs image the supporting structures of the teeth such as the periodontal ligament space and the surrounding bone tissues. Periapical radiographs may be exposed using film sizes #0, #1, or #2.
- **Occlusal radiographs** (see Figure 15–1) image a larger area than periapical radiographs. These projections are ideal for making a rapid survey of a large area of the maxilla, mandible, and floor of the mouth. They can reveal gross pathological lesions, root fragments, bone and tooth fractures, and impacted or supernumerary teeth and many other conditions. Occlusal radiographs may be used to make a rapid survey of an edentulous (without teeth) mouth. The size #4 film packet is especially designed as an occlusal film. Occlusal radiographs are usually exposed using film size #4. However, film size #2 may also be used with the occlusal radiographic technique. Size #2 film is commonly used for occlusal exposures on young children who may not be able to tolerate the film packet placement necessary for periapical radiographs.

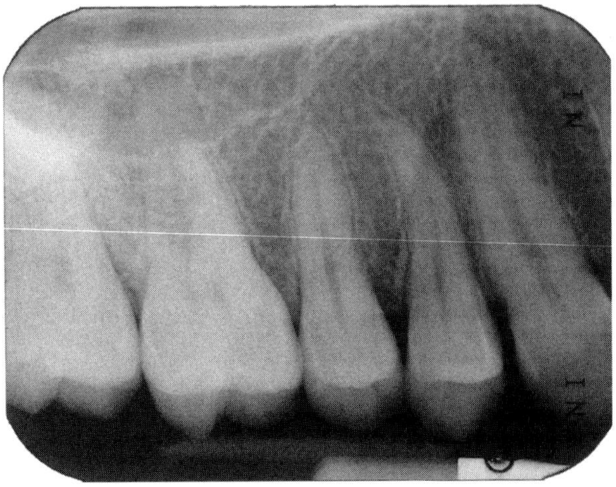

FIGURE 7-7 **Periapical radiograph.**

Extraoral Films

Extraoral films are designed for use outside the mouth. These large films are classified as screen film. **Screen film** (indirect-exposure film) is exposed primarily by a fluorescent type of light given off by special emulsion-coated **intensifying screens** that are positioned between the film and the x-ray source. The intensity of the fluorescent light emitted by the intensifying screens permits a significant reduction in the amount of radiation required to produce an image. The image produced on an extraoral film results from exposure to this fluorescent light, instead of directly from the x-rays.

Packaging

Larger extraoral films are generally packaged 25, 50, or 100 to a box (Figure 7–8). The films are sometimes sandwiched between two pieces of protective paper, and the entire group is wrapped in lead foil for protection. Because these films are designed for extraoral use with a cassette, which is discussed in detail in Chapter 27, they require neither individual lead backing nor moisture-resistant wrappings.

Film Size

Extraoral films vary in size. Different sizes can accommodate imaging the oral cavity and various regions of the head and neck. The most common sizes are:

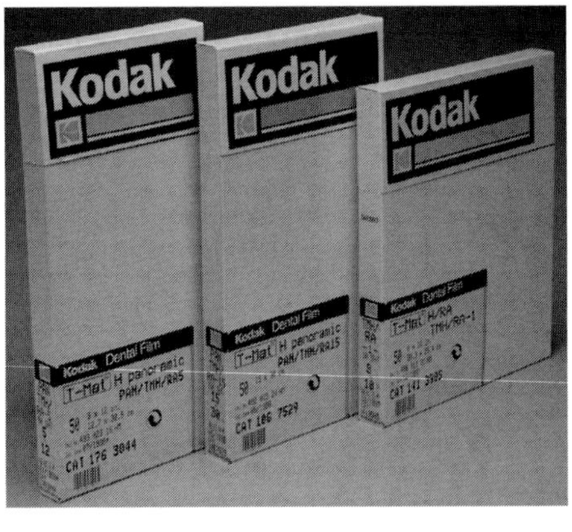

FIGURE 7-8 **Extraoral film packages.** 5 × 12-in. (13 × 30 cm), 6 × 12-in (15 × 30 cm) and 8 × 10 in. (20 × 26 cm) size extraoral film packages. (Used with permission of Eastman Kodak Company.)

- 5 × 7 in. (13 × 18 cm), used mainly for lateral views of the jaw or the temporomandibular joint (TMJ)
- 8 × 10 in. (20 × 26 cm), used for cephalometric profiles and posteroanterior views of the skull
- 5 or 6 in. × 12 in. (13 or 15 cm × 30 cm), used for panoramic radiographs of the entire dentition

Duplicating Film

When a duplicate radiograph, a copy identical to an original, is needed, oral health care practices often utilize two-film intraoral packets. However, if an additional copy is needed or a two-film packet was not utilized when taking the original radiograph, a duplicating machine with special duplicating film may be used.

Duplicating film is a type of photographic film that is similar to x-ray film, but is exposed by the action of infrared and ultraviolet light rather than by x-rays. Only one side of the duplicating film is coated with emulsion. The emulsion side appears dull and lighter under safe light conditions in the darkroom where it is used. The non-emulsion side is shiny and appears darker under safe light conditions. To make a copy of a radiograph, the emulsion side of the film is placed against the original radiograph with the non-emulsion side up (see Chapter 25). When the duplicating film is exposed to ultraviolet light in the duplicating machine, the **solarized emulsion** records the copy. Solarized emulsion is different than x-ray film emulsion in that the image produced in response to light exposure gets darker with less light exposure and lighter with more light exposure. The non-emulsion side contains an **antihalation coating.** The dye in the antihalation coating absorbs the ultraviolet light coming through the films to prevent back-scattered light from re-exposing the film and creating an unsharp image.

Duplication film, boxed in quantities of 50, 100, or 150 sheets, is available in periapical sizes and in 5 or 6 × 12 in. (13 or 15 × 30 cm) and 8 × 10 in. (20 × 26 cm) sheets.

Film Storage and Protection

All radiographic film is extremely sensitive to radiation, light, heat, humidity, chemical fumes, and physical pressure. Additionally, film is sensitive to aging; each film has a shelf life determined by the manufacturer. Precautions for safely storing and protecting films from these conditions must be followed. Film fogging is the darkening of the finished radiograph caused by one or more of these factors.

Radiation

Stray radiation, not intended for primary exposure, can fog film. Film should be stored in its original, lead-wrapped packaging in an area shielded from radiation. Individual film packets should also be kept in a shielded area. This is especially important while in the process of exposing several radiographs at one time, as is the case when exposing a set of bitewings or full mouth series on a patient. Once a film has been exposed to radiation, the crystals within the emulsion increase in their sensitivity. It should be placed in a shielded area while the next film is exposed. All exposed films should be kept safe from radiation until processing.

Light

Care should be taken when handling intraoral film packets so as not to tear the outer light-tight wrap. Extraoral cassettes must be closed tightly to prevent light leaks. Additionally, safe lighting in the darkroom must be periodically examined to ensure safe light conditions (see Chapter 17).

Heat and Humidity

To prevent fogging, film should be stored in a cool, dry place. Ideally, all unexposed film should be stored at 50°–70°F (10°–21°C) and 30–50 percent relative humidity.

Chemical Fumes

Additionally, film should be stored away from the possibility of chemical fumes contamination. Film should not be stored in the darkroom near processing chemicals.

Physical Pressure

Physical pressure and bending can fog film. When storing, boxes of film must not be stacked so high as to increase the pressure on the packets. Heavy objects should not be placed or stored on top of film.

Shelf Life

Dental x-ray film has a limited shelf life. The expiration date is printed on the film packaging (Figure 7–9). All intraoral film should be stored so that the expiration date can be readily seen and the appropriate films used first. Expired film compromises the diagnostic quality of the image and should not be used.

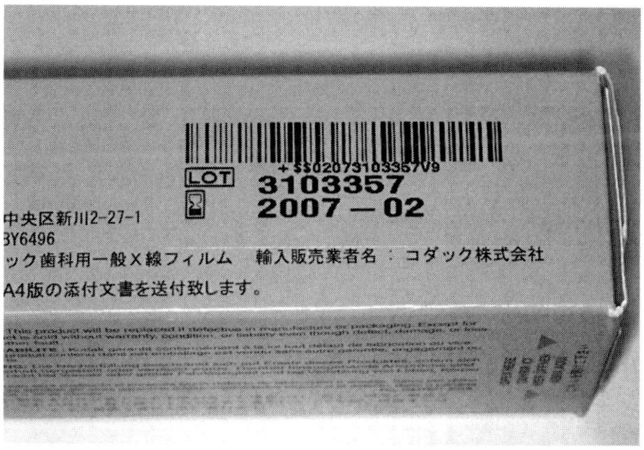

FIGURE 7–9 **Film package showing expiration date.**

REVIEW—Chapter Summary

X-ray film serves as a radiographic image receptor. The film used in dental radiography is photographic film that has been especially adapted in size, emulsion, film speed, and packaging for dental uses. All x-ray film has a polyester base that is coated with a gelatin emulsion containing silver halide (bromide and iodide) crystals.

During radiation exposure, the x-rays strike and ionize some of the silver halide crystals, forming a latent image. The image does not become visible until the film has undergone processing procedures.

An intraoral film packet consists of film, white-light tight black paper wrapping, lead foil, and a moisture-resistant outer wrapping.

Film speed (sensitivity) refers to the amount of radiation required to produce a radiograph of acceptable density. Film speed groups range from A (for the slowest) through F (for the fastest). Currently only D-, E-, and F-speed films are available for dental radiographs.

Intraoral films vary in size. Five sizes are available: #0, #1, #2, #3, and #4. There are three types of intraoral radiographic projections: bitewing, to image proximal tooth surfaces and alveolar bone crests; periapical, to examine the entire tooth and supporting structures; and occlusal, to survey larger areas of the maxilla and the mandible.

Extraoral films are designed for use outside the mouth and are much larger than intraoral films. Large extraoral films are classified as screen films because fluorescent light from intensifying screens is used to help the x-rays produce the image on the film. Extraoral films are used for lateral jaw exposures, cephalometric and panoramic radiographs.

Duplicating film is a special type of photographic film that is used to duplicate dental radiographs. The solarized emulsion is on one side only, and the non-emulsion side contains the antihalation coating.

All x-ray films are sensitive to radiation, light, heat, humidity, chemical fumes, physical pressure, and aging. Care must be exercised in storing and in handling the film before, during, and after exposure.

RECALL—Study Questions

1. Which of these provides support for the fragile film emulsion?
   a. Base
   b. Adhesive
   c. Silver halide crystals
   d. Protective coating
2. Which of these is light and x-ray sensitive?
   a. Lead foil
   b. Adhesive
   c. Gelatin
   d. Silver halide crystals
3. During x-ray exposure, crystals within the film emulsion become energized with a:
   a. Visible image.
   b. Slow image.
   c. Latent image.
   d. Intensified image.
4. What is the function of the lead foil in the x-ray packet?
   a. Moisture protection
   b. Absorb backscatter radiation
   c. Give rigidity to the packet
   d. Protect against fluorescence
5. All of the following can be found on the back side of an intraoral film packet *except* one. Which one is this *exception?*
   a. Film speed
   b. Film size
   c. Embossed dot location
   d. Number of films in packet
6. Which of these films has the greatest sensitivity to radiation?
   a. D-speed
   b. E-speed
   c. F-speed
7. A #4 intraoral film packet would most likely be used to expose a(n):
   a. Bitewing radiograph.
   b. Periapical radigraph.
   c. Occlusal radiograph.
   d. Pedodontic radiograph.
8. Which of these films will the dentist most likely prescribe for evaluation of a specific tooth and its surrounding structures?
   a. Bitewing radiograph
   b. Periapical radigraph
   c. Occlusal radiograph
   d. Panoramic radiograph
9. Intensifying screens will:
   a. Reduce exposure time.
   b. Decrease processing time.
   c. Increase x-ray intensity.
   d. Increase image detail.
10. Which of the following is considered to be a screen film?
    a. Occlusal
    b. Periapical
    c. Bitewing
    d. Panoramic
11. Which type of film is used to copy a radiograph?
    a. Duplicating film
    b. Screen film
    c. Non-screen film
    d. X-ray film
12. X-ray films should be stored:
    a. Away from heat and humidity.
    b. Near the source of radiation.
    c. In the darkroom.
    d. Stacked in columns.

REFLECT—Case Study

Utilize what you learned in this chapter about the sizes and types of projections to make a preliminary recommendation and/or to explain to the patient why the dentist has prescribed: (1) the type of projection; (2) the size of the film; and/or (3) the number of films to use for each of the following three cases.

1. An adult patient with suspected carious lesions on the proximal surfaces of posterior teeth. Additionally, this patient is considered to have a periodontal condition for which he is under maintenance treatment.
   a. The recommended type of projection will most likely be:
   b. The size of the film(s) will most likely be:
   c. The number of films to be exposed will most likely be:

2. An adult patient with a toothache in the area of the maxillary right molar.
   a. The recommended type of projection will most likely be:
   b. The size of film(s) will most likely be:
   c. The number of films to be exposed will most likely be:
3. An 8-year-old patient who, while skateboarding, seems to have suffered a traumatic injury to the anterior teeth.
   a. The recommended type of projection will most likely be:
   b. The size of film(s) will most likely be:
   c. The number of films to be exposed will most likely be:

RELATE—Laboratory Applicaton

Obtain one each of a size #0, size #1, size #2, size #3 and size #4 intraoral film packet. Beginning with the size #0 film packet, consider the following. Repeat with each of the film sizes. Write out your observations.

1. What is the film speed? How did you get the answer to this question?
2. What information is written on the outside of the film packet? Where is this information written: on the front or back of the film packet?
3. How many films do you expect to find inside this packet? How did you get the answer to this question?
4. Where is the embossed dot located? How did you find it? What is this used for?
5. What type of projection (bitewing, periapical, or occlusal) could be taken with this film size? Explain your answer.
6. What about this film packet's size makes it ideal; less than ideal; or not suited for the adult patient; child patient?
7. For what area(s) of the oral cavity will this film packet be best suited; not suited?
8. Now open the film packet. List the four parts of the packet and explain the purpose of each.
9. Next, hold the film up horizontal (parallel to the floor) at eye level and observe it from the edge. Can you see the film base with the emulsion coating on the top and the bottom?
10. Next, observe the metal foil. What is the reason for the embossed imprint?
11. When you opened the film packet, did you utilize the black paper's tab? The tab plays an important role in opening a contaminated film packet aseptically. This is discussed in detail in Chapter 9.

BIBLIOGRAPHY

Eastman Kodak. *Exposure and Processing for Dental Radiography.* Rochester, NY: Eastman Kodak, 1998.

8

Dental X-ray Film Processing

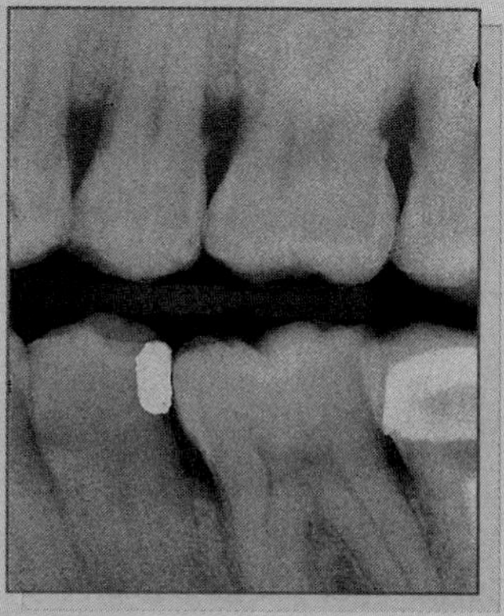

CHAPTER OUTLINE

■ OBJECTIVES

Following successful completion of this chapter, you should be able to:

1. Define the key words.
2. Explain how a latent image becomes a visible image.
3. List in sequence the steps in processing dental films.
4. List the four chemicals in the developer solution and explain the function of each ingredient.
5. List the four chemicals in the fixer solution and explain the function of each ingredient.
6. Discuss location, size and lighting as considerations for setting up a darkroom.
7. Discuss the five factors that affect safelighting.
8. Explain the role chemical replenishment and solution changes play in maintaining the darkroom.
9. List three radiographic wastes that are harmful to the environment.
10. Compare advantages and disadvantages of manual, automatic, and rapid film processing.
11. Identify the equipment needed for manual processing.
12. Demonstrate the step-by-step procedures for manual film processing.
13. Identify the parts of the automatic processing unit.
14. Demonstrate the step-by-step procedures for automatic film processing.
15. Identify when rapid film processing would be appropriate.

■ KEY WORDS

Acetic acid
Acidifier
Activator
Automatic processing unit
Chairside darkroom
Chairside processing
Darkroom
Daylight loader
Developer
Developing agent
Elon
Film feed slot
Film hanger
Film recovery slot
Fixer
Fixing agent
Halide
Hardening agent

Hydroquinone	Restrainer
Latent image	Reticulation
Light-tight	Roller transport system
Oxidation	Safelight
Potassium alum	Safelight filter
Potassium bromide	Selective reduction
Preservative	Sodium carbonate
Processing	Sodium sulfite
Processing tank	Sodium thiosulfate
Radiolucent	Time–temperature
Radiopaque	Viewbox
Rapid processing	Wet reading
Replenisher	Working radiograph

Introduction

Film **processing** is a series of steps that converts the invisible latent image on the dental x-ray film into a visible permanent image called a radiograph. The diagnostic quality of the visible image depends on strictly adhering to these processing steps. Film processing may be accomplished either manually or automatically. The purpose of this chapter is to explain the fundamentals of film processing; identify the roles processing solutions play in producing a visible image; and describe the need for proper chemical and film waste disposal. Because most processing is accomplished in a **darkroom** equipped with special lights, darkroom design and equipment will be described.

Overview of Film Processing

Processing transforms the **latent image** (latent means "hidden"), which is produced when the x-ray photons are absorbed by the silver **halide** crystals in the emulsion, into a visible, stable image by means of chemicals. The steps in manually (by hand) processing dental x-ray film are:

1. Developing
2. Rinsing
3. Fixing
4. Washing
5. Drying

Developing

The initial step in the processing sequence is the development of the film. The role of the **developer** solution is to reduce the exposed silver halide crystals within the film emulsion to black metallic silver. The unexposed silver halide crystals (in those areas of the film opposite metallic or dense structures that absorb and prevent the passage of x-rays) are unaffected at this time.

Rinsing

The purpose of the rinsing step is to remove as much of the alkaline developer as possible before placing the film in the fixer solution. Rinsing preserves the acidity of the fixer and prolongs its useful life.

Fixing

After brief rinsing, the film is immersed in the **fixer** solution. The role of the fixer solution is to remove the unexposed and/or undeveloped silver halide crystals from the film emulsion.

Washing

After the film is completely fixed, it is washed in running water to remove any remaining traces of the chemicals.

Drying

The final step is drying the film for storage as a part of the patient's permanent record. Films may be air-dried at room temperature or they may be dried in a heated cabinet especially made for this purpose.

The processed films are now called radiographs. The images on the radiograph are made up of microscopic grains of black metallic silver. The amount of silver deposited will vary with the thickness of the tissues penetrated. Soft tissues allow more radiation to reach the film emulsion, resulting in black areas on the film, while dense structures such as metal restorations will block the passage of x-rays, resulting in white areas on the film. As we saw in Chapter 4, the amount of light transmitted through the film varies according to the thickness of tissues penetrated by the radiation and accounts for the shades of black, gray, and white. Dark areas are referred to as **radiolucent** and light areas as **radiopaque.**

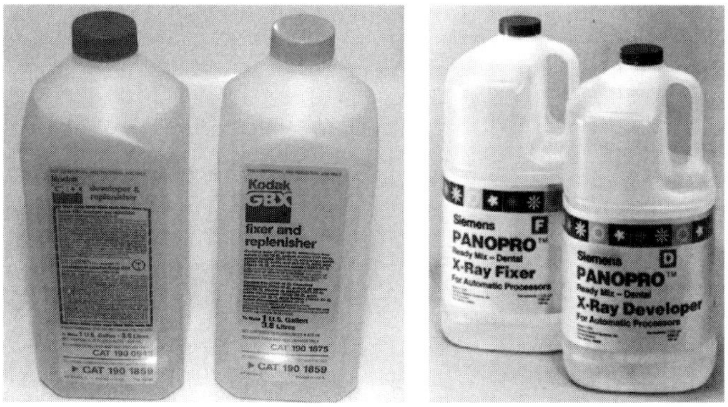

FIGURE 8–1 **Processing chemicals.** Liquid concentrate of developer and fixer for manual processing (*left*) and automatic processing (*right*). When mixed with distilled water, each bottle yields 1 gal (3.8 L) of solution, which is the normal capacity of an insert tank. (Courtesy of Siemens Medical Systems, Dental Division, Iselin, NJ)

Film Processing Solutions

Dental x-ray film processing requires the use of developer and fixer. These chemicals may be obtained in three forms:

- Powder
- Liquid concentrate
- Ready-to-use solutions

The powdered and liquid concentrate forms (Figure 8–1) must be mixed with water prior to using. Chemical manufacturers usually recommend the use of distilled water when mixing chemistry to avoid potential problems with other chemicals sometimes present in tap water.

Developer

The main purpose of the developer is to convert the exposed silver halide crystals into metallic silver grains.

There are four chemicals in the developer (Table 8–1):

1. Developing agents (also called reducing agents)
2. Preservative
3. Activator (also called alkalizer)
4. Restrainer

The **developing agent** reduces the exposed silver halide crystals to metallic silver but has no effect on the unexposed crystals at recommended time-temperatures. This is called **selective reduction,** meaning that only the non-metallic elements, the halides, are removed, and the exposed silver remains (Figure 8–2).

Developer contains two chemicals, **hydroquinone** and **elon.** The hydroquinone works slowly but steadily to build up density and contrast in the film. The elon works fast to bring out the gray shades (contrast) of the image. Both chemicals are affected by extreme temperatures. The higher the temperature, the less time required to develop the film; therefore, regulating the temperature of the developer is critical.

The **preservative, sodium sulfite,** protects the developing agents by slowing down the rapid oxidation rate of the developer.

The **activator,** usually **sodium carbonate,** provides the necessary alkaline medium required by the developing agents. It also softens and swells the gelatin, allowing more of the exposed silver halide crystals to come into contact with the developing agents.

The **restrainer, potassium bromide,** restrains the developing agents from developing the unexposed silver halide crystals and therefore inhibits the tendency of the solution chemically to fog the film.

Fixer

The fixer plays three roles: (1) stops further film development—thereby establishing the image permanently on the film; (2) removes (dissolves) the unexposed/undeveloped silver halide crystals (those that were not exposed to x-rays), and (3) hardens (fixes) the emulsion.

TABLE 8–1 **Composition of Developer**

Ingredient	Chemical	Action
Developing agents (reducing agents)	Hydroquinone	Reduces (converts) exposed silver halide crystals to black metallic silver. Slowly builds up black tones and contrast.
	Elon	Reduces (converts) exposed silver halide crystals to black metallic silver. Quickly builds up gray tones.
Preservative	Sodium sulfite	Prevents rapid oxidation of the developing agents.
Activator	Sodium carbonate	Activates developing agents by providing required alkalinity.
Restrainer	Potassium bromide	Restrains the developing agents from developing the unexposed silver halide crystals, which produce film fog.

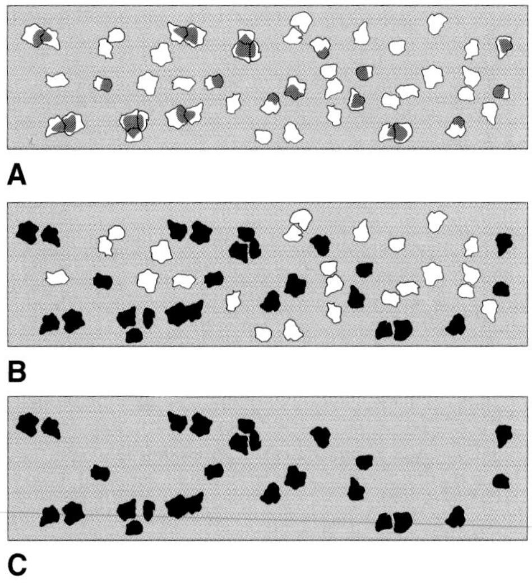

FIGURE 8–2 **Cross section of dental x-ray film emulsion.** (**A**) X-rays strike silver haldide crystals, forming latent image sites (shown in gray). (**B**) After development, crystals struck by x-rays (latent image sites) reduced to black metallic silver. (**C**) Fixer removes unexposed, undeveloped crystals, leaving the black metallic silver.

There are four chemicals in the fixer (Table 8–2):

1. Fixing agent (also called a clearing agent)
2. Preservative
3. Hardening agent
4. Acidifier

The **fixing** (clearing) **agent,** ammonium thiosulfate or **sodium thiosulfate,** also known as "hypo" or hyposulfate of sodium, removes all unexposed and any remaining undeveloped silver halide crystals from the emulsion.

The preservative, sodium sulfite (the same chemical as used in the developer), slows the rate of oxidation and prevents the deterioration of the hypo and the precipitation of sulfur.

The **hardening agent, potassium alum,** shrinks and hardens the gelatin emulsion. This hardening continues until the film is dry, thus protecting it from abrasion.

The **acidifier, acetic acid,** provides the acid medium to stop further development by neutralizing the alkali of the developer.

Hardening Agents

Depending on whether the chemicals are intended for use in manual, automatic, or rapid processors, special hardening agents are sometimes added to facilitate the transportation of the films through the roller systems of the automatic units.

Replenisher

Replenisher is a superconcentrated solution of developer or fixer. It is added to the developer or fixer in the processing tank to compensate for the loss of volume and strength from oxidation. Processing solutions lose their potency over time and with use. Adding replenisher helps to maintain solution strength.

Darkroom

The purpose of the **darkroom** is to provide an area where x-ray films can be safely handled and processed. A well equipped room with adequate safelighting aids in producing high quality radiographic images. Films can be processed outside the darkroom with **chairside** manual **processing** units (Figure 8–3) or **daylight loader**–equipped automatic processors (Figure 8–4). A darkroom remains the standard in most film-based practices, especially since safelight conditions are required to handle extraoral film cassette loading and processing. The darkroom should be located near the area where radiographs will be exposed and should be large enough to meet the requirements of the practice. The darkroom should be equipped with correct lighting, be well ventilated, and have adequate storage space for radiographic supplies.

The ability to store radiographic supplies such as extraoral film cassettes, duplicating film, and processing chemicals and cleaning supplies in the darkroom will add to the convenience of maintaining the ideal darkroom. Although storing unused film in the darkroom may seem convenient, it is not recommended. In addition to being sensitive to radiation and white light exposure, unexposed film is sensitive to heat, humidity and chemical fumes, all of which may be increased in the darkroom.

TABLE 8–2 Composition of Fixer

Ingredient	Chemical	Action
Fixing agent (clearing agent)	Ammonium thiosulfate or sodium thiosulfate	Removes the unexposed and any remaining undeveloped silver halide crystals.
Preservative	Sodium sulfite	Slows the rate of oxidation and prevents deterioration of the fixing agent.
Hardening agent	Potassium alum	Shrinks and hardens the gelatin emulsion.
Acidifier	Acetic acid	Stops further development by neutralizing the alkali of the developer.

Lighting

X-ray film is sensitive to white light. Any white light in the darkroom can blacken the film or cause film fog. Therefore, the darkroom must be **light-tight.** A light-tight room is one that is completely dark and excludes all light. Felt strips may have to be installed around the door(s) to the darkroom or any other area where a light leak is discovered. Although many darkrooms are painted black, this is not necessary. When completely sealed to white light, a lighter colored paint on the walls will reflect more usable safelight than black paint. The following forms of illumination are desirable in the darkroom.

1. **White ceiling light.** An overhead white ceiling light that provides adequate illumination for the size of the room will allow the clinician to perform equipment maintenance and other tasks requiring visibility. Fluorescent overhead lighting should not be used because of its tendency for afterglow that might contribute to film fog.
2. **Safelight.** Safelighting is achieved through the use of a special LED (light emitting diode) bulb or a filtered white light bulb that provides enough light in the darkroom to allow the clinician to perform activities without exposing or fogging the film.

   Recently new technology has made available LED bulbs safe for darkroom use. Traditional safelights consist of a 7 1/2 or 15 watt white incandescent light bulb with a **safelight filter** placed over it. The safelight filter removes the short wavelengths in the blue-green region of the visible light spectrum. The longer wavelength red-orange light is allowed to pass through the filter illuminating the darkroom. A variety of safelights with different types of filters are available. Some are designed to work best with intraoral films, others with extraoral films, and others are universal and can be used for both (Figure 8–5). The type of safelight required for film processing can usually be found written on the film package.

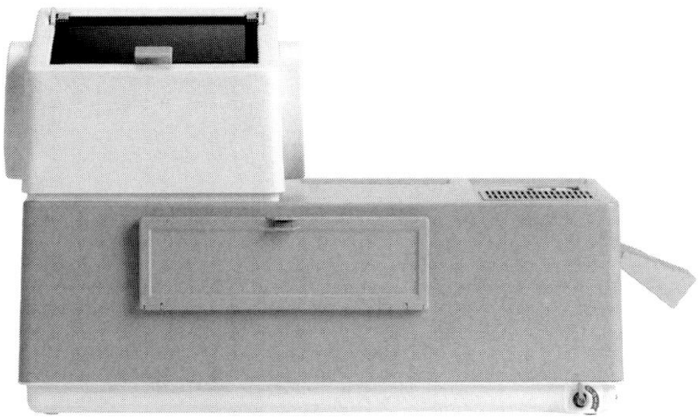

FIGURE 8-4 **Automatic processor with daylight loader attachment for use outside the darkroom.** (Courtesy of Air Techniques, Inc.)

   The term "safe" light is relative. Film emulsion can be damaged by prolonged exposure even to filtered safelight. Film handling should be limited to 2 1/2 minutes under safelight conditions or fogging (film darkening) may occur. Additionally, the distance between the lamp and the film is critical. The rule is 2 1/4 watts per ft (0.3 m) and a 4-ft (1.2 m) minimum distance from the source of light and the counter space where the film will be handled. A summary of the factors to be considered for safelighting are listed in Table 8–3.
3. **Viewbox.** A **viewbox** or illuminator is a light source (generally a lamp behind an opaque glass) used for viewing radiographs. A darkroom equipped with a wall-mounted or counter-top viewbox or illuminator will allow the clinician the opportunity for a quick reading, viewing the radiograph without leaving the darkroom. A viewbox emits considerable white light, and care must be taken not to turn it on when film packets are unwrapped. Additionally, if films are undergoing the developing process in a manual processor,

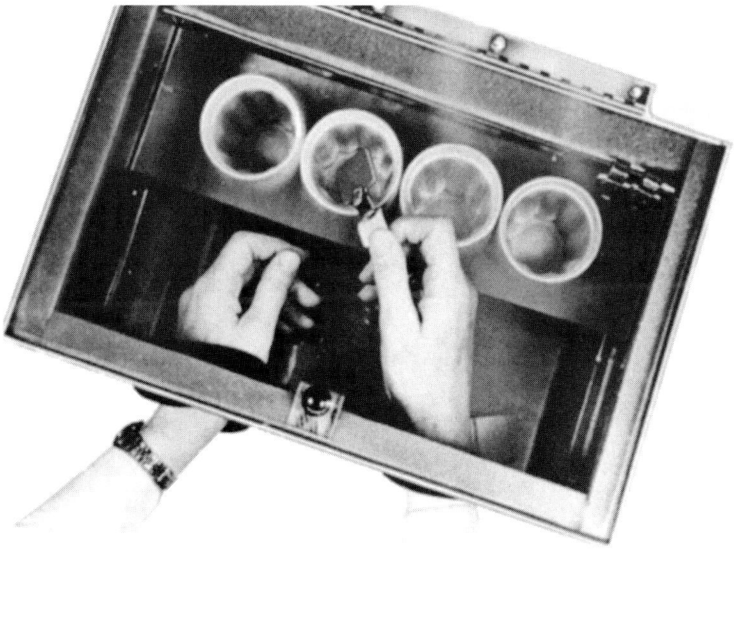

FIGURE 8-3 **Chair-side darkroom unit shown with view through plastic filtered top.** First cup is filled with developer, second cup with rinse water, third cup with fixer, and fourth cup with wash water. A heater with a thermostat keeps the solutions at optimum temperature for rapid processing. (Courtesy of Densply Rinn)

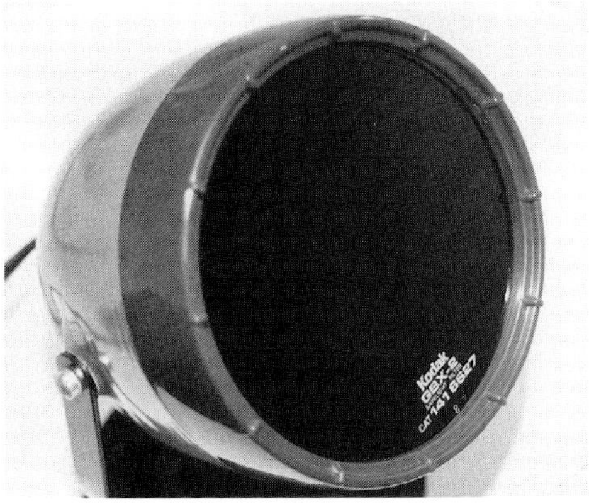

FIGURE 8-5 **Safelight.** A commercially available bracket-type lamp with safelight filter shielding the short wavelength, blue-green region of the visible light spectrum given off by the bulb. The light given off by this filter would appear dark red.

the manual processor tank cover must remain on during the use of a view box.

4. **In-use Light.** The darkroom door should be locked when processing films to prevent anyone from entering and inadvertently allowing white light into the darkroom. Some darkrooms are equipped with a warning light outside the darkroom, which indicates that it is not safe to open the door.

Maintenance

Cleanliness and orderliness are essential for the production of quality radiographs and the safety and health of the clinician using the area. Infection control protocol for opening film packets (Chapter 9) must be strictly adhered to. Because safelight conditions reduce visibility, the clinician must be skilled in the procedures to be performed. Needed materials should be within easy reach, and the person doing the processing should be familiar with where each item is located. The workspace counter must be free of substances that can contaminate films such as water, chemicals, and dust.

TABLE 8-3 Safelight considerations
• 7 1/2 or 15 watt white incandescent bulb.
• Darker red filters provide safer conditions for both intra and extraoral film handling than amber or yellow colored filters.
• Condition of the filter. Scratched or cracked filters allow white light to escape.
• 4 ft (1.2 m) minimum distance between lamp and counter surface where film is to be handled.
• Films should not be subjected to safelight exposure over a 2 1/2 minutes.

A utility sink large enough to accommodate cleaning the processing equipment should be available in the darkroom. A wastebasket should be placed in the darkroom for the disposal of general waste items. Lead foil is separated from other film wrappings and placed in an appropriate container for safe disposal, and the remainder of the film packet placed in a biohazard container for disposal.

Processing Chemical Maintenance

Both manual and automatic processing require chemical maintenance and solution replenishing and changing. A small amount of developer is lost daily through evaporation. Additional loss occurs when chemicals adhere to the film surfaces during transfer from solution to solution. Transfer of films between solutions slowly contaminates the chemicals and weakens them. All chemistry must be changed periodically to avoid diminishing quality. The useful life of the solutions is determined by:

- The original quality or concentration of the solution.
- The freshness of the solution.
- The number of films that are processed.
- Contamination of the chemicals.

Many chemical manufacturers recommend that processing solutions be changed at least every four weeks under "normal" use. Since normal use may be defined differently among different practices, one must refer to the manufacturer recommendations to determine reasonable intervals to change solutions. One way to maintain solution strength in between changes is through replenishment. Protective eyewear, mask, utility gloves, and a plastic or rubber apron should be worn when cleaning the processing tanks or changing the solutions.

Disposal of Radiographic Wastes

Disposal of biohazard wastes generated by the oral health care practice is often mandated by law. Equally important is the ethical responsibility to recycle or properly dispose of wastes that may be harmful to the environment. In many areas, it is against the law to discard used fixer into the municipal sewer system or to discard lead foil at municipal landfills. It is equally important to note that some state and local waste management regulations are more stringent than federal regulations. The radiographer must know what laws apply in the practice area.

Radiographic wastes that have the potential to harm the environment include used fixer chemicals, which contain silver halides removed from the film during processing; lead foil from inside intraoral film packets; and discarded radiographs, which contain silver in the emulsion. While the amount of these hazardous materials generated by a single oral health care practice is small, collectively, many practices generating these wastes begin to increase to a significant level. Therefore, alternative methods of discarding these materials should be sought.

The most common way to dispose of these hazardous materials appropriately is to contract with a waste disposal company

(Figure 8–6). Many practices already employ a waste management company to dispose of biohazard materials.

To manage used fixer waste, another method of disposal is the use of a silver recovery unit. Used fixer may be circulated through the silver recovery unit, which removes the hazardous silver ions from the used fixer before allowing the solution to go down the drain. Once the cartridge inside the silver recovery unit is saturated with silver ions, it can be removed by a commercial waste disposal company and replaced with a fresh cartridge.

Lead foil from inside intraoral film packets is sometimes collected for the purpose of recycling. However, it is important that the qualifications of the recycling agency used by the practice be investigated. If materials are disposed of inappropriately by the recycling company, it is possible that the oral health care practice would be partly liable for fines and costs incurred by faulty handling of materials by the disposal service.

Manual Film Processing

Manual processing is a method used to process films by hand in a series of steps, and requires the use of a processing tank. One of the advantages of manual film processing is that it is reliable and not subject to equipment malfunction. Additionally, the clinician has more control over the processing procedure, including the ability to adjust the time–temperature and the ability to read the radiographs prior to the end of the processing procedure (wet reading). The biggest disadvantage of manual processing is the time required to produce a finished radiograph.

Equipment

Manual processing requires the use of:

- Processing tank.
- Thermometer.
- Timer.
- Stirring paddles.
- Film hangers, drying racks, and drip pans

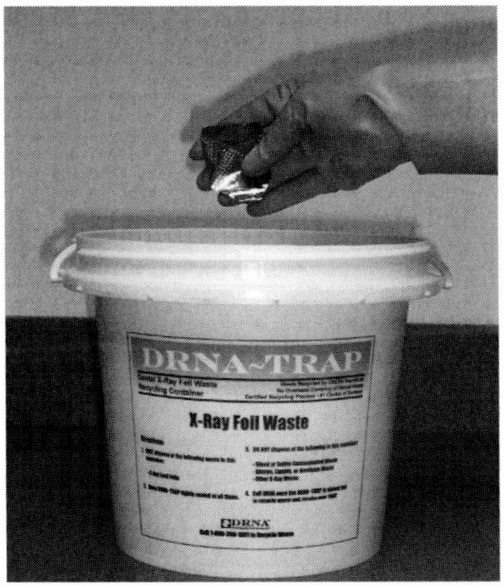

FIGURE 8–6 **Lead foil waste.** Radiographer collects lead foil waste for proper disposal.

1. **Processing tank.** A **processing tank** is a receptacle divided into compartments (for developer solution, rinse and wash water, and fixer solution) used to process radiographs. The processing tank has two insert tanks placed inside the master tank (Figure 8–7). The insert tanks hold the developer and fixer solutions. Usually, the left insert tank holds the developer solution, and the right insert tank contains the fixer solution. However, these tanks should be labeled to prevent confusion as to which tank contains which chemical. The area between the insert tanks holds water for rinsing and washing the films.

   Most tanks are made of stainless steel, which does not react with processing chemicals. Insert tanks are large enough to accept an 8 × 10 in. (20 × 26 cm) extraoral film. The capacity of an insert tank is 1 gallon (3.8 L).

   The insert tanks are removable to facilitate cleaning. A small hole at the bottom of the insert tank lets the solution drain into the master tank when a small rubber plug is pulled out. The master tank is connected to the water intake and to the drain. When in use, fresh water circulates constantly. An overflow pipe keeps the level of the water constant when the tank is full. Some tanks are equipped with a temperature control device, a water-mixing valve that mixes the hot and cold water in the pipes to any desired temperature. A close-fitting lightproof cover completes the tank assembly (Figure 8–8).
2. **Thermometer.** A thermometer is necessary to determine the temperature of the developing solution for time–tem-

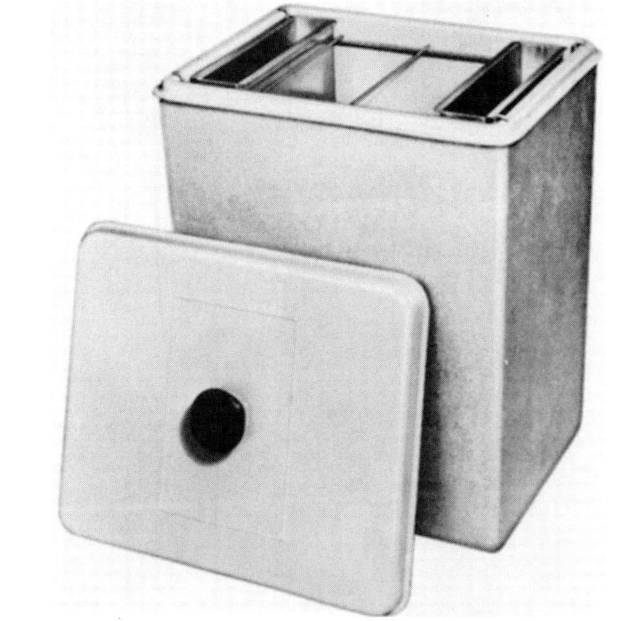

FIGURE 8–7 **Processing tank with removable inserts.** The central compartment holds the rinse/wash water. Usually, the insert on the left is filled with the developer solution, and the insert on the right is filled with the fixer solution.

perature manual processing. Both clip type and floating thermometers are available. Floating thermometers are preferred because they can be left floating in the developing tank and easily picked up for reading (Figure 8–9). Thermometers clipped to the side of the developing tank are more difficult to read.

3. **Timer.** An accurate interval timer is necessary for time–temperature manual processing. The timer is used to indicate how long the film is placed in the developing solution, the fixing solution, and the wash water. The timer must have an audible alarm to alert the radiographer to remove the films from each of the solutions.
4. **Stirring paddles.** Two stirring paddles, or rods, must be available for mixing and stirring the chemicals used for manual processing. To avoid contamination, the developer and the fixer each need their own stirring paddle. The paddles should be made of stainless steel or other material that will not corrode in the processing chemicals.
5. **Film hangers, drying racks, and drip pans.** A **film hanger** is a stainless steel frame to which the films can be attached. A film hanger allows the radiographer to transport the films to and from each of the processing solutions (Figure 8–10). Film hangers have an identification tag near the curved handle on which the patient's name can be written. Various film hanger sizes are available, holding up to 20 films. Films can be dried with a commercial film dryer that circulates warm air around the films. Film dryers are not as readily available commercially as they were when manual processing was the norm. Instead, drying racks (towel racks) can be mounted for hanging film hangers to air dry the films. Drip pans are

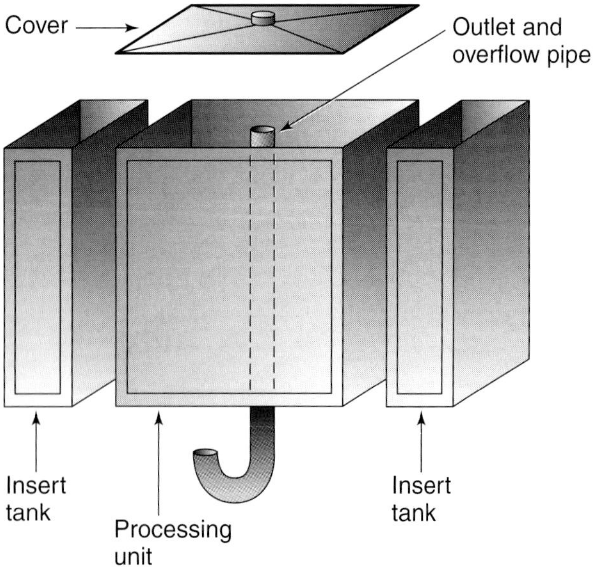

FIGURE 8–8 **Drawing showing the processing tank assembly.**

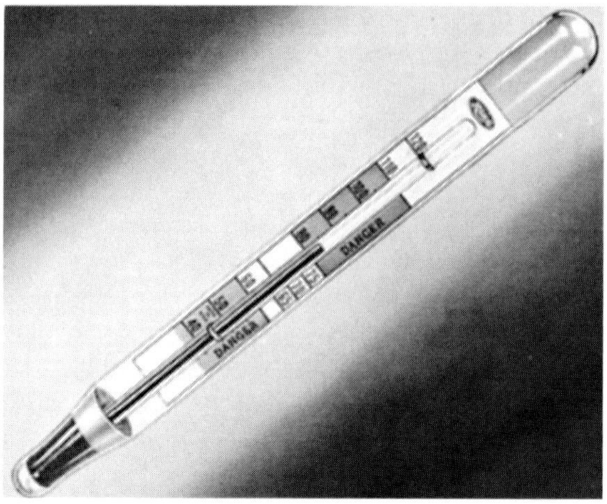

FIGURE 8–9 **Floating thermometer** for use in the developer insert. The ideal temperature for manually processing films is 68°F (20°C). (Courtesy of Dentsply Rinn)

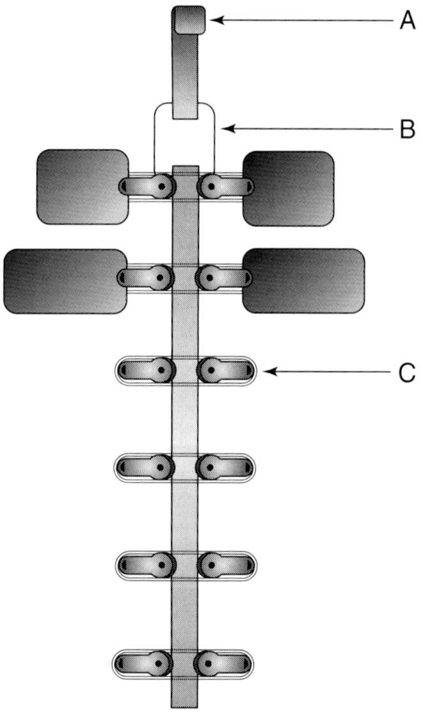

FIGURE 8–10 **Intraoral film hanger with 12 clips.** Various hangers ranging in capacity from a single film to 16 films are available. (**A**) Curved portion at the top of the hanger rests on upper rim of tank insert when films are immersed. (**B**) White plastic identification tag on which the patient's name can be written in pencil and later erased. (**C**) Clamps with three-point positive grip hold the firm securely in place. (Courtesy of Densply Rinn)

placed underneath the drying racks to catch water from wet films. To reduce drying time, an electric fan can be placed to blow air on the drying racks. A fan may also help to ventilate the darkroom air.

Maintenance

Oxidation makes manual processing maintenance especially important. **Oxidation** is the union of a substance—in this case, the developer—with the oxygen in the air. The developer is especially subject to oxidation in the presence of air and loses some of its effectiveness. Whenever possible, the processing tank should remain covered to prevent the possibility of oxidation and evaporation. The cover should be removed only when adding solutions to the proper level, when checking the temperature of the developer, and when inserting, removing, or changing the film hangers from one compartment or insert to another. The cover should be replaced immediately after any of these steps is completed.

Chemical contamination is the mixing of the alkali developer with the acidic fixer, an ever-present threat in film processing. Stirring paddles, thermometers, and film hangers must be cleaned after each use. Never use the same stirring paddle in both the developer and fixer without first cleaning it thoroughly. If the paddles are made of wood, separate ones must be used for each solution to prevent cross-contamination. Film hangers must be thoroughly rinsed to prevent chemicals from sticking to the clips for attaching the film. Make sure that the part of the tank cover over the developer is always placed there. Care must be taken not to rotate the cover when it is removed, causing a drop or two of condensed developer to fall into the fixer, or vice versa. The operator can minimize this threat by labeling the inserts and the cover.

The life of the processing solutions can be extended by replenishment. Replenishment consists of removing a small amount of developer and fixer and replacing with fresh chemistry, or chemical replenisher specifically made for this purpose. Based on a typical practice usage of processing 30 intraoral films per day, it is recommended that 6 to 8 ounces of developer and fixer be removed and discarded. Fresh chemicals should be added to raise the solution levels in the insert tanks to the full level. Manual processing solutions should be changed at least every 4 weeks regardless of usage, or as recommended by the chemical manufacturer.

The manual processing tank and its inserts should be scrubbed each time the solutions are changed. A solution made up of 1.5 oz (45 mL) of commercial hydrochloric acid, 1 qt (0.95 L) of cold water, and 3 qt (2.85 L) of warm water is sufficient to remove the deposits that frequently form on the walls of 1 gal (3.8 L) inserts. Commercial solutions for cleaning are also available. Cleansing powders should never be used, as they will leave a residue that contaminates the processing chemicals. If the inserts appear to be coated, fill them with acid-cleaning solution and let them soak for 30 minutes; then drain out the cleaning solution and rinse with plenty of water. All parts of the tank, including the cover, should be wiped clean before the plugs are replaced and the inserts filled.

Preparation

The key to manually processing dental radiographs is adequate preparation.

1. **Check the levels of the solution** to be sure the developer and fixer will cover the top clips of the film hanger. The tanks are full when the solution levels are about one inch from the top. Add fresh solution if necessary.
2. **Stir the developer and fixer** thoroughly to prevent the heavier chemicals from settling to the bottom and to equalize the temperature of the solution.
3. **Determine the temperature of the developing solution.** A floating thermometer should be kept in the developer tank for frequent temperature reading. The temperature of the developer should be read after stirring.

   When developing dental x-ray film, a **time–temperature** development chart (Table 8–4) must be used. The ideal (optimum) temperature for manual processing is 68°F (20°C) with a development time of five minutes. Temperature variations from the ideal of 68°F (20°C) are acceptable as long as the developing time is correspondingly adjusted. Lower temperatures make the chemical reaction sluggish, and higher temperatures increase film fog.

   The water should be allowed to circulate in the tank long enough before the films are processed to evenly adjust the temperature in all three compartments of the tank. Failure to do so may cause **reticulation**—a cracking of the film emulsion, producing a netlike pattern. Reticulation results when the film is removed from a warm solution (where the gelatin softens) and placed in a cold solution (cracking the gelatin).
4. **Select the proper film hanger** and examine the clips to ensure that they are in proper working order. Loose clips may cause films to be lost at the bottom of an insert tank. Extraoral film hangers have channels into which the film fits and is secured by a hinged retaining channel over the open end of the hanger.

TABLE 8–4 **Time–Temperature Chart**

Temperature		Development Time (min)
60°F (15.5°C)		9
65°F (18.3°C)		7
68°F (20°C)	**optimum**	**5**
70°F (21.1°C)		4.5
75°F (23.9°C)		4
80°F (26.7°C)		3

Procedure (Procedure Box 8–1)

The manual film processing sequence consists of five steps: developing, rinsing, fixing, washing, and drying.

1. **Developing.** The film hanger with the attached films should be immersed into the developer tank first. Gently agitating the hanger up and down a few times—taking care not to splash—will keep air bubbles from clinging to the film. Air bubbles prevent the developer from contacting all areas of the film. Safelight conditions must be maintained throughout the development step unless the light-tight cover is in place on the processing tank.
2. **Rinsing.** The purpose of the rinsing step is to remove as much of the alkaline developer as possible before placing the film into the fixer. When the timed developing step is complete, under safelight conditions, the film hanger should be lifted above the developing insert tank and allowed to drain a few seconds to minimize the amount of developer that will be removed from the tank. After gently agitating the film hanger in the rinse water, it should be held above the rinse water to drain for a few seconds to prevent diluting the fixer solution with excess water.
3. **Fixing.** The film hanger with the attached films should be immersed into the fixer insert tank next, gently agitating the hanger to keep air bubbles from clinging to the film. Safelight conditions must be maintained for the first two or three minutes of the recommended 10-minute fixing time. If the radiograph is needed immediately for a quick reading of the x-ray image, the film may be read under white light conditions after two or three minutes of fixing. This is called a **wet reading.** The film can be rinsed in water for a short interval and viewed on a viewbox. The film must be returned to the fixer as soon as possible to complete fixation and permit further shrinking of the emulsion. If this is not done, some of the unexposed silver halide grains may be left on the film, giving it a fogged and discolored appearance. Also, the emulsion may not completely harden.

   The recommended fixing time is 10 minutes. The fixing time is not as critical as the developing time, so films may remain in the fixer slightly longer. When the fixing time is too short, the result can be slow drying, poor hardening of the emulsion, a possible partial loss of detail, and the radiograph's darkening over time. When the fixing time is excessively long, the image will lighten.
4. **Washing.** Washing the film removes all chemicals left on the radiograph. When the fixing step is complete, the film hanger should be lifted above the fixer insert tank and allowed to drain a few seconds to minimize the amount of fixer that will be removed from the tank. The films should be placed in the circulating water for 20 minutes. Leaving the films in the water wash longer than 20 minutes is permissible, but leaving a film in water more than a few hours will begin to dissolve the emulsion. The processing tank cover should remain in place during the washing step; however, it is not necessary to maintain safelight conditions during this step.
5. **Drying.** Following the wash step, the film hanger should be lifted above the water tank and allowed to drain. Excess water may be removed by gently shaking the film hanger over the water tank. Films may be dried by one of the following methods.
   - Suspend the hanger from a drying rack. Take care that the film does not contact other films on adjacent racks or brush up against the wall.
   - Use a fan or blower to expedite the drying process.
   - Place the hanger in a commercial heated drying cabinet.

Following the Procedure

The steps taken to secure the darkroom are equally important to the preparation steps.

1. Check to see that none of the films have loosened from the clips and dropped on the floor or the bottom of the tank.
2. Clean the work area. Wipe up any moisture caused by dripping or accidental splashing of the water or chemical solutions. Use an EPA high-level disinfectant where necessary (see Chapter 9).
3. Remove the dry films from the hangers and place them in properly identified protective envelopes or on film mounts with identifying data (film mounting techniques are discussed in Chapter 18).
4. Remove or erase identification markings from the hangers. Clean, dry, and replace hangers, and any equipment used.

At the end of the working day, turn off the water to the tank, drain the water compartment, and turn off all lights in the darkroom.

Automatic Film Processing

Automatic processing is a simple method of processing dental x-ray film. Because of its ability to produce a large volume of radiographs in less time (usually five minutes from developer to dried finished radiograph), it is often preferred over manual processing. Another advantage of automatic processing is the unit's ability to regulate automatically the temperature of the processing solutions and the time of the development process. Automatic processing has several disadvantages, however, including initial unit expense, possible equipment malfunction, increased maintenance required for optimal output, and the fact that chemical depletion occurs more rapidly than with manual processing chemistry.

Equipment

Automatic processing requires the use of an automatic processor unit, which vary in size and complexity (Figures 8–4 and 8–11). Some have a limited capacity and process only intraoral or cer-

PROCEDURE 8–1

MANUAL FILM PROCESSING

1. Maintain infection control (see Chapter 9).
2. Select a film hanger and label with patient information.
3. Open the light-tight cover of the manual processing tank
4. Stir the developer and fixer solutions to ensure even concentration throughout the tank. (Use a different stirring paddle for each, developer and fixer, to prevent contamination of solutions.)
5. Check the developer temperature.
6. Refer to the time–temperature recommendations of the solution manufacturer and set timer. (Optimal time–temperature for manually processed radiographs is 68°F for five minutes.)
7. Lock the darkroom door, turn off the white light and turn on the safelight.
8. Open the film packets (see Procedure Box 9–5) and place films on hanger.
9. Immerse the films into the developer solution and agitate film hanger for five seconds to release trapped air bubbles.
10. Set the timer. (Time is dependent on temperature of the developer solution.)
11. Close the light-tight cover while the film is developing.
12. When the developing time is complete, under safelight conditions, open the light-tight cover and remove film hanger with films attached from developer solution.
13. Pause a few seconds over the developer tank to allow the excess solution to drain from the films.
14. Immerse the film hanger into the water rinse and agitate for 30 seconds.
15. Pause a few seconds over the water tank to allow the excess water to drain from the films.
16. Immerse the film hanger into the fixer solution and agitate for five seconds to release trapped air bubbles.
17. Activate the timer for 10 minutes.
18. Close the light-tight cover for the first three minutes of fixation. (It is safe to view the films under white light after two or three minutes of fixation for a wet reading, following which the films must be returned to the fixer solution for completion of the 10 minutes fixation time for archival quality.)
19. Remove the film hanger from the fixer solution when the time is up.
20. Pause a few seconds over the fixer tank to allow the excess solution to drain from the films.
21. Immerse the films into the water wash for 20 minutes.
22. Remove the film hanger from the water wash when the time is up.
23. Place the film hanger in a commercially made film dryer or hang to air dry when the wash is complete.
24. Mount and label the dried films.

tain sizes of extraoral films; others can handle any dental film regardless of size. Most are intended for use in the darkroom under safelight conditions. Automatic processors equipped with daylight loaders have a light-tight baffle for inserting the hands while unwrapping the film and can be used under normal white light conditions (Figure 8–4).

The automatic processor uses a roller transport system to move the film through the processing cycle. The typical automatic processor consists of three compartments: developing, fixing and water, and a drying chamber (Figure 8–12).

Unwrapped film is fed into the **film feed slot** on the outside of the processor. The **roller transport system** moves the film through the developer, fixer, water, and drying compartments. Motor-driven gears or belts propel the roller transport system. The film emerges from the processor through an opening on the outside of the processor called the **film recovery slot.**

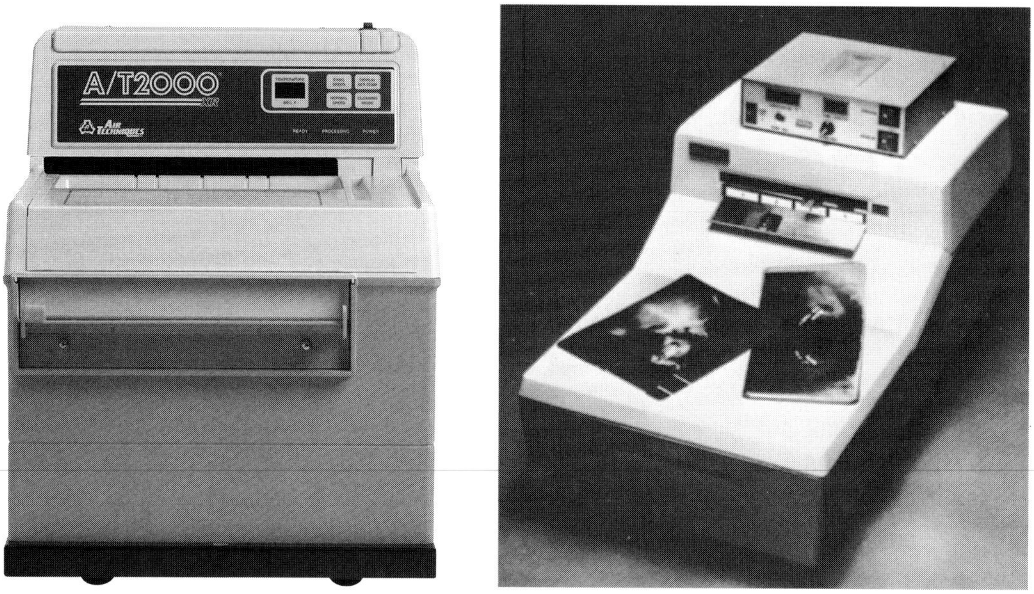

A B

FIGURE 8-11 **Automatic processors.** (**A**) Courtesy of Air Techniques, Inc.; (**B**) Courtesy of Philips Dental Systems.

All automatic processors require water. Some can be connected to existing plumbing, whereas other units have self-contained water. A heating unit warms the processing chemicals to the required temperature. As a rule, a 20-minute warming-up period is required before the unit is operational. Most units process a film in approximately five minutes. Some automatic processors have a two-minute setting for producing working radiographs for a quick reading.

Maintenance

The processing chemicals used in automatic processors differ from those used in manual procedures. Solutions are supersaturated and contain more hardener in the developer. The chemical solutions in automatic processors are heated to temperatures much higher than those used in manual processing—as high as 125°F (52°C) in some units. Fortunately, advanced film technology has produced film emulsions that can withstand these temperatures for the short times required in automated processing without excessive softening or melting. A recirculation system keeps the solutions agitated and distributed evenly in the compartments. Some units automatically replenish the solutions; others depend on the operator to keep them at the correct level.

Automatic processors require strict adherence to manufacturer's instructions for chemical replenishment and changes, and for cleaning the unit to maintain optimal performance. Few pieces of equipment in the oral health care practice require such diligence and regular care.

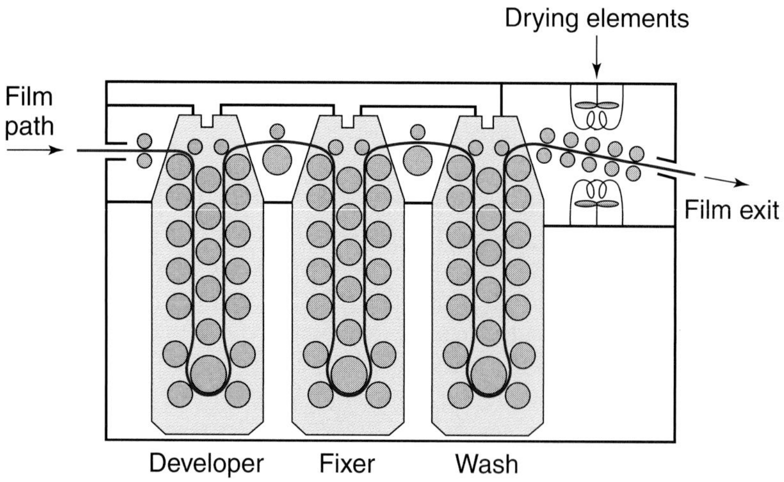

FIGURE 8-12 **Schematic illustration of automatic film processor.** Film is transported by roller assemblies through each of the processing steps.

Practice Point

In addition to being less effective, a breakdown in the integrity of the processing chemicals will occur if chemicals are not replenished or changed at the recommended intervals. This breakdown causes the solutions to become slick. Slick solutions cause the films to slide or slip through the rollers, making it difficult for the roller transports to advance the film through the processor, resulting in films that become stuck in the rollers.

Depending upon the workload, automatic processors require daily, weekly, or monthly cleaning. A specially made cleaning film may be run through the processor to remove any dirt and residual gelatin from the rollers daily. However, complete cleaning and maintenance of the roller transports and solution-holding tanks is also required. If the rollers are not kept clean, the radiographs emerge streaked. Most manufacturers recommend that the roller assembly be removed and cleaned weekly, in warm, running water and special cleansers. It is important to follow the manufacturer's instructions concerning care and maintenance.

Preparation

The automatic processor should be turned on and allowed to warm up according to the manufacturer's recommendations. Ensure that the water supply to the unit is also turned on. Chemicals should be replenished or changed as necessary. A special cleaning film designed to remove debris from the unit rollers should be run at the beginning of the day.

Procedure (Procedure Box 8–2)

The automatic film processing sequence usually consists of only four steps: developing, fixing, washing, and drying. The use of roller transports help "squeeze" excess solution from the film surface, allowing the automatic processor to omit the rinsing step between developing and fixing. Unless the automatic processor is equipped with daylight loader baffles, the processing procedure should begin under safelight conditions. Once unwrapped, the film is placed into the designated feed slot on the processor. Once the film is completely inside the automatic processing unit, safelighting is no longer necessary.

When processing multiple films, each should be placed into alternating feed slots, one at a time, to prevent the films from overlapping and getting stuck in the unit. Five to ten seconds should elapse between the insertion of each film. Inserting the films too rapidly after each other will also result in overlapping films.

When more than one operator uses the processor, or when processing more than one patient's films, a method of labeling the feed slots for film identification is necessary. Depending on the unit, the films will exit the processor in about five minutes, ready for mounting.

Following the Procedure

1. Check to see that all of the films have exited the processor.
2. Unless equipped with an automatic shutoff, the unit should be turned off or placed in stand-by mode to conserve water that would continue to run after the films have finished processing.
3. At the end of the working day, the main power and water supply to the unit should be turned off.

PROCEDURE 8–2

AUTOMATIC FILM PROCESSING

1. Maintain infection control (see Chapter 9).
2. Turn on the automatic processing unit.
3. Set the appropriate time/temperature as indicated by the unit.
4. Lock the darkroom door, turn off the white light and turn on the safelight.
5. Open the film packets (see Procedure Box 9–5) and place films into the automatic processor feed slot.
6. Allow the rollers to take the film before releasing.
7. Wait 10 seconds before placing an additional film into the same slot to avoid overlapping films.
8. Retrieve the processed films when the cycle is complete, usually about five minutes.
9. Mount and label the dried radiographs.

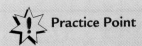

Rapid Processing (Chairside Processing) Procedure

A wet reading, which can be done during manual processing, is one way to obtain a diagnostic radiograph in minimal time. It is also possible to process intraoral films without a darkroom in about 30 seconds with the use of special, faster acting chemicals and a compact **chair-side darkroom** (Figure 8–3). **Rapid processing** is valuable in endodontic and oral surgery practices. A significant amount of chair time can be saved when it is necessary to expose a series of single films to check the progress in opening and cleaning out a root canal during endodontic treatment. Rapid processing enables the oral surgeon to determine instantly the extent or location of a fractured root. The general practitioner occasionally requires rapid confirmation of the success or failure of an operation performed. However, rapid processing has definite limitations and is not intended to replace conventional processing.

Equipment

Rapid processing requires the use of a chair-side darkroom and special developer and fixer chemicals.

The chair-side darkroom is a light-tight counter-top box that has two light-tight openings through which the hands can enter the working compartment when the lid is closed. The transparent plastic top functions to filter out unsafe light while permitting the operator to see into the box to unwrap the film packet and manually proceed through the processing steps. Four cups are set up inside the box containing developer, rinse water, fixer and wash water. Developing and fixing solutions made especially for rapid processing can be heated to 85°F (29.4°C) by a calibrated heater in the unit. A small film hanger with a single clip is used to transfer manually the film from solution to solution.

Maintenance and Preparation

Fresh developer and fixer are placed in the first and third cups, and distilled water is placed is the second and fourth cups, usually from left to right. Chemicals used for chairside processing are used for processing a limited number of films and then discarded. The cups of rinse water quickly become contaminated, so should be changed often. Once the solutions have reached the desired temperature, processing can begin.

Procedure

The steps for processing films using the rapid processing method are identical to the steps used for manual processing (see Procedure Box 8–1). The film is placed in the developer first, then rinsed and placed in the fixer, then washed and dried. The development time ranges from 5 to 15 seconds; the fix time is approximately 30 seconds.

Films processed in this manner are called **working radiographs** and are seldom suitable for filing with the patient's permanent record. Short developing and fixing times, combined with minimal washing, result in a substandard radiograph. Rapid processing chemistry does not produce archival results, and the films will eventually discolor. In the event that the film is to be retained with the permanent record, it should be refixed for 4 minutes and washed for 20 minutes at normal conventional darkroom temperatures and conditions. It must be recognized that while rapid processing fulfills the dentist's need to receive rapid information, it is at the expense of image quality.

Following the Procedure

1. Turn off the heater.
2. Empty, rinse, and dry each of the cups. Dispose of the used fixer appropriately.
3. Clean and disinfect the inside of the chairside darkroom. Wipe off the transparent plastic top as needed.
4. Continue fixing and complete the washing and drying steps to convert a working film to a permanent image.

REVIEW—Chapter Summary

Film processing is a series of steps that converts the invisible latent image on the dental x-ray film into a visible permanent image called a radiograph. The sequence of steps followed in manual processing is developing, rinsing, fixing, washing, and drying. Developing reduces the exposed silver halide crystals within the film emulsion to black metallic silver. Rinsing removes the alkaline developer before placing the film in the fixer solution. Fixing removes the unexposed and/or undeveloped silver halide crystals from the film emulsion. Washing removes any remaining traces of the chemicals. Drying preserves the film for storage as a part of the patient's permanent record.

Two processing chemicals are used—an alkaline developer and a slightly acidic fixer. There are four chemicals in the developer: developing agents (hydroquinone and elon), a preservative (sodium sulfite), an activator (sodium carbonate), and a restrainer (potassium bromide). The purpose of the developing solution is to reduce the exposed silver halide crystals to black metallic silver.

There are four chemicals in the fixer: a fixing agent (sodium thiosulfate), a preservative (sodium sulfite), a hardening agent (potassium alum), and an acidifier (acetic acid). The purpose of the fixing solution is to remove the undeveloped silver halide crystals and harden the emulsion.

A darkroom is a room completely devoid of white light, used to process x-ray film. With the exception of automatic processors equipped with daylight loaders and chairside rapid processing darkroom boxes, all processing must be done in the darkroom under safelight conditions. Safelighting is based on wattage, filter color and condition, distance from the work area, and the length of time the unwrapped film is exposed to the safelight.

Oxidation over time and chemical contamination through normal use prompt solution changes and regularly scheduled equipment maintenance and cleaning. The useful life of the solutions is determined by the original quality or concentration of the solution; the freshness of the solution; the number of films that are processed; and the contamination of the chemicals.

Oral health care practices have an ethical responsibility to dispose properly of used fixer, lead foil from intraoral film packets, and discarded radiographs.

Advantages of manual film processing include reliability, no equipment malfunction, control over the time and temperature, and the ability to produce a wet reading. The biggest disadvantage of manual processing is the long time required to produce a finished radiograph. Manual processing requires a processing tank, thermometer, timer, stirring paddles, film hangers and drying racks. The ideal time–temperature for manual processing is 68°F (20°C) for five minutes. Colder developer solution requires a longer developing time; warmer developer solution requires a shorter developing time.

The biggest advantage of automatic film processing is the short time required to produce a finished radiograph. Automatic processors equipped with daylight loader attachments can be used to process film without a darkroom. Disadvantages include initial unit expense, possible equipment malfunction, increased maintenance required for optimal output, and rapid chemical depletion. Automatic processors use a roller transport assembly to advance the films automatically from solution to solution, producing a finished radiograph in five minutes.

A chairside darkroom is utilized to produce working radiographs by the rapid processing method. Films are manually processed with special developer and fixer which produce a radiographic image in less than 1 minute. Rapid processing chemistry does not produce archival results, and the films will eventually discolor. The advantage of rapid processing is that it fulfills the need to receive rapid information. However, image quality will be diminished.

Step-by-step procedures for manual, automatic, and rapid processing are presented in this chapter.

RECALL—Study Questions

1. Which term best describes the process by which the latent image becomes visible?
   a. Reticulation
   b. Reduction
   c. Activation
   d. Preservation
2. Which of these is the correct processing sequence?
   a. Rinse, fix, wash, develop, dry
   b. Fix, rinse, develop, wash, dry
   c. Develop, rinse, fix, wash, dry
   d. Rinse, develop, wash, fix, dry
3. The basic constituents of the developer solution are:
   a. Reducing agent, activator, preservative, restrainer.
   b. Reducing agent, acidifier, preservative, restrainer.
   c. Clearing agent, activator, preservative, restrainer.
   d. Clearing agent, preservative, hardener, acidifier.
4. During which step of the processing procedure are the exposed silver halide crystals reduced to metallic silver?
   a. Developing
   b. Fixing
   c. Rinsing
   d. Washing
5. Which of the following removes the unexposed/undeveloped silver halide crystals from the film emulsion?
   a. Acetic acid
   b. Potassium bromide
   c. Sodium thiosulfate
   d. Hydroquinone
6. Which ingredient causes the emulsion to soften and swell?
   a. Acidifier
   b. Preservative
   c. Restrainer
   d. Activator
7. Which ingredient hardens the emulsion?
   a. Elon
   b. Potassium alum
   c. Sodium carbonate
   d. Sodium sulfite
8. Chemically, what is the major difference between solutions used for manual processing and those used for automatic and rapid processing?
   a. Manual processing solutions are more alkaline.
   b. There is more acid in rapid processing solutions.
   c. Manual processing solutions contain more preservative.
   d. Automatic and rapid processing solutions contain more hardener.
9. All of the following should be considered when setting up an ideal darkroom *except* one. Which one is this *exception?*
   a. Black walls
   b. Location
   c. Lighting
   d. Size
10. Which of the following filter colors would filter out the short-wavelength light that is unsafe for film processing?
    a. White
    b. Black
    c. Red
    d. Blue
11. How far above the work area in the darkroom should the safelight be located?
    a. 2 ft (0.6 m)
    b. 4 ft (1.2 m)
    c. 6 ft (1.8 m)
    d. 8 ft (2.4 m)
12. What is the appearance of the radiographic image when a film is exposed to a safelight too long?
    a. Oxidized
    b. Fogged
    c. Reticulated
    d. Attenuated
13. Replenisher is added to the developing solution to compensate for:
    a. Oxidation.
    b. Loss of volume.
    c. Loss of solution strength.
    d. All of the above.
14. Radiographic wastes include _____, _____, and _____.

15. The floating thermometer for manual processing should be placed in the:
    a. Developing solution.
    b. Water compartment.
    c. Fixing solution.
    d. Both a and c.
16. All of the following are necessary and required for manual processing *except* one. Which one is this *exception?*
    a. Thermometer
    b. Timer
    c. Film dryer
    d. Film hanger
17. What is the ideal temperature for processing film manually?
    a. 60°F (15.5°C)
    b. 68°F (20°C)
    c. 75°F (23.9°C)
    d. 83°F (28.3°C)
18. All of the following are advantages of automatic processing over manual processing *except* one. Which one is this *exception?*
    a. Less maintenance
    b. Decreased processing time
    c. Increased capacity for processing
    d. Self-regulation of time and temperature
19. Which of these is the biggest disadvantage of manual processing?
    a. Darkroom required
    b. Processing time is long
    c. Chemicals must be replenished
    d. Temperature must be regulated
20. A film may be exposured to white light for a wet reading after two or three minutes of:
    a. Developing.
    b. Rinsing.
    c. Fixing.
    d. Washing.
21. Manual and automatic processing tanks should be cleaned:
    a. Daily.
    b. Weekly.
    c. Monthly.
    d. Whenever the solutions are changed.

REFLECT—Case Study

You work for a temporary agency that provides staffing for oral health care practices in your area. Today your employer has sent you to a practice organized and set up for a left-handed practitioner. Your first patient requires a bitewing series of radiographs. You expose the films and proceed to the darkroom for processing. Unknown to you, this practice has set up the manual processing tanks with the developing solution tank on the right and the fixer tank on the left. You are used to working with processing tanks set up with the developing solution on the left and the fixer on the right, and you proceed to process your films in this manner. What effect will this have on the resultant radiographs? Why will they look this way? Explain why the processing solutions will produce this result. What can you do to avoid this mistake in the future? What can this practice do to prevent this mistake from happening again?

RELATE—Laboratory Application

For a comprehensive laboratory practice exercise on this topic, see E. M. Thomson, *Exercises in Oral Radiography Techniques: A Laboratory Manual,* 2nd ed. Upper Saddle River, NJ: Prentice Hall, 2007. Chapter 1, "Radiographic Film Processing and Darkroom Design and Maintenance."

BIBLIOGRAPHY

Eastman Kodak. *Exposure and Processing for Dental Radiography.* Rochester, NY: Eastman Kodak, 1998.

Thomson-Lakey, E. M. Developing an environmentally sound oral health practice. *Access* 10, no. 4, 19–26, 1996.

Part IV • Dental Radiographer Fundamentals

9

Infection Control

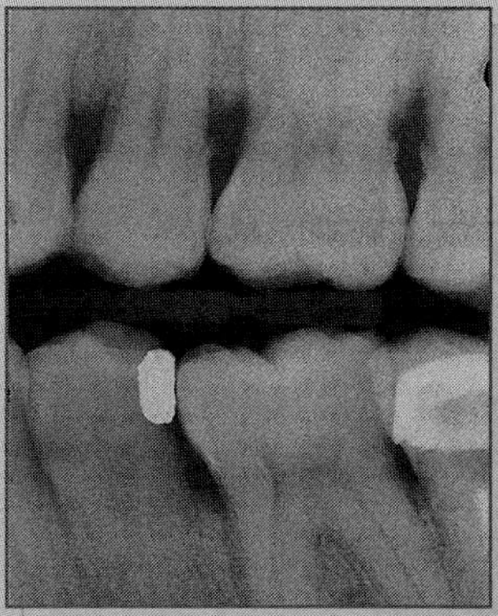

CHAPTER OUTLINE

■ OBJECTIVES

Following successful completion of this chapter, you should be able to:

1. Define the key words.
2. State the purpose of infection control.
3. Describe the possible routes of disease transmission.
4. Identify conditions for the chain of infection and methods of breaking the chain.
5. Advocate the concept of standard precautions.
6. List four personal protective barriers recommended for the dental radiographer.
7. Differentiate between semicritical and noncritical objects used during radiographic procedures.
8. Identify radiographic instruments and equipment requiring sterilization.
9. Identify radiographic instruments and equipment requiring disinfection.
10. List radiographic instruments or equipment that may be protected with a plastic barrier.
11. Demonstrate competency in following the infection control protocol used prior to radiographic procedures.
12. Demonstrate competency in following the infection control protocol used during radiographic procedures.
13. Demonstrate competency in following the infection control protocol used after radiographic procedures.
14. Demonstrate competency in following the infection control protocol used for processing intraoral film packets without barrier envelopes.
15. Demonstrate competency in following the infection control protocol used for processing intraoral film packets with barrier envelopes.

■ KEY WORDS

- Acquired immunodeficiency syndrome (AIDS)
- Antiseptic
- Asepsis
- Barrier
- Barrier envelope
- Bloodborne pathogens
- Contamination
- Cross-contamination
- Disinfect
- Disinfection
- Exposure incident
- Hepatitis B
- Human immunodeficiency virus (HIV)
- Immunization

Infection control	Sanitation
Infectious waste	Sepsis
Occupational exposure	Sharp
Parenteral exposure	Standard precautions
Pathogen	Sterilization
Protective barrier	Universal precautions

Introduction

The purpose of **infection control** procedures used in dentistry is to prevent the transmission of disease among patients and between patients and oral health care practitioners. Maintaining infection control throughout the radiographic process is a challenge; the radiographer must possess a thorough understanding of the recommended infection control protocols that should be followed before, during, and after radiographic exposures. The specific steps of these protocols require practice to achieve competency in skilled handling of contaminated radiographic equipment and supplies.

The purpose of this chapter is to identify infection control terminology, present the need for infection control during radiographic procedures, and to describe step-by-step infection control procedures used in dental radiology.

Purpose of Infection Control

Infectious diseases may be transmitted from patient to oral healthcare personnel, from oral healthcare personnel to patient, and from patient to patient. The primary purpose of infection control is to prevent the transmission of infectious diseases. People have always lived with the possibility of infection occurring through invasion of the body by pathogens such as bacteria or viruses. A **pathogen** is a microorganism capable of causing disease. Because of the special risk these diseases carry, of particular concern to the oral healthcare professional are **acquired immunodeficiency syndrome (AIDS),** the **human immunodeficiency virus (HIV),** viral hepatitis, including the highly infectious **hepatitis B** virus (HBV), tuberculosis (TB), and herpesvirus diseases.

Routes of infection transmission are:

- Direct contact with pathogens in open lesions, blood, saliva, or respiratory secretions.
- Direct contact with airborne contaminants present in aerosols of oral and respiratory fluids.
- Indirect contact with contaminated objects or instruments.

Chain of Infection

For infection to occur, four conditions must be present (Figure 9–1).

1. A susceptible (i.e., not immune) host
2. A disease-causing microorganism (pathogen)
3. Sufficient numbers of the pathogen to initiate infection
4. An appropriate route (portal of entry) for the pathogen to enter the host

The purpose of infection control is to alter one of these four conditions to prevent the transmission of disease.

Breaking the Chain of Infection

The chain of infection can be broken by:

1. **Immunization** of the susceptible host. The Centers for Disease Control and Prevention (CDC) recommends that den-

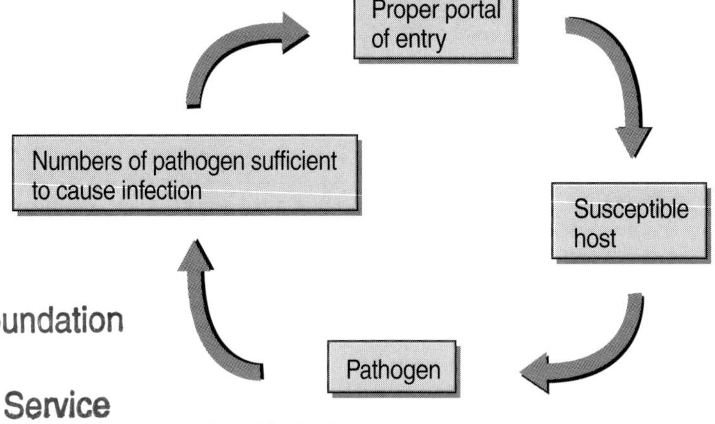

FIGURE 9–1 **Chain of infection.**

tal personnel working with blood or blood-contaminated substances be vaccinated for hepatitis B virus (HBV). Additionally, all dental healthcare workers should be vaccinated against influenza, measles, mumps, rubella, and tetanus.

2. **Removing the pathogen.** Use sterilization techniques and/or protective barriers.
3. **Reducing the sufficient numbers of pathogens.** Use disinfection and sterilization techniques and/or protective barriers.
4. **Blocking the portal of entry.** Use personal protective equipment (PPE) barriers such as protective clothes, masks, eyewear, and gloves.

Infection Control Terminology

The following terms are frequently used in infection control. They should be studied and understood.

Antiseptic: An agent used on living tissues to destroy or stop the growth of bacteria. An example would be antiseptic soaps used by oral health care personnel for washing hands and pre-procedural mouthrinses for reducing microorganisms present in aerosols.

Asepsis: The absence of septic matter or freedom from infection (*a* means without; *sepsis* means infection). The term is used to describe procedures that prevent infection of tissues by microorganisms.

Barrier: Used to describe any material that prevents the transmission of infective microorganisms. Barriers include protective clothing, masks, protective eyewear, gloves, and clinical contact surface covers.

Bloodborne pathogens: Pathogens present in blood that causes disease in humans.

Contamination: Soiling by contact or mixing.

Cross-contamination: To contaminate from one place or person to another place or person.

Disinfect: The use of a chemical or physical procedure to reduce the disease-producing microorganisms to an acceptable level on inanimate objects. This is done by wiping off those portions of the equipment that come into contact with the patient or operator with gauze saturated with a chemical disinfectant such as an EPA-registered surface disinfectant. Spores are not necessarily destroyed. Disinfecting agents are usually used only on surfaces and instruments because they are too toxic for use on living tissues.

Disinfection: The act of disinfecting.

Exposure incident: An incident that involves contact with blood or other potentially infectious materials and that results from procedures performed by oral health care personnel.

Immunization: The process of making someone immune to a disease. All dental personnel should have the recommended immunizations, including that for the hepatitis B virus.

Infection control: The prevention and reduction of disease-causing (pathogenic) microorganisms.

Infectious waste: Waste (such as blood, blood products, and contaminated sharps) that may contain pathogens.

Microbial aerosol: Suspension of microorganisms that may be capable of causing disease. Aerosols are produced during normal breathing and speaking, so are present during the radiographic procedure.

Occupational exposure: A worker (oral radiographer) coming in contact with blood, saliva, or other infectious material that involves the skin, eye, or mucus membrane.

Pathogen: A microorganism that can cause disease (*pathos* means disease). Infection control procedures are used to prevent the cross-contamination of pathogens.

Parenteral exposure: Exposure to blood that results from puncturing the skin barrier.

Sanitation: A term used when microorganisms are reduced to a level of concentration considered to be safe. Food-handling facilities are usually concerned about adequate sanitation.

Sepsis: Infection, or the presence of septic matter.

Sharp: Any object that can penetrate the skin, such as needles or scalpels.

Spatter: A heavier concentration of aerosols, such as visible particles from a cough or sneeze.

Standard precautions: A practice of care to protect persons from pathogens spread via blood or any other body fluid, excretion or secretion (except sweat).

Sterilize: The total destruction of spores and disease-producing microorganisms, accomplished by autoclaving or dry heat processes. If possible, all equipment and instruments should be sterilized.

Sterilization: The act of sterilizing. Cold sterilization is a term that has been commonly misused in medicine and dentistry for many years because it refers to procedures that result in disinfection, not sterilization.

Universal precautions: The concept of infection control where the focus was on bloodborne pathogens. The all-inclusive "standard precautions" has replaced this concept.

Guidelines for Infection Control

Research continues to update infection control guidelines. Currently the Centers for Disease Control and Prevention (CDC) publication *Guidelines for Infection Control in Dental Health-care Settings* (MMWR, 52, 2, RR-17, Dec. 19, 2003) has endorsed the standard precaution approach to infection control, whereas the recommendation is to "treat everyone as if known to be infectious."

It is a well known fact that some patients are reluctant to admit their infectious condition. In the past, there may have been a tendency to use a double standard where certain infection control precautions were used only if the patient was known to be infectious. Failure to use a single standard for all patients put everyone at risk. Taking a thorough medical history and performing an oral examination will not always identify potential infected patients. Therefore the use of **standard precautions,** where all body fluids (except sweat) of all patients, whether known to be infected or not, are assumed to be infected and the necessary infection control procedures must be applied to all.

Each oral health care practice should have written infection control protocols that are practical and compatible with local or state regulations. The dentist (or designated personnel) has the authority and the responsibility to see that the infection control policy is correctly carried out. The CDC's infection control guidelines that directly relate to dental radiology are listed in Table 9–1.

Personal Protective Equipment (PPE)

Personal protective equipment (clothing, masks, eyewear, and gloves) worn by dental personnel acts as a **protective barrier** (Figure 9–2). These prevent the transmission of infective microorganisms between oral healthcare practitioners and patients.

Protective Clothing

Protective clothing, such as gowns, uniforms, and lab coats, provides protection from exposure to body fluids. Protective clothing should be changed daily, or more frequently if soiled or wet. Protective clothing should be removed before leaving the treatment facility. Protective clothing should be laundered separately with bleach to prevent contamination of other items. Ideally, gowns and uniforms should be laundered by a commercial biohazard laundry service that can safely remove the items from the practice for laundering.

TABLE 9–1 The Centers for Disease Control and Prevention (CDC) Recommended Infection-Control Practices for Oral Radiography

- Wear patient treatment gloves when exposing radiographs and handling contaminated film packets.
- Use protective eyewear, mask, and gown as appropriate if spattering of blood or other body fluids is likely.
- Use heat-tolerant or disposable film holding devices whenever possible (at a minimum, high-level disinfect semicritical heat-sensitive devices such as digital radiographic sensors, according to the manufacturer's instructions).
- Clean and heat-sterilize film-holding devices between patients.
- Transport and handle exposed film packets in an aseptic manner to prevent contamination of processing equipment.
- Use FDA-cleared protective barriers on digitial radiographic sensors.

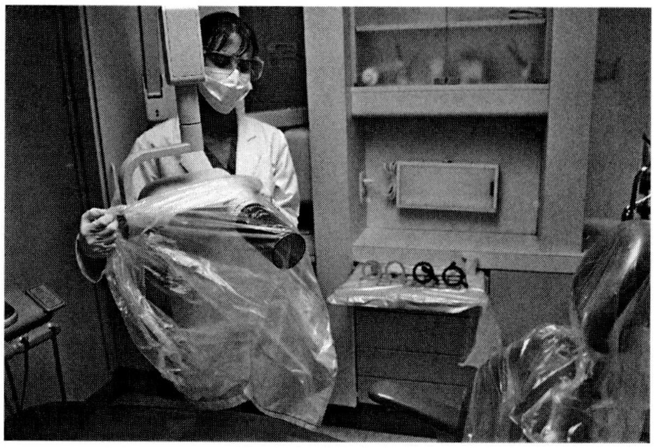

FIGURE 9–2 **Operator preparing x-ray equipment.** Operator wearing gloves, mask, and protective eyewear is placing barriers to cover PID, tube housing, and yoke of the x-ray unit.

Masks

While radiographic procedures are much less likely than other types of dental procedures to produce spatter, protection from aerosols may be achieved through the use of a mask. Masks should be changed when soiled or wet and between patients.

Protective Eyewear

While radiographic procedures are much less likely than other types of dental procedures to subject the radiographer to physical eye accidents, the use of protective eyewear will protect against aerosols and spatter. Types of protective eyewear include glasses with side shields, goggles, and full-face shields. Protective eyewear must be washed with appropriate cleaning agents following treatment and as needed.

The Centers for Disease Control and Prevention (CDC) publication *Guidelines for Infection Control in Dental Health-care Settings* (MMWR, 52, 2, RR-17, Dec. 19, 2003) considers the use of a mask and protective eyewear during radiographic procedures as appropriate if spattering of blood or other body fluids is likely. While some radiographers interpret this recommendation to be optional, they should be aware that there may be federal or state regulations requiring their use. The radiographer should be familiar with these regulations as well.

Gloves

Gloves must be worn at all times throughout the radiographic procedure. A variety of gloves are available for specialized uses. Sterile gloves are used for surgical procedures, non-sterile gloves are used for non-surgical procedures such as taking radiographs, plastic overgloves have temporary applications such as protecting or containing patient treatment gloves, and utility gloves are appropriate for cleaning and disinfection. Patient treatment gloves are made of latex or vinyl material. Powdered gloves should be avoided, as the powder residue can cause radiographic artifacts (see Chapter 16.) Gloves should never be washed with soap or disinfected for reuse. Soap may damage gloves in a way that would allow the flow of liquid through undetected holes. Punctured, torn, or cut gloves should be changed immediately. Gloves should always be changed and discarded between patients.

All personnel must be instructed to avoid touching areas such as doorknobs to access the darkroom, unexposed film packets, or patient records with contaminated gloves. Care should be taken to avoid touching anything that is not essential to the procedure being carried out.

Handwashing

Protective clothing, mask and eyewear should all be in place to prepare for handwashing prior to putting on patient treatment gloves. Hands should be cleaned thoroughly before and after treating each patient (before gloving and after removing gloves) (Procedure Box 9–1). Potentially infectious pathogens can grow rapidly inside a warm, moist glove.

When hands are visibly dirty they must be washed with an antimicrobial soap and water. If hands are not visibly soiled, an alcohol-containing preparation designed for reducing the number of viable microorganisms on the hands may be used. All jewelry including a watch and rings should be removed prior to handwashing. Long fingernails, false fingernails, and nail polish should be avoided as these may harbor pathogens and have the potential to puncture treatment gloves. Handwashing is most effective when nails are cut short and well manicured. Dry hands thoroughly before placing treatment gloves on.

Disinfection and Sterilization of Instruments and Equipment

Disinfection and sterilization of instruments break the chain of infection to prevent the transmission of infective microorganisms.

Disinfection

Disinfection is the use of a chemical or physical procedure to reduce the disease-producing microorganisms (pathogens) to an acceptable level on inanimate objects. Spores are not necessarily destroyed. Disinfecting agents are usually only used on surfaces and on some instruments that can not be sterilized because they are too toxic for living tissues.

One mandate of the U.S. Environmental Protection Agency (EPA) is the regulation and registration of surface disinfectants. EPA-registered sterilants-disinfectants are classified as:

- **High-level disinfectant.** Chemical germicides inactivate spores and can be used to disinfect heat-sensitive semicritical dental instruments.
- **Intermediate-level disinfectant.** Chemical germicides labeled as both hospital grade disinfectants and tuberculocidals. Examples are iodophors, phenolics, and chlorine-containing compounds. These do not destroy spores.
- **Low-level disinfectant.** Chemical germicides labeled as hospital grade disinfectants. Can not destroy spores, tubercle bacilli or nonlipid viruses.

Sterilization

Sterilization is the total destruction of spores and disease-producing microorganisms. Sterilization is usually accomplished by autoclaving or dry heat processes. Ideally, all equipment and instruments should be sterilized. Acceptable methods of sterilization in the dental office are:

- Steam under pressure (steam autoclave)
- Dry heat
- Heat/chemical vapor (chemical autoclave)
- Sterilant/disinfectant that has been registered by the EPA

PROCEDURE 9–1

PROCEDURE FOR HANDWASHING FOR RADIOGRAPHIC PROCEDURES

1. Put on protective gown, eyewear and mask.
2. Remove rings, wristwatch,* and other jewelry.
3. Wet hands with warm water and apply liquid antimicrobial soap.
4. Vigorously lather for 15 seconds; interlace fingers and thumbs and move hands back and forth; work lather under nails.
5. Rinse well, allowing water to run from finger tips.
6. Repeat the lather and rinse step two more times for an additional 15 seconds each.
7. Dry each hand thoroughly with a separate paper towel.
8. Unless equipped with a foot pedal, turn off the water by placing a clean paper towel between your clean, dry hand and the faucet.

* Wristwatch may be replaced after handwashing as long as it will remain protected under the gown or covered with the glove during the procedure.

Classification of Objects Used in Radiographic Procedures

Radiographic instruments and equipment are classified according to their risk of transmitting infection and to the need to sterilize them between uses (Table 9–2).

- Critical objects are those used to penetrate soft tissue or bone. Examples are needles, forceps, and scalers. Critical objects must be sterilized after each use. No critical instruments or equipment are used in dental radiology.
- Semicritical objects are those that contact but do not penetrate soft tissue or bone, such as intraoral dental mirrors and burrs. The instruments used for radiography procedures fall into this category. Semicritical instruments must be sterilized after use. While most quality-made film holders can be sterilized or are disposable, there may be devices on the market that are heat sensitive. While heat sensitive semicritical instruments may be sterilized with EPA-registered chemicals classified as high-level disinfectant, using instruments that can be heat sterilized or that are disposable is recommended.
- Noncritical objects are those that do not come into contact with the mucous membrane. Examples include the lead apron, the PID (position-indicating device), and the exposure button. Noncritical objects can be disinfected using EPA-registered chemicals classified as intermediate-level disinfectants.
- Clinical contact surfaces (or environmental surfaces) are those that do not contact the patient or contact is with the skin only. An example of a clinical contact surface is the head positioner guides of a panoramic x-ray machine. Clinical contact surfaces can be disinfected using EPA-registered chemicals classified as either intermediate-level or low-level disinfectants.

Cleaning and Disinfection of the X-ray Unit and Clinical Contact Surfaces

Prior to and following radiographic procedures, the treatment area and the equipment must be cleaned and disinfected. All surfaces that will be used for, or contacted during, the procedure must be cleaned and disinfected according to the object's classification as critical, semicritical or noncritical.

Protective barriers should be used whenever practical. Surfaces not covered must be cleaned and disinfected after the radiographic procedures are completed. It should be noted that disinfectants have several drawbacks. Like all liquids, disinfectants have the potential to affect electrical connections, so directly spraying or saturating the x-ray control panel, dials, or exposure button may damage the x-ray machine. Also, disinfecting solutions may not adequately reach irregular surfaces. For these reasons, the use of plastic wrap, plastic bags, paper towels, paper cups, aluminum foil, etc. may be used to cover appropriate surfaces, equipment and supplies. Barrier material is commonly placed over those surfaces most likely to be contaminated during the radiographic procedure such as the PID and tube head, control panel, exposure switch, and counter surfaces (Figures 9–3 to 9–5).

Infection Control Protocol Used for the Radiographic Procedure

Utilizing standard precautions, infection control procedures for radiography assume that all body fluids (except sweat) of all patients have the potential to be infectious. Infection control procedures for exposing radiographs can be divided into three categories: prior to, during, and after film exposure.

TABLE 9-2 Risk of Transmitting Disease Classification of Objects Used in Radiographic Procedures

Category	Radiographic Equipment	Sterilize or Disinfect
Critical	None	N/A
Semicritical	Film-holding instruments Panoramic biteblocks Digital sensor*	Sterilize or use disposable devices
Noncritical	X-ray tube head and PID X-ray tube head support arm & yoke Exposure controls** Exposure button** Lead apron and thyroid collar Extraoral radiographic head positioner guides: chin or forehead rest and side positioner guides on a panoramic unit; cephalostat	Clean and disinfect with an intermediate-level disinfectant
Clinical contact surface	Counter top in operatory Counter top in darkroom	Clean and disinfect with an intermediate- or low-level disinfectant

* Most digital radiographic sensor manufacturers recommend against sterilizing fragile digital sensors. Instead, these need to be covered with an FDA-cleared barrier and cleaned and disinfected as needed with a high-level disinfectant. Consult manufacturer's recommendations.

** Liquid disinfectants may damage the electrical components of the dental x-ray control panel. Therefore, most dental x-ray equipment manufacturers recommend covering the control panel exposure dials and exposure button with an FDA-cleared barrier. Consult manufacturer's recommendations.

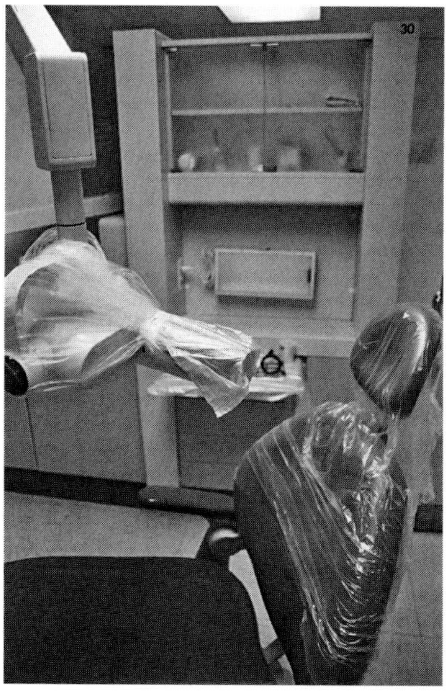

FIGURE 9-3 **Prepared dental x-ray equipment.** The PID, tube housing and yoke, and the operatory chair and head rest are protected with plastic barriers. In the background, note that film holders have been assembled and placed on a plastic barrier on the countertop.

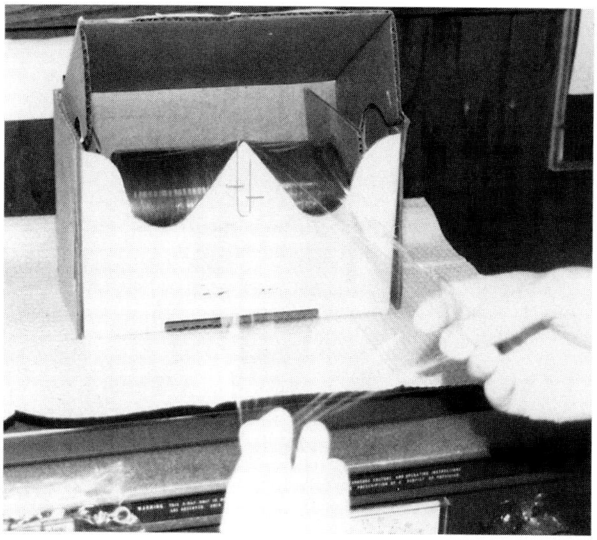

FIGURE 9-5 **Operator dispensing plastic barrier wrap.**

Protocol Prior to the Radiographic Procedure (Procedure Box 9-2)

Prepare the Treatment Area

All treatment area surfaces likely to come in contact with the patient either directly or indirectly must be sterilized, cleaned and disinfected or covered with a protective barrier. All supplies, film-holding devices, and films should be obtained and placed for easy access during the procedure.

Dental x-ray film should be dispensed in disposable containers such as a paper cup or small envelope. The film packet must be handled carefully to prevent cross-contamination. The film packet, with its heat-sensitive emulsion, cannot be sterilized and the liquid saturation required for disinfecting objects is not recommended for film packets, especially for paper film packets. Therefore the operator should contain used film packets in a cup until ready to develop. Another method used to prevent the transmission of microorganisms by the film packet is the use of **barrier envelopes.**

Barrier envelopes are commercially available for film sizes #0, #1, and #2. Film packets placed and sealed in these plastic envelopes (Figure 9–6) are protected from contact with fluids in the oral cavity during exposure. Film packets already sealed in barrier plastic envelopes by the manufacturer are also available commercially (Figure 9–7). Following removal from the patient's oral cavity, the barrier envelope is opened (Figure 9–8) and discarded appropriately. The film packet that was sealed in the barrier envelope may now be handled with clean hands (or new gloves) to complete the processing procedure.

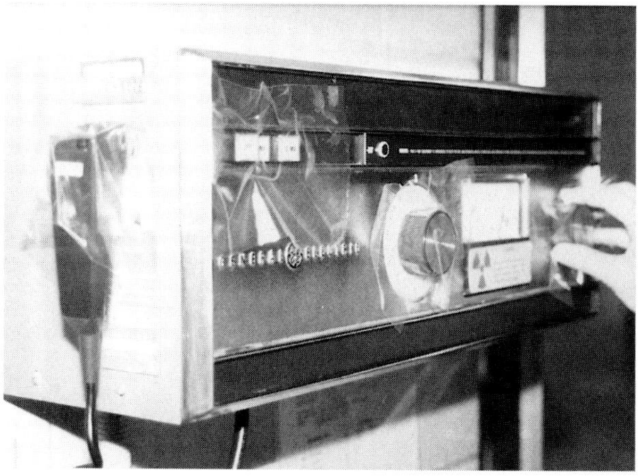

FIGURE 9-4 **Plastic barrier wrap covering exposure switch and controls on control panel.**

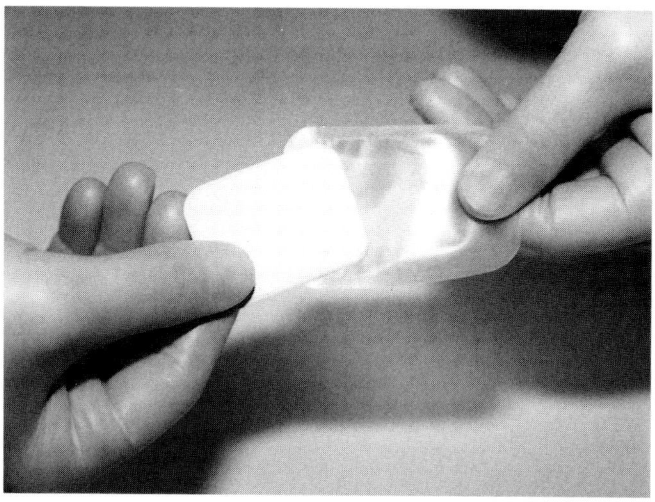

FIGURE 9-6 **Barrier protection.** Film packet is placed (and then sealed) in a plastic barrier envelope.

PROCEDURE 9-2

PROTOCOL PRIOR TO THE RADIOGRAPHIC PROCEDURE

1. Follow handwashing described in Procedure Box 9–1 or apply an antiseptic hand rub following the manufacturer's directions for use.*
2. Put on utility gloves.
3. Clean and disinfect with appropriate disinfectant all surfaces which will come in contact either directly or indirectly with the patient. See the following list:
   a. PID
   b. X-ray tube head
   c. Tube head support arms and handles
   d. Exposure button**
   e. Control panel dials (impulse timer, kVp, and MA controls)**
   f. Treatment chair including head rest, back support, arm rests, body and back of the chair
   g. Bracket table or counter top or other clinical contact surfaces that will be used during the procedure
   h. Lead apron/thyroid collar
4. Wash, dry, and remove utility gloves. Disinfect.
5. Wash hands with an antimicrobial soap or apply an antiseptic hand rub.*
6. Put on clean over gloves.
7. Obtain plastic or foil type barriers and cover all surfaces that will come in contact either directly or indirectly with the patient. See the following list:
   a. PID
   b. X-ray tube head (Figure 9–3)
   c. Tube head support arms and handles
   d. Exposure button (Figure 9–4)
   e. Control panel dials (impulse timer, kVp, and MA controls) (Figure 9–4)

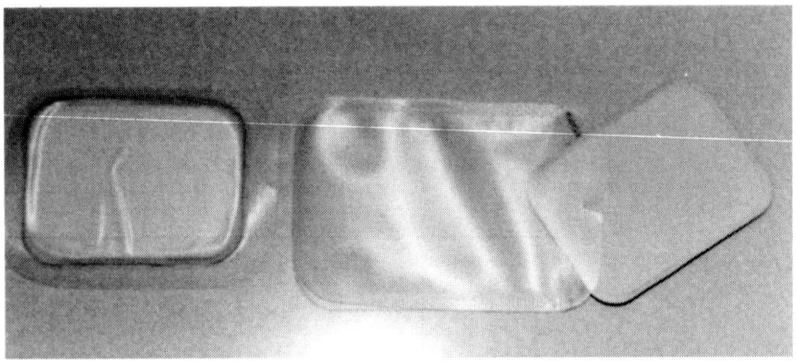

FIGURE 9-7 **Barrier envelope.** Left, film sealed in barrier packet ready to use from the manufacturer. Right, barrier envelope with film packet partially inserted.

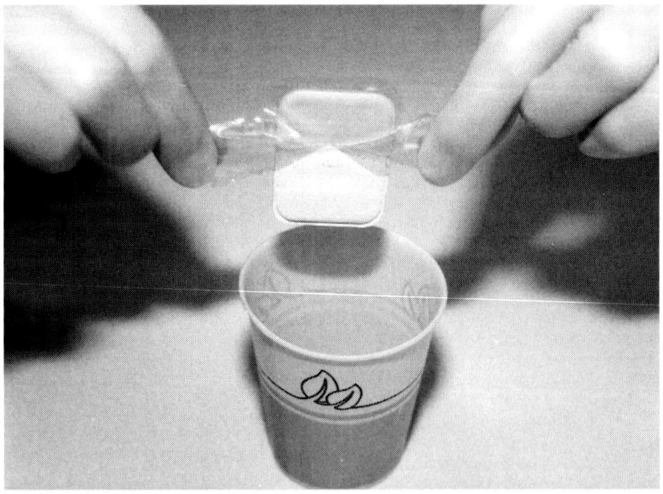

FIGURE 9-8 **Opening the barrier envelope.** A steady pull is used, allowing the film packet to drop in a clean cup.

PROCEDURE 9–2 *(cont.)*

f. Treatment chair including head rest, back support, arm rests, body and back of the chair
g. Bracket table or counter top or other clinical contact surface that will be used during the procedure
h. Lead apron/thyroid collar (optional)
i. Film packets (optional) (Figure 9–6)

8. Obtain radiographic supplies. See the following list:
   a. Film packets
   b. Sterile or disposable film-holding devices
   c. Film mount
   d. Disposable paper/plastic cup
   e. Paper towels
   f. Miscellaneous supplies (i.e., cotton rolls, extra disposable film-holding devices)
9. Place the film mount under the plastic barrier on the counter work space.
10. Place the film packets on the plastic barrier placed over the film mount.
11. Saturate a folded paper towel with disinfectant and place next to the film mount on top of the plastic barrier.
12. Prepare antimicrobial mouthrinse for patient use prior to procedure.***

* When hands are visibly dirty, they must be washed with an antimicrobial soap and water. If hands are not visibly soiled, an alcohol-containing preparation designed for reducing the number of viable microorganisms on the hands may be used. Refer to manufacturer's recommendations for use.

** Exposure switches and control panel dials may be damaged by the use of a disinfectant solution. Manufacturer's recommendations should be consulted. Saturating a paper towel with disinfectant and then carefully wiping the switches may be an option. Infection control may also be achieved through the use of a plastic or foil barrier (Figure 9–4). (Foot pedal exposure switches do not require disinfection.)

*** No scientific evidence indicates that pre-procedural mouth rinsing prevents the spread of infections. However, antimicrobial mouth rinses, e.g., chlorhexidine gluconate, essential oils, or povidone-iodine, can reduce the number of microorganisms the patient might release in the form of aerosols or spatter.

Protocol During the Radiographic Procedure (Procedure Box 9–3)

Patient Preparation

The patient is seated after the treatment area is prepared and supplies and film-holding devices have been dispensed. The patient may be asked to rinse with an anti-microbial mouthrinse to reduce oral microorganisms that contribute to infectious aerosols and draped with the lead or lead-equivalent apron and thyroid collar. Care must be taken when making adjustments to the treatment chair and head rest so as not to compromise the infection control process. Covering the treatment chair, including the head rest, with a plastic barrier will aid in the infection control process.

Any object that may interfere with film exposure, such as patient's eyeglasses, dentures, etc., should be removed by the patient and placed in an area so as not to become contaminated and so as not to contaminate other objects.

During Exposures

Once film exposures begin, care must be taken to touch only covered surfaces. The best way to minimize contamination is to touch as few surfaces as possible. If drawers or cabinets must be opened to retrieve additional supplies, or the radiographer must leave the treatment area during the procedure, the patient treatment gloves should be removed and the hands washed. New treatment gloves must be used when re-starting the procedure. Overgloves may also be used, if treatment must be interrupted. The patient treatment gloves may be rinsed briefly with water only (do not use soap, as it will compromise the integrity of the protection), dried, and covered with plastic overgloves. To restart the exposure procedure, the overgloves are removed.

Dry Exposed Film Packets

Immediately upon removing the film packet from the oral cavity, excess saliva should be removed. The most efficient way to do this while minimizing objects touched is to swipe the film packet across a disinfectant-soaked paper towel that was prepared during setup (Figure 9–9). The film should next be dropped into a paper cup without touching the outside edges of the cup. The cup will serve as the transport method of getting the contaminated film packets safely into the darkroom.

If using film packets with protective plastic barriers, the barrier should be opened immediately upon removing the film packet from the patient's oral cavity. Hold the film packet over the cup designated for containment and open the film packet

PROCEDURE 9–3

PROTOCOL DURING THE RADIOGRAPHIC PROCEDURE

1. Follow handwashing described in Procedure Box 9–1 or apply an antiseptic hand rub following the manufacturer's directions for use.
2. Put on patient treatment gloves.
3. Place overgloves over patient treatment gloves.
4. Place the lead apron and thyroid collar on the patient.
5. Remove over gloves and place on the counter.
6. Assemble the film packet into the appropriate film-holding device, place intraorally and position the x-ray tube head and PID.
7. Depress the exposure button and remove the film-holding device and film packet from the patient's oral cavity.
8. Remove the film packet from the film holding device.
9. Swipe the film packet across the disinfectant-soaked paper towel and drop into the containment cup.*
10. Proceed to place and expose all films in this manner.
11. If additional supplies are needed which require the operator to contact non-covered surfaces, or the procedure must otherwise be interrupted:
    a. Rinse treatment gloves with plain water (no soap) and dry.**
    b. Place overgloves over treatment gloves.
    c. To re-start the procedure, remove overgloves.

* Film packets sealed in plastic barrier envelopes should be opened immediately. Allowing the film packet to drop into the containment cup.

** If the procedure must be interrupted, the treatment gloves may be removed and discarded and the hands washed. Prior to restarting the procedure, the hands should be washed again and new treatment gloves put on.

(Figure 9–8), allowing the sealed film packet to drop into the cup untouched by gloved hands. Once all of the films are exposed and opened in this manner, the cup will contain uncontaminated film packets that are ready to be transported to the darkroom for processing.

Care of Film-holding Devices

The film-holding devices should be transferred from a barrier-protected surface to the patient's oral cavity and then back to the same covered surface. Never place contaminated instruments on an uncovered surface.

Protocol After the Radiographic Procedure (Procedure Box 9–4)

Once the radiographic procedure is complete, patient gloves should be removed and discarded, and hands washed with an antimicrobial soap or an alcohol-based hand rub. The lead apron can now be removed from the patient and the cup containing the exposed films, carried to the darkroom for processing.

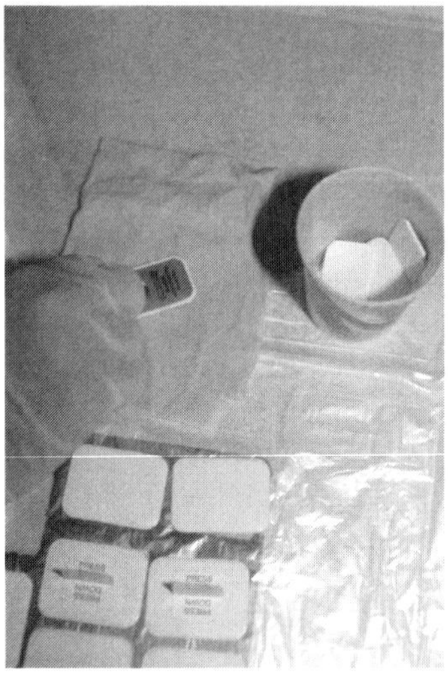

FIGURE 9–9 **Remove saliva.** Radiographer is swiping the film packet across a disinfectant-soaked paper towel prior to dropping the film into the containment cup.

PROCEDURE 9–4

PROTOCOL AFTER THE RADIOGRAPHIC PROCEDURE

1. Rinse, remove and discard patient treatment gloves and wash hands. Follow handwashing described in Procedure Box 9–1 or apply an antiseptic hand rub following the manufacturer's directions for use.
2. Remove lead apron with thyroid collar and dismiss patient.
3. Put on utility gloves.
4. Prepare and package film-holding devices for sterilization.*
5. Sterilize film-holding devices according to manufacturer's recommendations.
6. Discard all disposable contaminated items; i.e., disposable film-holding devices, paper towels, cotton rolls.
7. Remove and discard all plastic or foil barriers.
8. Clean and disinfect any uncovered surface.
9. Clean and disinfect lead apron and thyroid collar.
10. Wash, dry and remove utility gloves. Disinfect.
11. Wash hands with anti-microbial soap. Follow handwashing described in Procedure Box 9–1 or apply an antiseptic hand rub following the manufacturer's directions for use.

* Refer to manufacturer's recommendations for cleaning with soap and water or ultrasonic detergents.

Once the patient is dismissed, the radiographer should place utility gloves on for cleaning and disinfecting the treatment area. With utility gloves on, the film-holding devices are cleaned and prepared for sterilization according to the manufacturer's recommendations. Usually film holders can be washed with soap and water or ultrasonic cleaned in detergent and dried and packaged in an autoclave bag for sterilization. All disposable film holders and other disposable supplies, such as cotton rolls, should be discarded. Dispose of all contaminated items following local and state regulations. Plastic barriers should be carefully removed, making sure not to touch the surfaces underneath. All areas not covered should be cleaned and disinfected, including the lead apron and thyroid collar. When cleanup is complete, utility gloves may be washed with soap and water, removed and disinfected. The radiographer should wash hands again after removing utility gloves.

Infection Control Protocol Used for Radiographic Processing

Film-handling procedures for processing will depend upon whether or not barrier envelopes are used to protect the film packets.

Film Handling Without the Use of Barrier Envelopes (Procedure Box 9–5)

The use of commercial plastic film barrier envelopes protects the film packet from fluids in the oral cavity. Once the film packet is aseptically removed from the barrier envelope, it is safe to handle with clean, dry hands or clean treatment gloves. While readily available, the use of protective plastic envelopes for intraoral films is not universal. For this reason, it is important that the dental radiographer be skilled at handling film packets without barrier envelopes.

Once the film packets have been transported to the darkroom, the operator must put on treatment gloves, and proceed to open the packets aseptically (Figure 9–10). Skill in this procedure will help avoid dropping and potentially losing films in the darkroom's dim lighting. Additionally, the radiographer should be able to open all film packets, especially when processing a full mouth series, in two minutes or less to avoid prolonged exposure of the film to safelight. Prolonged exposure to light, even if it is called safelight, increases the risk of film fog (see Chapter 8.) After the last film is placed into the automatic processor or into the manual processing tank and the cover is closed, the darkroom must be cleaned and disinfected. Discard all materials appropriately, including the film packets, lead foil, and any materials used as protective barriers. Clean and disinfect darkroom counter surfaces and/or any other areas touched by gloved hands.

Film Handling with the Use of Barrier Envelopes

Although protected from contact with fluids in the oral cavity, film packets that were secured in barrier envelopes must still be handled carefully. Once the film packets have been removed from the plastic barrier envelopes they may be handled with clean, dry hands, or with new treatment gloves. To avoid fingerprints or other artifacts, handle films by the edges when feed-

PROCEDURE 9–5

PROTOCOL FOR PROCESSING RADIOGRAPHIC FILMS WITHOUT BARRIER ENVELOPES

1. Transport the contaminated film packets to the darkroom in the paper/plastic cup used for containment.
2. Place one paper towel on the counter work space and place the cup with contaminated films on this paper towel.
3. Place a second paper towel on the counter work space adjacent to the first paper towel and designate it as the uncontaminated area.
4. Secure darkroom door.
5. Turn off white overhead light and turn on safelight.
6. Put on clean patient treatment gloves.
7. Open each film packet (Figure 9–10).
   a. Peel back the outer plastic/paper wrap using the tab on the back of the packet.
   b. Grasp the black paper with film sandwiched in between, and pull straight out.
   c. Hold the black paper–film assembly over the designated uncontaminated paper towel and pull out slowly.
   d. Allow the film to drop out onto the paper towel. Do not touch the film with contaminated patient treatment gloves.
8. Drop the contaminated film packet outer plastic/paper wrap, black paper, and lead foil onto the contaminated paper towel.
9. Repeat steps 7 and 8 until all film packets have been opened.
10. Remove and discard patient treatment gloves and wash and dry hands.
11. With clean, dry hands, grasp by the edges and place films into the automatic processor feeder slots or load onto manual processing film racks for processing.
12. When the films are safely in the automatic processor, or the manual processing cover is securely closed, turn on the overhead white light.
13. Put on utility gloves.
14. Separate lead foil from film packets and discard into lead recycling waste.
15. Gather the contaminated paper towel with all waste and discard appropriately.
16. Clean and disinfect the counter work space and any other area that may have been touched during the procedure.
17. Wash, dry and remove utility gloves. Disinfect.
18. Wash and dry hands.*

* If hands are not visibly soiled, an alcohol-containing preparation designed for reducing the number of viable microorganisms on the hands may be used. Refer to manufacturer's recommendations for use.

ing into the automatic processor or placing on the manual processing film hangers. The use of powdered gloves should be avoided, since powder residue will leave artifacts on the radiograph (see Chapter 16).

Daylight Loader Attachments for Automatic Processors

Daylight loader attachments require special infection control considerations (Procedure Box 9–6). With strict adherence to proper infection control protocol, the use of daylight loaders should not compromise infection control. The radiographer should be discouraged from short-cutting these procedures, which would pose a health threat not only for the operator, but for others who use the device.

The key to infection control using the daylight loader is to remove the light-filter cover when placing and removing items (Figure 9–11). After removing the light-filter cover from the daylight loader, the cup containing the contaminated film packets, an additional, uncontaminated cup, and unused treatment gloves should be placed inside the unit on top of a plastic or paper towel barrier. With the light-filter cover replaced, clean, dry hands can be slid through the light-tight baffles to access the unit. With hands inside, the radiographer will place

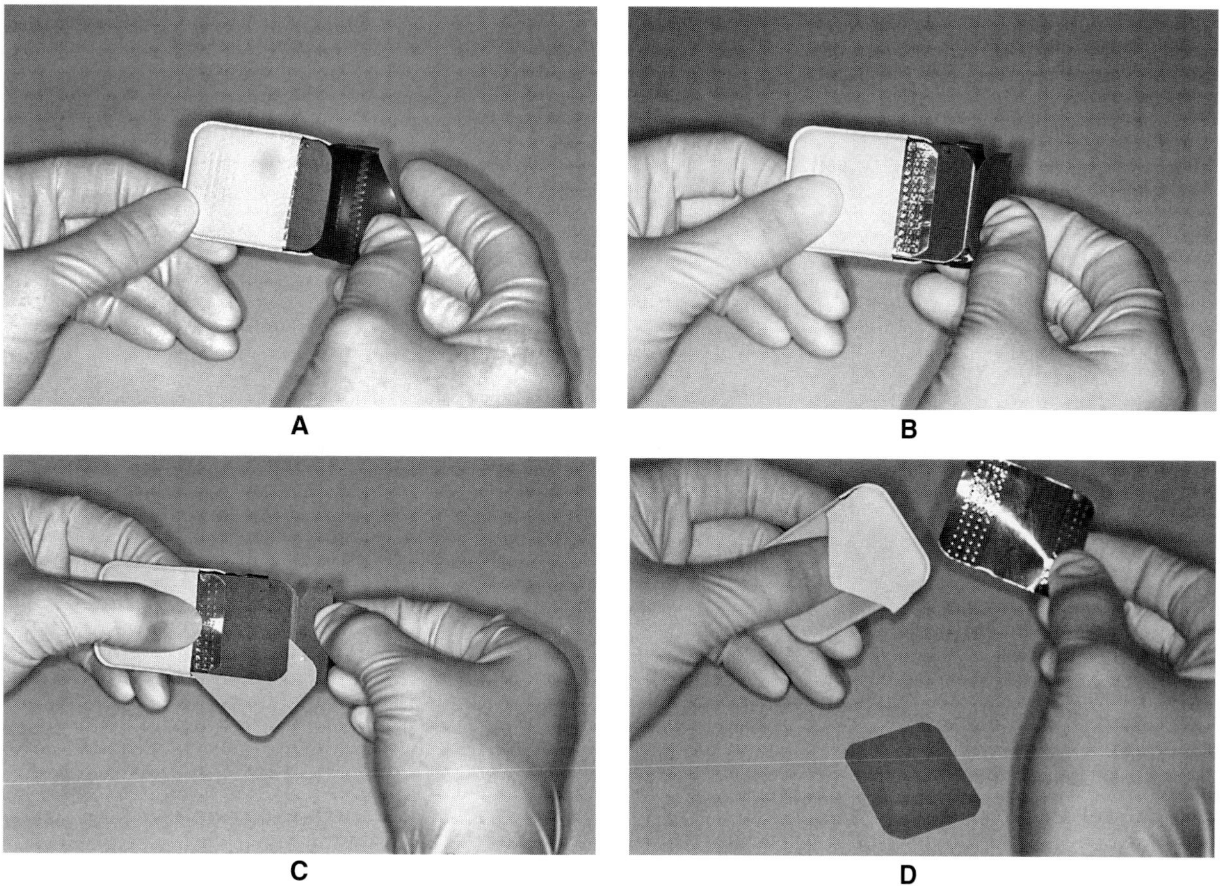

FIGURE 9–10 **Steps for removing film from packet without touching film with contaminated gloves.** (**A**) Open the film packet by lifting the plastic tab. (**B**) Locate the folded tab of black paper and grasp with finger and thumb. (**C**) Gently pull on the black paper tab sliding the film out of the packet. (**D**) Allow the film to drop out onto the plastic or paper towel barrier placed on the counter. Separate the lead foil from the rest of the packet and dispose of all materials appropriately.

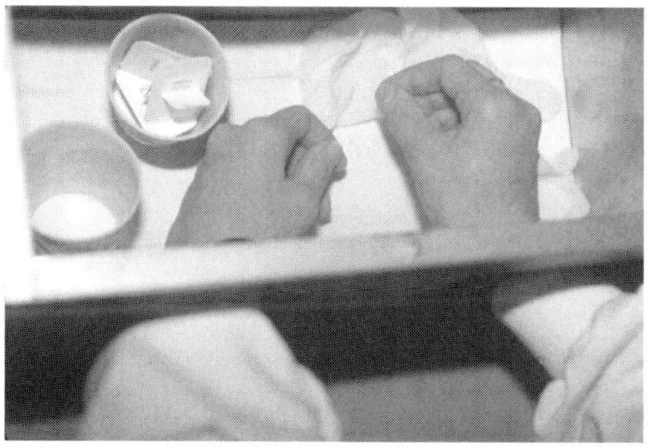

FIGURE 9–11 **Daylight loader with cover removed.** The operator placed clean, dry hands through the baffles. Note that gloves will be put on once the hands are inside the unit.

the treatment gloves on, open the film packets, separate the lead foil, and contain all contaminated items. Once all the film packets have been opened, the gloves are removed and placed with the contaminated items and the films can be loaded in the automatic processor with clean, dry hands. The ungloved hands are removed through the light-tight baffles and the light-filter cover is opened to remove the discarded items and clean and disinfect the inside of the unit. The key to infection control using the daylight loader is never to slide anything through the light-tight baffles except clean, dry hands.

Both film packets with barriers envelopes and without barrier envelopes may be processed via a daylight loader.

PROCEDURE 9–6

PROTOCOL FOR PROCESSING RADIOGRAPHIC FILMS USING A DAYLIGHT LOADER ATTACHMENT

1. Transport the contaminated film packets to the automatic processor equipped with the daylight loader attachment.
2. Obtain a clean pair of patient treatment gloves.
3. Open the light-filter cover and line the floor of the daylight loader compartment with a clean paper towel or plastic barrier. Designate one side as the contaminated side and the other side as uncontaminated.
4. Place the cup with the film packets on the contaminated side and a clean pair of patient treatment gloves on the uncontaminated side inside the daylight loader.
5. Replace the light-filter cover.
6. Slide clean, dry hands through the light-tight baffles.
7. Once inside, put on the pair of clean patient treatment gloves.
8. Open each film packet (Figure 9–10).
   a. Peel back the outer plastic/paper wrap using the tab on the back of the packet.
   b. Grasp the black paper with film sandwiched in between and pull straight out.
   c. Allow the film to drop onto the paper towel or plastic barrier on the uncontaminated side of the floor of the compartment. Do not touch the film with contaminated client gloves.
9. Drop the contaminated film packet onto the paper towel on the contaminated side of the floor of the compartment.
10. Repeat steps 8 and 9 until all film packets have been opened.
11. Remove patient treatment gloves and place on the contaminated side of the paper towel on the floor of the compartment.
12. With clean, dry hands, grasp by the edges and place films into the automatic processor feeder slots for processing.
13. When the films are safely in the automatic processor, remove ungloved hands through the light-tight baffles.
14. Wash and dry hands.*
15. Put on utility gloves.
16. Open the light-filter cover and separate the lead foil from the film packets, and dispose of appropriately. Remove the cup, contaminated film packet outer plastic/paper wrap, and paper towels or plastic barrier and discard appropriately.
17. Clean and disinfect the inside of the compartment.
18. Wash, dry and remove utility gloves. Disinfect.
19. Wash and dry hands.*

* If hands are not visibly soiled, an alcohol-containing preparation designed for reducing the number of viable microorganisms on the hands may be used. Refer to manufacturer's recommendations for use.

REVIEW—Chapter Summary

The purpose of infection control is to prevent the transmission of disease between patient and operators and between patients. Standard precautions must be taken to treat every patient as if known to be infectious.

The chain of infection involves a susceptible host, pathogens in sufficient numbers to initiate infection, and an appropriate route for the pathogen to enter the host. The oral healthcare practice should have a written infection control policy.

Personal protective equipment (PPE) is used to prevent the transmission of infective microorganisms. Protective clothing, masks, eyewear, and gloves worn by the oral healthcare professional act as barriers to prevent the transmission of infective microorganisms. Hands should be washed thoroughly before and after treating each patient.

Disinfection and sterilization breaks the "chain of infection" to prevent the transmission of infective microorganisms. Radiographic equipment and instruments may be classified as semicritical or noncritical, and should be sterilized or disinfected accordingly. Specific step-by-step infection control procedures are carried out prior to, during, and after film exposure.

Recommended step-by-step procedures for handling film with and without barrier envelopes is presented. Darkroom infection control protocol must be mastered by the radiographer to prevent lost or fogged radiographs. Strict infection control protocol must be followed when using daylight loaders.

RECALL—Study Questions

1. The purpose of infection control is to prevent the transmission of disease between:
   a. Patients.
   b. Patient and operator.
   c. Operator and patient.
   d. All of the above.
2. All of the following will break the chain of infection *except* one. Which one is this *exception?*
   a. Increasing the number of pathogens
   b. Use of sterilizaton
   c. Immunization of oral health care practitioners
   d. Use of personal protective equipment
3. An approach to infection control protection that states that the body fluids of all patients should be treated as if infected is:
   a. Universal precautions.
   b. Standard precautions.
   c. Parenteral exposures.
   d. Occupational exposures.
4. List 4 items of personal protective equipment recommended for the dental radiographer:
   a. ____________________
   b. ____________________
   c. ____________________
   d. ____________________
5. Which of the following is the correct order for maintaining infection control when applying personal protective equipment?
   a. Gloves, mask, eyewear, gown
   b. Gloves, eyewear, gown, mask
   c. Gown, mask, eyewear, gloves
   d. Gown, gloves, eyewear, mask
6. Film-holding instruments are classified as:
   a. Critical objects.
   b. Semicritical objects.
   c. Noncritical objects.
   d. Environmental objects.
7. After use the lead apron should be:
   a. Sterilized.
   b. Disinfected with a low-level disinfectant..
   c. Disinfected with an intermediate-level disinfectant.
   d. Disinfected with a high-level disinfectant.
8. All of the following may be protected with a plastic barrier to maintain infection control during the radiographic procedure *except* one. Which one is this *exception?*
   a. Film packet
   b. Film holder
   c. Exposure button
   d. PID and tube head
9. Following the radiographic procedure, the patient treatment area may be cleaned and disinfected using:
   a. Clean, dry hands.
   b. Patient treatment gloves.
   c. Plastic overgloves.
   d. Utility gloves.
10. Which of the following is the correct order for maintaining infection control after the radiographic procedure?
    a. Remove patient treatment gloves, remove lead apron, put on utility gloves, clean and disinfect
    b. Remove lead apron, remove patient treatment gloves, put on utility gloves, clean and disinfect
    c. Remove lead apron, clean and disinfect, remove patient treatment gloves, put on utility gloves
    d. Put on utility gloves, remove lead apron, clean and disinfect, remove patient treatment gloves

REFLECT—Case Study

While exposing a full mouth series of radiographs on your patient, you accidentally drop the film-holding device on the floor. Since you still have additional exposures to complete, you need the use of this device. Explain in detail what infection control protocol you would follow to deal with this dilemma.

RELATE—Laboratory Application

For a comprehensive laboratory practice exercise on this topic, see E. M. Thomson, *Exercises in Oral Radiography Techniques: A Laboratory Manual,* 2nd ed., Upper Saddle River, NJ: Prentice Hall, 2007. Chapter 6, "Infection Control and Student Partner Practice."

BIBLIOGRAPHY

Brand, J., Benson, B., & Ciola, B. American Academy of Oral and Maxillofacial Radiology infection control guidelines for dental radiographic procedures. *Oral Surg. Oral Med. Oral Pathol.* 3:48–249, 1992.

Cottone, J. A., Terezhalmy, G. T., & Molinari, J. A. *Practical Infection Control in Dentistry,* 2nd ed. Philadelphia: Lippincott Williams & Wilkins,1996.

Dietz-Bourguignon, E., & Badavinac, R. *Safety Standards and Infection Control for Dental Hygienists.* Albany: Delmar, Thomson Learning, 2002.

Huber, M. A., Holton, R. H., & Terezhalmy, G. T. Cost analysis of hand hygiene using antimicrobial soap and water versus an alcohol-based hand rub. *Oral Surg. Oral Med. Oral Pathol.* 99:4, 2005.

Karpay, R. I., Plamondon, T. J., & Dove, S. B. Infection control in dental radiology. *Operatory Infection Control Update.* 5:1–6, 1997.

Kohn, W. G., Harte, J. A., Malvitz, D. M., Collins, A. S., Cleveland, J. L., & Eklund, K. J. Guidelines for infection control in dental health care settings—2003. *JADA* 135:33–47, 2004.

Proceedings of the National Symposium on Hepatitis B and the Dental Profession. *JADA* 110:613–650, 1995.

Puttaiah, R., Langlais, R. P., Katz, J. O., & Langland, O. E. Infection control in dental radiology. *J. Calif. Dent. Assoc.* 23:21–28, 1995.

U.S. Dept. of Health and Human Services for Disease Control and Prevention, Centers for Disease Control and Prevention. *Guidelines for Infection Control in Dental Health-Care Settings. MMWR* 52(RR17), 1–61, Dec. 19, 2003.

U.S. Dept. of Health and Human Services for Disease Control and Prevention, Centers for Disease Control and Prevention. *Guideline for Hand Hygiene in Health Care Settings: Recommendations of the Healthcare Infection Control Practices Advisory Committee and the HICPAC/SHEA/APIC/IDSA Hand Hygiene Task Force. MMWR 51*(RR16);1–44, Oct. 25, 2002.

Wilkins, E. M. *Clinical Practice of the Dental Hygienist,* 9th ed. Philadelphia: Lippincott Williams & Wilkins, 2005.

10

Legal and Ethical Responsibilities

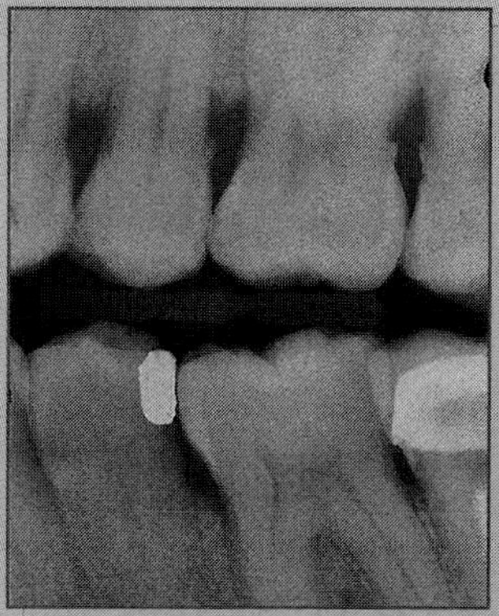

CHAPTER OUTLINE

■ OBJECTIVES

Following successful completion of this chapter, you should be able to:

1. Define the key words.
2. Discuss the federal and state regulations concerning the use of dental x-ray equipment.
3. Describe licensure requirements for exposing dental radiographs.
4. Identify specific risk management strategies for radiography.
5. Recognize negative remarks about radiographic equipment that should be avoided.
6. List the five aspects of informed consent.
7. List the radiographic items that must be documented in the patient's record.
8. Explain what should be said to patients who refuse radiographs.
9. Identify the role professional ethics play in guiding the radiographer's behavior.

■ KEY WORDS

American Dental Assistants Association (ADAA)
American Dental Association (ADA)
American Dental Hygienists' Association (ADHA)
Code of Ethics
Confidentiality
Consumer-Patient Health and Safety Act
Direct supervision
Disclosure
Ethics
Federal Performance Act of 1974
Health Insurance Portability and Accountability Act (HIPAA)
Informed consent
Liable
Malpractice
Negligence
Risk management
Self-determination
Statute of limitations

Introduction

Legal and ethical issues directly relate to radiation safety. The dental radiographer must understand and respect the law governing the use of ionizing radiation. Additionally, the radiographer should be aware of the dental profession's codes of ethics that guide decisions regarding the use of ionizing radiation. The purpose of this chapter is to discuss regulations that apply to dental radiography and to present the ethical use of dental radiographs.

Regulations and Licensure

To perform radiographic services for patients safely and legally, the dental radiographer should be aware of the laws and regulations pertaining to dental radiology. This is especially important since laws vary from state to state and often change to meet the changing needs of society.

Equipment Regulations

There are both federal and state regulations that control the manufacture and use of x-ray equipment. The **Federal Performance Act of 1974** requires that all x-ray equipment manufactured or sold in the United States meet federal performance standards. These standards include safety requirements for filtration, collimation, and other x-ray machine characteristics.

In addition to federal regulations, there are city, county, and state laws that affect the use of dental x-ray equipment. Most state laws require registration and inspection of x-ray machines. Inspections are conducted every 2 to 4 years, and usually fees are collected for this service. Because laws and regulations vary for each state and are subject to change, the dental radiographer should contact the state's bureau of radiological health for specific information.

Licensure Requirements

Additionally, there are laws that establish guidelines regarding who can place and expose radiographs. In 1981, then updated in 1991, the federal **Consumer-Patient Radiation Health and Safety Act** was passed and signed into law to protect patients from unnecessary radiation. This act established minimum standards for state certification and licensure of personnel who administer radiation in medical and dental radiographic procedures. The intent of the act was to minimize unnecessary exposure to potentially hazardous radiation.

Adoption of the act's standards was made discretionary with each state. As a result, not all states have voluntarily established licensure laws for personnel who place and expose dental radiographs. Nevertheless, most state laws require that operators of x-ray equipment be trained and certified or licensed to take dental radiographs. Many states consider dental hygienists and dental assistants who have passed the National Board Dental Hygiene Examine (NBDHE) and the Dental Assisting National Board Examination (DANB) respectively, and hold a license to practice in the state as a Registered Dental Hygienist or Certified Dental Assistant, respectively, to meet this requirement. However, there are states that require dental hygienists and dental assistants to take an additional examination, or to fulfill continuing education requirements annually to be certified specifically in radiation safety or radiographic technique competency.

State laws regulating personnel who expose dental radiographs vary considerably for on-the-job trained dental assistants. Whereas many states have a mandatory state examination or a continuing education requirement, some states allow these uncertified dental assistants with proper training to take radiographs under the direct supervision of a dentist without certification. **Direct supervision** means the dentist is present in the office when the radiographs are taken. Each state's Dental Commission controls the scope of practice for assistants and hygienists. Because laws and regulations vary for each state and are subject to change, the dental radiographer should contact the state's Dental Commission directly to learn about legal requirements for placing and exposing dental radiographs in that state. A complete list of state Dental Commisions can be viewed on the American Dental Association's website (www.ada.org) (Table 10–1).

Legal Aspects

To aid in ensuring that one is practicing within the scope of the law, the dental radiographer should be familiar with all laws and regulations pertaining to dental radiography.

Risk Management

The most important legal aspect of dental radiology is **risk management.** Risk management can be defined as the policies and procedures to be followed by the radiographer to reduce the

TABLE 10-1 **Web Sites for Professional Organizations**

American Dental Assistant Association (ADAA)	www.dentalassistant.org
American Dental Hygienists' Association (ADHA)	www.adha.org
American Dental Association (ADA)	www.ada.org
Hispanic Dental Association (HDA)	www.hdassoc.org
National Dental Association (NDA)	www.ndaonline.org
National Dental Assistants Association (NDAA)	Link from www.ndaonline.org
National Dental Hygienists Association (NDHA)	www.ndhaonline.org

chances that a patient will file legal action against the dentist and oral healthcare team. Malpractice actions have increased in number and amount of awards in recent years. All members of the oral healthcare team must participate to make an effective risk management program. Following standard procedures and performing procedures correctly will help reach the goal of providing quality care and minimizing risk. (See Table 10–2 for a radiography mini-audit for avoiding risk.)

Specific risk management procedures that can be a good defense when performed correctly or a liability if performed poorly include: attempting to obtain a duplicate copy of a new patient's radiographs before re-exposing the patient to ionizing radiation; using the best equipment currently available, including fast speed film, leaded aprons and thyroid collars, film-holding devices, collimination; and establishing a written quality assurance system for the darkroom to include daily, weekly, and monthly evaluation. Providing all radiographers with a radiation monitoring badge, whether required by law or not, is also a good risk management tool (Figure 10–1). Monitoring radiation exposure, or more precisely the lack of exposure, will provide the practice with documentation of safe work habits.

TABLE 10-2 **Radiography Safety Audit for Risk Management**

- Are all radiographers legally licensed, or certified, or properly trained to work with the x-ray equipment?
- Are radiographers' licenses, registrations, certificates, and continuing education achievements posted for public view?
- Are equipment inspection certificates posted near or on the x-ray equipment as may be required by law?
- Are accident prevention signs in place as needed? (i.e., to watch head when pulling x-ray tube head away from the wall)
- Are signs posted regarding the use of ionizing radiation as may be required by law?
- Does the radiographer wear personal protective equipment (PPE) during the procedure?
- Are all radiographers required to wear a radiation dosimeter?
- Are radiation safety rules posted near the x-ray units?
- Are exposure settings for types of projections and patients posted near the control panel?
- Is a signed informed consent from the patient secured prior to radiography procedure?
- Are adequate records kept on patient exposures? (consent, assessment of need, number and type of exposures, re-takes, name of radiographer who took the radiographs)
- Are patient radiographs kept confidential? How?
- Will patient radiographs be interpreted thoroughly and findings documented and communicated to the patient following the appointment?
- Is x-ray equipment up to date on all required inspections?
- Is documentation on quality control tests performed on all darkroom equipment kept?
- Does the radiographer wear impervious gloves and gowns and safety goggles when handling processing chemistry?
- Is an emergency eye wash station near where processing chemistry is handled?
- Do all radiographers or handlers of chemicals know the location of the hazardous chemicals lists?
- Is emergency spill equipment available?

Patient Relations

Patient relations refers to the relationship between the patient and the dental radiographer. It is important to make the patient feel comfortable by establishing a relaxing and confident chairside manner (see Chapter 11). Always explain to the patient what and how procedures are to be performed. Answer all questions the patient may have concerning the procedures. Good patient relations reduces the risk of possible legal actions.

Avoid negative remarks about procedures, equipment, and the dental staff. Statements like, "The films got stuck in the processor again" or "This tube head always drifts" should never be made to the patient or in front of the patient. These statements imply that you have chosen to use known defective equipment on a patient. This is not the same as saying, "The films got stuck in the processor. They must be re-taken. However, we will not process the new films until a thorough investigation is made to correct the problem with the processor." or "This tube head is drifting. Since this is a problem, we can not use it to take your x-rays until it is repaired. Let's move to another room for your procedure." If equipment is not working properly, it should be repaired or serviced.

Informed Consent

Informed consent is the consent the patient gives for treatment after being informed of the nature and purpose of all treatment procedures.

All patients have the legal right to make choices about the health care they receive. This is called **self-determination.** Self-determination includes the right to refuse treatment. To make a

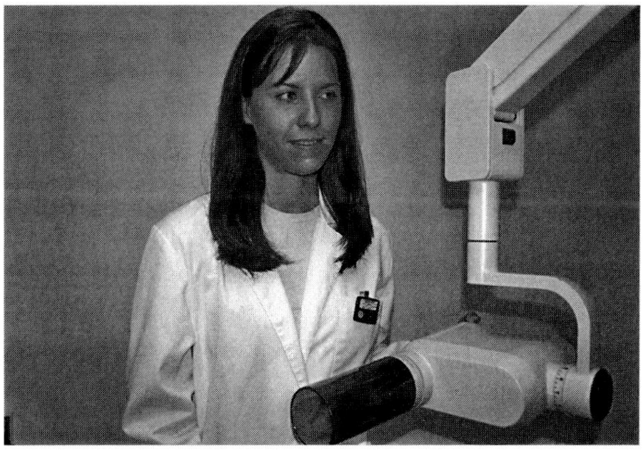

FIGURE 10-1 **Radiographer wearing a radiation monitoring badge.**

decision regarding informed consent, the patient must be informed of the following:

- The purpose of taking radiographs
- The benefits the radiographs will supply
- The possible risks of radiation exposure
- The possible risks of refusing the radiographs
- The person who will perform the procedure

It is the responsibility of the dentist to explain the nature and purpose of all treatment procedures. When taking radiographs, the risks and benefits must be explained in lay terms. The informing process is called **disclosure.** The patient should be given the opportunity to ask questions prior to radiography. Answer all questions completely in terms the patient understands. State laws vary concerning informed consent. Be sure to become familiar with your state laws.

Liability

Liable means to be legally obligated to make good any loss or damage that may occur. Many states have laws that require dentists to supervise the performance of dental radiographers. Both dentists and dental radiographers are liable for procedures performed by the dental radiographer. Therefore, it is important to understand that even though radiographers work under the supervision of the dentist, they are legally liable for their own actions. In malpractice cases, both the supervising dentist and the dental radiographer may be sued for the actions of the radiographer.

Patient Records

A record of all aspects of dental care must be kept for every patient. Dental radiographs are considered a part of the patient's record and are therefore legal documents.

Documentation

The exposure of dental radiographs should be documented in the patient's record. Entries in the patient's record should be made by the dentist or under the dentist's supervision. The following items must be documented in the patient's record.

- The patient's informed consent
- The number and type of radiographs, including re-takes
- The date the radiographs are taken and the name of the radiographer who took them
- The reason for taking the radiographs
- The interpretive results

Confidentiality

State laws have always governed **confidentiality** to protect the patient's privacy. On April 14, 2003, the federal government signed into law privacy standards to protect patients' medical records and other health information, including radiographs. Developed by the Department of Health and Human Services (HHS) as part of the **Health Insurance Portability and Accountability Act** of 1996 **(HIPAA),** this new federal law is designed to provide patients with more control over how their personal health information is used and disclosed. Radiographs are confidential and should never be shown or discussed with anyone outside of the oral healthcare practice without first obtaining a current, signed release form from the patient. A patient will usually be asked to sign a notice that indicates how their radiographs may be used and their privacy rights under this new law.

Ownership

The courts have ruled that radiographs are the property of the dentist. The patient pays for the dentist's ability to interpret the radiographs and to arrive at a diagnosis. However, patients may have reasonable access to their radiographs. They may request a copy of their radiographs if they decide to change dentists or request a consultation with a dental specialist (Procedure Box 10–1). The original radiographs, however, belong to the dentist. Because of statute of limitation laws, it is recommended that all records (including radiographs) be retained indefinitely.

Retention

Dental radiographs must be retained for seven years after the patient ceases to be a patient. Legal actions that can be brought against the dentist depend on the malpractice and limitation statues that vary from state to state.

For adult patients, the statute of limitations generally begins to run at the time of the injury, or when the injury should have reasonably been discovered. For children, the statute of limitations does not begin until the child reaches the age of majority

PROCEDURE 10–1

PROCEDURE FOR RELEASING A COPY OF THE PATIENT'S RADIOGRAPHS

1. Patient requests copy of radiographs in writing.
2. Keep the letter requesting radiographs in the patient's record.
3. Duplicate the original radiographs.
4. Send the duplicate radiographs by registered or certified mail.
5. Keep the postal receipt in the patient's record.

(18 to 21 years old, depending on the state). If you work for a governmental entity, the statute of limitations may be affected by certain notice statutes, which may greatly reduce the time in which a suit may be brought. Because the time period is so indefinite, it is recommended that radiographs be retained forever.

Insurance Claims

Insurance companies have the right to request pretreatment radiographs to evaluate the dental treatment plan that they will be paying for. Again, only duplicate radiographs should be sent. The oral healthcare practice should keep the originals.

Malpractice Issues

Malpractice results when one is negligent. Negligence occurs when the dental diagnosis or treatment is below the standard of care provided by dentists in a similar locality and under similar conditions.

Negligence

Negligence is defined as the failure to use a reasonable amount of care when failure results in injury or damage to another. Negligence may result from the care (or lack of care) of either the dentist or the dental radiographer.

Statute of Limitations

Statute of limitations is the time period during which a patient may bring a malpractice action against a dentist or radiographer. State laws govern this time period, which begins when the patient discovers, or should have discovered, an injury due to negligent dental treatment.

Sometimes negligence is not discovered until years later, when a patient changes dentists and discovers an injury has occurred. In such cases, the statute of limitations begins years after the negligent dental treatment occurred. An example would be where appropriate radiographs were not taken on a patient with periodontal disease. Years later, the patient is examined by another dentist and is informed of the irreversible periodontal condition that might have been prevented if detected earlier.

Besides the statute of limitations, many states have separate malpractice laws that may limit damages or, in the case of governmental entities, may provide limited or complete immunity from suit, under certain circumstances. Because the laws vary greatly from state to state, it is desirable to consult a lawyer experienced in this area to provide training and answer questions for the entire oral healthcare practice team, as part of the risk management program.

Patients Who Refuse Radiographs

Occasionally, for a variety of reasons, patients express opposition to the dentist's proposal that x-rays be taken. Often these patients believe that such radiographs are unnecessary or that they will add to the cost of treatment, or the patient may be fearful that dental x-ray exposure will be hazardous to their health. When this happens, the dentist and radiographer must carefully explain in clear terms why the radiographs are needed to supplement the diagnosis, prognosis, or treatment plan and therefore benefit the patient.

Frequently a patient may offer to sign a paper to assume the responsibility for not taking radiographs. The patient must be informed in a diplomatic manner that legally, such documents to release the dentist from liability are not valid because the patient cannot legally consent to negligent care. If the patient still refuses the radiographs, the dentist must carefully decide whether treatment can be provided. Usually, in such cases, the dentist cannot treat the patient.

Ethics

In addition to the law, the ethics of a profession also guide the behavior of the healthcare practitioner. **Ethics** is defined as a sense of moral obligation regarding right and wrong behavior. Professional ethics define a standard by which all members of the profession are obligated to conform. These professional rules of conduct are called a profession's **Code of Ethics.** See Table 10–1 for a list of Web sites where you can locate the Code of Ethics for the **American Dental Association (ADA), American Dental Hygienists' Association (ADHA),** and **American Dental Assistants Association (ADAA).** A professional Code of Ethics helps to define the rules of conduct for its members.

Goals

Managing risk, knowing the law, and applying ethics, the dental radiographer should strive for practice that is safe, professional, and places the patient's well-being first. One achieves this by setting goals. Such goals are closely related, and all are equally important. Goals of the dental radiographer:

- **Achieve perfection with each radiograph.** This is accomplished by careful attention to details. Each step in the process, whether in film placement, exposure technique, or processing and identification is significant.
- **Perform confidently and with authority.** Patients are more likely to cooperate with someone who demonstrates self-confidence. Communicate with patients in a respectful manner.
- **Take pride in services rendered and professional advancement.** Obtain certification in radiation safety, whether or not required by law. Improve skills and update techniques by attending continuing education lectures and workshops, participating in professional association meetings, and reading professional journals and books.
- **Keep radiation exposure as low as possible.** Take the time to use protective devices that minimize radiation to the patient and follow strict protocols to protect yourself during exposures. Maintain an environment that minimizes the risk of harm.
- **Avoid retakes.** Be familiar with common errors to avoid them. Do not retake any exposure when you are not sure

of the corrective action. If the patient can not tolerate film packet placement or can not cooperate with the procedure, stop and get assistance, or try an acceptable alternative procedure.

- **Develop integrity, dedication, and competence** that promotes ethical behavior and high standards of care. Provide patients with information to assist them in making informed decisions regarding their consent to radiographic procedures. Serve all patients without discrimination.

REVIEW—Chapter Summary

The dental radiographer should be aware of the laws and regulations pertaining to dental radiography. There are both federal and state regulations that control the manufacture and use of x-ray equipment.

State laws require that operators of x-ray equipment be trained and certified or licensed to take dental radiographs. Some states may require the registered dental hygienist and the certified dental assistant to take an additional examination or continuing education course to be certified to take radiographs. Other states allow an on-the-job-trained dental assistant with proper training to place and expose radiographs under the direct supervision of the dentist.

Risk management strategies and good patient relations reduce the risk of possible legal actions. Informed consent allows the patient to make decisions regarding the procedure. Disclosure informs the patient about the radiographic procedure and answers all questions the patient may have concerning the procedures. Both the dentist and the dental radiographer are liable for procedures performed by the dental radiographer.

The patient's records, including the radiographs, are confidential. The courts have ruled that radiographs are the property of the dentist; the patient pays only for the diagnosis. However, patients may have access to their films via copies.

When an individual ceases to be a patient, the radiographs should be retained for seven years. Risk management and the statutes of limitation suggests that radiographs should be retained indefinitely.

The patient who refuses radiographs may not legally consent to negligent care. The professional's code of ethics guides the behavior of the radiographer. Goals for the dental radiographer are presented.

RECALL—Study Questions

1. Registration and inspection of x-ray machines is regulated by the:
   a. Federal government
   b. State government
   c. Local government
   d. Any of the above
2. The laws allowing individuals to place and expose dental radiographs vary from state to state.
   a. True
   b. False
3. Which of the following is a risk management strategy?
   a. The use of fast speed film, film-holding devices, and collimation
   b. Monitoring the dental radiographer with radiation dosimeters
   c. Obtaining a copy of a new patient's radiographs from a previous dentist
   d. All of the above
4. Which of these comments should be avoided when talking to the patient?
   a. "We have switched to a fast speed film."
   b. "This exposure button sticks sometimes."
   c. "You must stay still during the exposure."
   d. "I'm certified to take your radiographs."
5. List five aspects of informed consent.
   a. ____________________
   b. ____________________
   c. ____________________
   d. ____________________
   e. ____________________
6. Every patient has the legal right to make choices about the health care they receive. This is called:
   a. Disclosure.
   b. Informed consent.
   c. Self-determination.
   d. Liability.
7. List five items regarding the radiographic procedure that should be documented in the patient's record?
   a. ____________________
   b. ____________________
   c. ____________________
   d. ____________________
   e. ____________________
8. Legally dental radiographs should be retained for an individual who ceases to be a patient for:
   a. Three years.
   b. Five years.
   c. Seven years.
   d. Nine years.
9. Both the dentist and the dental radiographer are liable for procedures performed by the dental radiographer.
   a. True
   b. False
10. Failure to use a reasonable amount of care that results in injury is termed:
    a. Risk.
    b. Liability.
    c. Confidentiality.
    d. Negligence.
11. The courts have ruled that radiographs are the property of the:
    a. Patient.
    b. Dentist.
    c. Dental radiographer.
    d. The state.
12. When patients express opposition to having dental radiographs taken, the radiographer should:
    a. Ask the patient to sign a document to release the dentist of liability.
    b. Consult the professional code of ethics about what to do next.
    c. Postpone the procedure and ask the patient to return at a later date.

   d. Explain why the radiographs are needed and what the benefits will be.

13. A professional code of ethics:
   a. Makes the laws that govern the use of dental radiographs.
   b. Establishes the time frame for taking dental radiographs.
   c. Helps to define the rules of conduct for its members.
   d. Protects the dental radiographer in cases of legal action.
14. All of the following are goals of the radiographer *except* one. Which one is this *exception?*
   a. Increasing the demand for dental x-ray services
   b. Reducing the radiation dose used during an exposure
   c. Professional improvement and advancement
   d. Presenting confidence to gain patient acceptance

REFLECT—Case Study

Consider the following scenario.

You have been working in a practice for over a year and have developed a friendship with another dental assistant. You often socialize together outside of work, and your children play together. One evening during dinner, your dental assistant friend tells you that even though she has been exposing dental radiographs on patients since she was hired by the practice over two years ago, she does not have the state-required radiation safety certification. She tells you that the dentist never asked to see her certificate during the job interview. She wasn't planning to "break the law" but the first day on the job, the dentist explained to a patient that she would be taking the full mouth series, and "not to worry, because she was a competent clinician." Your friend explains to you that it would have been embarrassing to tell the dentist at that point that she was not certified, so she exposed the films. After that, she thought about taking a course to prepare for the state examination, but didn't want to get "caught" taking the exam after she had already been placing and exposing radiographs all this time. She hopes you will keep her confidence, since you are friends.

Reflect on this scenario and answer the following questions.

1. How has your friend broken the law?
2. How has this behavior endangered the patient? Your friend? Your employer?
3. Describe the legal and/or ethical situation she faces.
4. Describe the legal and/or ethical dilemma you face.
5. How could your employer have prevented this situation?
6. What aspects of the Dental or Dental Assisting Code of Ethics apply to this situation?
7. Take the role of your friend; what would you have done if you were she?

RELATE—Laboratory Practice

Using the computer, visit the Web sites for the board of radiological health or the board of dentistry in all 50 states and the District of Columbia. Compile a listing of states with certification requirements for dental radiographers and answer the following questions.

1. How many states require all radiographers to be certified for performing radiographic procedures?
2. What states accept a registered dental hygienist's or certified dental assistant's credentials as certification for performing radiographic procedures?
3. Are there states that require additional tests or continuing education classes for a dental assistant or dental hygienist to maintain radiographic certification?
4. Why do you think some states do not require certification for those individuals who place and expose dental radiographs?
5. What are the advantages to the oral healthcare practice to hire only certified radiographers?
6. How should the public be educated on these laws governing the certification of individuals to place and expose dental radiographs?

BIBLIOGRAPHY

Bundy, A. L. *Radiology and the Law.* Rockville, MD: Aspen, 1988.

Darby, M. L. & Walsh, M. M. *Dental Hygiene Theory and Practice,* 2nd ed. St. Louis: Saunders, 2003.

Davison, J. A. *Legal and Ethical Considerations for Dental Hygienists and Assistants.* St. Louis: C.V. Mosby, 2000.

U.S. Dept. of Health and Human Services. *Fact Sheet: Protecting the privacy of patients' health information.* www.hhs.gov/news/facts/privacy.html.

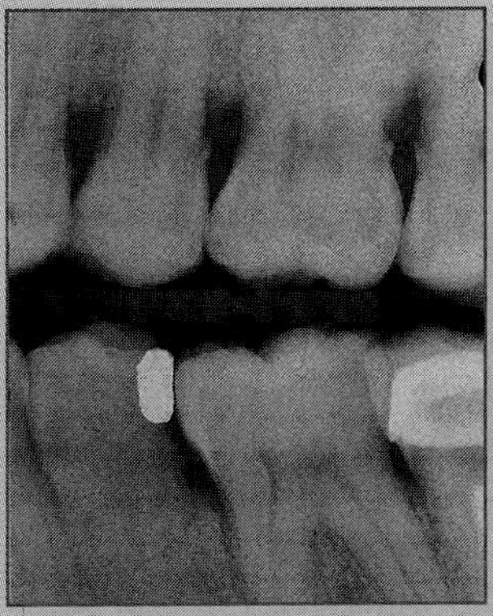

11

Patient Relations and Education

CHAPTER OUTLINE

■ OBJECTIVES

Following successful completion of this chapter, you should be able to:

1. Define key words.
2. Value the need for patient cooperation in producing quality radiographs.
3. List the aspects of patient relations that help to gain confidence and cooperation.
4. Explain how appearance and first impression affect patient relations.
5. Identify five areas where the radiographer's positive attitude will foster patient confidence.
6. State examples of interpersonal skills that are used to communicate effectively.
7. Explain the relationship between verbal and nonverbal communication.
8. Give an example of a negative-sounding word that should be avoided when explaining the radiographic procedure.
9. Explain the communication method show-tell-do and give three examples of when this method would be effective.
10. State the two reasons patient education in radiography is valuable.
11. Respond to a patient's concern regarding unnecessary exposure to x-rays.
12. Describe two methods by which the patient can be educated to appreciate the value of dental radiographs.

■ KEY WORDS

Attitude
Chairside manner
Communication
Empathy
Frequently asked questions (FAQs)
Interpersonal skills
Nonverbal communication
Patient education
Patient relations
Show-tell-do
Verbal communication

Introduction

Effective communication is essential to producing quality radiographic images. The radiographic procedure requires that the patient understand and cooperate with the process. The radiographer must be able to communicate specific directions for success of the procedure. Precise patient positioning, the sometimes difficult placement of film packets in the oral cavity, and the potentially harmful nature of ionizing radiation make clear communication and good interpersonal skills especially important. The purpose of this chapter is to discuss how interpersonal skills affect the radiographic process, present guidelines for effective communication, and to investigate the role the dental assistant and the dental hygienist play in educating the patient regarding the need for dental radiographs.

Practice Point

Always greet the patient by name. Address the patient using their proper title (Miss, Mrs., Ms., Mr., Dr., etc.) and last name. If you are uncertain of the correct pronunciation of the patient's name, ask the patient to pronounce it for you. Always introduce yourself to the patient, using both your name and title. For example: "Good morning, Ms. Washington. My name is Maria Melendez. I'm the dental assistant who will be taking your radiographs today. Please follow me to the x-ray room and we will get started."

Patient Relations

Patient relations refers to the relationship between the patient and the oral healthcare professional. Appearance, attitude, interpersonal skills, and communication help gain patient confidence and cooperation, the outcome of which will be the production of quality radiographs.

Appearance

The patient's first impression of the dental radiographer is important. The first impression is often made based on the radiographer's **appearance.** The dental radiographer should always maintain a professional appearance. The careful attention given to personal hygiene and grooming such as trimmed nails, clean hands, and fresh breath convey an understanding of the importance of maintaining all aspects of infection control. A clean, neat appearance builds confidence in patients.

Attitude

Attitude is defined as the position assumed by the body in connection with a feeling or mood. Attitude will play a significant role in gaining the patient's trust in the radiographer's ability. The attitude of the radiographer toward the procedure will be conveyed to the patient. If the radiographer feels that the procedure is uncomfortable or unnecessary, these feelings will be conveyed to the patient. The radiographer should not impose his/her own feelings onto the patient. While the radiographer may have had a less than ideal experience with a certain procedure, this does not necessarily mean that the patient will experience the same discomfort. For example, the radiographer may have experienced a gag reflex when posterior periapicals were taken on him/her. If this radiographer approaches the patient with the attitude that posterior periapicals will excite a gag reflex, the outcome is likely to be just that. A fresh, positive attitude with each, new patient will more likely produce a cooperative patient. This is especially true if the patient perceives the radiographer as possessing a non-judgmental attitude.

The radiographer's attitude toward his/her own technical ability will also be conveyed to the patient. Because a demonstration of technical skill will build patient confidence, the radiographer should feel that his/her training and education adequately prepared him/her for this role. Having confidence in oneself fosters confidence in others.

Additionally, the unique close working relationship of the oral healthcare team requires that everyone work well together. Attitudes toward an employer and co-workers also play a role in determining the degree of successful patient management. Patients can sense the professional's attitude by the way he/she walks, talks, and behaves. For example, the patient will easily sense a disgruntled dental assistant who had to interrupt what he/she was doing to take radiographs for a dental hygienist who was running behind in the schedule. Maintaining a pleasant, positive attitude will help generate the same from patients.

Interpersonal Skills

Interpersonal skills are used to communicate with others successfully. Respectfulness, courtesy, empathy, patient, honest and tactful communication are examples of interpersonal skills. When explaining the need for radiographs, consider how the patient will feel. If the patient has concerns regarding the need for x-ray exposure, respect their views. Statements such as "Don't worry" and "Everything will be okay" may convey an attitude of apathy, or imply that the patient's apprehensions don't matter. If film packet placement during the radiographic procedure is uncomfortable, show empathy. **Empathy** is defined as the ability to share in another's emotions or feelings. Be courteous and polite at all times even in difficult situations. However, if discomfort must be tolerated to produce the necessary radiograph, empathetic, yet direct and tactful communication can help bring about the desired result.

An important aspect of interpersonal skills is the radiographer's chairside manner. **Chairside manner** refers to the conduct of the radiographer while working at the patient's chairside. The radiographer should strive to always make the patient feel comfortable. Working in a confident manner will help put the patient at ease. Comments that indicate a lack of control, such as "Oops!," must be avoided. An important consideration during the radiographic procedure is to praise the patient for any assistance they may give. Positive reinforcement and feedback that the procedure is going well will help foster even more cooperation. For example, letting a patient know that you appreciated their ability to hold the film holder in place long enough to make the exposure will help to motivate the patient to continue working together with you to complete the procedure. Likewise, showing frustration with a patient who is having difficulty managing the film packet placement will most likely only increase the patient's anxiety.

Practice Point

If it is necessary to place a film packet into a particularly sensitive area, encourage the patient to cooperate and praise him/her for the willingness to tolerate the difficult placement. Show empathy, but let the patient know that the placement is correct and if he/she can tolerate the discomfort for the short time required for exposure, the result will be a diagnostic quality radiograph. Avoid asking, "Does that feel okay?" The patient will perceive this to mean that discomfort equals incorrect film packet and will feel obligated to inform you of any and all feelings associated with the packet placement. The patient will now be acutely aware of the feeling of the packet in the mouth and continue to inform you regarding the "feeling" of each subsequent film, possibly making the procedure more difficult. Saying "Are you doing okay so far?" is a better way to let the patient know you are aware of their efforts to cooperate.

Communication

Communication is defined as the process by which information is exchanged between two or more persons. This may be accomplished verbally (with words) or non-verbally (without words). Effective communication is communication that works (Table 11–1).

Honesty

Verbal and nonverbal communication is essential to building patient confidence. Patient questions must be answered honestly. It is very important the radiographic procedure be explained honestly, including any possible discomfort anticipated, to gain cooperation and assistance. Honesty develops trust. When a patient trusts the dental radiographer, the patient is more likely to cooperate with the radiographic procedure.

TABLE 11–1 **Guidelines for Effective Communication**

- Introduce yourself and show interest.
- Face the patient and make eye contact.
- Lean forward to demonstrate listening.
- Be honest to build trust.
- Show courtesy and respectfulness.
- Maintain a positive attitude.
- Demonstrate empathy when appropriate.
- Use clear commands.
- Make nonverbal communication in agreement with verbal communication.

Verbal Communication

Effective use of words in **verbal communication** begins with facing the patient directly and maintaining eye contact. Since a face mask is recommended PPE (personal protective equipment) (see Chapter 9) during radiographic procedures, it is very important that the verbal requests and commands used to communicate specific directions during the radiographic procedures be understood by the patient. Once the film packet is in place, the operator needs to give explicit directions to complete the procedure quickly. For example, once the film packet is placed, the patient must be requested to bite firmly and to hold completely still while the operator leaves the area to make the exposure. The process will be hindered and prolonged if the patient does not understand the requests or the operator must repeat the commands.

Practice Point

Always give a command, and not a question, to request that the patient hold still during the exposure. For example, asking the patient "Can you hold still, please?" will most likely cause the patient to attempt to move to answer you, defeating the purpose of your request. The command, "Hold still, please" is less likely to prompt the patient to move.

The radiographer's choice of words and sentence structure are also important. Words used should be at a level the patient can understand. For example, young children may better understand, "These are pictures of the teeth made with a special dental camera" (Table 11–2). An adult would appreciate hearing a more professional sounding "Here's a radiograph showing your periodontal condition." However, too many highly technical words may confuse the patient and result in misunderstandings. Words that imply negative images such as "zap," "shot," and "irradiate" are better avoided.

TABLE 11-2 Guidelines for Communicating with Children

- Use guidelines for effective communication.
- Use age-level appropriate language.
- Do not talk down or use baby talk.
- Avoid threatening-sounding words.
- Expain the procedure simply and clearly.
- Use show-tell-do.
- Tell the truth whenever possible.

TABLE 11-3 Guidelines for Communicating with the Elderly

- Use guidelines for effective communication.
- Address by the person's title unless they instruct you otherwise.
- Avoid condescending salutations such as "Honey" and "Dear."
- Be aware of generational differences.
- Be aware of sensory or cognitive impairments such as hearing loss, effects of stroke.
- Encourage the use of eyeglasses and hearing aids during the procedure and especially when showing radiographs during patient education.

Practice Point

Sentence structure is important for the short, precise directions needed for radiographic procedures. For example, requesting that the patient bite down on the film holder by saying, "Close slowly, please" may prompt the patient to close before the operator says the word "slowly." Rearranging the words to say "Slowly close, please" may be more likely to produce the desired result.

Nonverbal Communication

Nonverbal communication includes gestures, facial expressions, body movement, and listening. A nod of the head indicates yes or agreement, while a shake of the head indicates no or disagreement. We usually use a combination of verbal and nonverbal communication. Nonverbal communication is very believable. When verbal and nonverbal communications are not in synch, it is often the nonverbal communication that conveys the strongest message. For example, if you tell the patient that you don't mind that they have to stop and take a break in between each radiographic exposure, but you roll your eyes or tap your foot while waiting for them to feel ready to begin again, the patient will probably not believe you, because your actions speak louder than your words. Facial expressions strongly convey the attitude of the radiographer. A smile by the radiographer will likely relax the patient and reduce apprehension.

It is just as important that the radiographer practice good listening skills. Careful attention to listening results in fewer misunderstandings. Eye contact and attentive body posturing communicates warmth and caring to the patient. Additionally, the radiographer should listen to the patient's nonverbal communication. There is most likely something wrong with a patient who is clutching the arms of the treatment chair with tears in her eyes, even if she has not verbally communicated with you.

The use of **show-tell-do** as a method of combined verbal and nonverbal communication is useful in dental radiography, especially when barriers to communication exist such as in the case of a language or cultural difference, a sensory impairment, or a cognitive impairment (Tables 11–3 and 11–4). Showing a radiograph to the patient will help to explain what the procedure is. A film holder can be used to show and demonstrate PID placement. Showing all patients the film and film-holding devices can help alleviate apprehension regarding the procedure.

Patient Education in Radiography

Educating patients about the importance of dental radiographs in comprehensive oral health care depends on the radiographer's ability to communicate (Figure 11–1). This communication ability is based on the radiographer's knowledge, education and training in the area of dental radiology. It is surprising how many patients, even today, do not comprehend the enormous value of a radiographic examination of their teeth and the supporting oral structures.

Value of Patient Education

The value of **patient education** is twofold. First is the understanding that dental radiographs disclose pathology (disease) that might otherwise go undetected, and become an increasing threat to the patient's health if not treated in a timely manner. Second is that the educated patient is more inclined to understand and accept dental treatment plans and embrace suggestions for oral health promotion and disease prevention. Such patient acceptance helps to develop a spirit of confidence and mutual trust in the oral healthcare practice.

TABLE 11-4 Guidelines for Communicating with People of Different Cultures

- Use guidelines for effective communication.
- Learn about the cultures in your community.
- Be accepting and non-judgmental.
- Be aware that gestures may be interpreted differently.
- Be aware that touch and personal space are sometimes considered differently by different cultures.
- Speak slowly and avoid the use of slang or uncommon terms.
- Verify that the listener has understood what you said.

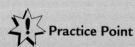

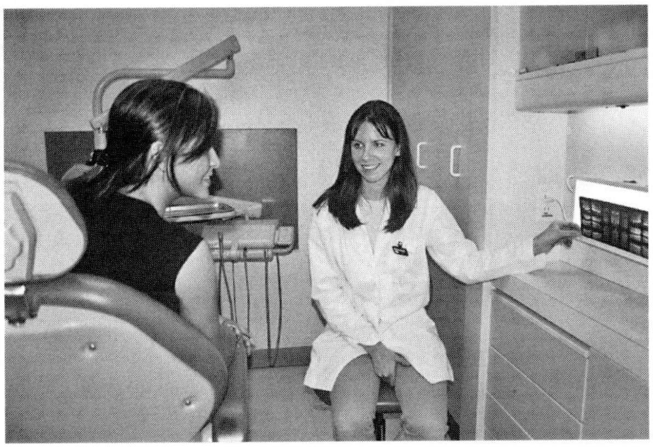

FIGURE 11–1 **Patient education. The dental radiographer educates the patient on the value of radiographs.**

Necessity for Patient Education

Most people have heard negative reports regarding the effects of overexposure to radiation. The dental patient, when faced with a treatment plan recommending radiographs, will rightfully question the necessity of being exposed to x-radiation. It is the responsibility of the entire dental team to provide the patient with clear, concise, and satisfactory answers regarding any questions or concerns he/she may have. Acceptance of the dental treatment plan is more likely not only when a satisfactory explanation of need is presented, but when the patient is given an explanation of the ethical safeguards the practice has adopted to reduce the risk of harm.

Identifying with the patient's concerns is the first step to open communication. The radiographer can verbally agree with the patient that excess radiation exposure is a concern and that the practice has adopted a strict radiation safety program. Patient acceptance and confidence increase when he/she is made aware of the many safety protocols the practice has put into place.

To begin the conversation, the patient should be told about the evidenced-based selection criteria guidelines developed by an expert panel of health care professionals and recently updated (2004) by the American Dental Association that aid the dentist in deciding when, what type, and how many radiographs should be taken (see Chapter 6). These evidenced-based guidelines are the single biggest factor in eliminating unnecessary radiographs.

Further, the patient should be informed that all standard safety protocols as suggested by federal agencies, such as the National Council on Radiation Protection and Measurements, and the state and local laws governing inspections, calibrations and the use of radiological equipment are being adhered to. Many people may not realize that x-ray equipment is strictly regulated by law.

In some locations, laws also regulate who can operate the dental x-ray machine. Where applicable, individuals who place and expose radiographs must be educated and trained, and pass an examination prior to being certified as "radiation-safe" to place and expose dental radiographs. If the state issues a license or a certificate of compliance to show that a radiation safety examination has been passed, that can be offered in evidence. Many radiographers display their certificates near the x-ray machine. Patient confidence in the radiographer increases when he/she knows that the professional has been educated or trained and has passed a certification exam in the safety protocols governing the use of x-radiation.

The patient should be assured that everyone in the office who works with the dental x-ray machine, regardless of state-mandated certification, is trained in its use and the safety aspects of radiation. Continuing education courses in radiology taken by the radiographer also boost patient confidence and elevate the practice as one that values competency.

Finally, the patient and radiographer may have a discussion about equipment specially designed to reduce radiation exposure, such as collimated position indicating devices (PIDs), thyroid collars and protective lead aprons, fast speed film, and modern equipment that is better constructed to prevent unnecessary radiation. The patient may not be aware of the reasoning behind the use of these devices. Many patients assume the lead apron is only for pregnant females and may be unaware that utilizing a film holder prevents them from having to hold the film in their mouth and unnecessarily expose their fingers.

Methods of Patient Education

The patient can be educated on the value of radiographs through verbal discussion or via printed literature, or a combination of both. Backing up your verbal explanation with a printed brochure is very effective at getting the message across. Literature may be obtained from professional organizations and commercial dental product companies, and off the Web. However, care should be taken to use reliable sources of literature. The radiographer should be aware of misleading sources of information, especially those readily available to patients on the Web. The radiographer should be prepared to help the patient separate correct information from incorrect or misleading information.

Oral Presentation

An effective method of educating the patient is to give an oral presentation using a series of radiographs showing typical dental conditions, both normal and abnormal. Placed in convenient mounts, the radiographs are shown to the patient on a screen or an illuminated viewer (Figure 11–1).

The viewer-enlargers shown in Figures 11–2 and 11–3 are well suited for enlarging radiographs. Patients are generally able to identify the areas that are pointed out to them on the radiographs better if the images are magnified and the brightness of the light is controlled. A sample set of radiographs will allow the radiographer to explain the value of the use of radiographs in the patient's oral care plan. When viewing the patient's own radiographs, the radiographer should remember that all members of the oral health care team can interpret radiographs, but it is the dentist's responsibility to make the final interpretation and diagnosis. The difference between interpretation and diagnosis is discussed in Chapter 18.

Printed Literature

An effective education method is to place printed literature in the reception area or to give it to patients before their x-ray appointment. Giving pamphlets to the patient opens the door for

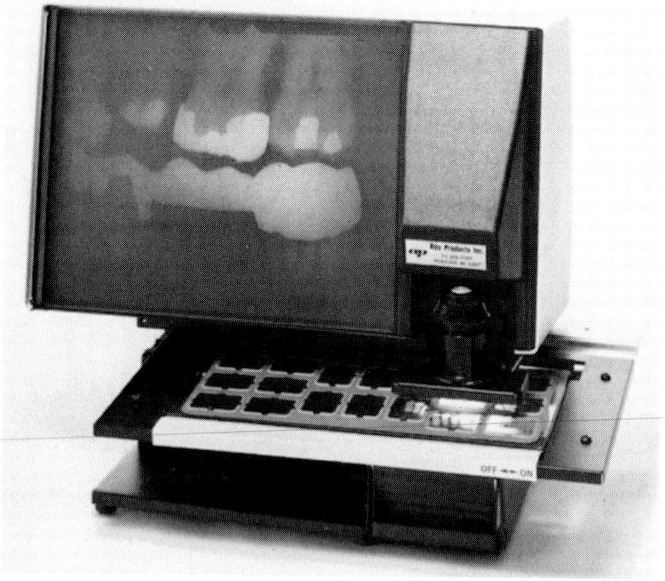

FIGURE 11-2 **Viewer-enlarger.** (Courtesy of Ada Products, Inc.)

two-way communication on the advisability and necessity of regular radiographic examinations. All too often the patient is simply told that the doctor requires radiographs and will not treat the patient unless they are taken, or else the explanation is limited to a few short and often unsatisfactory answers.

Literature may be obtained from one's professional association (American Dental Association, American Dental Hygienists' Association, American Dental Assistants Association) or can be custom produced to meet the needs of the practice (Table 11–5).

Frequently Asked Questions

Here are some examples of **frequently asked questions (FAQs)** and answers reprinted from the American Dental Association brochure Dental X-ray Examinations: Your Dentist's Advice and Web site (www.ada.org/public/topics/xrays_Faq.asp) and from the Academy of General Dentistry's Web site (www.agd.org/consumer/topics/xrays/main.asp).

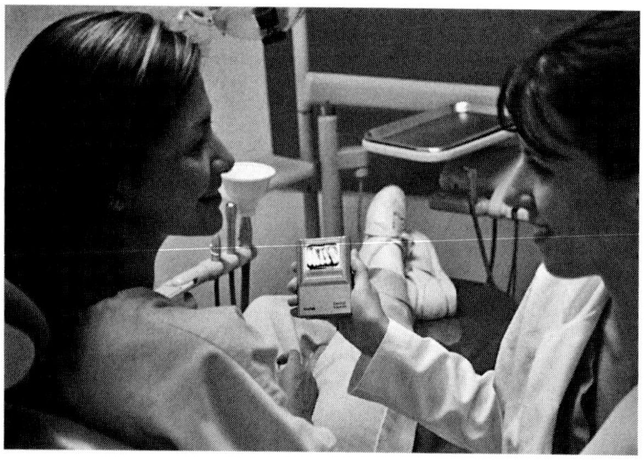

FIGURE 11-3 **Handheld viewer-enlarger** is a helpful adjunct to patient education.

QUESTION: What are the benefits of dental x-rays?

ANSWER: Many diseases of the teeth and surrounding tissues cannot be seen through a visual examination alone. An x-ray examination may reveal:

- Small areas of decay between the teeth.
- Infections in the bone.
- Abscesses or cysts.
- Developmental abnormalities.
- Some types of tumors.

Finding and treating oral health problems at an early stage can save time, money, and unnecessary discomfort. Radiographs can detect damage to oral structures not visible during a regular exam. If you have a hidden tumor, radiographs may even help save your life.

QUESTION: How often should x-rays be taken?

ANSWER: How often radiographs (dental x-rays) should be taken depends on the patient's individual health needs. It is important to recognize that just as each patient is different from the next, so should the scheduling of x-ray exams be individualized for each patient. The dentist will review your history, examine your mouth and then decide whether you need radiographs and what type. If you are a new patient, the dentist may recommend radiographs to determine the present status of the hidden areas of your mouth and to help analyze changes that may occur later.

The schedule for needing radiographs at recall visits varies according to your age, risk for disease, and signs and symptoms. Recent films may be needed to detect new cavities, to determine the status of gum disease, or for evaluation of growth and development. Children may need x-rays more often than adults. This is because their teeth and jaws are still developing and because their teeth are more likely to be affected by tooth decay than those of adults.

QUESTION: Can I refuse dental x-rays and still be treated?

ANSWER: No. Treatment without necessary radiographs is considered negligent care. Even if you signed a paper stating that you refused radiographs and released the dentist from all liability, you would be consenting to negligent care. You cannot, legally, consent to negligent care. (Negligent care is discussed in Chapter 10.)

QUESTION: What kind of radiographs does my dentist usually take?

ANSWER: Typically, most dental patients have periapical or bitewing radiographs taken. These require patients to hold or bite down on a film packet and film holder. Bitewing radiographs typically determine the presence of decay in between teeth, while periapical radiographs show root structure, bone levels, cysts and abscesses.

TABLE 11-5 **Web Site Resources for Patient Education Materials**

Source	URL
American Dental Association	www.ada.org/public/topics/xrays_faq.asp
Academy of General Dentistry	www.agd.org/consumer/topics/xrays/main.asp
U.S. National Library of Medicine	www.nlm.nih.gov/medlineplus/ency/article/003801.htm
Nova Scotia Dental Association	www.healthyteeth.org/about.html (children)
WebMD Health	www.my.webmd.com/hw/health_guide_atoz/hw211991.asp

QUESTION: My dentist has prescribed a panoramic radiograph. What is that?

ANSWER: Just as a panoramic photograph allows you to see a broad view such as the Grand Canyon, a panoramic radiograph allows your dentist to see the entire structure of your mouth in a single image. Within one large film, panoramic radiographs reveal all of your upper and lower teeth and parts of your jaw.

QUESTION: Why do I need both types of radiographs?

ANSWER: What is apparent through one type of radiograph often is not visible on another. The panoramic radiograph is a comprehensive view of your entire mouth on a single film, which a periapical or bitewing radiograph can not show. On the other hand, periapical or bitewing radiographs show a highly detailed image of a smaller area, making it easier to see decay or cavities between your teeth. Radiographs are not prescribed indiscriminately. Your dentist has a need for the different information that each radiograph can provide to formulate a diagnosis.

QUESTION: How is x-ray exposure measured?

ANSWER: Special units are used to measure x-rays. When human tissue or other materials are exposed to x-rays, some of the energy is absorbed and some passes through without effect. The amount of energy absorbed by the tissue is the dose. The dose is often measured in sieverts (Sv). In modern diagnostic dental x-ray procedures, the exposures are usually so small that they are expressed in "milli" units—that is, units that are equal to one-thousandth of a Sv, or mSv.

QUESTION: What effects can x-rays have on the body?

ANSWER: Scientists have known for some time that exposure to very large amounts of x-radiation is harmful. Changes can occur in the reproductive system, altering the genetic material that determines the health of future generations. Large amounts of radiation can cause changes in the tissues of the body, including the possibility of cancer.

On the other hand, diagnostic procedures involve very low doses. With modern techniques and equipment, the amount of radiation received in a dental exam is minuscule. Also only a small part of the body is exposed (approximately the region corresponding to the size of the film). Therefore, the risk of harmful effects from dental x-ray exams is extremely small.

QUESTION: How do dental x-rays compare to other sources of radiation?

ANSWER: We are exposed to radiation every day from various sources, including outer space, minerals in the soil, and appliances in our homes (like smoke detectors and television screens). Here is a sample of a comparison of radiation doses from different sources:

Source	Estimated Exposure (mSv*)
Dental radiographs	
Bitewings (4 films)	0.038
Full-mouth series (about 19 films)	0.150
Medical radiographs	
Lower GI series	4.060
Upper GI series	2.440
Chest	0.080
Average radiation from outer space In Denver, CO (per year)	0.510
Average radiation in the United States from natural sources (per year)	3.000

*The term millisievert (mSv) is a unit of radiation measurement that allows for comparisons between different types of radiation.
Source: Adapted from N. L. Frederiksen, X-rays: What is the risk? *Texas Dental Journal, 1995;112(2):68–72.*

QUESTION: Why do you use a lead apron?

ANSWER: Because a lead apron and thyroid collar absorbs the x-rays and protects you from unnecessary radiation.

QUESTION: Why does the radiographer leave the room when x-ray exposures are taken?

ANSWER: If the radiographer did not leave the room or stand behind a barrier, he/she would be exposed many times a day to radiation. Although the amount of radiation he/she would receive each time is quite small, over a long period of time they would receive a needless dose that provides no benefit to them.

QUESTION: If I am pregnant or think I may be pregnant, should dental x-ray exams be postponed?

ANSWER: A recent study (*JAMA* 291:16, 2004) suggests that dental radiography during pregnancy is associated with low birth weight specifically with full-term pregnancies. It is currently unclear whether dental radiation affects the reproductive organs directly; or exposure to the head and neck area affects the thyroid function and thereby indirectly affects pregnancy outcomes; or whether factors unrelated to radiation are responsible for the low birth weight. Currently, the American Dental Association recommends that pregnant women postpone elective dental x-rays until after delivery and reinforces the importance of using leaded thyroid collars in addition to abdominal shielding (e.g., protective aprons). (Radiographs for the pregnant patient are discussed in Chapter 24.)

QUESTION: If I have had radiation therapy for cancer of the head or neck, should I avoid dental x-rays?

ANSWER: No. The dose of radiation required for dental x-rays is extremely small compared to that used for radiation therapy. The effects of very high doses involved in therapeutic radiation may increase your susceptibility to diseases, such as tooth decay. This can occur as a result of a decrease in secretions of the salivary glands. It is especially important for you to have x-ray exams as needed, to detect problems at an early stage. (Radiographs for the cancer patient are discussed in Chapter 24.)

QUESTION: Can dental x-rays cause skin cancer?

ANSWER: There have been no recorded cases of patients developing cancer from modern diagnostic dental x-rays. In the early days, prior to radiation safety standards, dentists who repeatedly held the film in the patient's mouth during exposures developed cancer on their fingers.

QUESTION: What special precautions will you take to minimize the amount of radiation I receive?

ANSWER: There are several ways we minimize the amount of radiation that you receive. First and foremost, only necessary radiographs are taken. We use the fastest type of x-ray film currently available, and use equipment that restricts the beam to the area that needs to be examined. A lead apron and thyroid shield will be placed on you during the exposure, and the films will be developed according to the manufacturer's recommendations, to produce a high quality image.

QUESTION: Who owns my dental radiographs?

ANSWER: The dentist owns all your dental records, including the radiographs. You have the right of reasonable access to your dental records, but they remain the property of the dentist.

QUESTION: Should I have my previous radiographs sent to my new dentist?

ANSWER: Yes, if possible. These radiographs can reveal your previous disease activity and may assist in determining the need for a new x-ray exam. Although the dentist who treated you in the past is considered the owner of your records, including your x-rays, arrangements can usually be made to have x-rays duplicated and sent to your new dentist. You should contact your former dentist and request that this be done.

REVIEW—Chapter Summary

Effective communication is the key to producing quality radiographs. The radiographer must be a skilled communicator.

Patient relations affect the confidence level of the patient and help the radiographer gain trust. The radiographer's appearance and attitude play a significant role in conveying professionalism.

The attitude of the radiographer toward the patient, the radiographic procedure and his/her own technical ability, coworkers, and employer will be conveyed to the patient. A positive, empathetic attitude will most likely generate a cooperative patient who will accept treatment recommendations and embrace oral health promotion and disease prevention. The radiographer should be cognizant of the roles interpersonal skills and chairside manner play in producing quality radiographs.

Honesty in verbal and nonverbal communication develops trust. Nonverbal communication is often stronger than verbal communication. Show-tell-do is an effective method of communication for all patients, especially when barriers to communication exist such as a language or cultural difference, a sensory impairment, or a cognitive impairment.

Patient education is valuable in securing acceptance of treatment and in addressing concerns about the safety of the radiographic procedures. The entire oral health care team must be able to provide the patient with complete explanations regarding the need for radiographs. The methods of patient education include oral presentations and the distribution of printed materials.

Examples of FAQs (frequently asked questions) and answers are provided.

RECALL—Study Questions

1. The key to producing quality radiographic images is:
   a. Gaining patient trust and cooperation.
   b. Presenting a confident, caring image.
   c. Communicating effectively.
   d. All of the above.
2. List four aspects of patient relations that help to gain confidence:
   a. ____________________
   b. ____________________
   c. ____________________
   d. ____________________
3. Dental radiographers with a positive attitude are more likely to produce high-quality radiographs.
   a. True
   b. False
4. When a patient trusts the radiographer, the patient is more likely to cooperate with the radiographic procedures.
   a. True
   b. False

5. The ability to share in the patient's emotions and feelings is called:
   a. Chairside manner.
   b. Atitude.
   c. Empathy.
   d. Verbal communication.
6. All of the following will enhance verbal communication *except* one. Which one is this *exception?*
   a. Face the patient.
   b. Look the patient in the eyes.
   c. Use clear commands.
   d. Use slang words.
7. Which of the following words should be avoided when discussing the radiographic procedure?
   a. Picture
   b. Zap
   c. X-ray
   d. Radiograph
8. The use of highly technical words may confuse the patient and result in miscommunication.
   a. True
   b. False
9. The method of show-tell-do is a beneficial way of communicating with:
   a. Cultures different from your own.
   b. Children.
   c. Hearing impaired patients.
   d. All of the above.
10. What is the value of patient education regarding dental radiographs?
    a. Radiographer is more likely to spend less time exposing radiographs.
    b. Radiographer is more likely to develop a positive attitude.
    c. Patient is more likely to accept the treatment plan.
    d. Patient is more likely to request radiographs at each appointment.
11. Patient education in radiography is necessary to:
    a. Increase the demand for oral health services.
    b. Increase acceptance of oral healthcare recommendations.
    c. Assure the patient that the radiographer is licensed.
    d. Meet legally required mandates for it.
12. List four things you could tell the patient in response to his/her concerns regarding the necessity of dental x-rays and the reduction of excess radiation exposure:
    a. ____________________
    b. ____________________
    c. ____________________
    d. ____________________

REFLECT—Case Study

A new patient to your practice has just been examined by the dentist, who has prescribed a set of vertical bitewings and a panoramic radiograph. You escort the patient to the x-ray room to prepare to expose the radiographs. At this time, the patient is having second thoughts about consenting to the radiographic surveys. She begins to question you about the procedure. Respond to the questions listed below. Write out your answers. Together with a partner, role play this scenario.

"Why do I need x-rays?"
"Why do I have to have bitewings and a panoramic x-ray?"
"How often should I have x-rays taken?
"Are you going to take the x-rays, or will the dentist take them?"
"I'm a little nervous about having this done."
"How long will it take?"
"What will you do to protect me from excessive exposure?"

RELATE—Laboratory Application

Produce your own brochure for the purpose of educating patients about the radiographic procedure. Give your brochure a title, for example "Dental X-Rays for Your Health," or something similar. The narration should be simple and in language that is professional, yet not overly technical. You may direct your brochure to a target population. For example your brochure may be for children or for a particular culture (e.g., for Spanish speakers). Include pictures of radiographs illustrating conditions that can be identified easily. Search the Web for information and pictures to download (Table 11–5).

BIBLIOGRAPHY

American Dental Association. *The Benefits of Dental X-ray Examinations.* Chicago: ADA, 2000.

American Dental Association. *Answers to Common Questions about Dental X-rays.* Chicago: ADA; 2000.

Grubbs, P. A. *Essentials for Today's Nursing Assistant.* Upper Saddle River, NJ: Prentice Hall, 2003.

Hujoel, P. P., Bollen, A. M., Noonan, C. J., & del Aguila, M. A. Antepartum dental radiography and infant low birth weight." *JAMA* 291(16): 1987–1993, 2004.

Pulliam, J. L. *The Nursing Assistant: Acute, Sub-Acute and Long-Term Care,* 4th ed. Upper Saddle River, NJ: Prentice Hall, 2006.

Thunthy, K. H. X-rays: Detailed answers to frequently asked questions. *Compendium of Continuing Education in Dentistry,* 14:394–398, 1993.

PART V • INTRAORAL TECHNIQUES

12

Intraoral Radiographic Procedures

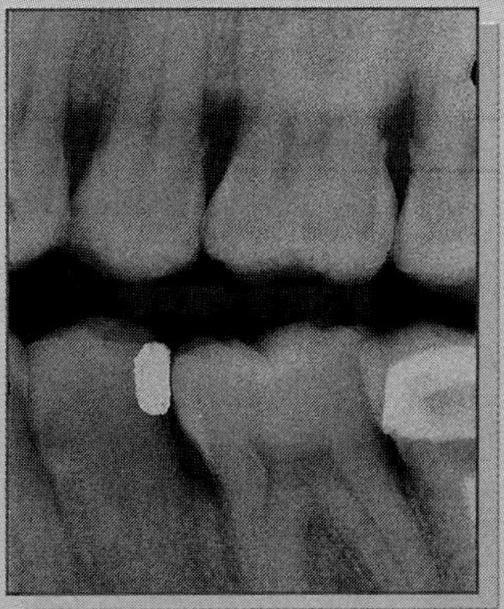

CHAPTER OUTLINE

■ OBJECTIVES

Following successful completion of this chapter, you should be able to:

1. Define the key words.
2. Identify the three intraoral x-ray examinations.
3. List the five rules for shadow casting.
4. Discuss the principles of the bisecting technique.
5. Discuss the principles of the paralleling technique.
6. Compare the paralleling and bisecting techniques.
7. List at least five contraindications for using the patient's finger to hold the film packet during exposure.
8. Explain the proper patient seating position.
9. Locate the facial points of entry.
10. Explain horizontal and vertical angulation.

■ KEY WORDS

Ala
Ala–tragus line
Angulation
Bisecting technique
Bisector
Biteblock
Bitewing radiograph
Canthus
Film holder
Horizontal angulation
Intraoral
Midsaggital plane
Negative angulation
Occlusal plane
Occlusal radiograph
Paralleling technique
Periapical radiograph
Point of entry
Positive angulation
Rule of isometry
Shadow casting
Tragus
Vertical angulation

Introduction

Intraoral radiography consists of methods of exposing dental x-ray films within the oral cavity. Producing diagnostic quality dental radiographs depends on knowledge of and attention to:

- Positioning the patient in the chair.
- Selecting a film packet of suitable size.
- Determining how the film is to be positioned and held in place while the exposure is made.
- Setting the control devices correctly to make the exposure.
- Aiming the position indicating device (PID).

Each of these steps have specific applications for each of the three types of intraoral examinations and when utilizing the bisecting technique or the paralleling technique. The purpose of this chapter is to introduce the three types of intraoral examinations, describe the fundamentals of producing intraoral images (shadow casting), and explain the principles of the bisecting and paralleling techniques.

Intraoral Procedures

The three types of intraoral radiographic examinations each use a slightly different film and technique, and each has a different objective.

1. **Bitewing examination.** Shows the coronal portions of the teeth and the alveolar crests of bone of both the maxilla and mandible of a given area on one film. The technique used to image **bitewing radiographs** is unique to the bitewing exam. However, because of the almost parallel placement of the film packet, the bitewing technique could be considered to be a modification of the paralleling technique.
2. **Periapical examination.** The fundamental purpose of periapical radiographs is to show the apices of the teeth and the surrounding bone. **Periapical radiographs** may be taken utilizing the bisecting technique or the paralleling technique.
3. **Occlusal examination.** The purpose of occlusal radiographs is to show the entire maxillary or mandibular arch, or a portion thereof, on a single film. The technique used to image **occlusal radiographs** is unique to the occlusal exam. However, because of the film packet placement required, the occlusal technique could be considered a modification of the bisecting technique.

Techniques

There are two basic techniques employed in intraoral radiography, bisecting and paralleling. Either technique can be modified to meet special conditions and requirements. While each technique will produce diagnostic quality radiographic images if the fundamental principles of the technique are followed, paralleling is the technique of choice.

The concept of the **bisecting technique** (also called the bisecting-angle or short-cone technique) originated in 1907 through the application of a geometric principle known as the **rule of isometry.** This theorem states that two triangles having equal angles and a common side are equal triangles (Figure 12–1). The bisecting technique was the only method used for many years. However, since many radiographers experienced difficulties and obtained unsatisfactory results, the search for a less complicated technique that would produce better radiographs more consistently resulted in the development of the paralleling technique in 1920. The **paralleling technique** (also called right-angle, extension-cone, or long-cone technique) is considered to be the technique of choice because better quality radiographs are produced with this technique.

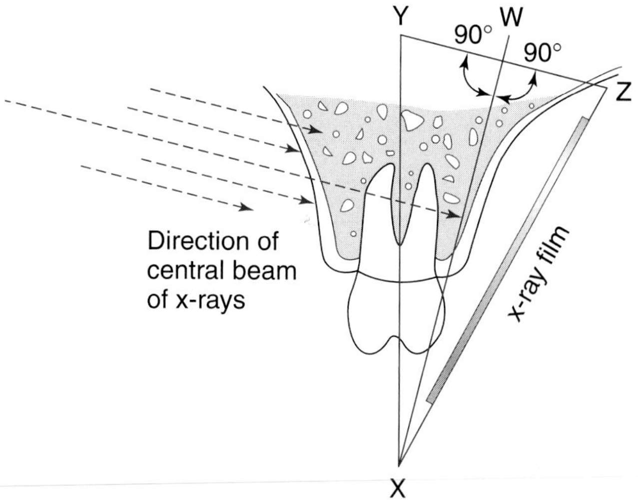

FIGURE 12–1 **Rule of isometry applied to the bisecting technique.** Line XY passes through the long axis of a maxillary first premolar while the film is positioned along line XZ. The central beam of radiation is directed perpendicularly through the apical area of the tooth toward the bisector XW. Because triangles WXY and WXZ are equal, the shadow image cast on the film will be approximately equal to the length of the film, provided that the bisector line is correctly estimated. Most errors in foreshortening and elongation are traceable to estimating incorrectly the location of the bisector line.

Fundamentals of Shadow Casting

X-rays producing an image on a film is similar to light casting a shadow of an object. When a hand is placed between a nearby light source such as an electric bulb and a flat object such as a tabletop, the shadow of the hand is seen on the tabletop. The same happens in dental radiography, where x-rays cast a shadow of the tooth on the film.

The radiograph is a film with a shadow image. To produce an image that represents the teeth and supporting structures accurately, the x-ray beam must be directed at the structures and the film at certain angles. The function of the film is to record the shadow image. To produce the best image, it is important to understand the fundamentals of **shadow casting.** Shadow casting refers to five basic rules for casting a shadow image (see Chapter 4).

1. Use the smallest possible source (focal spot) of radiation.
2. The object (tooth) should be as far as practical from the source of radiation.
3. The object (tooth) and the recording plane (film) should be as close to each other as possible.
4. The object (tooth) and the recording plane (film) should be parallel to each other.
5. The radiation (central ray) must strike both the object (tooth) and the recording plane (film) at right angles (perpendicularly).

Neither the bisecting nor the paralleling technique completely meets all five requirements for accurate shadow casting. With the bisecting technique, the object and film are not parallel to each other and the radiation does not strike the object and the film at right angles. In the paralleling technique, the distance between the object and the film is greater than ideal in most film placement areas. However, the rules met by the paralleling technique make it less likely to produce image distortion. For this reason, the paralleling technique is the recommended technique.

Principles of the Bisecting Technique

The bisecting principle is applied when the film packet is not, or cannot, be placed parallel to the long axes of the teeth. This is often the case with children, adults with a shallow palatal vault or a torus present, or when edentulous regions exist. If the irregularities of the oral tissues and the curvature of the palate will not allow the film packet to be placed parallel to the long axis of the tooth, the bisecting technique is employed.

To cast a shadow of a tooth onto a film, the angle formed by the long axis of the tooth and the plane of the film must be bisected. One must first find the long axis of the tooth and then find the long axis of the film packet as it is placed next to the tooth. After visualizing these two planes, one must imagine a line, called the **bisector,** which bisects the angle where the long axis of the tooth and the long axis of the film plane meet. The radiation beam is directed perpendicular to the imaginary bisector and not to the long axis of the tooth or the film plane (Figure 12–2).

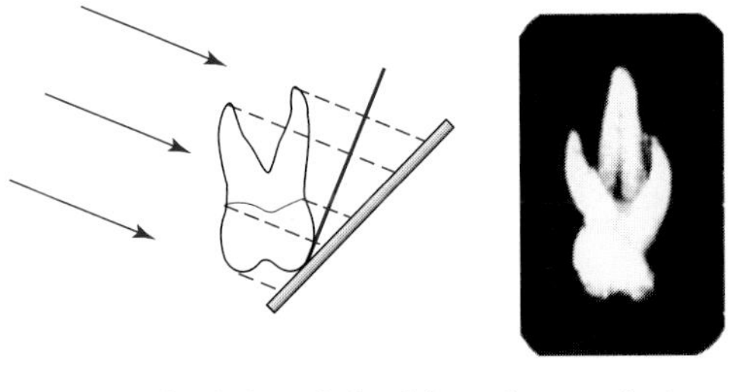

FIGURE 12–2 **Principle of the bisecting technique.** The x-ray beam is directed perpendicular to the imaginary line that bisects the angle formed by the recording plane of the dental x-ray film and the long axis of the tooth. (Courtesy of Dentsply Rinn)

Practice Point

To aid in estimating the imaginary bisector, utilize the two *visible planes:* the teeth and the film packet. Looking at the teeth, locate the long axes. Then align the x-ray beam to intersect the long axes of the teeth perpendicularly. Study the PID and make a mental note of this angle. Next look at the film packet. Note the plane of the film packet as it is placed against the teeth. Then shift the PID so that the x-ray beam is aligned to intersect the film packet plane perpendicularly. Note this angle while recalling the angle at which the x-ray beam intersected the long axes of the teeth. If you need to, repeat this process, shifting the PID to allow the x-ray beam to intersect the long axes of the teeth and then the film plane perpendicularly until you can estimate a position halfway in between these two angles. This halfway point is the imaginary bisector.

Theoretically, two isometric triangles (triangles having equal measurements) are formed when the central ray is directed perpendicularly toward the bisector, and the film image that results should be the same size as the tooth. In practice, this does not always happen. The diagnostic quality of the image is usually compromised, with some dimensional distortion that is inherent in the bisecting technique.

Principles of the Paralleling Technique

The basic principles of the paralleling technique are:

- The film is placed parallel to the long axes of the teeth being radiographed.
- The central ray is directed at right angles to both the teeth and film (Figure 12–3).

Oral structures, particularly the curvature of the palate, make it difficult to place the film parallel to the long axes of the teeth.

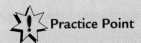

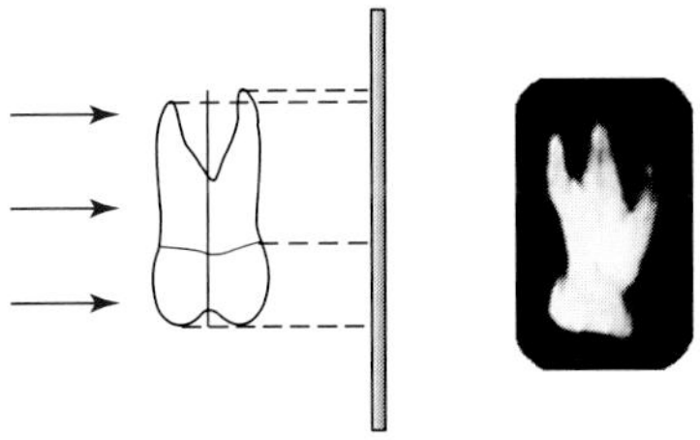

FIGURE 12–3 **Principle of the paralleling technique.** The x-ray beam is directed perpendicular to the recording plane of the film, which has been positioned parallel to the long axis of the tooth. (Courtesy of Dentsply Rinn)

TABLE 12-1 **Advantages and Disadvantages of the Paralleling Technique**

Advantages	Disadvantages
• Produces images with minimal dimensional distortion. • Minimizes superimposition of adjacent structures. • Tooth and film packet planes can be visually located making it easier to direct the x-rays appropriately. • Many choices of film holders on the market with external aiming devices specifically designed to make paralleling simple and easy to learn. • With appropriate film holding devices, takes less time than trying to locate the position of an imaginary bisector. • When using a long PID (16 in./41 cm), patient radiation dose may be reduced.	• Parallel film packet placement is difficult to achieve on certain patients: children, adults with small mouths, low palatal vaults, or the presence of tori, patients with sensitive oral mucosa or an exaggerated gag reflex, edentulous regions. • These same conditions may increase patient discomfort when the film packet impinges on oral tissues. • A short PID (8 in./20.5 cm) should not be used. (A long PID may be more difficult to maneuver.)

The paralleling technique achieves parallelism by placing the film away from the crowns of the teeth. Paralleling is accomplished by using a **film holder** specifically designed to allow the patient to stabilize the film packet in this position away from the crowns of the teeth. To compensate for the increased object–film distance, the target–film distance should also be increased. Ideally, the target–film distance used in paralleling is 16 in. (41 cm) or at least 12 in. (30 cm). The PID length contributes to the target–film distance.

Comparing the Paralleling and Bisecting Techniques

While the paralleling technique is the recommended technique, its greatest disadvantage is that parallel film packet placement is difficult to achieve on some patients (Table 12–1). For this reason, the bisecting technique still plays a valuable role in imaging acceptable quality radiographs for those patients. Proficiency should be developed in both techniques (Table 12–2). An operator using the paralleling technique may change to the bisecting method for one or two exposures during a full-mouth series because of anatomical limitations such as heavy muscle attachments or the shape of the palate. So it is important to compare the paralleling and bisecting techniques to fully understand if and when to use each. Important differences include the use of distance, angles, and film-holding devices.

Distances

Target–film and object–film distances differ in the two techniques.

Target–Film Distance

The shorter 8 in. (20.5 cm) target–film distance is generally, but not necessarily, used in the bisecting method. Because the long axis of the tooth and the film plane are not parallel, a shorter target–film distance will limit magnification and distortion (see Figures 4–11 and 4–12). An x-ray unit with an 8 in. (20.5 cm) PID is best suited for the bisecting method. The paralleling method should be matched with a longer target–film distance to compensate for the greater object–film distance. While the 8 in. (20.5 cm) target–film distance is the minimum

TABLE 12-2 **Advantages and Disadvantages of the Bisecting Technique**

Advantages	Disadvantages
• Film packet placement may be easier with certain patients: children, adults with small mouths, low palatal vaults, or the presence of tori, patients with sensitive oral mucosa or an exaggerated gag reflex, edentulous regions. • A short PID (8 in./20.5 cm) may be used. (Some operators find a short PID easier to manuver.)	• Produces images with dimensional distortion. (Some elongation or foreshortening will occur even when the technique is performed correctly.) • Often superimposes adjacent structures. (The necessary vertical angle increase often causes a shadow of the zygomatic process of the maxilla to be superimposed over the molar roots in the maxillary areas.) • Estimating the location of the imaginary bisector may be difficult. • When using a short PID (8 in./20.5 cm), patient radiation dose may be increased.

distance one should use with the paralleling technique, a longer 12 in. (30 cm) or ideally, 16 in. (41 cm) is preferred.

Object–Film Distance

A shorter object–film distance is used in bisecting procedures, with the exception of the mandibular molar areas, where film placement is almost identical with both techniques. In the bisecting technique, the film is placed as close to the teeth as possible. However, because of the supporting structures in the oral cavity, this close film packet placement results in a film packet that is not parallel to the long axes of the teeth. Instead, an angle is formed between the long axes of the teeth and the film packet. In the paralleling technique, the film packet is placed parallel to the long axes of teeth. Because of the supporting structure in the oral cavity, to accomplish a parallel relationship between the long axes of the teeth and the film plane, the film must be placed farther away from the teeth.

Vertical Angle of Beam to Object and Film

With the bisecting method, the central rays of the x-ray beam are aimed perpendicularly to the imaginary bisector in the vertical dimension and do not strike either the tooth or the film at a right angle. This positioning produces more dimensional distortion (Figure 12–4).

With the paralleling method, the central rays are directed at a right angle (perpendicularly) to both the long axes of the teeth and to the film plane. The paralleling technique uses a parallel relationship between the film and the tooth structures for a more accurate image (Figure 12–5).

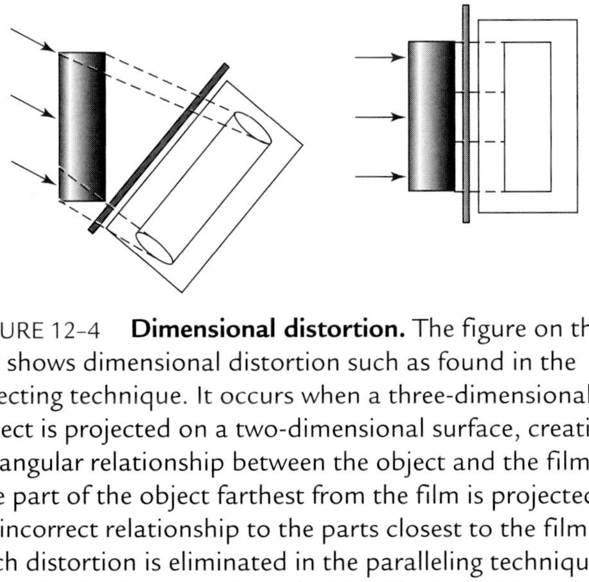

FIGURE 12-4 **Dimensional distortion.** The figure on the left shows dimensional distortion such as found in the bisecting technique. It occurs when a three-dimensional object is projected on a two-dimensional surface, creating an angular relationship between the object and the film. The part of the object farthest from the film is projected in an incorrect relationship to the parts closest to the film. Such distortion is eliminated in the paralleling technique, shown in the figure on the right. The film is positioned parallel to the object, so that all parts of the object are in their true relationship to one another. (Courtesy of Dentsply Rinn)

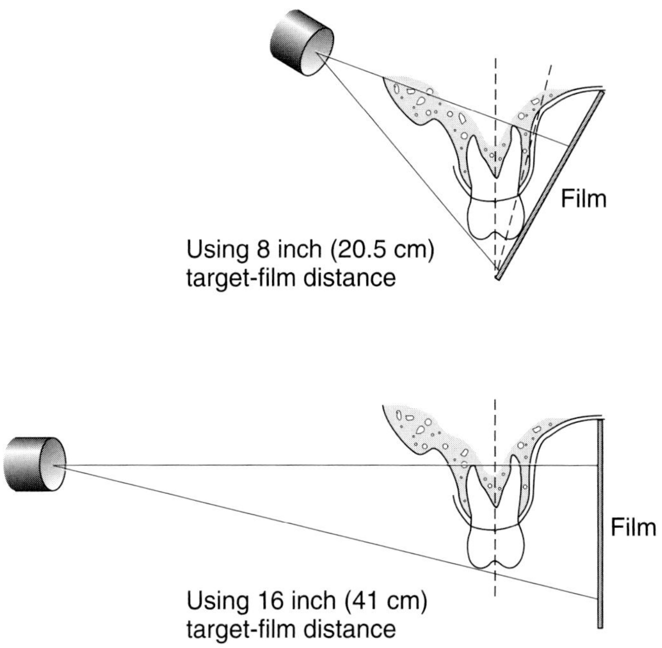

FIGURE 12-5 **Comparison of the bisecting and paralleling methods.** In the bisecting method, the film is positioned adjacent to the tooth, and the target-film distance is approximately 8 in. (20.5 cm). In the paralleling method, the film is positioned near the center of the oral cavity, where it must be retained in a position parallel to the long axes of the teeth, and the target-film distance is approximately 16 in. (41 cm). (Courtesy of Dentsply Rinn)

Film-holding Method

Film holders are used to hold the film packet in place when using either the bisecting method or the paralleling method. When the bisecting technique was first introduced in 1907 film holders did not yet exist. Instead, the patient was directed to hold the film in the mouth using a finger or thumb. Asking the patient to hold the film in this manner has many disadvantages, and this practice is no longer acceptable (Table 12–3). Film holders vary from simple disposable **biteblocks** that require no sterilization to complex devices that position the film at the correct angles for directing the x-ray beam in relation to the teeth and film (see Figure 6–13.) Commercially manufactured film holders are designed specifically for the bisecting technique or the paralleling technique. Some holders may be slightly altered to accommodate both techniques (Figures 12–6 and 12–7).

Patient Seating Position

If the film holder utilized has an external aiming device, the patient's head can be in any position. Without these special holders that indicate x-ray beam positions, patients must be seated upright with their head straight. This position is necessary for consistent results in determining the best horizontal and vertical angulations of the x-ray beam. With the correct patient

TABLE 12-3 **Contraindications for Using the Patient's Finger to Hold the Film Packet in Place**

Potential for film bending.	Radiation exposure of the patient's fingers.
Potential to move the film from the correct position.	No external aiming device to assist with aligning the x-ray beam to the correct position.
Increased patient instruction and cooperation required.	Potential to be viewed by the patient as unprofessional and unsanitary.
Potential patient objection to placing the fingers in the mouth.	

seating position, the horizontal angulation is determined in the same manner in both the bisecting and the paralleling techniques. However, the specific vertical angulations required when utilizing the bisecting technique differ when utilizing the paralleling technique. When utilizing the bisecting technique, the x-rays are directed at the bisector. When utilizing the paralleling technique, the x-rays are directed at the long axes of the teeth and film plane.

The recommended position is to seat the patient upright and adjust the headrest so that the **occlusal plane** for the arch being examined is parallel to the floor. The **midsagittal plane** that divides the patient's head into a right and left side should be positioned perpendicular to the floor (Figure 12–8). Although an experienced radiographer can expose radiographs with the patient either upright or supine, the use of predetermined head positions is recommended to standardize the procedure.

> **Practice Point**
>
> Seating the patient with the head against the headrest not only helps position the occlusal and midsaggital planes, but the patient is much less likely to move during the exposures when his/her head is firmly supported by the head rest. Additionally, Chapter 24 states that directing the patient's attention to the back of the head where it touches the head rest (the occipital protuberance) can serve as a distraction technique when needed (for example, when an exaggerated gag reflex presents).

Points of Entry

The point of entry is the spot on the surface of the face at which the central ray is directed (Figure 12–9). Points of entry are most helpful when using a film holder without an external aiming device. Points of entry are located at the level of the apices of the teeth. When the patient is seated in the recommended position, the apices of the maxillary teeth are located along an imaginary line drawn from the **ala** of the nose to the **tragus** of the ear. Chapter 19 refers to anatomical landmarks that can be used to determine the location of the apices of the teeth.

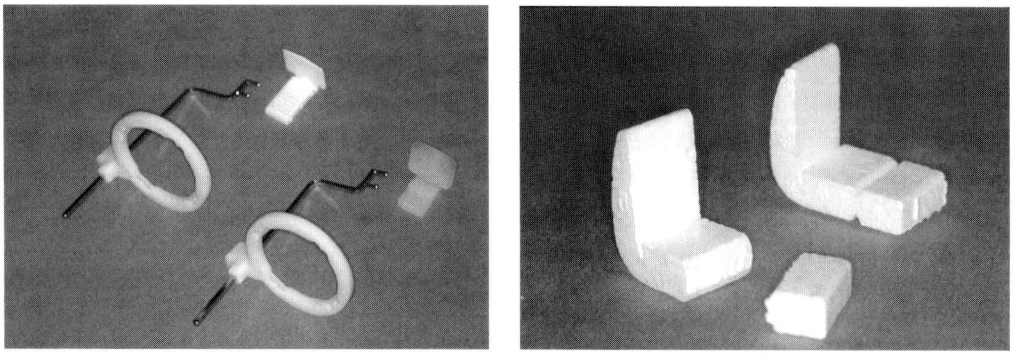

A B

FIGURE 12-6 **Film holders.** (**A**) Rinn XCP® (Dentsply Rinn) instruments with a plastic external aiming device. Available in both the paralleling technique version (on the left: XCP®—Extension Cone Paralleling) and the bisecting version (on the right: BAI®—Bisecting Angle Instrument) instruments. (**B**) Disposable Stabe® (Dentsply Rinn) biteblocks may be used with the bite extension broken off for use with the bisecting technique (on the left) or intact for the paralleling technique (on the right).

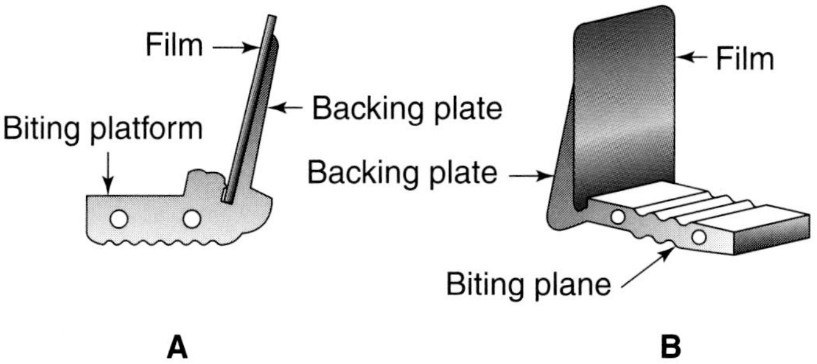

FIGURE 12-7 **Film holders.** (**A**) Anterior biteblock of BAI®. The raised platform on which the patient bites is close to the backing plate. The 105° angle of the backing plate keeps the film close to the lingual surface of the tooth. (**B**) Anterior biteblock of XCP®. The biting plane is at a right angle (90°) with the backing plate. The patient bites down far enough back on the bite extension to keep film and teeth parallel. (Courtesy of Dentsply Rinn)

The following landmarks are helpful in determining the **point of entry.** For maxillary teeth these are located along an extension of the **ala–tragus line** as follows:

1. The tip of the nose for the incisors.
2. The depression formed by the ala of the nose for the canines.
3. A point below the pupil of the eye for the premolars.
4. A point below the outer **canthus** of the eye for the molars.

A point directly below the same landmarks and approximately 1/2 inch (1.3 cm) above an imaginary line parallel to the lower border of the mandible is used to locate the point of entry for the corresponding mandibular teeth. These points of entry are only approximations. With a little practice, the point of entry for each maxillary and mandibular tooth position can be determined at a glance.

The truest image is produced when the central rays are directed through the point of entry toward the apices of the roots. However, the increased use of smaller beam diameters and film holders with collimating devices that limit the size of the beam makes it preferable to direct the central rays through the middle of the teeth instead of through the apices. The end of the PID should almost touch the face, with its midpoint centered over the point of entry. Failure to project the central ray through this point and toward the middle of the film packet results in cone cutting error.

Horizontal and Vertical Angulation Procedures

Angulation is defined as the procedure by which the tube head and PID are aligned to obtain the optimum angle at which the radiation is to be directed toward the film. Angulation is changed by rotating the tube head horizontally and vertically. The x-ray machine is constructed with three swivel joints to support the yoke and tube head. One of these, located at the top and center of the yoke where it attaches to the extension arm, permits

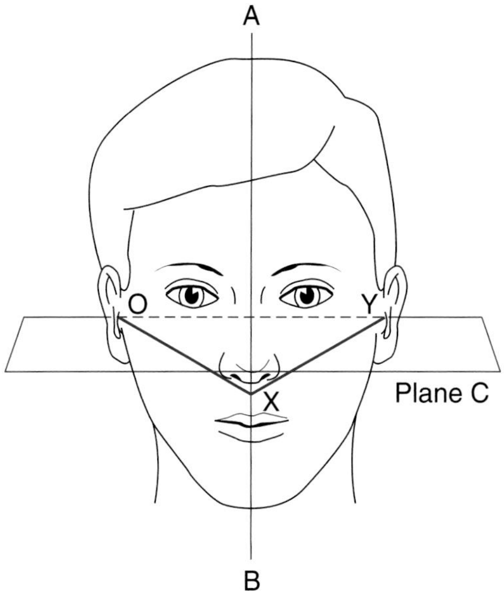

FIGURE 12-8 **Head divided by midsagittal plane and occlusal plane.** The midsagittal plane (**A–B**) must be perpendicular to the floor, and the occlusal plane (**C**) must be parallel with the floor unless special film-holding devices are used. The **O–X** and **X-Y** are the lines of orientation for the maxillary teeth, also known as the ala–tragus line. The apices of the roots of the maxillary teeth are located close to this line.

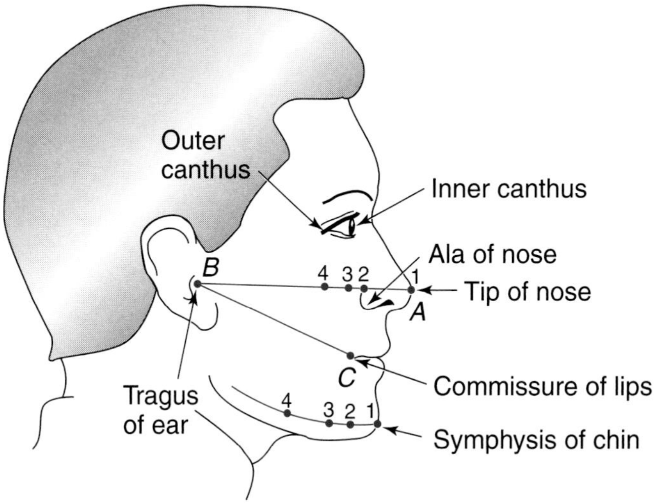

FIGURE 12-9 **Points of entry.** The facial landmarks that provide the radiographer with a quick reference for the positioning of the PID and the directing of the central beam of radiation. Unless special film holders are used that eliminate the need for positioning, the patient is seated upright with the midsagittal plane perpendicular to the floor.

horizontal movement of the tube head to control the anterior–posterior dimensions. The other two swivel joints are located at either side of the yoke. These permit the tube head to be rotated up or down in a vertical direction to control the longitudinal dimensions of the resulting image. Determining the correct direction of the central beam in the horizontal and vertical planes requires practice.

Horizontal Angulation

Horizontal angulation is achieved by directing the central rays perpendicularly (at a right angle) toward the film surface in a horizontal plane (Figure 12–10). The steps to determining correct horizontal angulation are the same for both the bisecting and paralleling methods. To change direction, swivel the tube head from side to side. The objective is to permit the central rays to pass directly through the interproximal spaces. Incorrect alignment in the horizontal plane caused by incorrect angulation toward the mesial or the distal results in an overlapping of adjacent tooth structures shown on the radiograph.

Vertical Angulation

Vertical angulation is accomplished by directing the central rays perpendicularly toward the film surface in a vertical plane. Because the film position, with the exception of the mandibular molar area, is not the same in bisecting and paralleling, the technique procedures differ. The direction of the central ray is changed by swiveling the tube head vertically so that the tip of the PID is raised or lowered (Figure 12–11).

Vertical angulation is customarily described in degrees. On most x-ray machines the vertical angles are scaled in intervals of 5 or 10 degrees on both sides of the yoke where the tube head is connected. The vertical angulation of the tube head and the PID begins at zero. In that position the PID is parallel to the plane of the floor. All deviations from zero in which the PID is tilted downward to direct the x-rays toward the floor are called **positive** (plus) **angulations.** Those in which the PID is tipped upward to direct the x-rays toward the ceiling are called **negative** (minus) **angulations.**

Average Vertical Angles for the Bisecting Technique

When the bisecting technique is used, the central ray—in the vertical plane—must be directed through the roots of the teeth perpendicularly toward the bisector (Figure 12–2). When the patient's head is in the recommended position, predetermined vertical angulations can often be used. Obviously, such angulations will vary from patient to patient. The average vertical angulations suggested in Table 12–4 are intended only as a guide and should not replace visual judgment.

Sometimes it may be necessary to increase or to decrease the vertical angulation. For example, a change from +40 to +50 degrees or from −10 to −20 degrees is called an increase in vertical angulation; the reverse, a change from +50 to +40 degrees or from −20 to −10 degrees is called a decrease in vertical angulation.

The operator should be alert to observe anatomical variations and to understand what change in angulation is required in each instance. For example, Table 12–4 suggests that the average vertical angulation for the maxillary molars is +20 degrees. Changes are indicated when the patient's vault (palate) is high or low. When the vault is high, the angulation is decreased to +15 degrees or less because the film packet now lies in a more vertical plane in the mouth. Conversely, when the vault is low, an increase to +25 degrees or more should be made, since the film packet now assumes a more horizontal position. In the mandibular region, if the floor of the mouth is shallow or the teeth are facially inclined, the vertical angulation should be increased by 5 to 10 degrees. Vertical angulation should be decreased by 5 to 10 degrees when the floor of the mouth is very deep or the teeth

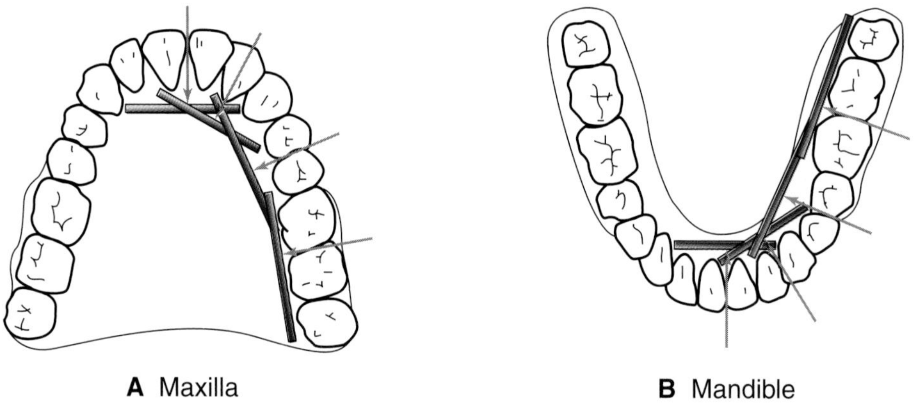

A Maxilla **B** Mandible

FIGURE 12–10 **Horizontal angulation.** Horizontal angulation is determined by directing the x-ray beam perpendicularly to the mean tangent of the teeth being radiographed, which is also the corresponding position of the film. The beam passes directly through the interproximal spaces. Standard #2 film is shown; however, the narrow #1 film is recommended for the incisor and canine region.

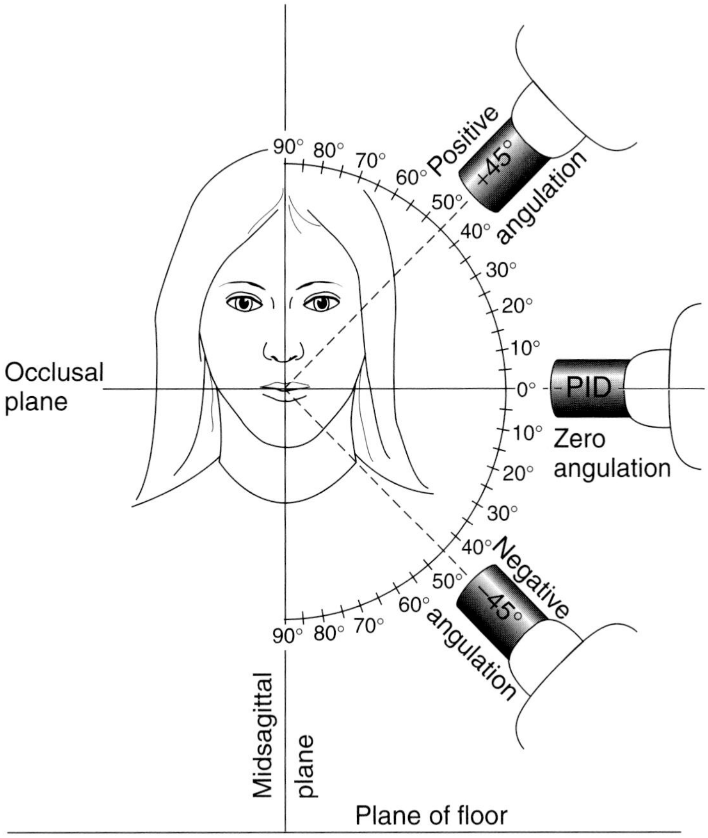

FIGURE 12-11 **Vertical angulation.** Diagram showing patient sitting in the recommended position upright in dental chair with midsagittal line perpendicular and occlusal plane parallel with the floor. Zero angulation is achieved when the long axis of the PID is directed parallel to the floor. All vertical angulations above the occlusal plane are called positive, or plus (+), angulations. These are used for all maxillary and bitewing exposures. Vertical angulations below the occlusal plane are negative, or minus (−), angulations. These are used for all mandibular exposures. There are suggested average vertical angulations that can be set when using the bisecting technique (Table 12-4). When using a film holder with an external aiming device, the need for numerically setting the angulations and positioning the patient's head in a predetermined position is eliminated.

incline lingually. Again, the suggested average vertical angulations do not take the place of visually determining the location of the imaginary bisector and directing the central ray toward it perpendicularly.

When the vertical angle is correctly estimated and the rays are directed perpendicularly to the bisector, no appreciable distortion results. Excessive vertical angulation when utilizing the bisecting technique will foreshorten the image. Insufficient vertical angulation when utilizing the bisecting technique will elongate the image.

When the paralleling technique is employed, the central ray in the vertical plane must be directed perpendicularly (at a right angle) through the roots of the teeth toward the film packet. Excessive vertical angulation when utilizing the paralleling technique will result in the loss of the image of the crown, and insufficient vertical angulation will result in the loss of the image of the apex. Errors made with incorrect horizontal and vertical angulations is explained in Chapter 16.

TABLE 12-4 **Suggested Average Vertical Angulations When Utilizing the Bisecting Technique**

Maxillary incisors	+40 degrees
Maxillary canines	+45 degrees
Maxillary premolars	+30 degrees
Maxillary molars	+20 degrees
Mandibular incisors	−15 degrees
Mandibular canines	−20 degrees
Mandibular premolars	−10 degrees
Mandibular molars	−5 degrees

REVIEW—Chapter Summary

The three types of intraoral radiographic procedures are the bitewing, periapical, and occlusal surveys. Each of these examinations differs in purpose, and a variety of film sizes may be used to achieve the desired result.

Both the bisecting and the paralleling techniques are used to produce a shadow image of the tooth onto the radiograph. While neither technique completely satisfies all the requirements for accurate shadow casting, the paralleling technique produces superior results. Each technique has advantages and disadvantages. The skilled operator, within the limits of the equipment available, must select the technique that fits the situation. The method of positioning and holding the film packet in place in the oral cavity differs between the bisecting and the paralleling techniques. In bisecting, the film is positioned closer to the teeth. In paralleling, the film is positioned farther from the teeth to achieve parallelism to the long axes of the teeth.

Horizontal angulation is achieved in the same manner in both techniques. The central ray is directed perpendicularly to the film in the horizontal plane.

Vertical angulation is achieved for bisecting and paralleling differently. In bisecting, the central ray is aimed perpendicularly at the imaginary bisector of the planes of the long axes of the teeth and the plane of the film. In paralleling the central ray is directed perpendicularly to the long axes of the teeth and perpendicularly to the film plane.

Unless the film holder has an external aiming device to indicate the correct angulation, care must be taken to seat the patient so that the occlusal plane is parallel with the floor and that the midsaggital plane is perpendicular to the floor.

RECALL—Study Questions

1. Which of these is not an intraoral survey?
   a. Bitewing
   b. Occlusal
   c. Panoramic
   d. Periapical
2. All of the following are shadow casting rules *except* one. Which one is this *exception?*
   a. Object and film should be perpendicular to each other.
   b. Object and film should be as close as possible to each other.
   c. Object should be as far as practical from the source of radiation.
   d. Radiation should strike the object and film perpendicularly.
3. What term describes the imaginary line between the long axis of the tooth and the film plane?
   a. Tangent
   b. Median
   c. Midsagittal
   d. Bisector
4. When utilizing the bisecting technique, the film is placed:
   a. Parallel to the tooth.
   b. As close as possible to the tooth
   c. As close as possible to the bisector.
   d. Parallel to the bisector.
5. When utilizing the bisecting technique, the central ray is directed:
   a. Perpendicular to the bisector.
   b. Parallel to the bisector.
   c. Perpendicular to the film.
   d. Parallel to the film.
6. The bisecting technique satisfies more shadow casting rules. A better image results when the shadow casting rules are followed.
   a. The first statement is true; the second statement is false.
   b. The first statement is false; the second statement is true.
   c. Both statements are true.
   d. Both statements are false
7. Which of these target-film distances is recommended for use with the paralleling technique?
   a. 8 in. (20.5 cm)
   b. 12 in. (30 cm)
   c. 16 in. (41 cm)
8. When utilizing the paralleling technique, the film is placed:
   a. Parallel to the tooth.
   b. As close as possible to the tooth.
   c. As close as possible to the bisector.
   d. Parallel to the bisector.
9. All of the following are advantages of the paralleling technique *except* one. Which one is this *exception?*
   a. Produces images that are less likely to be distorted.
   b. The choice of film holders for this method is great.
   c. Superimposition of adjacent structures is reduced.
   d. Patient comfort is increased during film packet placement.
10. All of the following are disadvantages of the bisecting technique *except* one. Which one is this *exception?*
    a. Produces images with dimensional distortion.
    b. Often superimposes adjacent structures.
    c. Estimating the location of the bisector is difficult.
    d. May not be used with children or adults with small oral cavities.
11. List five contraindications for using the patient's finger to hold the film packet in position during exposure.
    a. ____________________
    b. ____________________
    c. ____________________
    d. ____________________
12. Which of the following is the correct seating position for the patient during radiographic examinations when a film holder with an external aiming device is not utilized?
    a. Occlusal and midsaggital planes parallel to the floor
    b. Occlusal and midsaggital planes perpendicular to the floor
    c. Occlusal plane parallel and midsaggital plane perpendicular to the floor
    d. Occlusal plane perpendicular and midsaggital plane parallel to the floor
13. Which of the following is the suggested point of entry for exposing the maxillary incisors?
    a. The tip of the nose
    b. The depression formed by the ala of the nose
    c. A point below the pupil of the eye
    d. A point below the outer canthus of the eye

14. What is the result of incorrect horizontal angulation?
    a. Image cut off
    b. Overlapping
    c. Elongation
    d. Foreshortening
15. At which of the following settings would the PID be pointing to the floor?
    a. −30
    b. 0
    c. +20
16. What change in angulation should be made when a patient has an unusually low vault?
    a. Horizontal angulation is shifted mesially.
    b. Horizontal angulation is shifted distally.
    c. Vertical angulation is increased.
    d. Vertical angulation is decreased.
17. With the bisecting technique, what is the effect on the radiographic image if the vertical angulation is 15° greater than necessary?
    a. Overlapping
    b. Cone cutting
    c. Elongating
    d. Foreshortening

REFLECT—Case Study

Imagine that you are about to expose a full mouth series of periapical and bitewing radiographs on your patient. The dentist has prescribed the radiographs especially to image the patient's periodontal condition. This means that imaging the alveolar bone is critical. The patient's record indicates that several molars are missing. A cursory exam reveals the presence of bilateral lingual tori and a moderately large palatal torus. As you prepare for the exposures, the patient nervously tells you that he is a "gagger." Consider the following and write out your answers:

1. Which radiographic technique for exposing periapical radiographs will you choose for this exam? Why?
2. What conditions exist that may prompt you to alter your technique?
3. What are the limitations of the technique you chose? What are the advantages and disadvantages?
4. Why didn't you choose the other technique? What are the advantages and disadvantages of the other technique?
5. Are any errors more likely to occur on this patient than another patient? Why?
6. What can be done to prevent these errors?
7. Describe the film holder that you would use for these radiographs.
8. Why would you choose this holder?
9. How will your patient be seated for the exposures? Why?
10. Summarize the steps you would take to locate the vertical and horizontal angulations.

RELATE—Laboratory Application

For a comprehensive laboratory practice exercise on this topic, see E. M. Thomson, *Exercises in Oral Radiography Techniques: A Laboratory Manual,* 2nd ed., Upper Saddle River, NJ: Prentice Hall, 2007. Chapter 5, "Radiographic Techniques with Supplemental Film Holders."

BIBLIOGRAPHY

Eastman Kodak. *Successful Intraoral Radiography.* Rochester, NY: Eastman Kodak, 1998.

Rinn Corporation. *Intraoral Radiography with Rinn XCP/BAI Instruments.* Elgin, IL: Dentsply/Rinn Corporation, 1983.

White, S. C. & Pharoah, M. J. *Oral Radiology Principles and Interpretation,* 5th ed. St. Louis: Elsevier, 2004.

13

The Periapical Examination

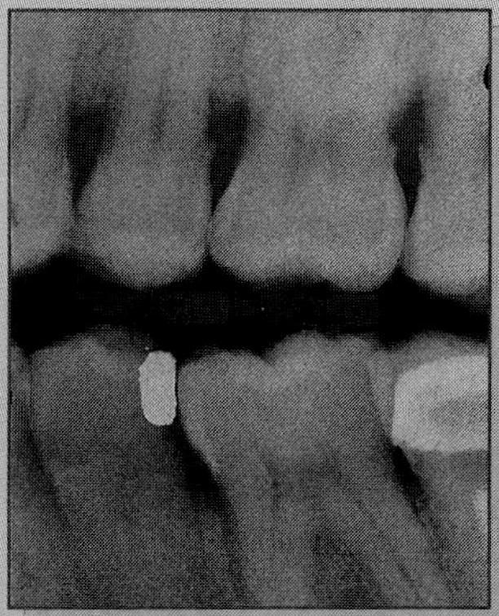

CHAPTER OUTLINE

■ OBJECTIVES

Following successful completion of this chapter, you should be able to:

1. Define the key words.
2. Select the type and number of films required for a full mouth survey.
3. Differentiate between the vertical angulation errors made when using the paralleling and bisecting techniques.
4. Identify and be able to assemble and position film holders for the paralleling and bisecting techniques.
5. Explain the importance of film placement sequencing.
6. Describe patient preparation for periapical exposures.
7. Demonstrate the method of positioning the film packet for maxillary and mandibular periapical exposures when using the paralleling technique.
8. Demonstrate the method of positioning the film packet for maxillary and mandibular periapical exposures when using the bisecting technique.

■ KEY WORDS

Bisector
Bite extension
Biteblock
Dot in the slot
External aiming device
Film holder
Full-mouth survey (full-mouth series)
Horizontal placement
Identificaton dot
Indicator ring
Mean tangent
Periapical radiograph
Vertical placement

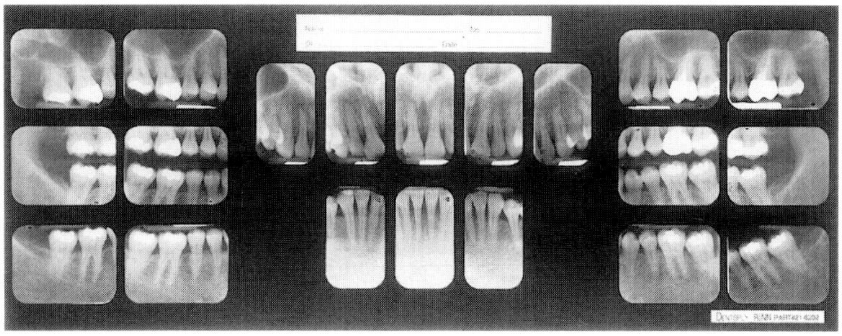

FIGURE 13–1 **Full-mouth radiographic survey.** The 20-film radiographic series shown includes 4 bitewing films in addition to the 8 anterior and 8 posterior periapical films.

Introduction

The purpose of the periapical examination is to view the entire tooth and surrounding bone. The word periapical is derived from the Greek word *peri* (meaning around) and the Latin word *apex* (meaning highest point). Therefore, as the word suggests, the **periapical radiograph** shows the entire tooth including the root end and surrounding bone.

The purpose of this chapter is to present the step-by-step procedures for exposing a full-mouth series of periapical radiographs using both the paralleling and bisecting techniques.

Fundamentals of Periapical Radiographs

The periapical radiograph may be used to examine a single tooth or condition, or may be used in combination with other periapical and bitewing radiographs to image the entire dentition and supporting structures (full mouth series) (Figure 13–1). Conditions prompting the exposure of a periapical radiograph include apical pathology (abscesses), fractures, large carious lesions (Figure 13–2), extensive periodontal involvement (Figure 13–3), examination of developmental anomalies such as missing teeth and abnormal eruption patterns, and any unexplained pain or bleeding. Periapical radiographs may be taken utilizing the paralleling or the bisecting technique. A film-holding device should be used to position the film packet in the oral cavity. A **film holder** with an **external aiming device** will assist the radiographer with directing the x-ray beam at the correct angles. It is important, however, that the radiographer possess the ability to evaluate the correct placement of these devices to avoid errors that result when incorrect angles are used.

Film Requirements

When the periapical examination includes a series of films that image all of the teeth, the term **full-mouth survey** is used to describe the collection of films (Figures 13–1 and 13–4). Bitewing radiographs are often included in the full mouth series (see Chapter 14). Periapical radiographs can be made with any of the three periapical film sizes (#0, #1, #2) or any combination of these films. Film size depends on:

- The age of the patient.
- The size of the oral cavity.
- The shape of the dental arches.

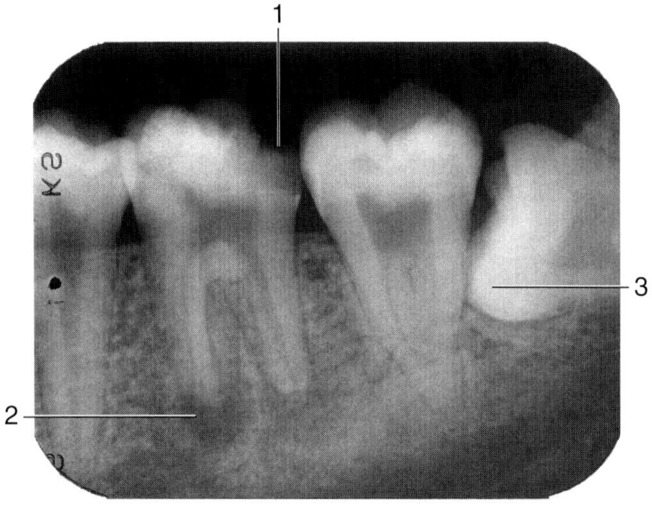

FIGURE 13–2 **Periapical radiograph.** Posterior periapical radiograph showing (**1**) extensive caries and (**2**) apical pathology, and (**3**) impacted third molar. Note the horizontal positioning of the long dimension of the film packet for imaging the posterior regions.

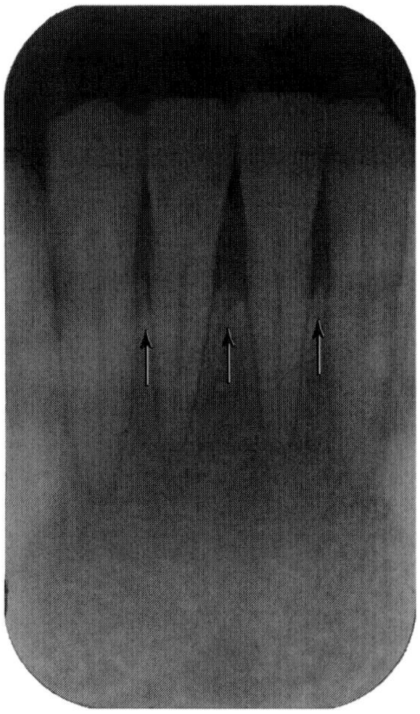

FIGURE 13–3 **Periapical radiograph.** Anterior periapical radiograph showing extensive periodontal involvement. Note the vertical positioning of the long dimension of the film packet for imaging the anterior regions.

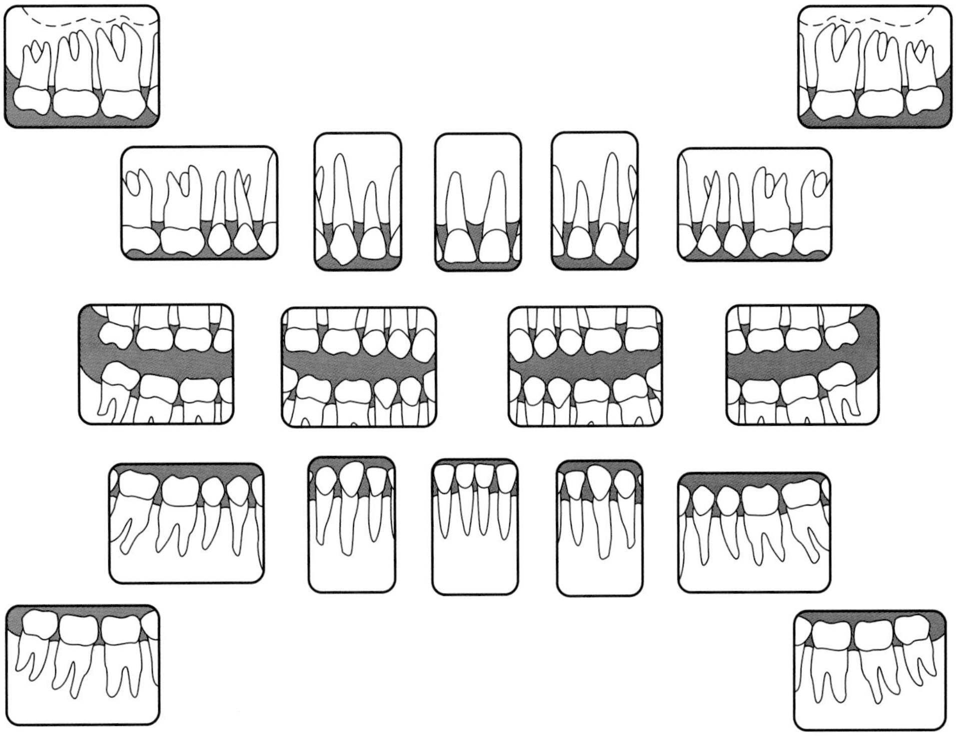

FIGURE 13–4 **Full-mouth survey.** Drawing of 18-film full-mouth survey using 14 periapical and 4 bitewing films.

- The presence or absence of unusual conditions or anatomical limitations.
- The film holder and technique used.
- The patient's ability to tolerate the film packet placement.

The number and size films used for a full mouth series of periapical radiographs varies among oral healthcare practices. A minimum of 14 periapical films (Figure 13–4) make up a full-mouth survey for most adult patients. These 14 films are used to image the following areas:

- One film each for the maxillary and mandibular incisor area
- One film in each of the canine areas (two maxillary and two mandibular)
- One film in each of the premolar areas (two maxillary and two mandibular)
- One film in each of the molar areas (two maxillary and two mandibular)

While most all practices will use eight size #2 films for the exposure of the posterior periapicals on an adult patient, the number and size of films used for the exposure of the anterior teeth varies. The general rule is to use the largest film that can readily be positioned to minimize the number of exposures. However, more films may be required for unusual conditions or for narrow arches requiring small films. A size #1 film is often used instead of the size #2 film for exposures of the anterior teeth. However, the narrow size #1 film may require the use of additional films in order to completely image the area. Three examples of film combinations for the use of anterior periapicals using the narrow #1 film or the standard #2 film are:

- **Eight anterior films.** Five size #1 films may be used for the exposure of the maxillary anterior teeth (Figure 13–5A). One film is centered at the midline behind the central incisors; one film each is centered behind the right and left lateral incisors; and one film each is centered behind the right and left canines. Three size #1 films are used for the exposure of the mandibular arch where the teeth are smaller. One film is centered behind the central and lateral incisors, and one film each is centered behind the right and left canines.
- **Eight anterior films.** Four size #1 films may be used for the exposure of the maxillary anterior teeth (Figure 13–5B). One film each is centered behind the right and left central and lateral incisors, and one film each is centered behind the right and left canines. Four size #1 films are used for the exposure of the mandibular anterior teeth in much the same way as for the maxilla. One film each is centered behind each of the right and left central and lateral incisors, and one film each is centered behind the right and left canines.
- **Six anterior films.** Three size #1 or three size #2 films may be used for the exposure of the maxillary anterior teeth (Figure 13–5C). One film is centered at the midline behind the central and lateral incisors and one film each is centered behind each of the right and left canines. The three size #1 or three size #2 films used for the exposure of the mandibular arch are positioned in the same manner as

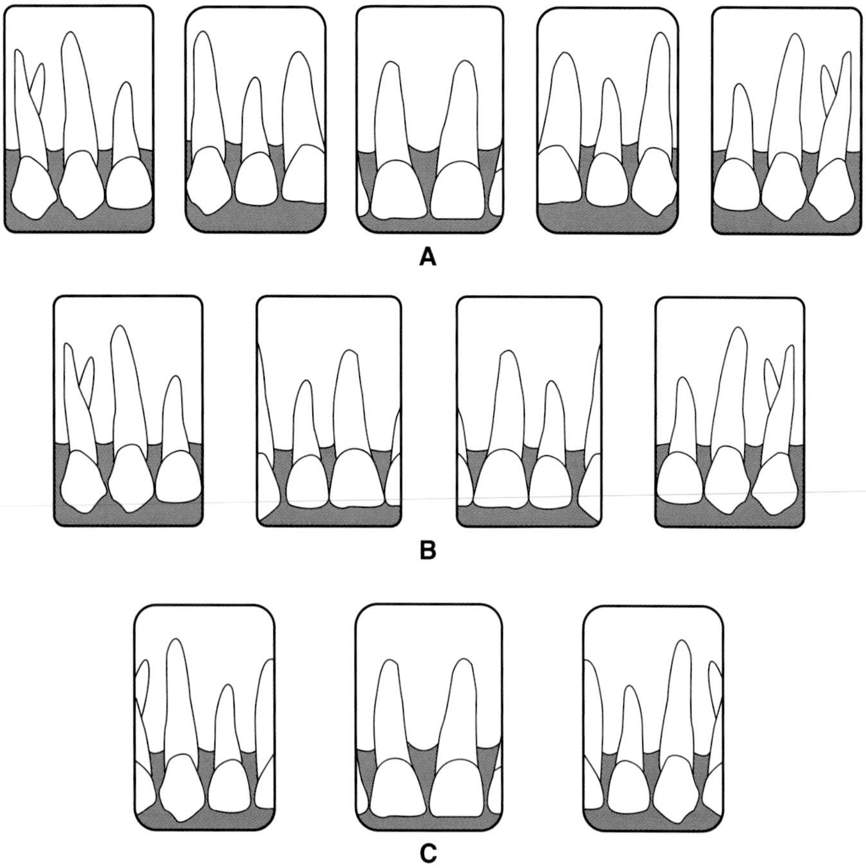

FIGURE 13–5 **Maxillary anterior film placement.** (**A**) Five-film survey. (**B**) Four-film survey. (**C**) Three-film survey.

described above, where one film is centered behind the central and lateral incisors and one film each is centered behind the right and left canines. While the use of size #2 film for anterior periapical radiographs is acceptable, the narrower size #1 film usually fits this area better. When using the size #2 film in the anterior region, there is a tendency to bend the film corners to make it fit more comfortably. Bending the film will result in a distorted image and/or radiolucent or radiopaque creases. Some practices utilize one size #2 film for the exposure of the maxillary central and lateral incisors, where the area is the widest, and use size #1 films to expose the remaining five areas.

See Table 13–1 for a list of all the various combinations of standard placements of the film packet for each of the periapical radiographs of a full-mouth survey.

Orientation of the Film Packet

With few exceptions, film packets for exposure of the anterior areas are placed with the longer dimension of the film vertically (described as **vertical placement**) (Figure 13–3). Film packets for exposure of the posterior areas are placed with the longer dimension horizontally (described as **horizontal placement**) (Figure 13–2). The white, unprinted side of the film packet (front side) must face the source of radiation.

When placing the film packet for periapical radiographs, it is important to make note of where the identification dot is located. The **identification dot,** embossed into the film by the manufacturer, will be utilized during interpretation of the radiograph to distinguish between the patient's right and left sides (see Chapter 18). There is a tendency for the embossed identification dot to distort images, so during film packet placement it is important to position the identification dot away from the area of interest. In the case of periapical radiographs, the identification dot should be positioned toward the occlusal or incisal edges, where it is least likely to interfere with diagnostic information.

Practice Point

When using a film-holding device with a film slot, it is helpful to remember that "dot in the slot" will position the embossed identification dot away from the apices of the teeth where it could interfere with diagnosis. **Dot in the slot** will position the identification dot toward the incisal or occlusal edges for both maxillary and mandibular periapical radiographs.

Angulations

The correct horizontal and vertical angulations are critical to producing a quality periapical radiograph.

TABLE 13-1 **Standard Film Packet Placements for Periapical Radiographs of a Full Mouth Series**

Periapical Radiograph	Film Packet Placement
Maxillary central incisors (Film size #1 or size #2)	Center the film packet to line up behind the central and lateral incisors; if using a size #2 film, include the mesial halves of the canines.
Maxillary central and lateral incisors (Film size #1)	Center the film packet to line up behind the central and lateral incisors; include the distal half of the central incisor on the opposite side and the mesial half of the canine.
Maxillary lateral incisor (Film size #1)	Center the film packet to line up behind the lateral incisor; include the distal half of the central incisor and the mesial half of the canine.
Maxillary lateral incisor and canine (Film size #1)	Center the film packet to line up behind the lateral incisor and canine; include the distal half of the central incisor and the mesial half of the premolar.
Maxillary canine (Film size #1 or size #2)	Center the film packet to line up behind the canine; include the distal half of the lateral incisor and the mesial half of the first premolar.
Mandibular central incisors (Film size #1 or size #2)	Center the film packet to line up behind the central and lateral incisors; if using a size #2 film, include the mesial halves of the canines.
Mandibular central and lateral incisors (Film size #1)	Center the film packet to line up behind the central and lateral incisors; include the distal half of the central incisor on the opposite side and the mesial half of the canine.
Mandibular canine (Film size #1 or size #2)	Center the film packet to line up behind the canine; include the distal half of the lateral incisor and the mesial half of the first premolar.
Maxillary and mandibular premolar (Film size #2)	Align the anterior edge of film packet to line up behind the distal half of the canine; include the entire first and second premolars and mesial half of the first molar.
Maxillary and mandibular molar (Film size #2)	Align the anterior edge of film packet to line up behind the distal half of the second premolar; include the entire first, second, and third molars.

Horizontal Angulation

Horizontal angulation, the positioning of the central ray (PID) in a horizontal (side-to-side) plane, is determined in the same manner as that used for bitewing radiographs of the same area (see Chapter 14). The central ray (PID) should be directed perpendicular to the curvature of the arch, through the contact points of the teeth. The horizontal angulation is established by directing the central rays perpendicularly through the **mean tangent** of the embrasures between the teeth of interest (see Figure 12–10 and Table 13–2). Incorrect horizontal angulation results in overlapped contact points (see Figure 14–6).

Vertical Angulation

Vertical angulation is the positioning of the central ray (PID) in a vertical (up and down) plane. Positive (+) angulation, the positioning of the central ray (PID) downward toward the floor, is generally used for the exposure of the maxillary arch. Negative (−) angulation, the positioning of the central ray (PID) upward toward the ceiling, is generally used for the exposure of the mandibular arch.

The precise vertical angulation setting for periapical radiographs is determined differently depending on the technique used. When utilizing the paralleling technique, the correct vertical angulation is achieved by directing the central rays of the x-ray beam perpendicular to the film and perpendicular to the long axes of the teeth in the vertical plane (see Chapter 12). A film-holding device, when used to position the film packet parallel to the long axes of teeth, will aid the radiographer in determining the correct vertical angulation. Incorrect vertical angulation when utilizing the paralleling technique results in cutting off a portion of the area of interest from the image. When the vertical angulation is excessive (greater than perpendicular to the film plane), the incisal or occlusal edges of the teeth will most likely be cut off and when the vertical angulation is inadequate (less than perpendicular to the film plane), the root apices of the teeth will most likely be cut off (Figure 13–6).

When utilizing the bisecting technique, the correct vertical angulation is achieved by directing the central rays of the x-ray beam perpendicular to the imaginary **bisector** between the long

TABLE 13-2 **Determining the Horizontal Angulation**

Periapical	Horizontal Angulation
Maxillary and mandibular central and lateral incisors	Direct the central rays perpendicularly through the left and right central incisor embrasure.
Maxillary and mandibular canines	Direct the central rays perpendicularly at the center of the canine.
Maxillary and mandibular premolars	Direct the central rays perpendicularly through the first and second premolar embrasure.
Maxillary and mandibular molars	Direct the central rays perpendicularly through the first and second molar embrasure.

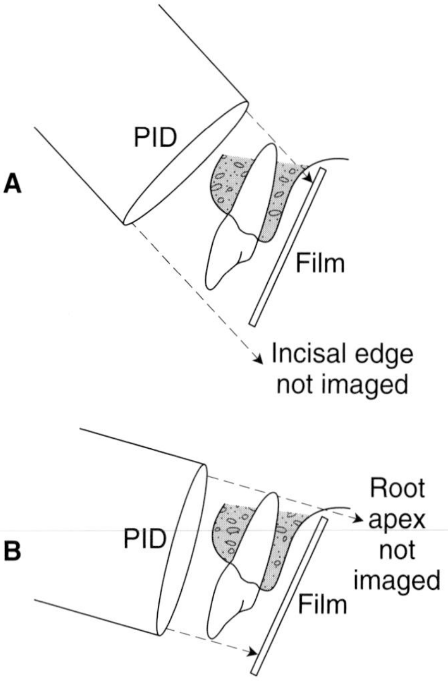

FIGURE 13-6 **Vertical angulation error–paralleling technique.** (**A**) Excessive vertical angulation results in incisal/occlusal edges being cut off the image. (**B**) Inadequate vertical angulation results in the apices being cut off the image.

axes of the teeth and the film plane in the vertical plane. If the patient is seated with the head positioning correct, the occlusal plane parallel to the floor, and the mid-saggital plane perpendicular to the floor, predetermined vertical settings may be utilized to position the PID at the correct vertical angulation (see Table 13–3). It is important to check that the occlusal plane of the arch being imaged is parallel to the floor. Incorrect vertical angulation when utilizing the bisecting technique results in elongated or foreshortened images. When the vertical angulation is excessive (greater than perpendicular to the imaginary bisector)

TABLE 13-3 **Recommended Vertical Angulation Settings for Periapical Radiographs of a Full Mouth Series when Utilizing the Bisecting Technique**

Periapical	Recommended Vertical Setting*
Maxillary central and lateral incisors	+40 degrees
Maxillary canines	+45 degrees
Maxillary premolars	+30 degrees
Maxillary molars	+20 degrees
Mandibular central and lateral incisors	−15 degrees
Mandibular canines	−20 degrees
Mandibular premolars	−10 degrees
Mandibular molars	−5 degrees

*The patient must be seated in the correct position, with the occlusal plane of the arch being imaged parallel to the floor and the midsaggital plane perpendicular to the floor.

the image will be foreshortened, and when the vertical angulation is inadequate (less than perpendicular to the imaginary bisector), the image will be elongated (Figure 13–7). Vertical angulation error is explained in Chapter 16.

Point of Entry

The point of entry for the central ray for periapical radiographs may be located with the use of a film holder with an external aiming device. Without an external indicator, care should be taken to center the film packet within the beam of x-radiation. Use the portion of the film holder, or biteblock, that extends from the oral cavity to estimate the center of the film. Incorrect point of entry, or not centering the film packet within the x-ray beam, will result in cone cut error.

When utilizing the bisecting technique, if the patient is seated with the correct head position, the point of entry may be estimated with the use of recommended landmarks (Table 13–4). (See Figure 12–9.)

The open end of the PID should be placed as close to the patient's skin as possible without touching. Failure to bring the end of the PID in close to the patient will result in an underexposed radiograph. As the beam of radiation spreads out, less radiation is available to strike the film and produce a diagnostic quality image.

Holding the Periapical Film Packet in Position

The choice of film holder for stabilizing the film packet for periapical exposures depends on the method to be used to expose the radiographs. Many film holders are designed for use with the paralleling technique only, or the bisecting technique only. There

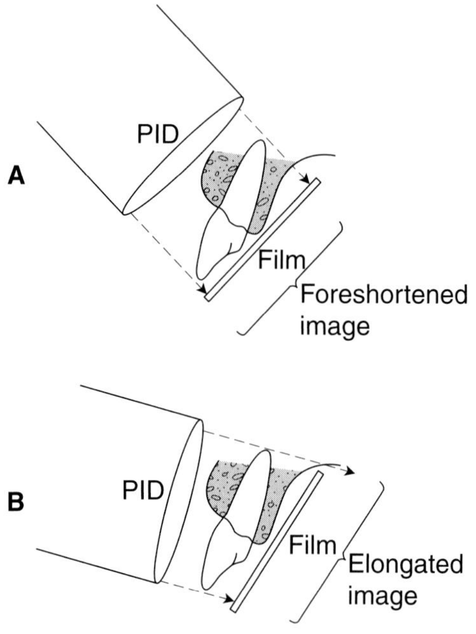

FIGURE 13-7 **Vertical angulation error—bisecting technique.** (**A**) Excessive vertical angulation results in foreshortening of the image. (**B**) Inadequate vertical angulation results in elongation of the image.

TABLE 13-4 **Recommended Landmarks for Locating the Point of Entry When Utilizing the Bisecting Technique**

Periapical	Recommended Point of Entry*
Maxillary central and lateral incisors	At a point near the tip of the nose
Maxillary canines	At the root of the canine; at the ala of the nose
Maxillary premolars	At a point on the ala-tragus line directly below the pupil of the eye
Maxillary molars	At a point on the ala-tragus line directly below the outer canthus of the eye
Mandibular central and lateral incisors	At a point on the center of the chin, 1 in. (2.5 cm) above the lower border of the mandible
Mandibular canines	At the center of the root of the canine, 1 in. (2.5 cm) above the inferior border of the mandible
Mandibular premolars	At a point on the chin, 1 in. (2.5 cm) above the lower border of the mandible, directly inferior to the pupil of the eye
Mandibular molars	At a point on the chin, 1 in. (2.5 cm) above the lower border of the mandible, directly below the outer canthus of the eye

*The patient must be seated in the correct position with the occlusal plane of the arch being imaged parallel to the floor and the midsagittal plane perpendicular to the floor.

are also film holders that, with minor adaptation, can be used with either technique. It is important that the radiographer match the film holder with the technique for which it was designed, to achieve optimal results.

Film holders designed for use with the paralleling technique must be able to achieve a parallel relationship between the film packet and the long axes of the teeth. Oral structures, particularly the curvature of the palate, make it difficult to place the film packet close to the teeth and, at the same time, remain parallel to the long axes of the teeth. To achieve parallelism, the film packet must be placed a greater distance from the teeth. The paralleling technique film holder's long **biteblock** area will allow for a parallel film packet to teeth relationship. Additionally, a film holder designed for the paralleling technique will often have an L-shaped backing to help support the film and keep it in position. Examples of paralleling film holders are the Rinn XCP® (Extension Cone Paralleling) (see Figure 6–14) and the Isaac Masel Company Precision® (see Figure 6–7). These two instruments have an external aiming device to assist the radiographer in locating the correct angles and points of entry, making errors less likely. The external aiming device also eliminates the need to position the patient's head precisely.

It should be noted, however, that the extra size and weight of the external aiming device may make placement of a film packet difficult or uncomfortable for the patient. If film packet placement is compromised, not positioned correctly, the aiming device will indicate directing the x-ray beam to the wrong place.

Holders designed with a short biteblock should be considered bisecting technique holders even if not labeled as such. Typically, a shorter biteblock will allow the film packet to be placed close to the lingual surface of the teeth. However, when the film packet is placed close to the teeth, it is important to remember that it is probably not parallel to the long axes of the teeth and therefore, the technique used to make the exposures should be altered to the bisecting technique. Examples of film holders designed for the bisecting technique are the Rinn BAI® (Bisecting Angle Instrument) (Figure 13–8) and the Rinn Snap-A-Ray® (Figure 13–9).

Examples of film holders that may be used with both the paralleling and the bisecting technique are the Stabe® (Dentsply Rinn Corporation) and the SUPA® (Single Use Positioning Aid manufactured by Flow X-Ray Corporation). These film holders provide a long biteblock and L-shaped back support for the film

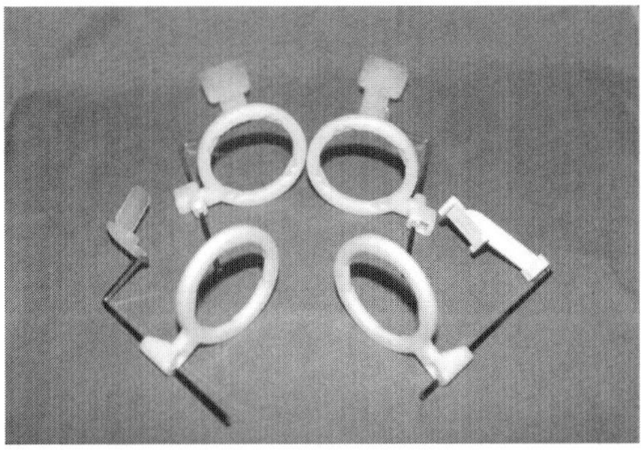

FIGURE 13-8 **Rinn BAI® bisecting technique film holders.** Note that these instruments are similar to the Rinn XCP® holders. The BAI® film holder replaces the paralleling L-shaped backing of the film-holder biteblock with a biteblock with a 105 degree slanted back to accommodate placing the film close to the teeth.

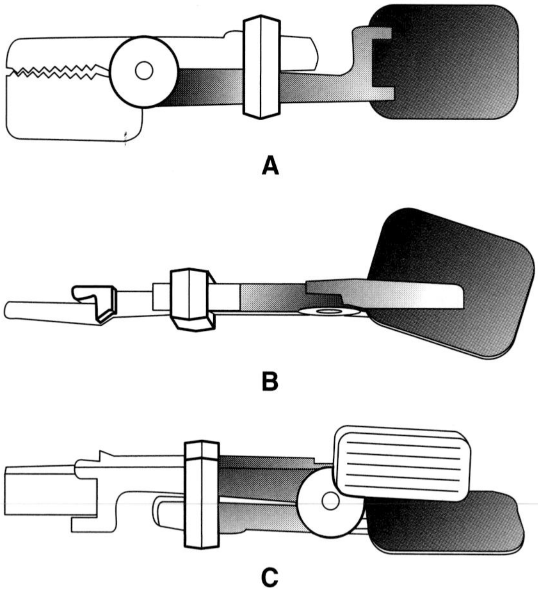

FIGURE 13-9 **Rinn Snap-A-Ray® film holder.** While many clinicians observe the versatility this autoclavable film holder provides, its short biteblock does not allow for parallel placement of the film packet in all areas of the oral cavity. For this reason, one should be cautioned that the Snap-A-Ray® should be used when employing the bisecting technique. This illustration shows the film packet positioned to image (**A**) the anterior areas, (**B**) the mandibular third molar area, and (**C**) the posterior areas. (Courtesy of Dentsply Rinn)

packet for use with the paralleling technique. However, these manufacturers have designed the film holder with a scored groove that allows the radiographer to break off the bite extension and use the holder with the bisecting technique as well (Figure 13–10). The light, polystyrene single-part construction makes these film holders comfortable, easy to place, and versatile. The radiographer must be skilled in estimating the correct angles and point of entry to utilize these devices. For this reason, it is important that the radiographer develop the skills necessary to evaluate film packet placement for correctness, regardless of the holder used.

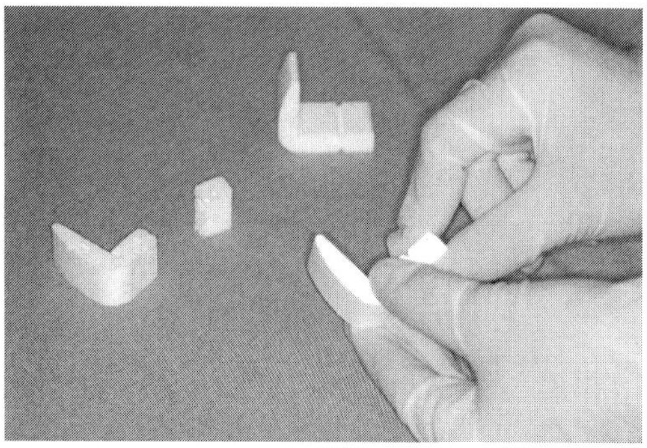

FIGURE 13-10 **Stabe®.** The bite extension may be broken off the Stabe® film holder for use with the bisecting technique.

It is beneficial to have a variety of film holders available, because one type of holder may not be suitable for all patients, or even all areas of the same patient's mouth. Additionally, the operator may have to alternate between the paralleling and the bisecting technique to complete a full mouth series on a patient. Because of its ability to produce superior diagnostic quality radiographs, the paralleling technique should be the technique of choice when exposing periapical radiographs. However, the radiographer who is skilled in both paralleling and bisecting techniques will be better prepared to produce quality radiographs in most all situations.

Sequence of Film Placement

A definite sequence of film positioning should be followed to prevent omitting an area or exposing an area twice. Develop a set routine to prevent errors and save time.

Opinions differ as to which region should be exposed first when taking a full-mouth survey. Some radiographers prefer to begin in the right maxillary molar region and continue in sequence to the left maxillary molar region, drop down to the left mandibular molar region, and finish in the right mandibular molar region.

Others begin with the anterior exposures, on the theory that the film packet placement is more comfortable here and less likely to excite a gag reflex than when it is placed in the maxillary molar region, where the tissues are more sensitive (see Chapter 24). If the first few films produce no discomfort, the patient will become used to the feel of the film and will more readily accept it.

For an experienced radiographer who can place the film skillfully and rapidly, it probably makes little difference which area is exposed first. However, the same order of film placement should always be followed to make sure that all regions are exposed. The following sequence of film positioning is suggested to help the student adopt a systematic routine:

- Maxillary anterior periapicals
- Mandibular anterior periapicals
- Maxillary posterior periapicals
- Mandibular posterior periapicals
- Anterior bitewings
- Posterior bitewings

Anterior film placements are usually more comfortable and allow the patient to become accustomed to the procedure. The bitewing examination (see Chapter 14) is last because the patient tolerates these fairly well and the radiographic procedure can end pleasantly. Additionally, it may be helpful for the radiographer not to have to break the sequence of exposing periapical radiographs by switching to a bitewing holder and changing techniques.

PROCEDURE 13-1

PROCEDURE FOR EXPOSING PERIAPICAL RADIOGRAPHS

1. Perform infection control procedures (see Procedure Box 9–2).
2. Prepare unit. Turn on and set exposure factors.
3. Seat patient and explain the procedure.
4. Request that the patient remove objects from the mouth that can interfere with the procedure and remove eyeglasses.
5. Adjust chair to a comfortable working level.
6. Adjust the head rest to position the patient's head so that the occlusal plane of the maxilla is parallel to the floor and the midsagittal plane (midline) is perpendicular to the floor.
7. Place the lead apron and thyroid collar on the patient.
8. Perform a cursory inspection of the oral cavity and note possible obstructions (tori, shallow palatal vault, mal-aligned teeth) that may require an alteration of technique or number of films exposed.
9. Place the film packet into the film-holding device. Place such that the embossed dot will be positioned toward the occlusal/incisal edge ("dot in the slot"). Position anterior film packets vertically and posterior film packets horizontally.
10. Insert the film and film holder into the patient's oral cavity and center the film packet behind the area to be imaged. (See Table 13–1 for the exact film packet placements for each of the maxillary and mandibular periapical radiographs in the procedure.) Visually locate the contact points of the teeth to be imaged and place the film packet perpendicular to the embrasures.
11. Hold the film holder against the occlusal/incisal surface of the maxillary/mandibular teeth while asking the patient to bite firmly onto the biteblock of the film holder. (Use a sterilized cotton roll for stabilization if needed.)
12. Release the film holder when the patient has closed firmly, holding it in place.
13. Set the vertical angulation:
    a. To intersect the film plane and the long axes of the teeth perpendicularly when utilizing the paralleling technique. If using a film holder with an external aiming device, align the open end of the PID with the indicator ring.
    b. To intersect the imaginary bisector of the film plane and the long axes of the teeth perpendicularly when utilizing the bisecting technique. (See Table 13–3 for the recommended vertical angulation setting for the area being imaged.)
14. Determine the correct horizontal angulation by directing the central ray of the x-ray beam perpendicular to the film in the horizontal plane through the contact point of the teeth of interest. (See Table 13–2 for the exact embrasure space through which to direct the central ray for each of the periapical radiographs in the procedure. Horizontal angulation is determined the same for both paralleling and bisecting techniques.) If using a film holder with an external aiming device, align the open end of the PID with the indicator ring.
15. Center the PID over the film packet. If using a film holder with an external aiming device, align the open end of the PID with the indicator ring. (See Table 13–4 for point of entry recommendations when utilizing the bisecting technique.)
16. Make the exposure.
17. Remove the film packet and holder from the patient's oral cavity.
18. Repeat steps 9–17 until all maxillary films in the series have been exposed.
19. Re-adjust the head rest to position the patient's head so that the occlusal plane of the mandible is parallel to the floor. Ensure that the midsagittal plane (midline) is perpendicular to the floor.
20. Repeat steps 9–17 until all mandibular films in the series have been exposed
21. Remove the lead apron and thyroid collar from the patient.
22. Perform infection control procedures following the exposures (see Procedure Box 9–4).

The Periapical Examination: Paralleling Technique

Unit Preparation

Prior to placing the film packet intraorally, the unit should be turned on and the exposure settings selected. It is helpful to place the tube head and PID in the approximate position for this first exposure to limit the time required for this step once the film packet has been placed into the patient's oral cavity.

Patient Preparation

To help gain patient cooperation and confidence, it is important to explain the procedure to the patient. Include specific instructions regarding the need for patient cooperation and be honest about any difficulties anticipated (see Chapter 11). Perform a cursory oral inspection and ask the patient to remove any objects from the mouth that would interfere with the procedure, such as removable dentures or orthodontic appliances, chewing gum, etc. Ask the patient to remove eyeglasses; if any metal or thick plastic parts of the eyeglasses remain in the path of the x-ray beam, they will be imaged onto the radiograph. Protect the patient with the lead apron and thyroid collar barriers.

Position the patient's head so that the occlusal plane of the arch to be imaged is parallel to the floor and the midsagittal plane (midline) is perpendicular to the floor (see Figure 14–15). Use the head rest to adjust the patient's position. When using a film holder with an external aiming device, the patient's head position is not as critical. However, stabilizing the patient's head against the head rest is important to prevent movement during the exposure. Place the head rest against the occipital protuberance (the back, base of the skull) for greatest stability.

Managing Exposures

As described in Chapter 12, the basic principles of the paralleling technique are:

- The film is placed parallel to the long axes of the teeth being radiographed.
- The central ray is directed at right angles to both the teeth and film (see Figure 12–3).

To achieve parallel placement of the film packet, the film holder selected must have a long biteblock. For illustration purposes, the Rinn XCP® film holder is described here because its external aiming device attachment aids in directing the central ray at the teeth and film perpendicularly (Figure 13–11). While the radiographer should refer to the manufacturer's instructions for use, important key points regarding the Rinn XCP® are:

- The patient must bite down on the biteblock as far away from the teeth as possible, utilizing the full extent of the biteblock. (The exception to this rule is for the mandibular premolar and molar regions, where the film can be close to the teeth and still remain parallel).
- The patient must bite down on the biteblock firmly enough to hold the film packet in place. A sterilized cotton roll may be placed on the opposite side of the biteblock to provide stablization and add to patient comfort.
- The external **indicator ring** attachment must be slid all the way down the metal arm of the device to be as close to the patient's skin as possible without touching the patient prior to the exposure.
- The open end of the PID is aligned to the indicator ring to achieve correct horizontal and vertical angulations and correct point of entry.

To compensate for the increased object–film distance needed when using the paralleling technique, the target–film distance is also increased to a 12 in. (30 cm) or 16 in. (41 cm) PID.

Figures 13–12 through 13–19 illustrate the precise film packet positions and the required angulations for each of the periapical radiographs in a basic 14-film full mouth series utilizing the paralleling technique. See Table 13–5 for a summary of the technique.

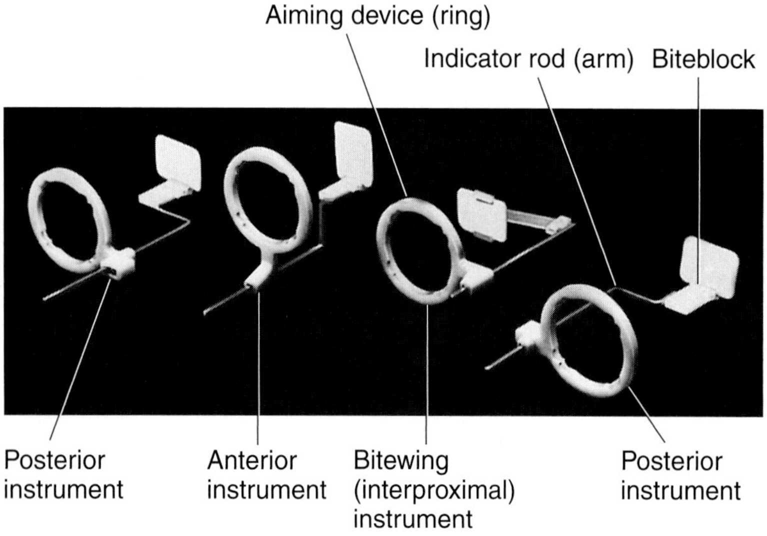

FIGURE 13–11 **Rinn XCP® paralleling technique film holders.** Note that these instruments require assembly of multiple parts. Note the mirror-image assembly of these posterior periapical film holders. The holder assembly on the left is used for exposures on the maxillary right and the mandibular left, while the holder assembly on the right is used for exposures on the maxillary left and on the mandibular right. (Courtesy of Dentsply Rinn)

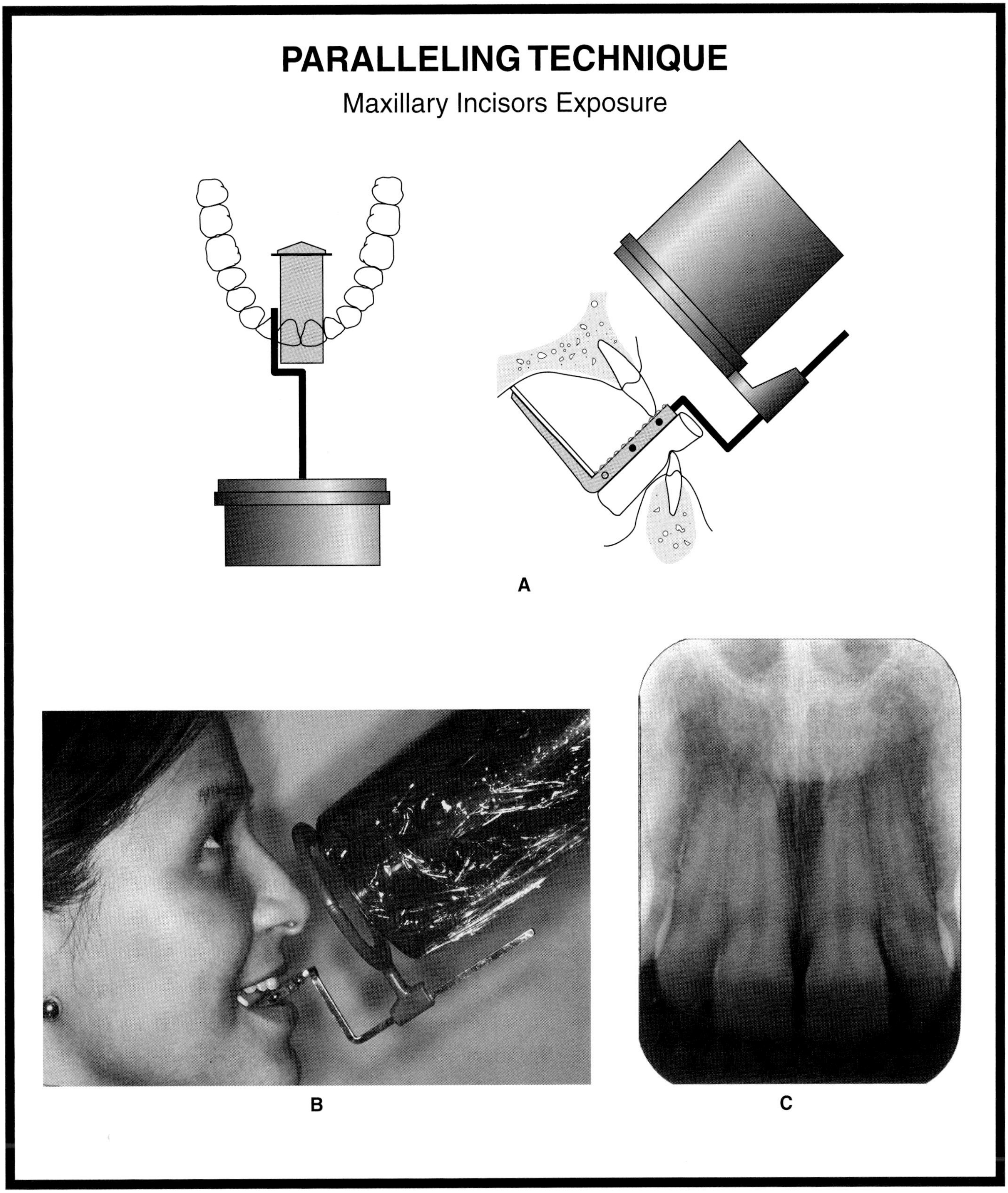

FIGURE 13-12 **Maxillary incisors exposure.** (**A**) Diagrams show the relationship of film, teeth, XCP® instrument, and PID. As in all anterior areas, the film is positioned with the long dimension vertically. Film is parallel to the teeth with the biteblock inserted to its full length to position the film back toward the region of the first molars to achieve parallelism with the long axes of the incisors. A sterile cotton roll may be placed on the biteblock on the opposite side from the film to help stabilize the placement. (**B**) Patient showing position of XCP® instrument and 12 in. (30 cm) circular PID. (**C**) Maxillary incisors radiograph.

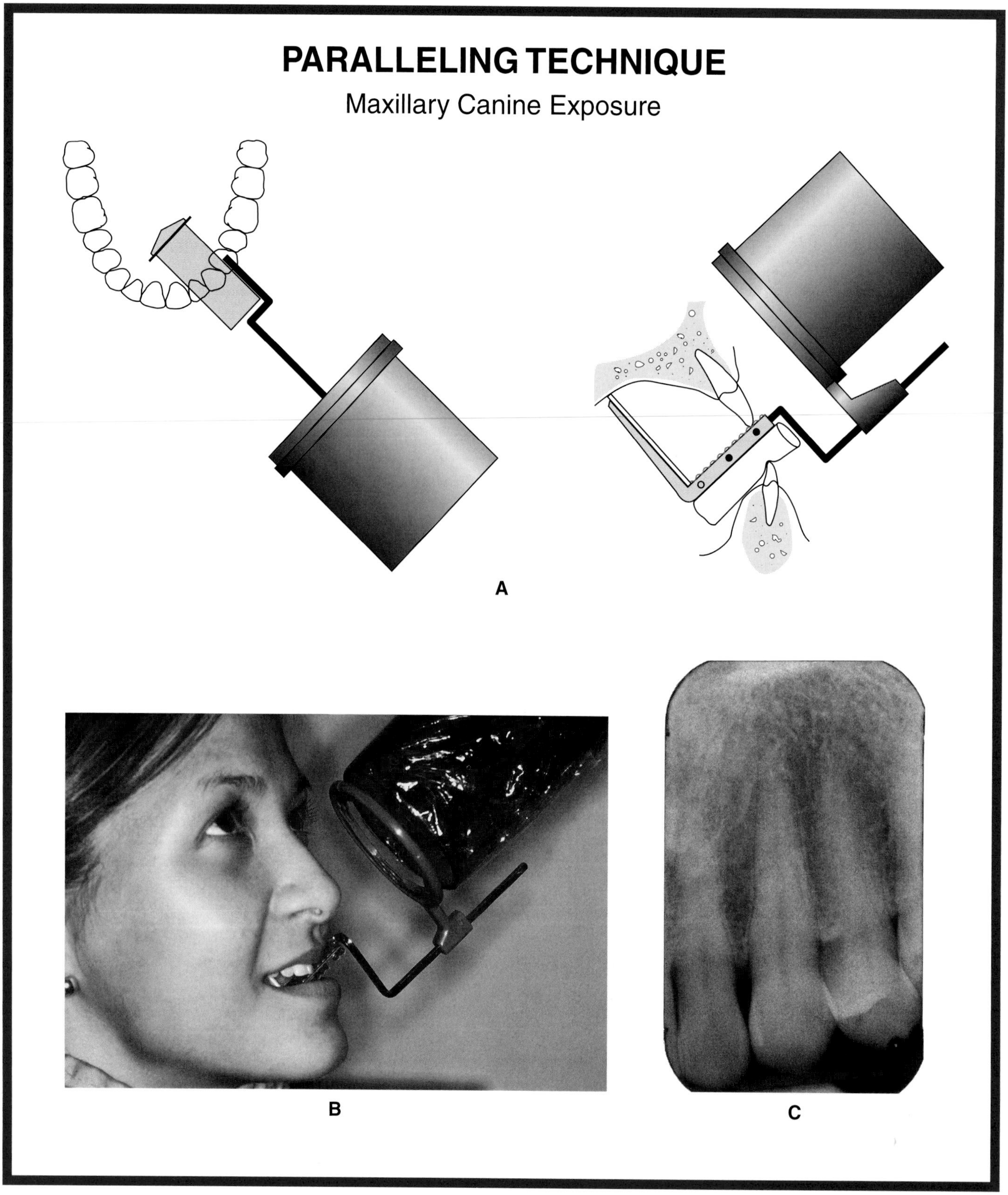

FIGURE 13–13 **Maxillary canine exposure.** (**A**) Diagrams show the relationship of film, teeth, XCP® instrument, and PID. As in all anterior areas, the film is positioned with the long dimension vertically. Film is parallel to the teeth with the biteblock inserted to its full length to position the film up into the midline of the palate to take advantage of the highest point and achieve parallelism with the long axis of the canine. A sterile cotton roll may be placed on the biteblock on the opposite side from the film to help stabilize the placement (**B**) Patient showing position of XCP® instrument and 12 in. (30 cm) circular PID. (**C**) Maxillary canine radiograph.

PARALLELING TECHNIQUE

Maxillary Premolar Exposure

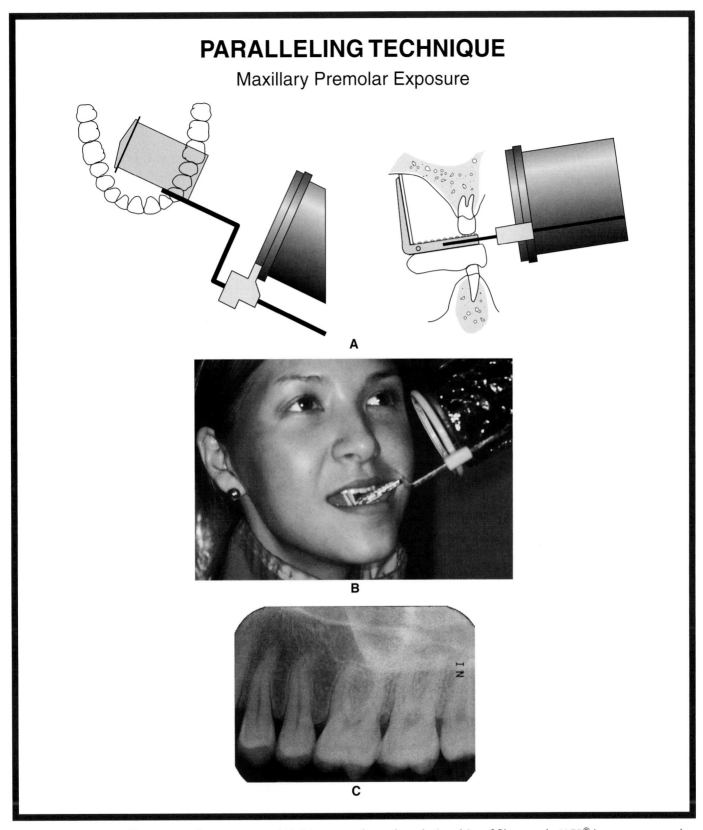

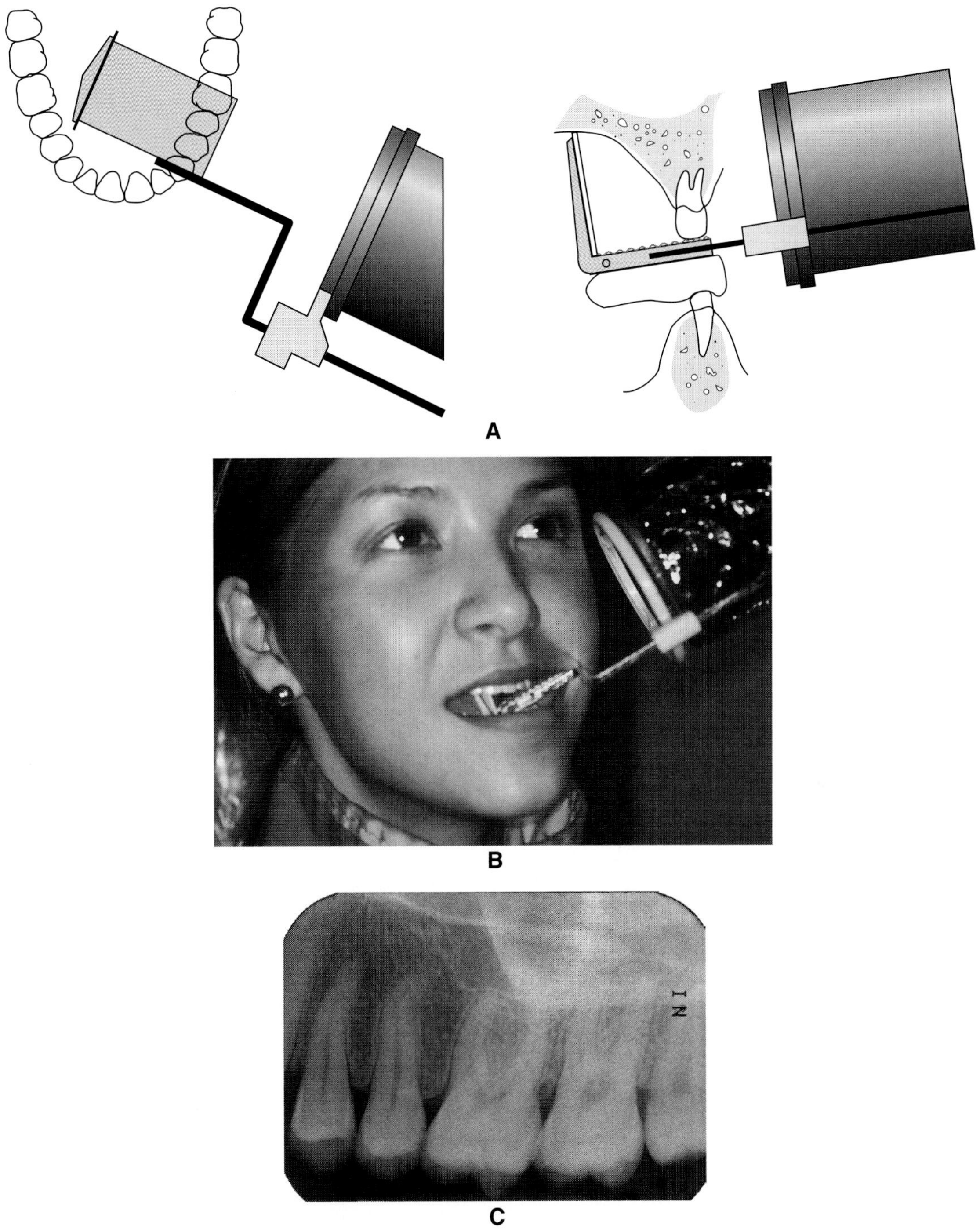

FIGURE 13-14 **Maxillary premolar exposure.** (**A**) Diagrams show the relationship of film, teeth, XCP® instrument, and PID. As in all posterior areas, the film is positioned with the long dimension horizontally. Film is parallel to the teeth with the biteblock inserted to its full length to position the film up into the midline of the palate to take advantage of the highest point and achieve parallelism with the long axes of the premolars. A sterile cotton roll may be placed on the biteblock on the opposite side from the film to help stabilize the placement. (**B**) Patient showing position of XCP® instrument and 12 in. (30 cm) circular PID. (**C**) Maxillary premolar radiograph.

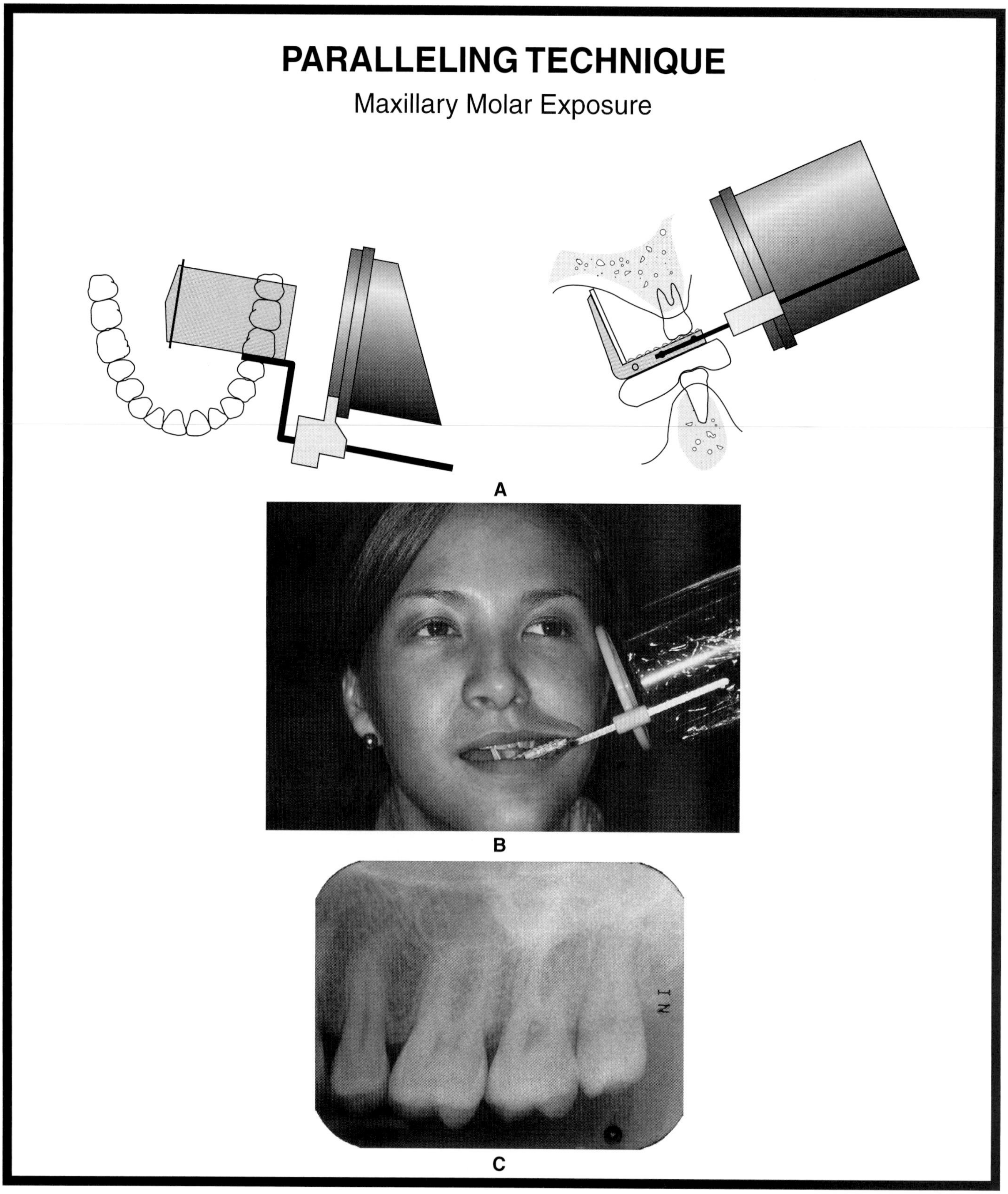

FIGURE 13-15 **Maxillary molar exposure.** (**A**) Diagrams show the relationship of film, teeth, XCP® instrument, and PID. As in all posterior areas, the film is positioned with the long dimension horizontally. Film is parallel to the teeth with the biteblock inserted to its full length to position the film up into the midline of the palate to take advantage of the highest point and achieve parallelism with the long axes of the molars. A sterile cotton roll may be placed on the biteblock on the opposite side from the film to help stabilize the placement. (**B**) Patient showing position of XCP® instrument and 12 in. (30 cm) circular PID. (**C**) Maxillary molar radiograph.

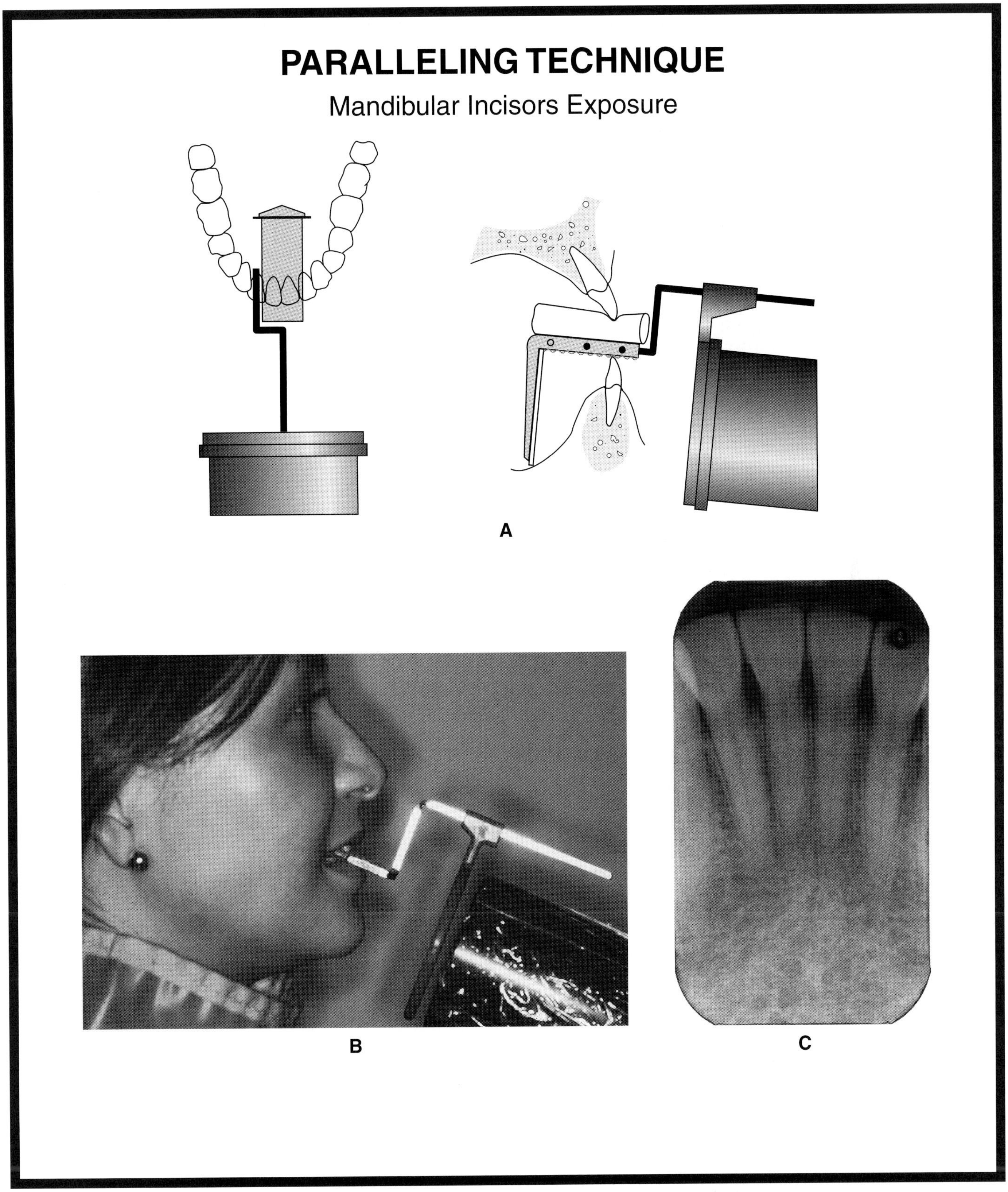

FIGURE 13–16 **Mandibular incisors exposure.** (**A**) Diagrams show the relationship of film, teeth, XCP® instrument, and PID. As in all anterior areas, the film is positioned with the long dimension vertically. Film is parallel to the teeth. A sterile cotton roll may be placed on the biteblock on the opposite side from the film to help stabilize the placement. This will aid in forcing the biteblock down into position when the opposing teeth occlude. (**B**) Patient showing position of XCP® instrument and 12 in. (30 cm) circular PID. (**C**) Mandibular incisors radiograph.

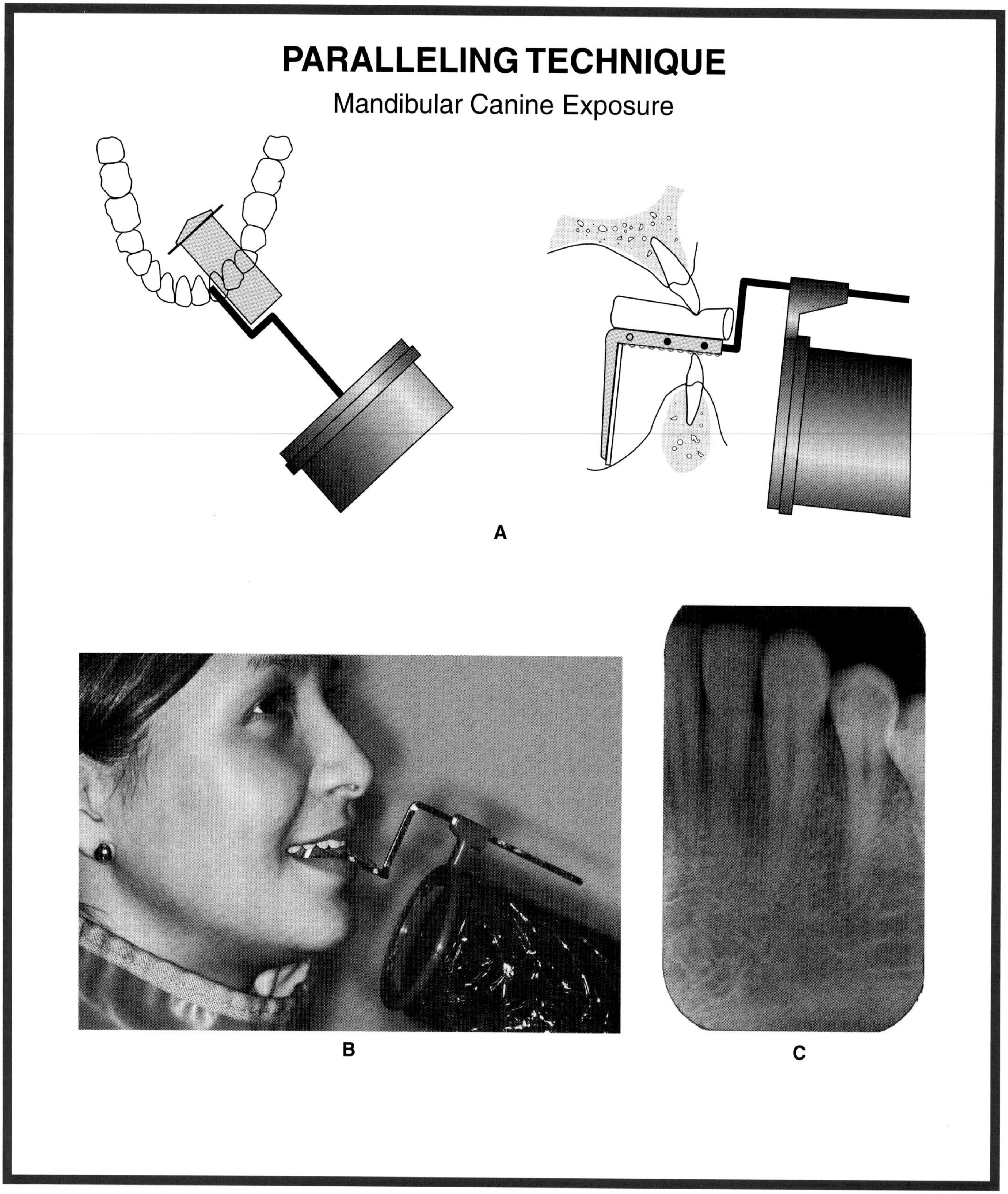

FIGURE 13-17 **Mandibular canine exposure.** (**A**) Diagrams show the relationship of film, teeth, XCP® instrument, and PID. As in all anterior areas, the film is positioned with the long dimension vertically. Film is parallel to the teeth. A sterile cotton roll may be placed on the biteblock on the opposite side from the film to help stabilize the placement. This will aid in forcing the biteblock down into position when the opposing teeth occlude. (**B**) Patient showing position of XCP® instrument and 12 in. (30 cm) circular PID. (**C**) Mandibular canine radiograph.

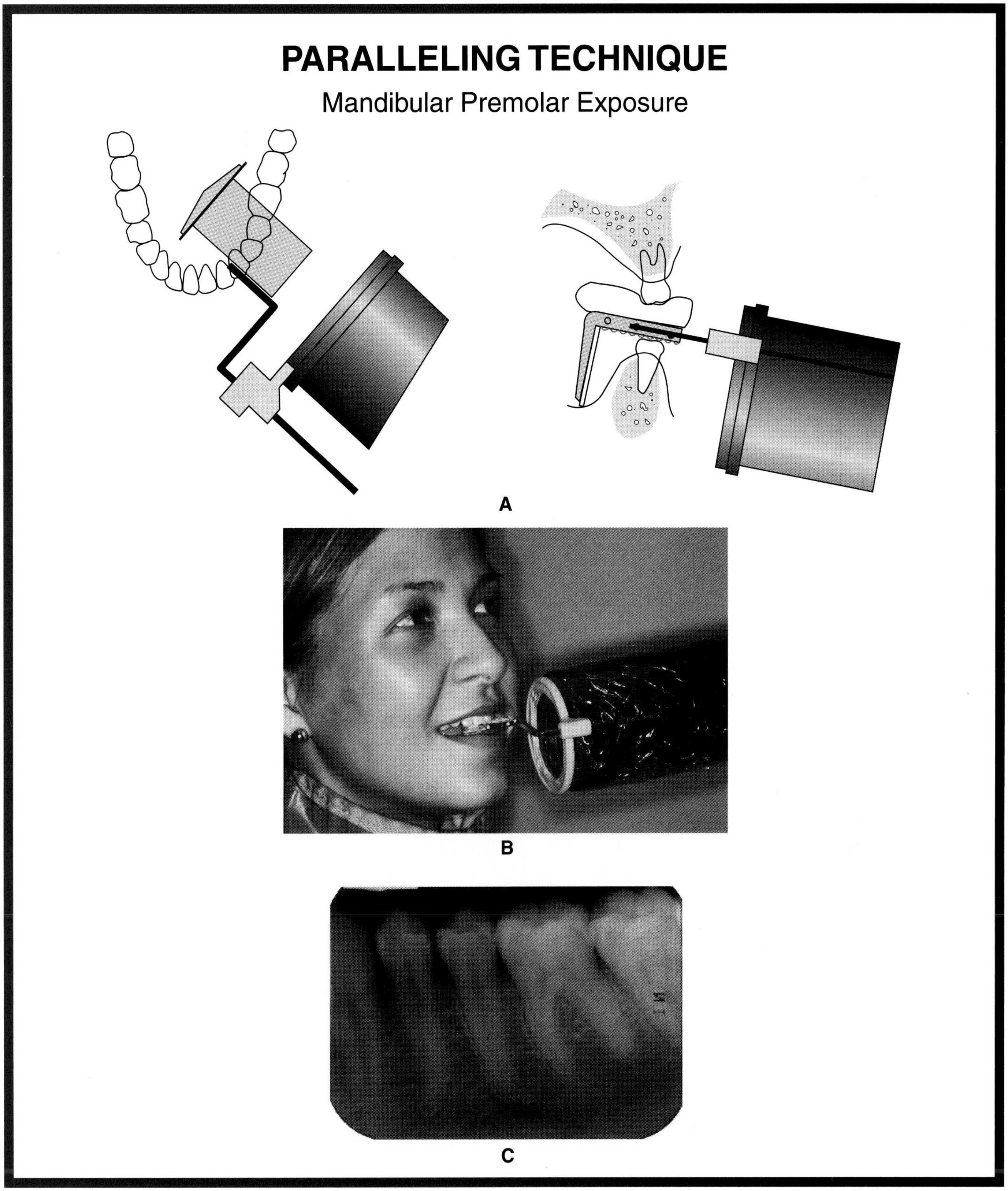

FIGURE 13-18 **Mandibular premolar exposure.** (**A**) Diagrams show the relationship of film, teeth XCP® instrument, and PID. As in all posterior areas, the film is positioned with the long dimension horizontally. Film is parallel to the teeth. A sterile cotton roll may be placed on the biteblock on the opposite side from the film to help stabilize the placement. This will aid in forcing the biteblock down into position when the opposing teeth occlude. (**B**) Patient showing position of XCP® instrument and 12 in. (30 cm) circular PID. (**C**) Mandibular premolar radiograph.

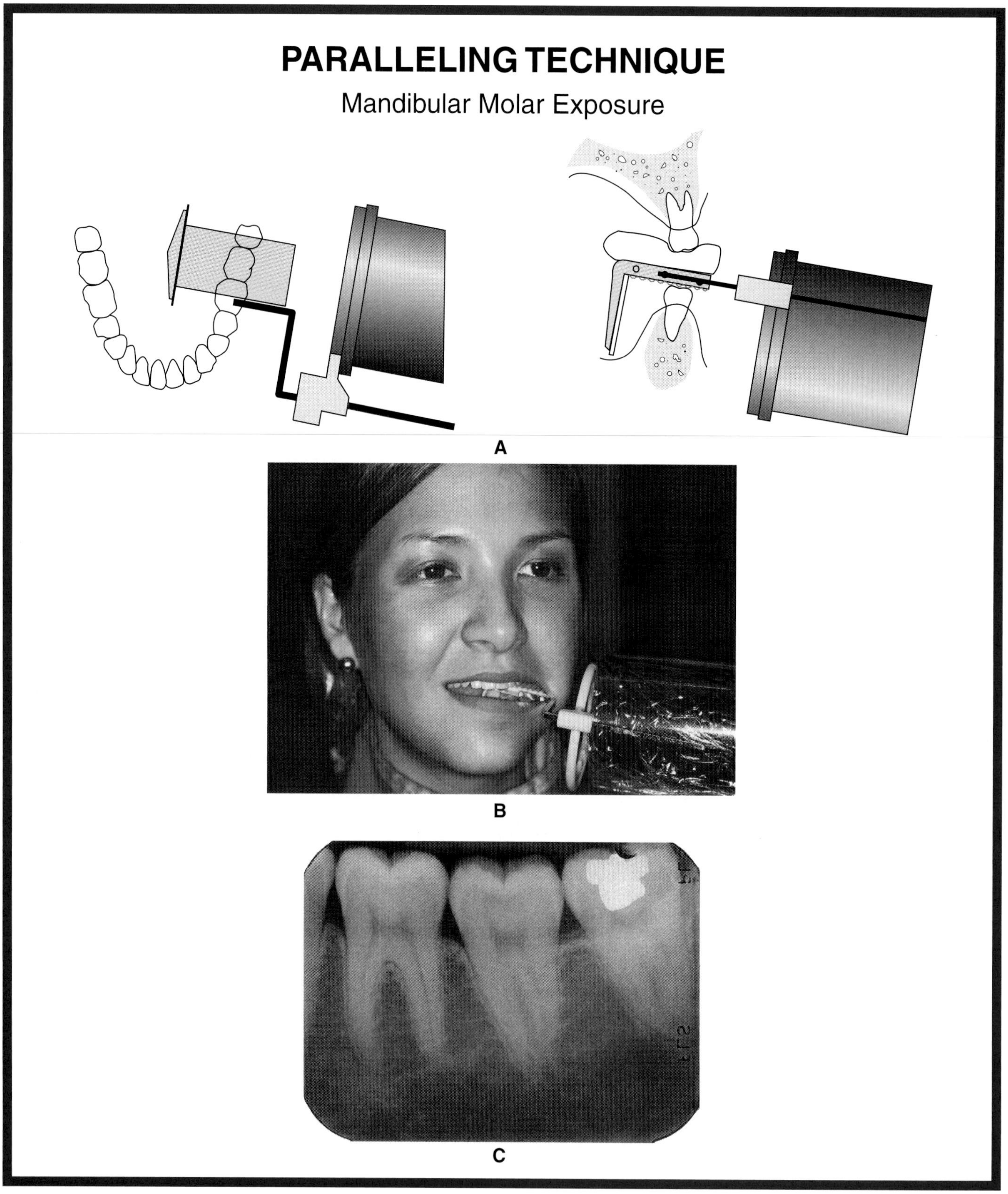

FIGURE 13-19 **Mandibular molar exposure.** (**A**) Diagrams show the relationship of film, teeth, XCP® instrument, and PID. As in all posterior areas, the film is positioned with the long dimension horizontally. Film is parallel to the teeth. A sterile cotton roll may be placed on the biteblock on the opposite side from the film to help stabilize the placement. This will aid in forcing the biteblock down into position when the opposing teeth occlude. (**B**) Patient showing position of XCP® instrument and 12 in. (30 cm) circular PID. (**C**) Mandibular molar radiograph.

TABLE 13-5 **A Summary of Periapical Radiographic Techniques**

Periapical Radiograph	Film Packet Placement	Vertical Angulation	Horizontal Angulation	Point of Entry
Maxillary incisors (Film size #1 or size #2)	Center the film packet to line up behind the central and lateral incisors; if using a size #2 film, include the mesial halves of the canines.	*Paralleling technique* Direct the central rays toward the film perpendicularly in the vertical dimension. PID will be pointing down. *Bisecting technique* Direct the central rays toward the imaginary bisector between the long axes of the teeth and the film in the vertical dimension, +40°.	Direct the central rays perpendicularly through the left and right central incisor embrasure.	*Paralleling technique* Center the film packet within the x-ray beam. Direct the central ray at the center of the film. *Bisecting technique* Direct the central rays at point near the tip of the nose.
Maxillary canine (Film size #1 or size #2)	Center the film packet to line up behind the canine; include the distal half of the lateral incisor and the mesial half of the first premolar.	*Paralleling technique* Direct the central rays toward the film perpendicularly in the vertical dimension. PID will be pointing down. *Bisecting technique* Direct the central rays toward the imaginary bisector between the long axis of the tooth and the film in the vertical dimension, +45°.	Direct the central rays perpendicularly in the horizontal direction at the center of the canine.	*Paralleling technique* Center the film packet within the x-ray beam. Direct the central rays at the center of the film. *Bisecting technique* Direct the central rays at the root of the canine, at the ala of the nose.
Maxillary premolar (Film size #2)	Align the anterior edge of the film packet to line up behind the distal half of the canine; include the first and second premolars and mesial half of the first molar.	*Paralleling technique* Direct the central rays toward the film perpendicularly in the vertical dimension. PID will be pointing down. *Bisecting technique* Direct the central rays toward the imaginary bisector between the long axes of the teeth and the film in the vertical dimension, +30°.	Direct the central rays perpendicularly through the first and second premolar embrasure.	*Paralleling technique* Center the film packet within the x-ray beam. Direct the central rays at the center of the film. *Bisecting technique* Direct the central rays at a point on the ala–tragus line directly below the pupil of the eye.
Maxillary molar (Film size #2)	Align the anterior edge of the film packet to line up behind the distal half of the second premolar; include the first, second, and third molars.	*Paralleling technique* Direct the central rays toward the film perpendicularly in the vertical dimension. PID will be pointing down. *Bisecting technique* Direct the central rays toward the imaginary bisector between the long axes of the teeth and the film in the vertical dimension; +20°.	Direct the central rays perpendicularly through the first and second molar embrasure.	*Paralleling technique* Center the film packet within the x-ray beam. Direct the central rays at the center of the film. *Bisecting technique* Direct the center rays at a point on the ala–tragus line directly below the outer canthus of the eye.

(continued)

TABLE 13-5 **A Summary of Periapical Radiographic Techniques** (*cont.*)

Periapical Radiograph	Film Packet Placement	Vertical Angulation	Horizontal Angulation	Point of Entry
Mandibular incisors (Film size #1 or #2)	Center the film packet to line up behind the central and lateral incisors.	*Paralleling technique* Direct the central rays toward the film perpendicularly in the vertical dimension. PID will be pointing up. *Bisecting technique* Direct the central rays toward the imaginary bisector between the long axes of the teeth and the film in the vertical dimension, −15°.	Direct the central rays perpendicularly through the left and right central incisor embrasure.	*Paralleling technique* Center the film packet within the x-ray beam. Direct the central rays at the center of the film. *Bisecting technique* Direct the central rays at a point on the chin, 1 in. (2.5 cm) above the lower border of the mandible.
Mandibular canine (Film size #1 or #2)	Center the film packet to line up behind the canine; include the distal half of the lateral incisor and the mesial half of the first premolar.	*Paralleling technique* Direct the central rays toward the film perpendicularly in the vertical dimension. PID will be pointing up. *Bisecting technique* Direct the central rays toward the imaginary bisector between the long axis of the tooth and the film in the vertical dimension, −20°.	Direct the central rays perpendicularly in the horizontal direction at the center of the canine.	*Paralleling technique* Center the film packet within the x-ray beam. Direct the central rays at the center of the film. *Bisecting technique* Direct the central rays at the center of the root of the canine, 1 in. (2.5 cm) above the inferior border of the mandible.
Mandibular premolar (Film size #2)	Align the anterior edge of the film packet to line up behind the distal half of the canine; include the first and second premolars and mesial half of the first molar.	*Paralleling technique* Direct the central rays toward the film perpendicularly in the vertical dimension. PID will be pointing up. *Bisecting technique* Direct the central rays toward the imaginary bisector between the long axes of the teeth and the film in the vertical dimension; −10°.	Direct the central rays perpendicularly through the first and second premolar embrasure.	*Paralleling technique* Center the film packet within the x-ray beam. Direct the central rays at the center of the film. *Bisecting technique* Direct the central rays at a point on the chin, 1 in. (2.5 cm) above the border of the mandible, directly inferior to the pupil of the eye.
Mandibular molar (Film size #2)	Align the anterior edge of the film packet to line up behind the distal half of the second premolar; include the first, second, and third molars.	*Paralleling technique* Direct the central rays toward the film perpendicularly in the vertical dimension. PID will be pointing up. *Bisecting technique* Direct the central rays toward the imaginary bisector between the long axes of the teeth and the film in the vertical dimension, −5°.	Direct the central rays perpendicularly through the first and second molar embrasure.	*Paralleling technique* Center the film packet within the x-ray beam. Direct the central rays at the center of the film. *Bisecting technique* Direct the central rays at a point on the center of the chin 1 in. (2.5 cm) above the lower border of the mandible, directly below the outer canthus of the eye.

The Periapical Examination: Bisecting Technique

When irregularities or obstructions of the oral tissues and the curvature of the palate prevent a parallel film packet to long axes of the teeth placement, an acceptable diagnostic quality radiograph may be obtained utilizing the bisecting technique. Although the bisecting technique is not recommended, because images produced utilizing the bisecting technique contain inherent dimensional distortion, careful attention to the steps of the technique can produce an acceptable image when needed. The radiographer who possesses knowledge of both the paralleling and the bisecting techniques is better able to serve all patients.

Unit and Patient Preparation

The unit and patient preparation for exposing periapical radiographs utilizing the bisecting technique is the same as those used with the paralleling technique. Of particular importance is the patient's head positioning. The patient's occlusal and midsaggital planes must be correctly positioned to allow for use of pre-determined set vertical angulations and points of entry often used with the bisecting technique.

Managing Exposures

As explained in Chapter 12, the bisecting principle is applied to cast a shadow of the teeth onto the film. The x-ray beam must be directed perpendicularly through the apex of the tooth toward the imaginary bisecting line (see Figure 12–2). A variety of holders, ranging in complexity from polystyrene biteblocks (Figure 13–10) to the Rinn BAI® (Bisecting Angle Instrument) (Figure 13–8) may be selected for use with the bisecting technique. These holders will allow for a close, but not parallel, relationship between the film packet and the teeth.

Figures 13–20 through 13–27 illustrate the precise film packet positions and the required angulations for each of the periapical radiographs in a basic 14-film full mouth series utilizing the bisecting technique. See Table 13–5 for a summary of the technique.

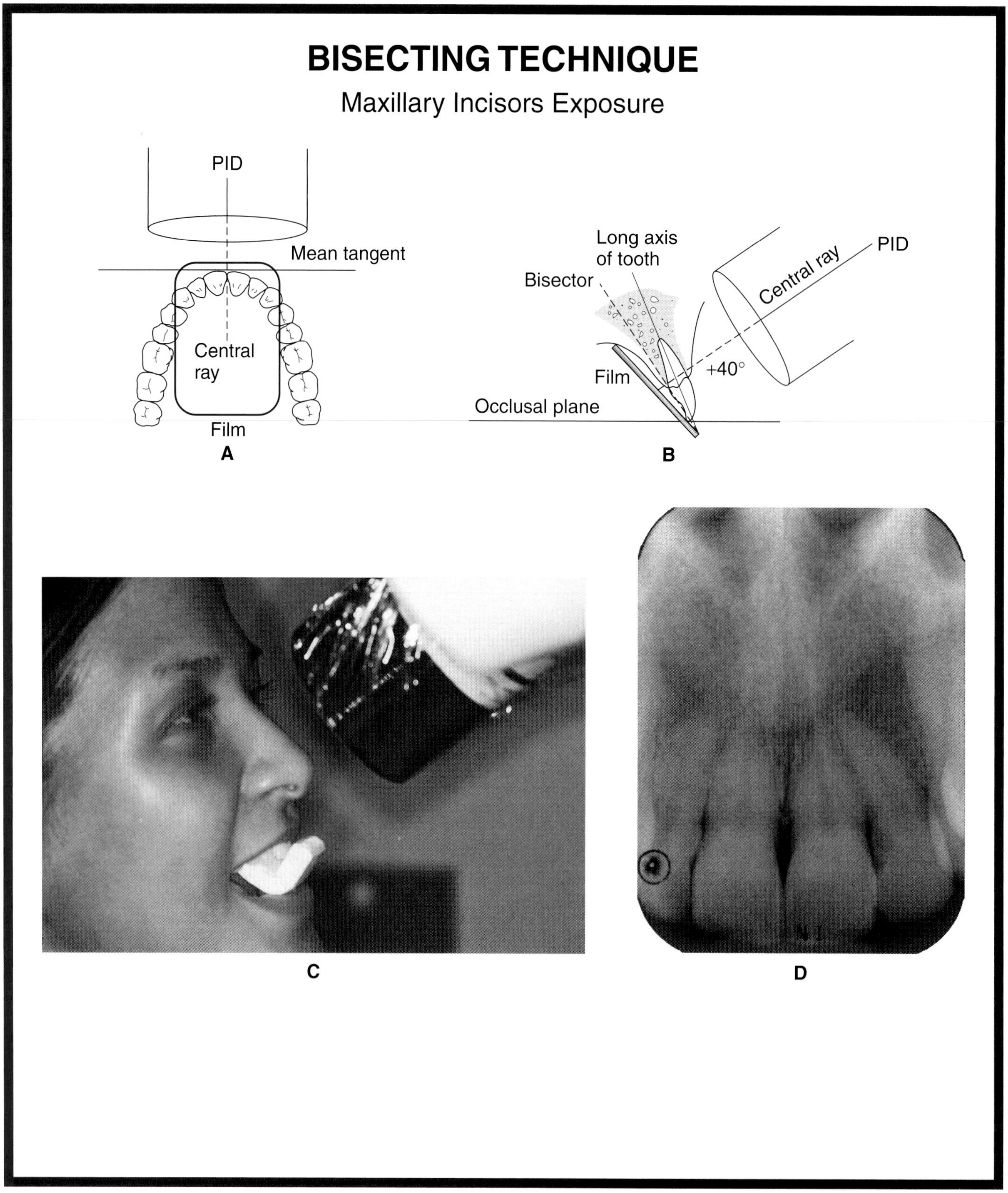

FIGURE 13-20 **Maxillary incisors exposure.** (**A**) Diagram shows horizontal projection is through the midline embrasure and perpendicular to the mean tangent. (**B**) Vertical projection is directed perpendicular to the bisector at approximately + 40 degrees with the PID tilted downward. (**C**) Patient showing position of Stabe® and 8 in. (20.5 cm) circular PID. (**D**) Maxillary incisors radiograph.

BISECTING TECHNIQUE

Maxillary Canine Exposure

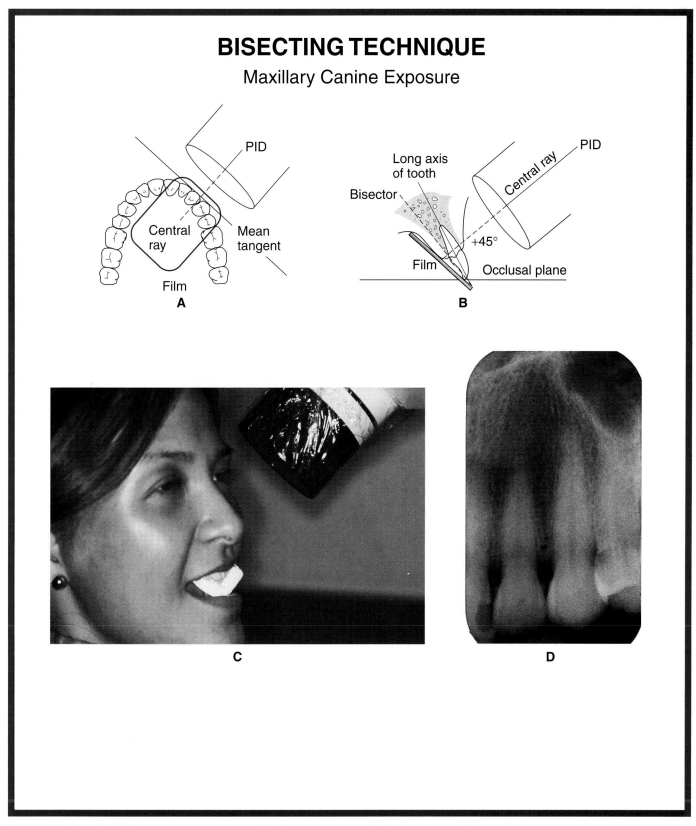

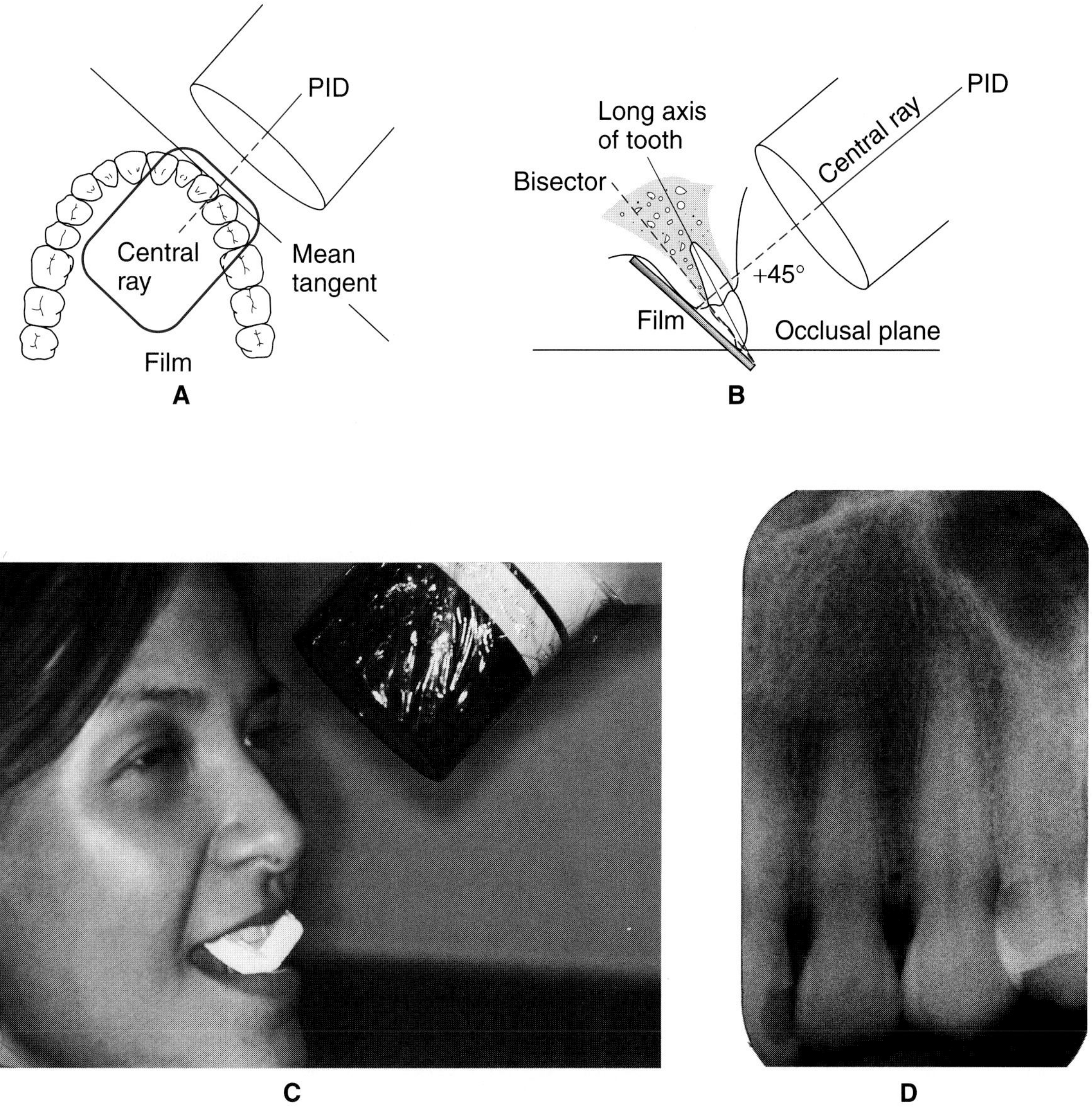

FIGURE 13–21 **Maxillary canine exposure.** (**A**) Diagram shows horizontal projection is through the canine and perpendicular to the mean tangent. (**B**) Vertical projection is directed perpendicular to the bisector at approximately + 45 degrees with the PID tilted downward. (**C**) Patient showing position of Stabe® and 8 in. (20.5 cm) circular PID. (**D**) Maxillary canine radiograph.

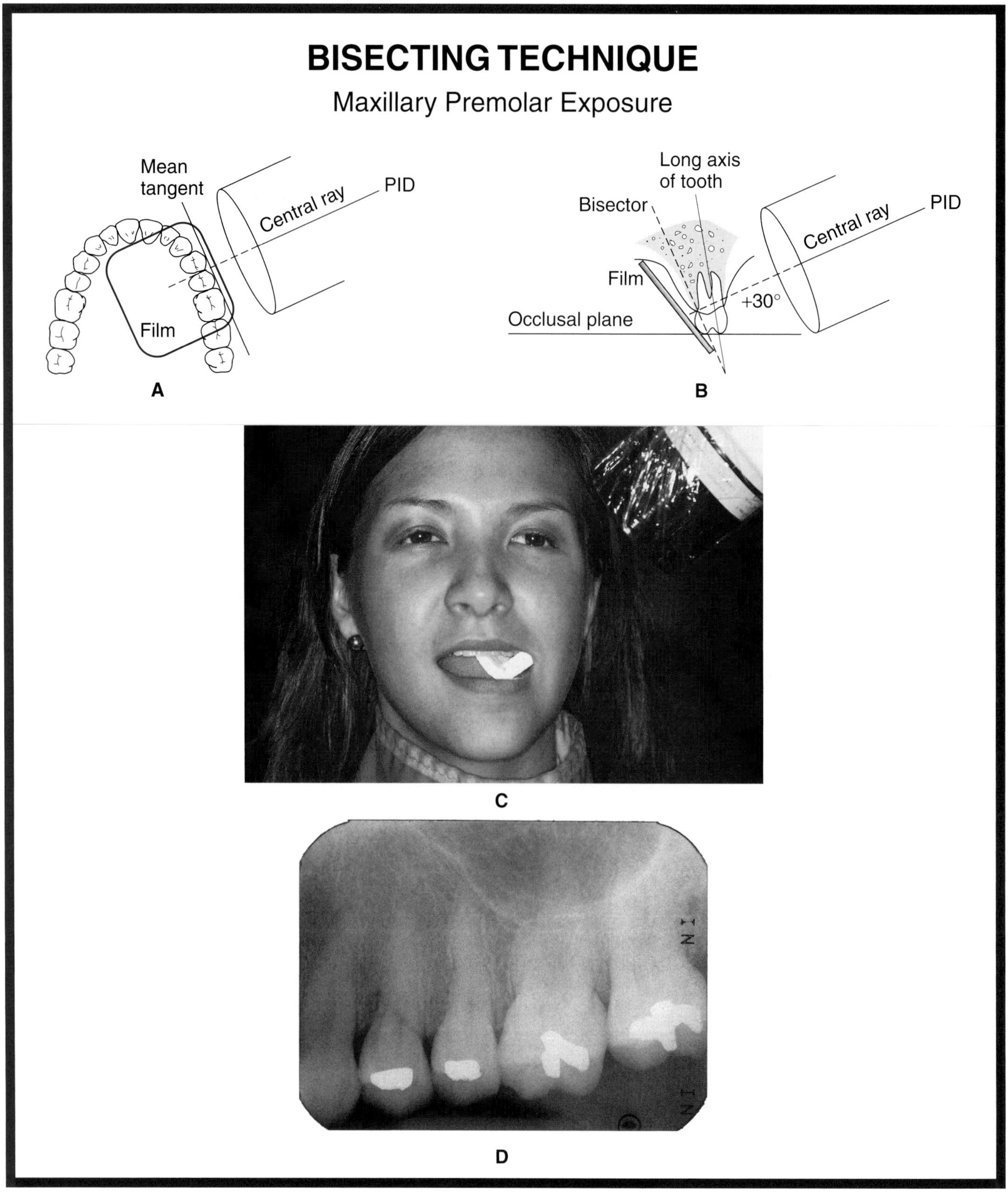

FIGURE 13-22 **Maxillary premolar exposure.** (**A**) Diagram shows horizontal projection is through the embrasure between the premolars and perpendicular to the mean tangent. (**B**) Vertical projection is directed perpendicular to the bisector at approximately +30 degrees with the PID tilted downward. (**C**) Patient showing position of Stabe® and 8 in. (20.5 cm) circular PID. (**D**) Maxillary premolar radiograph.

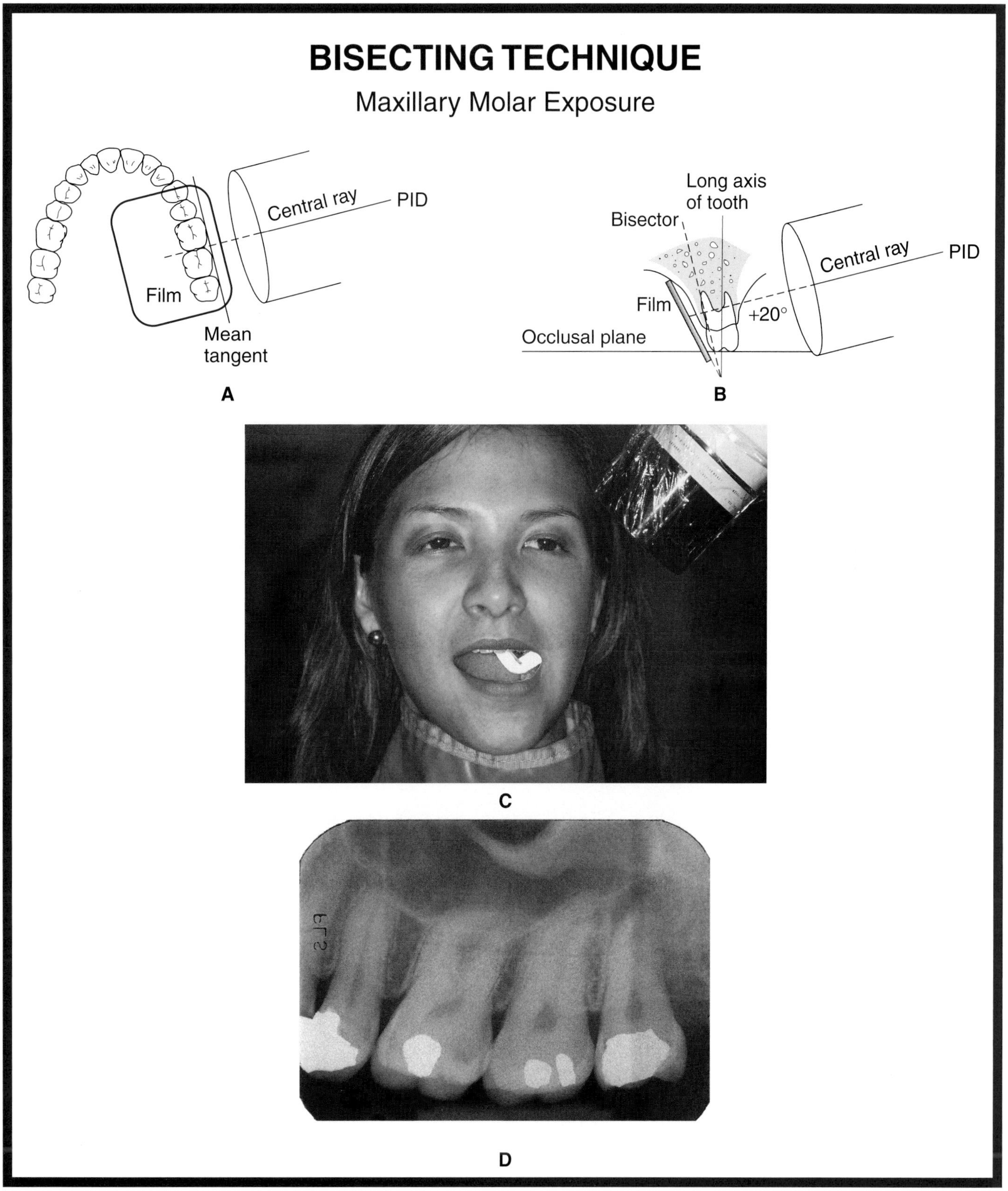

FIGURE 13–23 **Maxillary molar exposure.** (**A**) Diagram shows horizontal projection is through the embrasure between the first and second molars and perpendicular to the mean tangent. (**B**) Vertical projection is directed perpendicular to the bisector at approximately +20 degrees with the PID tilted downward. (**C**) Patient showing position of Stabe® and 8 in. (20.5 cm) circular PID. (**D**) Maxillary molar radiograph.

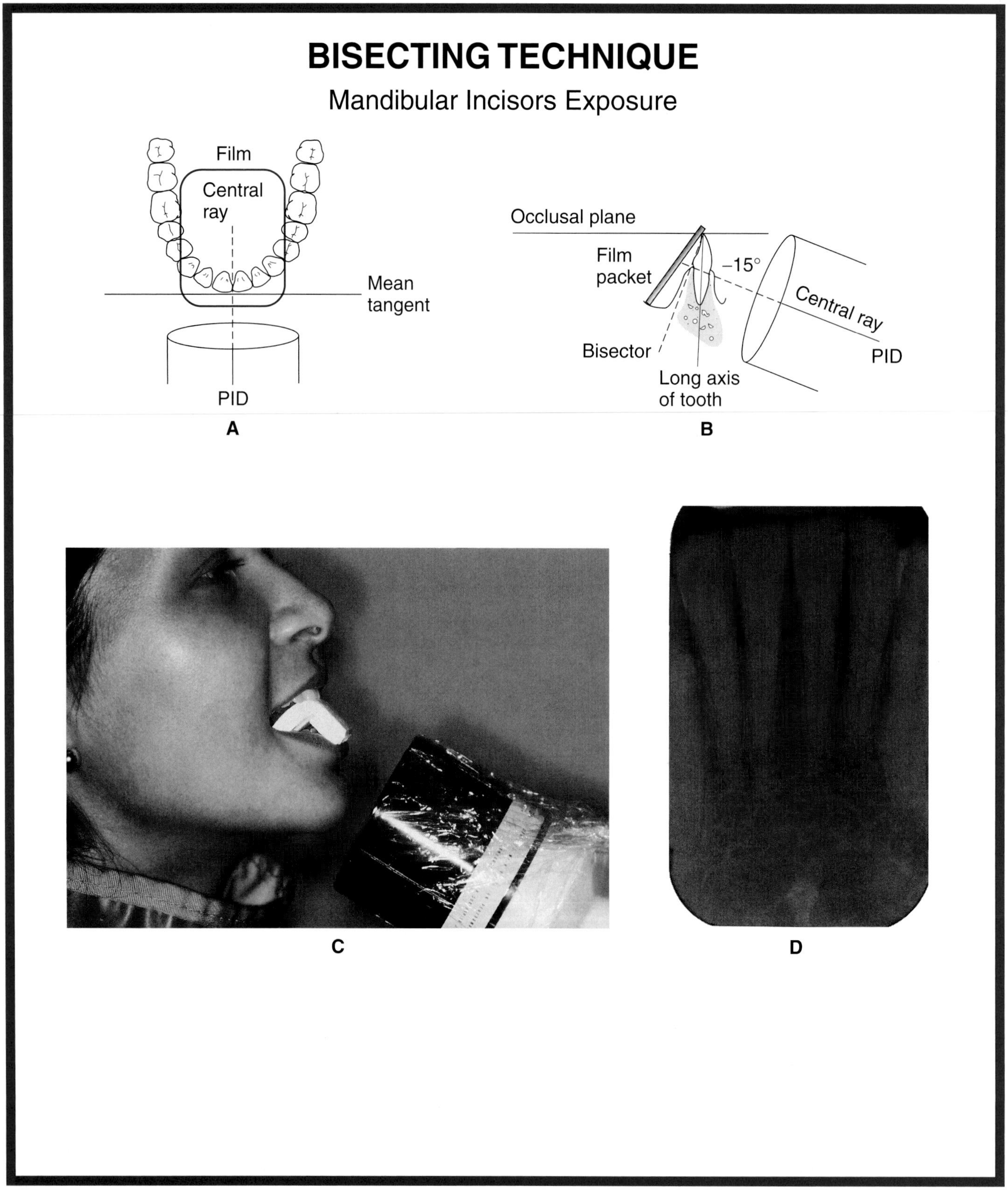

FIGURE 13-24 **Mandibular incisors exposure.** (**A**) Diagram shows horizontal projection is through the midline embrasure and perpendicular to the mean tangent. (**B**) Vertical projection is directed perpendicular to the bisector at approximately −15 degrees with the PID tilted upward. (**C**) Patient showing position of Stabe® and 8 in. (20.5 cm) circular PID. (**D**) Mandibular incisors radiograph.

BISECTING TECHNIQUE

Mandibular Canine Exposure

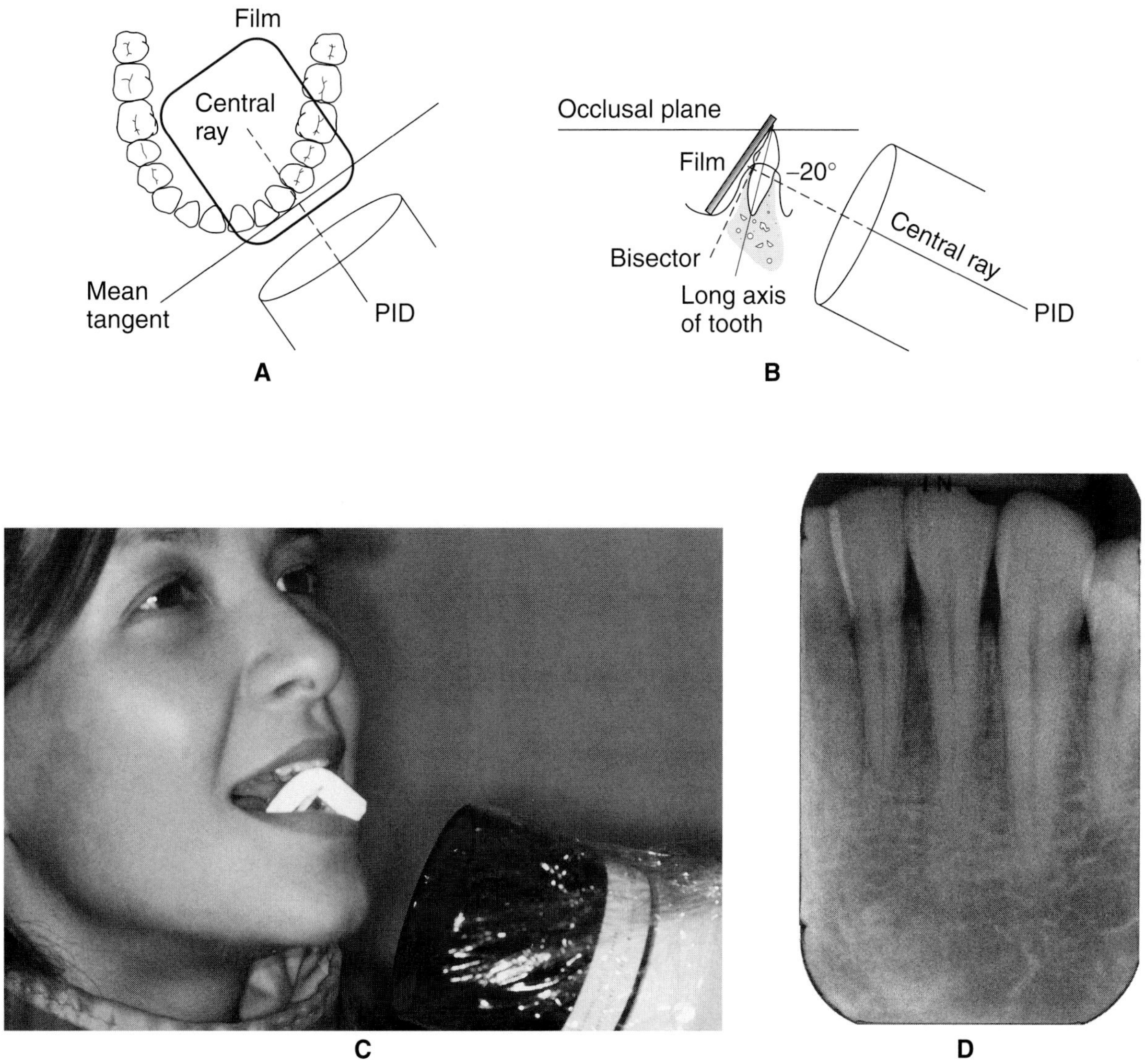

FIGURE 13-25 **Mandibular canine exposure.** (**A**) Diagram shows horizontal projection is through the canine and perpendicular to the mean tangent. (**B**) Vertical projection is directed perpendicular to the bisector at approximately −20 degrees with the PID tilted upward. (**C**) Patient showing position of Stabe® and 8 in. (20.5 cm) circular PID. (**D**) Mandibular canine radiograph.

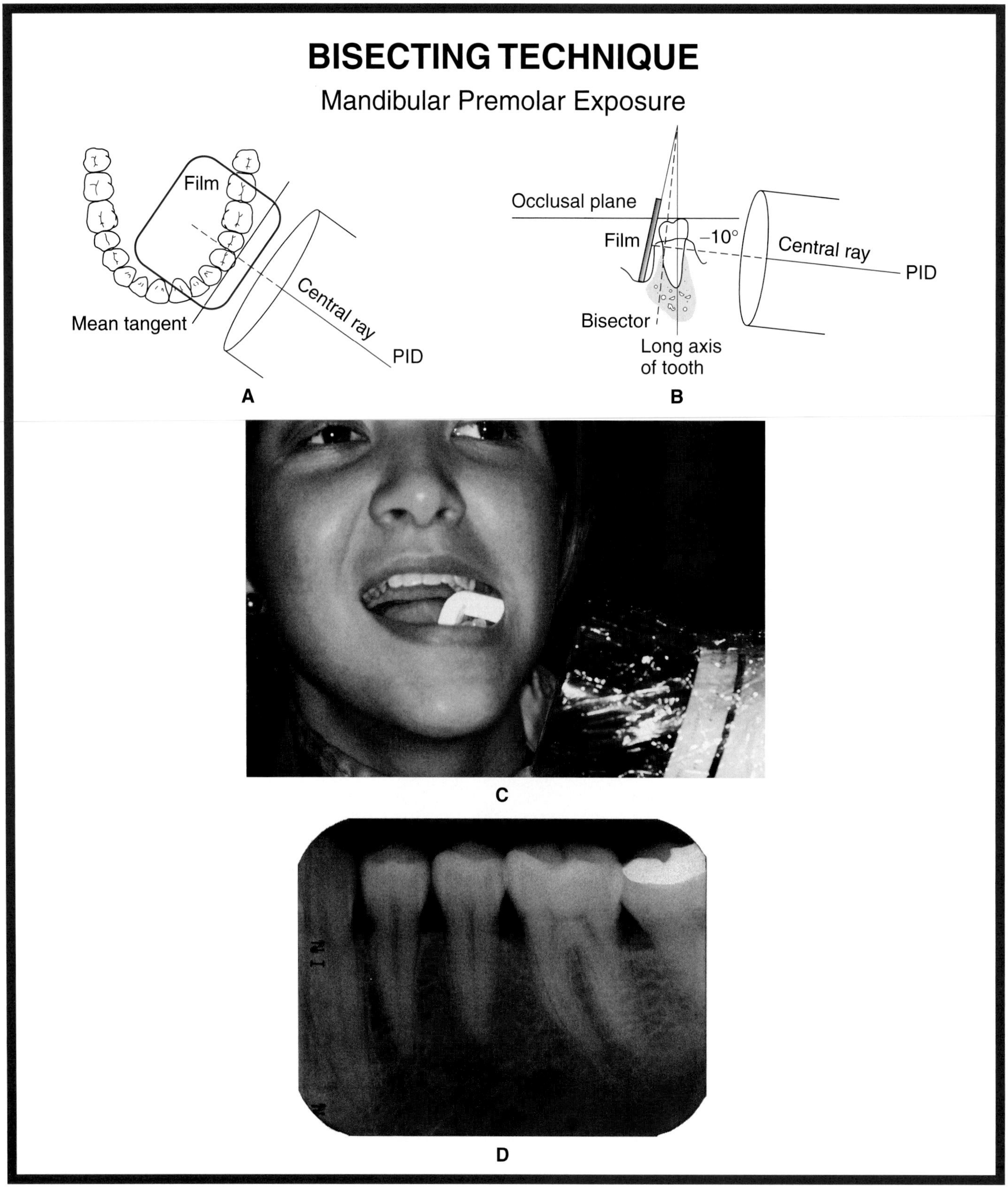

FIGURE 13-26 **Mandibular premolar exposure.** (**A**) Diagram shows horizontal projection is through the embrasure between the premolars and perpendicular to the mean tangent. (**B**) Vertical projection is directed perpendicular to the bisector at approximately −10 degrees with the PID tilted upward. (**C**) Patient showing position of Stabe® and 8 in. (20.5 cm) circular PID. (**D**) Mandibular premolar radiograph.

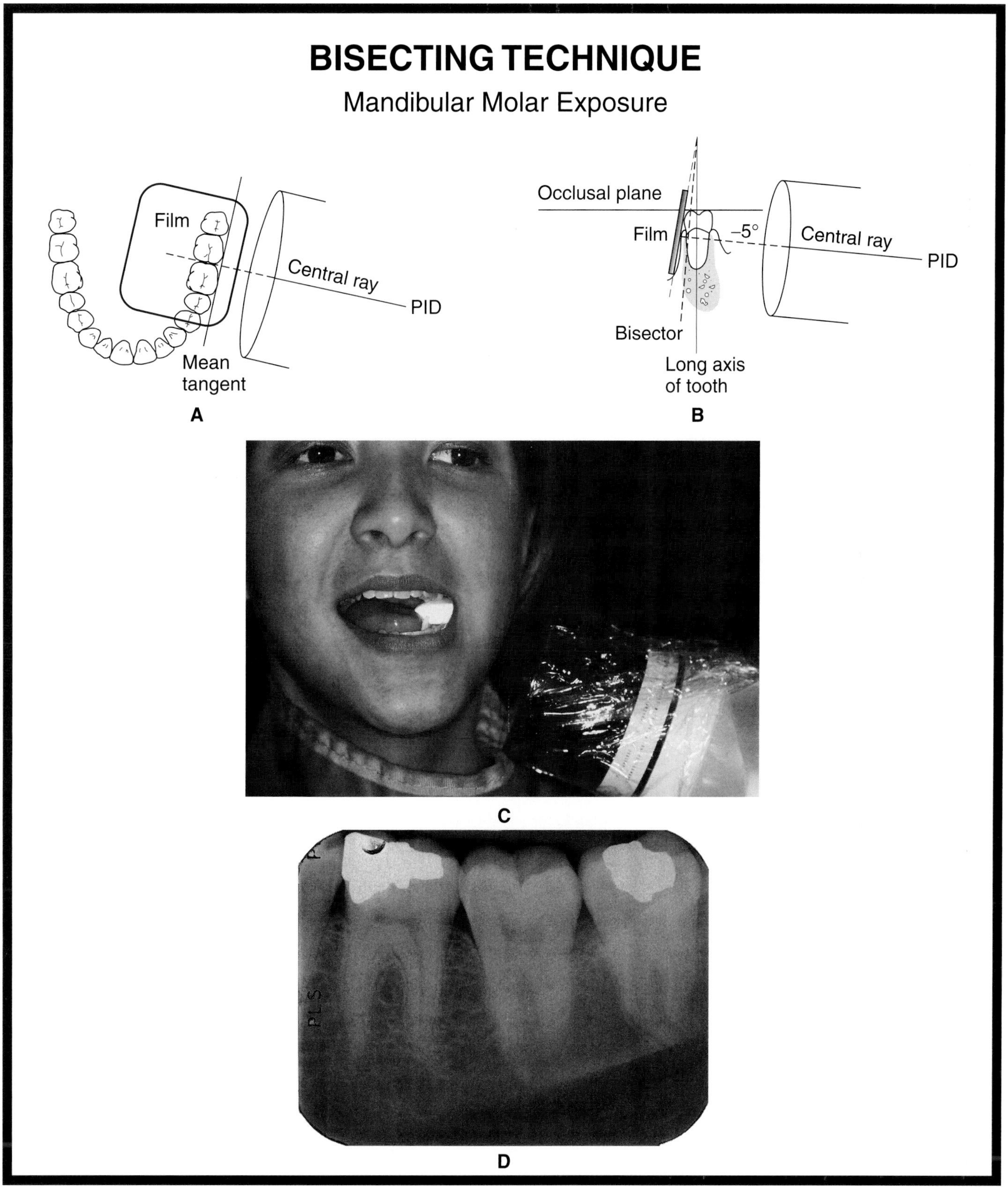

FIGURE 13-27 **Mandibular molar exposure.** (**A**) Diagram shows horizontal projection is through the embrasure between the first and second molar and perpendicular to the mean tangent. (**B**) Vertical projection is directed perpendicular to the bisector at approximately −5 degrees with slight upward tilt of the PID. (**C**) Patient showing position of Stabe® and 8 in. (20.5 cm) circular PID. (**D**) Mandibular molar radiograph.

REVIEW—Chapter Summary

The size and number of films to include in a full-mouth radiographic survey depends on several factors. A minimum of 14 periapical films are required for a full-mouth series of an adult patient—additional films may be needed if narrow size #1 films are used in the anterior regions. Exposures include the central incisors, canine, premolar, and molar areas of the right and left maxilla and mandible.

The horizontal angulation is determined by directing the central rays of the x-beam perpendicular to the film plane through the mean tangent of the embrasures between the teeth of interest. Both paralleling and bisecting techniques determine horizontal angulation in the same manner.

The vertical angulation is determined by directing the central rays of the x-beam perpendicular to the film plane and the long axes of the teeth when utilizing the paralleling technique. When utilizing the bisecting technique, the vertical angulation is determined by directing the central rays of the x-ray beam perpendicular to the imaginary bisector. If the patient's head position is correct, predetermined vertical angle settings may be used.

The film packet must be centered within the beam of radiation. When using the bisecting technique, if the patient's head position is correct, predetermined landmarks may be used to estimate the point of entry.

Because the film is positioned farther from the teeth in the paralleling technique, a film-holding device with a long biteblock is required. Film holders may be designed for use with the paralleling or the bisecting technique only, or may be modified to use with both techniques.

An exposure sequence is recommended. Step-by-step illustrated instructions for exposing a full-mouth series of periapical radiographs utilizing both the paralleling and the bisecting techniques are presented.

RECALL—Study Questions

1. Which of these factors does *not* need to be considered when deciding which film size to use when making the full-mouth survey?
   a. Age of the patient
   b. Shape of the dental arches
   c. Previous accumulated exposure
   d. Patient's ability to tolerate the film packet
2. What is the minimum film requirement for an adult full-mouth survey of periapical radiographs?
   a. 12
   b. 14
   c. 16
   d. 18
3. Anterior periapical film packets are placed ____________ in the oral cavity. Posterior periapical film packets are placed ____________ in the oral cavity.
   a. vertically; horizontally
   b. horizontally; vertically
   c. vertically; vertically
   d. horizontally; horizontally
4. Where should the embossed identification dot be positioned when taking periapical radiographs?
   a. Toward the midline of the oral cavity
   b. Toward the incisal or occlusal edge of the tooth
   c. Toward the palate or floor of the mouth
   d. Toward the distal or back of the arch
5. When the patient's head is in the correct position, a ________ vertical angulation is used when exposing maxillary periapicals and a ____________ vertical angulation is used when exposing mandibular periapicals.
   a. positive, positive
   b. negative, negative
   c. positive, negative
   d. negative, positive
6. Elongation results from:
   a. Excessive horizontal angulation.
   b. Inadequate horizontal angulation.
   c. Excessive vertical angulation.
   d. Inadequate vertical angulation.
7. Cutting off the root apex portion of the image on a periapical radiograph results from:
   a. Excessive horizontal angulation.
   b. Inadequate horizontal angulation.
   c. Excessive vertical angulation.
   d. Inadequate vertical angulation.
8. The most important reason for using a film holder when utilizing the paralleling technique is to stabilize the film packet in a position:
   a. Parallel to the teeth.
   b. At a right angle to the teeth.
   c. Perpendicular to the teeth.
   d. Parallel to the imaginary bisector.
9. Which of the following is an example of a film holder that can be used with both the paralleling technique and the bisecting techniques?
   a. Snap-A-Ray.
   b. Precision.
   c. Stabe.
   d. XCP.
10. All of the following are parts of the assembled XCP® holder *except* one. Which one is this *exception?*
    a. Indicator ring
    b. 105-degree angled backing
    c. Long biteblock
    d. Metal arm
11. Which of the following is the best sequencing for exposing a full-mouth survey of periapical radiographs?
    a. Mandibular posteriors, maxillary posteriors, mandibular anteriors, maxillary anteriors
    b. Mandibular anteriors, maxillary anteriors, mandibular posteriors, maxillary posteriors
    c. Maxillary anteriors, mandibular anteriors, maxillary posteriors, mandibular posteriors
    d. Maxillary posteriors, mandibular posteriors, maxillary anteriors, mandibular anteriors

12. Centering the film packet behind the left and right central and lateral incisors describes the film packet placement for which of the following periapical radiographs?
    a. Central incisors
    b. Canine
    c. Premolar
    d. Molar
13. Lining the film packet up behind the distal half of the canine to include the first and second premolars and mesial half of the first molar describes the film packet placement for which of the following periapical radiographs?
    a. Central incisors
    b. Canine
    c. Premolar
    d. Molar
14. When utilizing the bisecting technique, the recommended vertical setting for the maxillary premolar periapical radiograph is:
    a. +45 degrees
    b. +30 degrees
    c. −10 degrees
    d. −5 degrees
15. When utilizing the bisecting technique, the recommended vertical setting for the mandibular canine periapical radiograph is:
    a. +40 degrees
    b. +20 degrees
    c. −15 degrees
    d. −20 degrees
16. To determine the horizontal angulation for the maxillary molar periapical radiograph, the central rays of the x-ray beam should be directed at the film perpendicularly through the embrasures of the:
    a. Canine and first premolar.
    b. First and second premolars.
    c. Second premolar and first molar.
    d. First and second molars.
17. To determine the horizontal angulation for the mandibular premolar periapical radiograph, the central rays of the x-ray beam should be directed at the film perpendicularly through the embrasures of the:
    a. Canine and first premolar.
    b. First and second premolars.
    c. Second premolar and first molar.
    d. First and second molars.
18. When utilizing the bisecting technique, the recommended point of entry for the maxillary central incisors periapical radiograph is:
    a. At a point near the tip of the nose.
    b. At the ala of the nose.
    c. At a point on the ala–tragus line directly inferior to the pupil of the eye.
    d. At a point on the ala–tragus line directly inferior to the outer canthus of the eye.
19. When utilizing the bisecting technique, the recommended point of entry for the mandibular canine periapical radiograph is:
    a. At a point on the center of the chin 1 in. (2.5 cm) above to the inferior border of the mandible.
    b. At the center of the root of the canine 1 in. (2.5 cm) above the inferior border of the mandible.
    c. At a point on the chin 1 in. (2.5 cm) above the inferior border of the mandible directly below the pupil of the eye.
    d. At a point on the chin 1 in. (2.5 cm) above the inferior border of the mandible directly below the outer canthus of the eye.

REFLECT—Case Study

You have recently accepted a position in a general practice dental office. This week you discovered that the film-holding device for exposing a full-mouth survey is the one pictured in Figure 13–9. You have always used the film-holding device pictured in Figure 13–11, and are unfamiliar with the device in Figure 13–9. Based on what you have learned about film holders designed for use with the paralleling and bisecting techniques, answer the following questions:

1. Which technique are these holders designed to be used with? How can you tell?
2. How are the holders similar? Different?
3. Which film holder would it be best to know how to use? Why?
4. What are the advantages of the film holder used at this practice? (Figure 13–9)
5. What are the disadvantages of the film holder used at this practice? (Figure 13–9)
6. What are the advantages of the film holder you are used to using? (Figure 13–11)
7. What are the disadvantages of the film holder you are used to using? (Figure 13–11)
8. What is your recommendation for the practice? Should they continue to use this film holder (Figure 13–9) or should they purchase the film holder you are familiar with? (Figure 13–11)

RELATE—Laboratory Application

For two comprehensive laboratory practice exercises on this topic, see E. M. Thomson, *Exercises in Oral Radiography Techniques: A Laboratory Manual,* 2nd ed., Upper Saddle River, NJ: Prentice Hall, 2007. Chapter 3, "Periapical Radiographs—Paralleling Technique" and Chapter 4, "Periapical Radiographs—Bisecting Technique."

BIBLIOGRAPHY

Eastman Kodak. *Successful Intraoral Radiography.* Rochester, NY: Eastman Kodak, 1998.

Rinn Corporation. *Intraoral Radiography with Rinn XCP/BAI Instruments.* Elgin, IL: Dentsply/Rinn Corporation, 1983.

White, S. C., & Pharoah, M. J. *Oral Radiology Principles and Interpretation,* 5th ed. St. Louis: Elsevier, 2004.

14

The Bitewing Examination

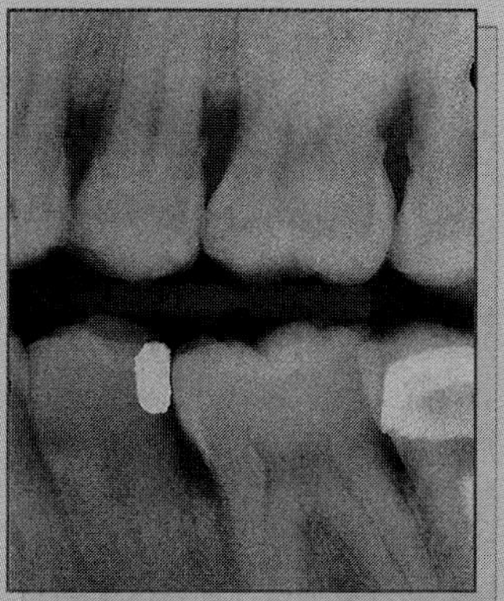

■ OBJECTIVES

Following successful completion of this chapter, you should be able to:

1. Define the key words.
2. List two purposes of the bitewing examination.
3. Compare and contrast periapical and bitewing radiographs.
4. List the four sizes of film that can be used for bitewing surveys.
5. Identify the type, size, and number of films best suited for an adult posterior bitewing survey.
6. Identify the type, size and number of films best suited for a periodontally involved adult bitewing survey.
7. Identify the type, size and number of films best suited for a child bitewing survey.
8. Explain the effect of horizontal angulation on the resultant bitewing image.
9. Identify positive and negative vertical angulations.
10. State the recommended vertical angulation for bitewing exposures.
11. Compare methods used for holding the bitewing film in position.
12. Differentiate between horizontal and vertical bitewing radiographs.
13. Describe the film packet placement, horizontal and vertical angulation, and point of entry for horizontal and vertical posterior bitewing examinations.
14. Describe the film packet placement, horizontal and vertical angulation, and point of entry for a vertical anterior bitewing examination.

■ KEY WORDS

Bitetab
Bitewing radiograph
Contact points
Embrasures
External aiming device
Film loop
Horizontal angulation
Horizontal bitewing radiograph
Interproximal radiograph
Negative angulation
Overlap
Point of entry
Positive angulation
Vertical angulation
Vertical bitewing radiograph

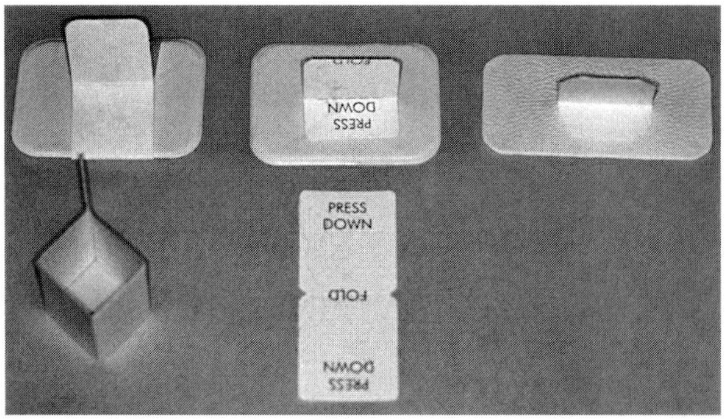

FIGURE 14-1 **Bitewing tabs and loops. (A)** Loop tabs; **(B)** Stick-on tabs; **(C)** Size #3 film packet with manufacturer-attached tab.

Introduction

Bitewing radiographs are probably the most frequently performed intraoral dental radiographic technique. **Bitewing radiographs** image the crowns and alveolar bone of both the maxillary and mandibular teeth on a single radiograph. The bitewing examination, sometimes referred to as an **interproximal radiograph,** is especially useful in detecting caries (dental decay) in posterior teeth. Bitewing radiographs are also used to examine crestal bone of patients with periodontal disease.

The name bitewing is descriptive. Traditionally, the bitewing film had a wing, or tab that was either attached to the film by the manufacturer or attached by the radiographer as a film holder (Figure 14–1). The patient bites on this tab to hold the film in place. Additionally, there are a variety of film holding devices that may or may not resemble the original paper bitetabs.

The purpose of this chapter is to explain the bitewing examination and to describe the step-by-step procedures for conducting bitewing examinations.

Fundamentals of Bitewing Radiography

Bitewing (interproximal) radiographs may be taken as a bitewing series or in conjunction with a full mouth series of periapical radiographs or with a panoramic survey. Bitewings are most often exposed at the time of regularly scheduled recare or recall appointments. Bitewing radiographs showing the crowns and alveolar crests of both the maxillary and mandibular teeth on the same film are ideal for examining dental caries that begin on the proximal surfaces of the teeth (where adjacent teeth contact each other in the arch) and periodontal bone loss near the gingival line (Figure 14–2).

To expose a bitewing radiograph, the film packet is positioned near and almost parallel to the teeth of both arches when the patient's teeth are occluded (closed). Bitewing film packet placement is closer to the teeth and the central ray of the x-ray beam can be directed at a more ideal angle than for periapical radiographs (Figure 14–3). With this ideal film packet placement, the bitewing radiograph often images decay and the height of the alveolar bone crest better than periapical radiographs. It is because of this improved imaging for these conditions that bitewing radiographs are taken in conjunction with periapical radiographs of the same area when exposing a full mouth series.

The true value of the bitewing radiograph is that it reveals caries in the earliest stages. This is particularly important in the premolar and molar regions, where small carious lesions are often concealed by the wide bucco-lingual diameters of these teeth.

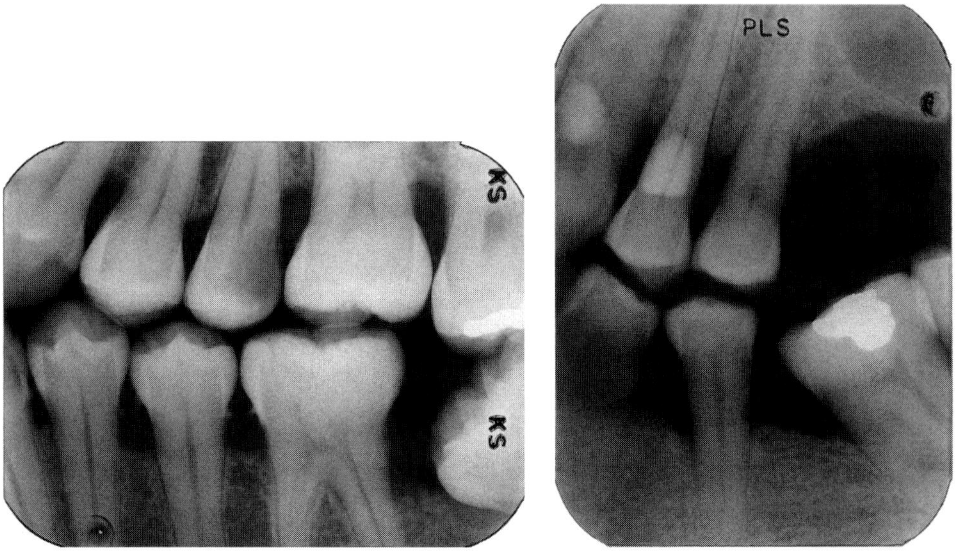

A B

FIGURE 14-2 **Horizontal and vertical bitewing radiographs.** Bitewing radiographs are ideal at imaging the interproximal areas of the teeth to show caries and alveolar bone crests. Note the increased coverage of the alveolar bone imaged on the vertical bitewing radiograph.

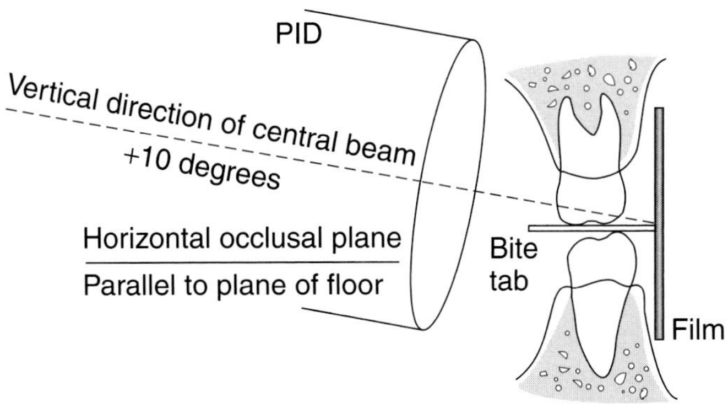

FIGURE 14-3 **Bitewing placement.** The bitewing film packet placement is such that the coronal portion of both the maxillary and the mandibular teeth will be recorded on the film. The close relationship between the teeth and the film and the ideal angle of the x-ray beam often make bitewings a better choice for imaging caries and alveolar bone crests than periapical radiographs.

Such lesions are frequently unnoticed in a visual inspection. Bitewing radiographs do not image the entire tooth and therefore will not reveal apical conditions or lesions.

Film

The bitewing survey can be made with two to eight films, using size #0, #1, #2, or #3. The number and size of films to use depends on the type of survey required and the size and shape of the patient's oral cavity (Table 14–1). A complete set of seven or eight **vertical bitewing radiographs** may be exposed for the examination of a periodontally involved patient. This vertical bitewing set will include both posterior and anterior bitewings. When the patient does not require anterior bitewings, two or four posterior bitewing radiographs positioned either vertically or horizontally are usually taken.

Additional factors to be considered when deciding how many and what size film to select is the length and curvature of the arches, which vary in all individuals. A single film placed on each side of the mouth often provides adequate coverage for children, prior to the eruption of the permanent second molars. While a size #0 or #1 is usually used for a child with primary teeth, the preferred size for mixed dentition is standard #2 film. However, tissue sensitivity or anatomical limitations must be taken into consideration and film size based on the individual. The advantage to using the largest size film possible is that the amount of structures imaged, including the developing permanent teeth, will be increased. For most adults, four #2 films (two on each side) are generally preferred.

Size #3 (extra-long) film with pre-attached tabs are especially made for taking **horizontal bitewing radiographs**. The advantage of these film packets is that only one film needs to be exposed on each side. However, when compared with the standard #2 film, the #3 film has two serious disadvantages. One is that in most dental arches there are two slightly divergent pathways of the posterior teeth, one for the premolars and the other for the molars. As the central rays pass through these divergent **embrasures**, some of the interproximal structures **overlap** on the radiograph compromising the image. The other disadvantage is that the long film is narrower in the vertical dimension than size #2 film and will reveal less of the periodontal crestal bone level (Figure 14–4).

Film Packet Placement

The goal of film packet placement is to image all contacts (mesial and distal surfaces) of all of the teeth of interest. It is important to remember that each bitewing—molar, premolar, canine, and incisors—has a standard film packet placement. This means that a premolar bitewing taken at one oral health practice will most likely image the same teeth as a premolar bitewing exposed in every other practice. This standardization is important.

TABLE 14-1 **Suggested Film Size and Number to Use for Bitewing Radiographs**

Film Size	Recommended for Use with These Patients	Number of Films and Orientation of Film Packet
#0	Child with primary dentition	2 horizontal posterior
#1	Child with primary or mixed dentition	2 horizontal posterior
	Adult for caries detection or the presence of periodontal disease	3 or 4 vertical anterior
#2	Child with mixed dentition, prior to the eruption of the permanent second molars	2 horizontal posterior
	Adolescent after the eruption of the permanent second molars	4 horizontal posterior
	Adult	4 horizontal posterior
	Adult with periodontal disease	4 vertical posterior
#3	Adolescent after the eruption of the permanent second molars	2 horizontal posterior
	Adult	2 horizontal posterior

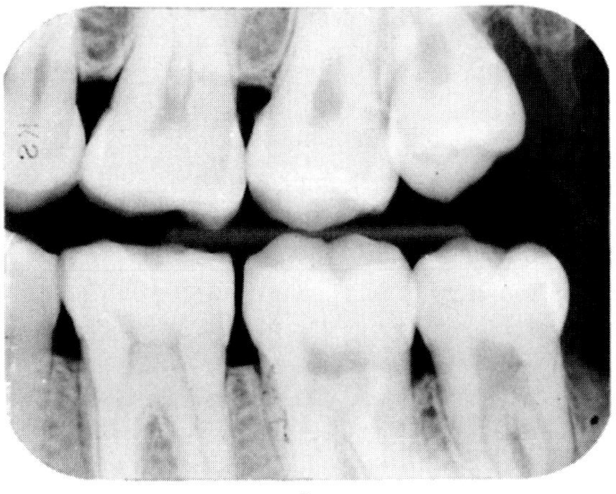

A

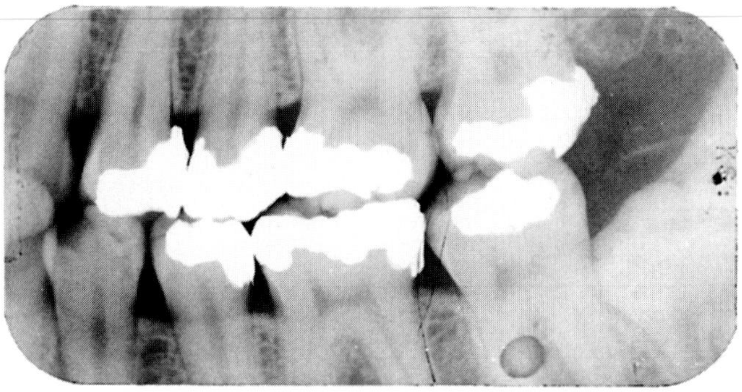

B

FIGURE 14-4 **Comparison of size #2 and size #3 films.** Size #3 film **(B)** is shorter in the vertical dimension than the size #2 film **(A)** and therefore images slightly less of the crowns of the teeth and less of the alveolar bone crest.

While instructions for imaging a bitewing radiograph will call for the film packet to be placed such that the teeth of interest are centered in the middle of the film, it is equally important to focus on imaging the distal and mesial halves of the teeth adjacent to those of interest. For example, when placing a film packet to image a premolar horizontal or vertical bitewing radiograph, the first and second premolars will mostly likely be centered on the film. However, the distal half of the canine and mesial half of the first molar must also be imaged. Imaging the distal half of the canine and the mesial half of the first molar will ensure that the proximal surfaces of the premolars are recorded as well. During film packet placement, the radiographer should focus on placing the anterior edge of the film so that it lines up behind the distal half of the canine, and the rest of the teeth should be imaged correctly.

It is important to visually inspect the patient's occlusion to determine which canine, maxillary or mandibular, to use when aligning the film packet. The premolar bitewing must image the distal portion of both the maxillary and the mandibular canines. The radiographer should align the anterior edge of the film packet behind the canine that is further forward in the mouth (the most mesial canine).

When placing a film packet to image a molar horizontal or vertical bitewing radiograph, the radiographer should focus on placing the anterior edge of the film so that it lines up behind the distal half of the second premolar. Again, a visual inspection of the patient's occlusion will determine whether or not to line up the film packet with the maxillary or the mandibular second premolar.

Generally, in Class I and III occlusal relationships, the radiographer will choose to align the anterior edge of the film packet behind the distal half of the mandibular canine for a premolar bitewing radiograph, and behind the distal half of the mandibular second premolar for a molar bitewing radiograph. When a Class II occlusal relationship presents, the radiographer will most likely choose to align the anterior edge of the film packet behind the distal half of the maxillary canine for a premolar bitewing radiograph and behind the distal half of the maxillary second premolar for a molar bitewing radiograph (Figure 14–5). However, it should be noted that individuals often present with different occlusal relationships on the right and left sides or individual teeth that are mal-aligned or missing. It is important to perform a visual inspection prior to each film packet placement.

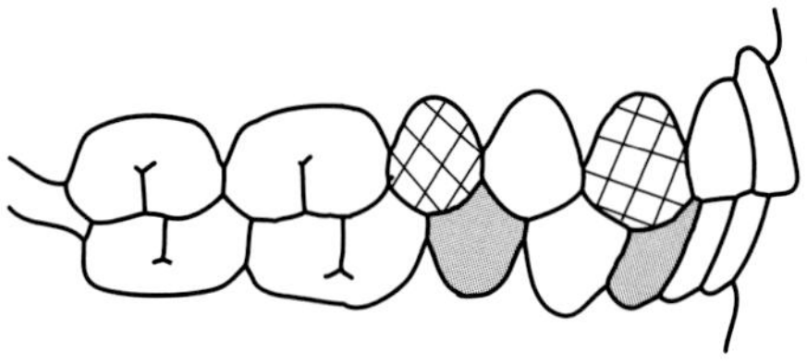

A

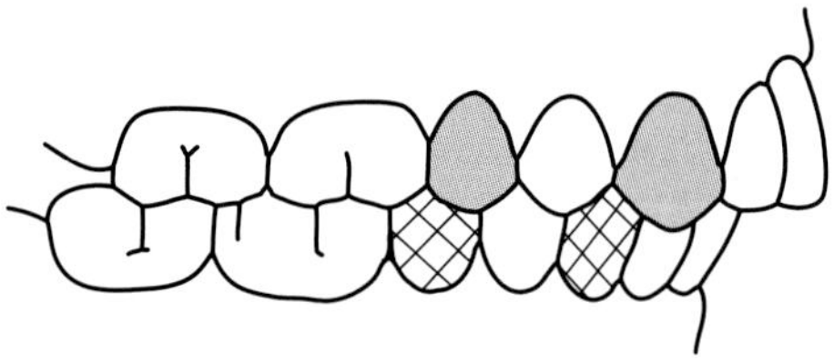

B

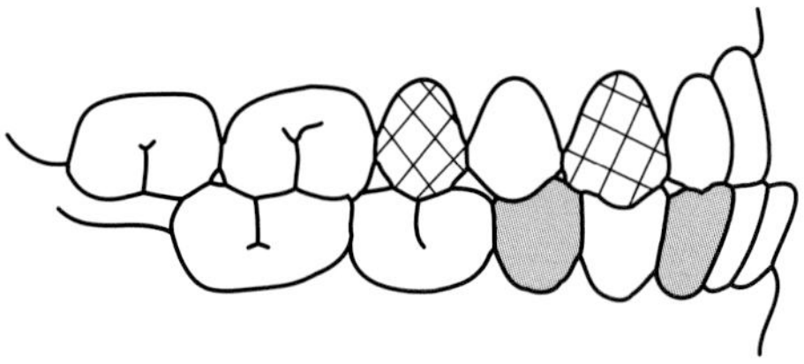

C

FIGURE 14-5 **Occlusal relationships.** (**A**) **Class I occlusion** demonstrating that the mandibular canine and second premolar are located further forward in the oral cavity. (**B**) **Class II occlusion** demonstrating that the maxillary canine and second premolar are located further forward in the oral cavity. (**C**) **Class III occlusion** demonstrating that the mandibular canine and second premolar are located further forward in the oral cavity.

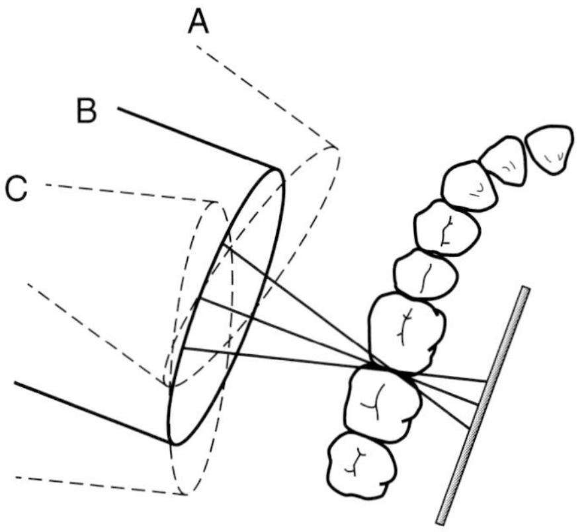

FIGURE 14-6 **Horizontal angulation.** (**A**) Mesiodistal projection shown here is deviated from a right angle by about 15°, resulting in overlap of the contacts in the distal areas of the radiograph. (**B**) Correct horizontal projection of x-ray beam resulting in no overlapping. (**C**) Distomesial projection shown here is deviated from a right angle about 15°, resulting in overlap in the mesial areas of the radiograph.

Angulations

The correct horizontal and vertical angulations are critical to producing a quality bitewing radiograph.

Horizontal Angulation

Horizontal angulation is the positioning of the central ray (PID) in a horizontal (side-to-side) plane. The horizontal angulation for bitewing exposures is the same as that used for periapical radiographs of the same area (see Chapter 13). The central ray (PID) should be directed perpendicular to the curvature of the arch, through the **contact points** of the teeth. The horizontal angulation is established by directing the central rays perpendicularly through the mean tangent of the embrasures between the teeth of interest (see Figure 12–10). The contact points should appear open or separate from each other on the resultant radiograph. Incorrect horizontal angulation results in overlapped contact points. Overlapped contacts result when the images of adjacent teeth are superimposed onto one another (Figure 14–6). When the horizontal angulation is directed obliquely from the mesial, the overlapping will be more severe in the distal or posterior region of the image; when the horizontal angulation is directed obliquely from the distal, the overlapping will be more severe in the mesial or anterior region of the image (Figure 14–7). Since bitewing radiographs are taken to reveal information about the interproximal areas of the teeth, radiographs with overlapping error are undiagnostic.

Vertical Angulation

Vertical angulation is the positioning of the central ray (PID) in a vertical (up and down) plane. Vertical angulation is measured in degrees as indicated on a dial on the side of the tube head (Figure 14–8). **Positive (+) angulation** is the positioning of the central ray (PID) downward toward the floor. **Negative (−) angulation** is the positioning of the central ray (PID) upward toward the ceiling.

The correct vertical angulation for bitewing radiographs is +10 degrees because the maxillary posterior teeth have a slight buccal inclination and the mandibular posterior teeth have a slight lingual inclination. Additionally, adjusting the vertical angulation of the PID to a +10 degrees will match the slight angle the film packet takes on when the patient closes and the palate pushes down against the film packet (Figure 14–9). Incorrect vertical angulation results in an unequal distribution of the arches on the radiograph. A quality bitewing radiograph should image an equal portion of the maxillary and mandibular teeth plus a portion of the supporting bone. When the vertical angulation is excessive

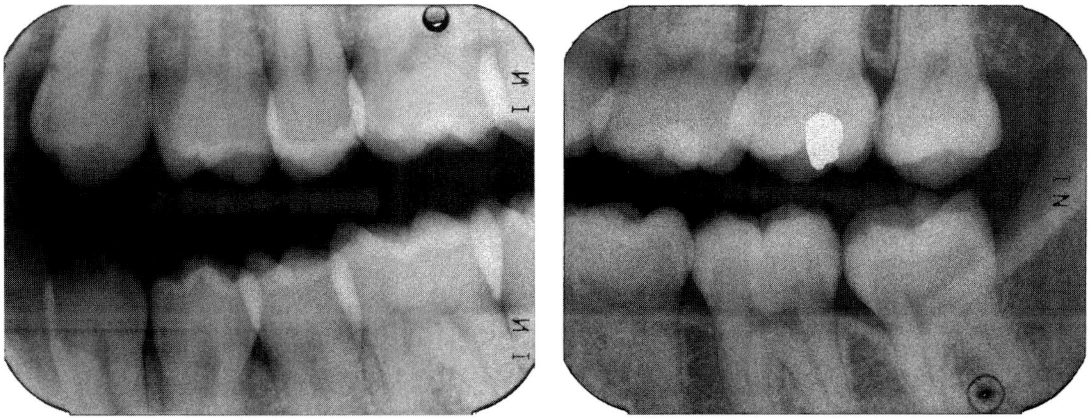

A B

FIGURE 14-7 **Horizontal overlap error.** (**A**) When the PID is directed obliquely from the mesial, the overlapping will be more severe in the distal or posterior region of the image. (**B**) When the horizontal angulation is directed obliquely from the distal, the overlapping will be more severe in the mesial or anterior region of the image.

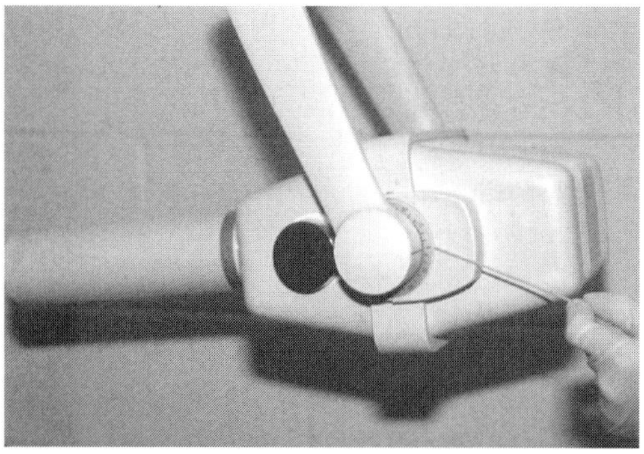

FIGURE 14-8 **Vertical angulation.** Vertical angulation may be indicated on the dial on the side of the tube head.

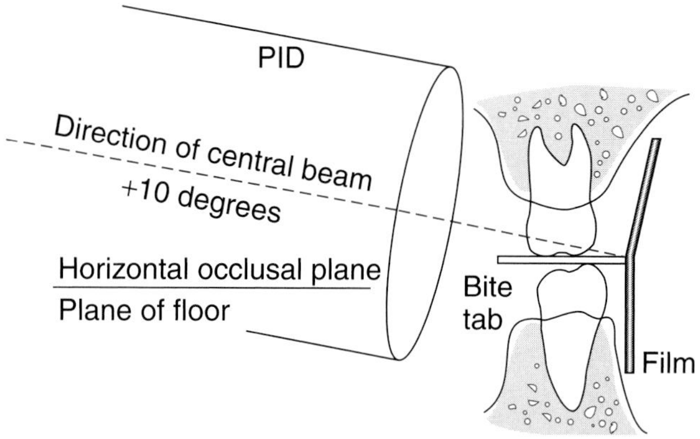

FIGURE 14-9 **Vertical slant of the film packet.** The film packet may slant lingually when contacted by the palate.

(greater than +10°), more of the maxillary teeth and bone is imaged, cutting off a portion of the mandibular structures; when the vertical angulation is inadequate (less than +10°) more of the mandibular teeth and bone is imaged, cutting off a portion of the maxillary structures (Figure 14–10).

Point of Entry

The **point of entry** for the central ray for all bitewing exposures is on the level of the incisal or occlusal plane (near the lip line) at a point opposite the center of the film and through the interproximal spaces of the teeth being x-rayed (see Figure 14–3). Incorrect point of entry, or not centering the film packet within the x-ray beam will result in cone cut error, where the portion of the film that was not in the path of the x-ray beam will be clear or blank on the resultant radiograph (see Figures 16–5 and 16–6).

The open end of the PID should be placed as close to the patient's skin as possible without touching. Failure to bring the end of the PID in close to the patient will result in an underexposed radiograph. As the beam of radiation spreads out, less radiation is available to strike the film and produce a diagnostic quality image.

Holding the Bitewing Film Packet in Position

There are many commercially made film holders for stabilizing the film packet for bitewing exposures. Stick-on paper **bitetabs** have the most versatility because they can be fastened to the film packet for both horizontal and vertical bitewings. The paper **film loop** into which the film can be slid is limited to horizontal bitewings. Bitetabs and loops are easy to use, disposable, and easily tolerated by the patient. Bitetabs must be attached to the white unprinted side (front) of the film packet. When using film loops and other film-holding devices, the film packet must be placed so that the white unprinted side will face the PID (x-rays) when placed intraorally.

Generally the bitetab or loop is visible after the film is placed and the patient bites down. This serves as a guide for directing the central rays toward the center of the film. Without a significantly visible **external aiming device**, some operators find it difficult to determine the correct horizontal and vertical angulations and centering of the film packet within the x-ray beam.

An example of a bitewing film holder with an external aiming device is the Rinn bitewing instrument (Figure 14–11). The external aiming device is the greatest advantage of this film holder. By eliminating the necessity for numerical angulation or specific

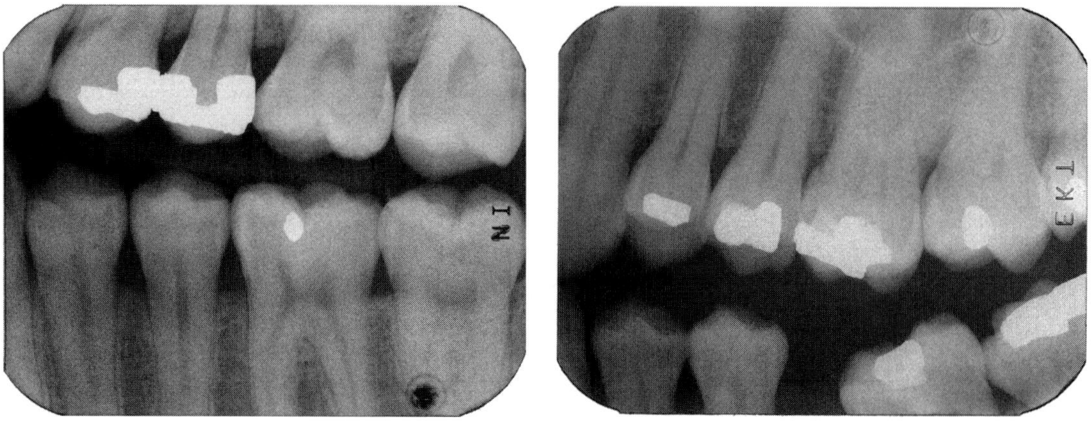

FIGURE 14-10 **Vertical angulation error.** (**A**) Inadequate vertical angulation results in imaging more of the mandible, while (**B**) excessive vertical angulation results in imaging more of the maxilla.

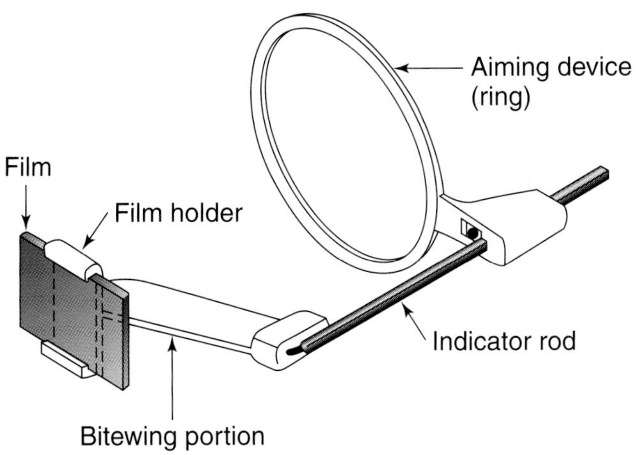

FIGURE 14-11 **The Rinn bitewing instrument.** This instrument consists of a plastic biteblock that supports the film-holding device at one end and a receptacle for insertion of the metal indicator arm at the other end. A ring slides over the arm. (Courtesy of Dentsply Rinn)

head positioning, many of the common errors such as overlapped interproximal spaces, unequal distribution of the arches, and cone cutting are reduced. The Rinn bitewing film holder is autoclavable and now comes with color-coded pieces to make assembly easy (see Figure 6–14). Biteblock film holder attachments are available for both horizontal and vertical bitewings. The biggest disadvantage of this film holding device is that the size and weight of the device may make film packet placement uncomfortable and difficult to tolerate. Additionally, the plastic biteblock is wider than paper bitetabs and loops, preventing the patient from biting down far enough to image the greatest amount of alveolar bone (Figure 14–12). This is especially important when periodontal disease is suspected or present. To overcome this disadvantage, the vertical bitewing biteblock film holder attachment can be substituted for the horizontal holder.

When difficulties arise during the placement of a film packet because the film-holding device is uncomfortable, there is a tendency to compromise placement. If a film holder with an external aiming device is not positioned correctly, the aiming device will indicate directing the x-ray beam to the wrong place. For this reason, it is important that the radiographer develop the skills necessary to evaluate film packet placement for correctness, regardless of the holder used. The technique procedures that follow are based on the use of bitetabs to help the radiographer develop the skill needed to evaluate angles and direction of the x-ray beam.

Regardless of the film holder used, care should be taken to ensure that the film packet is positioned in such a manner that it is evenly divided between the maxillary and mandibular teeth. The curvature of the palate or tongue interference has a tendency to disorient the film packet in its horizontal plane. Once the film is satisfactorily positioned, the patient must close down on the tab or biteblock in an edge-to-edge relationship and hold it there for the duration of the exposure.

The Bitewing Examination

The posterior bitewing examination consists of either two (one on the left and one on the right) or four (two on the left and two on the right) films (Figure 14–13A,B). The film packet orientation in the oral cavity may be such that the longer dimension is placed horizontally or vertically. Traditionally, the film packet has been placed horizontally in the posterior region. This remains the placement of choice for children. However, if there is a need to image more of the supporting bone, as is the case in periodontally involved patients, a vertical placement of the film packet is recommended.

The anterior bitewing examination consists of either three (one just left of center, one centered behind the central incisors, and one just right of center) (Figure 14–13C) or four (two just left of center and two just right of center) films. The film packet orientation in the oral cavity is usually such that the longer dimension is placed vertically. For ease of placement and to avoid bending the film packet, the narrow size #1 film is recommended, especially for imaging the lateral-canine region. However, a size

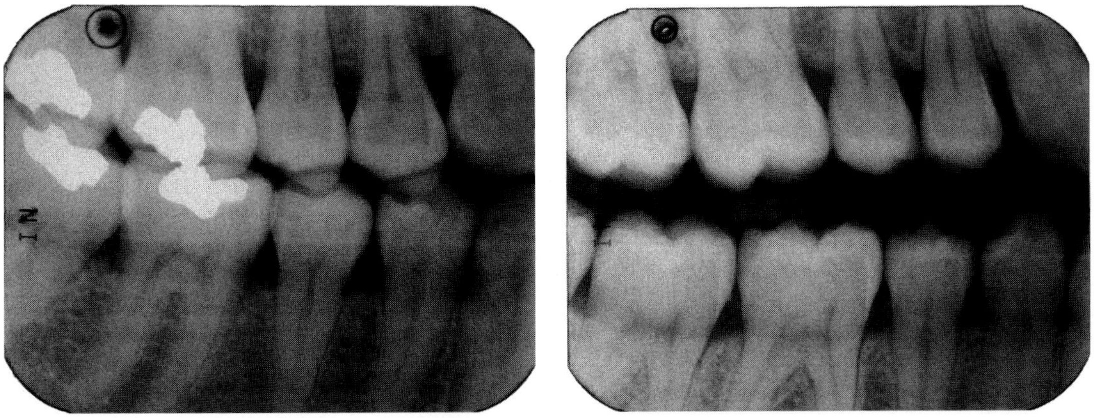

FIGURE 14-12 **Holder comparison.** (**A**) This bitewing was taken using the disposable paper stick-on bitetab. Notice the increased alveolar bone imaged, versus (**B**) the bitewing taken using a thicker plastic, autoclavable film-holding device.

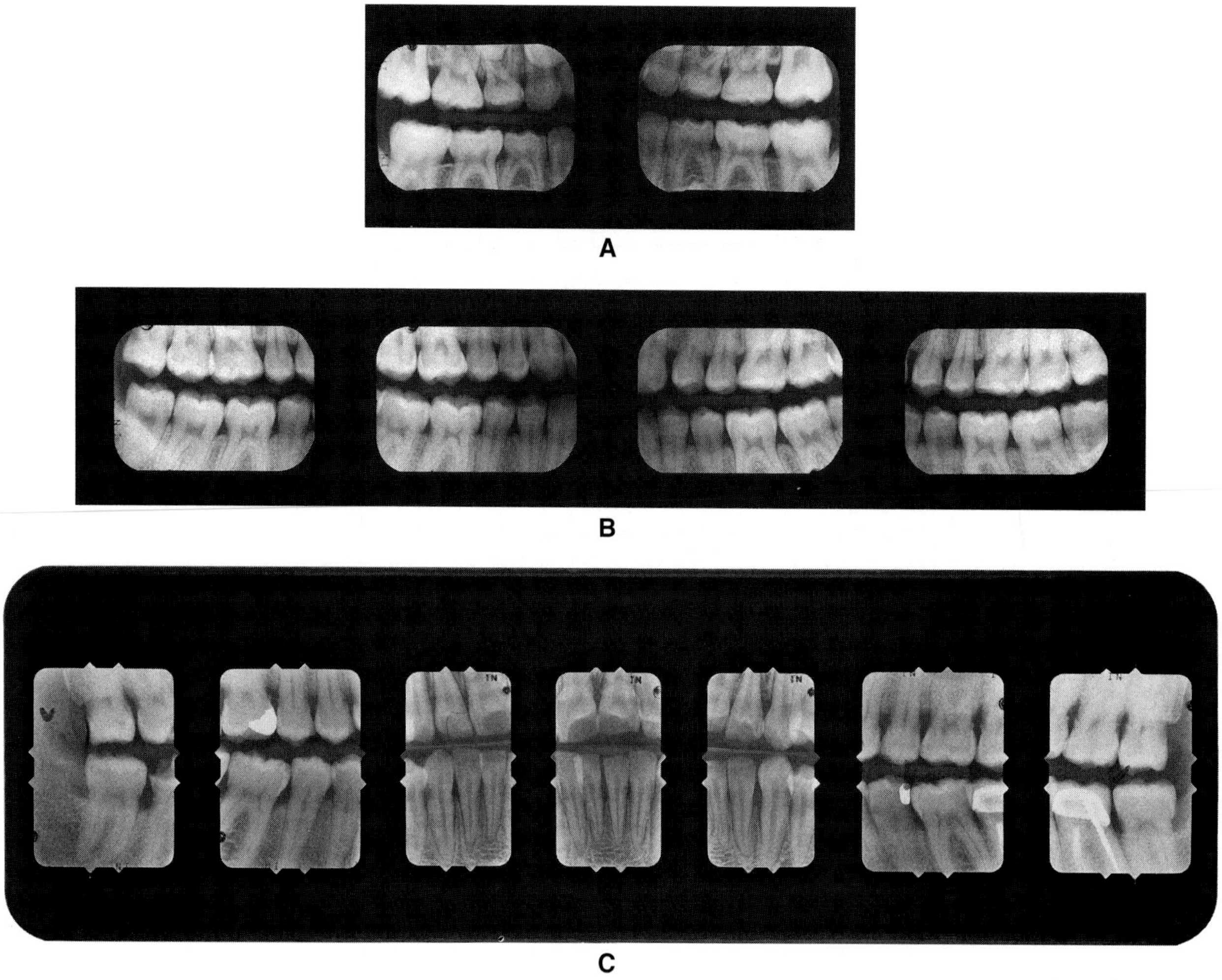

FIGURE 14-13 **Horizontal and vertical bitewing series.** (**A**) Set of two horizontal posterior bitewing series. (**B**) Set of four horizontal posterior bitewing series. (**C**) Set of seven vertical bitewing series, including posterior and anterior radiographs.

#2 may be used for the central incisors when the arch permits. Using a longer bitetab than that used for the posterior exposures will allow the film to be placed further lingually in the mouth. This will prevent the film from bending in the middle as the tab is pulled forward when the patient is asked to bite down. Two stick-on paper bitetabs may be attached in such a way as to lengthen the bitetab for this purpose (Figure 14–14).

The technique for posterior horizontal and vertical bitewings and for anterior vertical bitewings is the same for all patients, adults and children. Although vertical angulations may vary slightly from patient to patient, the average vertical angulation used should be +10 degrees and the horizontal angulation is directed perpendicularly through the embrasures toward the film (Procedure Box 14–1).

Sequence of Film Placement

It is recommended always to follow a systematic order for film packet placement when taking radiographs, to prevent errors and to utilize time more efficiently. At what point to take bitewing

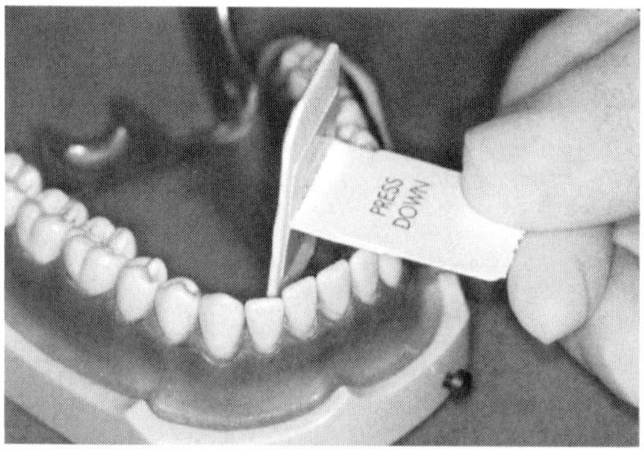

FIGURE 14-14 **Two stick-on bitetabs for anterior bitewings.** Using two stick-on paper bitetabs to lengthen the holder for use in the anterior region.

PROCEDURE 14–1

PROCEDURE FOR EXPOSING BITEWING RADIOGPRAPHS

1. Perform infection control procedures (see Procedure Box 9–2).
2. Prepare unit. Turn on and set exposure factors.
3. Seat patient and explain the procedure.
4. Request that the patient remove objects from the mouth that can interfere with the procedure and remove eyeglasses.
5. Adjust chair to a comfortable working level.
6. Adjust head rest to position patient's head so that the occlusal plane is parallel to the floor and the midsagittal plane (midline) is perpendicular to the floor.
7. Place the lead apron and thyroid collar on the patient.
8. Perform a cursory inspection of the oral cavity and note possible obstructions (tori, shallow palatal vault, mal-aligned teeth) that may require an alteration of technique or number of films exposed. Note the patient's occlusion to assist with aligning the film packet with the maxillary or mandibular teeth.
9. Attach a bitetab or loop to the film packet or place the film packet into the film-holding device.
10. Insert the film into the patient's oral cavity and center the film behind the area to be imaged. (See Table 14–3 for the exact film packet placements for each of the bitewing radiographs in the procedure.) Visually locate the contact points of the teeth to be imaged and place the film perpendicular to the embrasures.
11. Hold the tab or film holder firmly against the occlusal/incisal surface of the mandibular teeth while asking the patient to close the mouth so that the teeth occlude normally.
12. Release the bitetab or film holder when the patient has closed firmly, holding it in place.
13. Set the vertical angulation to +10° or align as indicated by the external aiming device of the film holder.
14. Determine the correct horizontal angulation by directing the central ray of the x-ray beam perpendicular to the film in the horizontal plane through the contact point of the teeth of interest. (See Table 14–3 for the exact embrasure space through which to direct the central ray for each of the bitewing radiographs in the procedure.) Or align as indicated by the external aiming device of the film holder.
15. Center the PID over the point of entry, a spot on the occlusal plane between the maxillary and mandibular teeth of interest. (See Table 14–3 for the exact entry point to direct the central ray for each of the bitewing radiographs in the procedure.) Or align as indicated by the external aiming device of the film holder.
16. Make the exposure.
17. Remove the film packet and holder from the patient's oral cavity.
18. Repeat steps 9–17 until all films in the series have been exposed. (See Table 14–2 for reccommanded sequence.)
19. Remove the lead apron and thyroid collar from the patient.
20. Perform infection control procedures following the exposures (see Procedure Box 9–4).

radiographs when exposing a full mouth series is explained in Chapter 13. When exposing a set of four posterior bitewings alone, it is recommended that the premolar bitewing on one side be exposed first, followed by the molar bitewing on the same side. Placing the premolar film packet intraorally may be more comfortable for the patient and less likely to excite a gag reflex, gaining the patient's confidence for the more difficult molar film packet placement. Then the premolar and molar bitewing on the opposite should be exposed. Completing both the premolar and molar bitewing radiographs on one side first will avoid shifting the tube head back and forth across the patient.

When exposing a series of seven or eight posterior and anterior bitewings, exposing the less uncomfortable anterior bitewings first will again allow the patient to adapt to the procedure, permitting the radiographer to continue with the posterior bitewings. After exposing the three or four anterior bitewings, the same sequence as posterior bitewings should be followed, exposing the premolar and molar bitewing on one side first and then proceeding to the other side (Table 14–2).

Unit Preparation

Prior to placing the film packet intraorally, the unit should be turned on and the exposure settings selected. It is helpful to place the tube head and PID in the approximate position to limit the time required for this step once the film packet has been placed into the patient's oral cavity. Because the vertical angulation is the same for all bitewing radiographs (+10°), it may be set at this time.

TABLE 14-2 **Recommended Sequence for Exposing Bitewing Radiographs**

Bitewing Series	Recommended Sequence
2 posterior	1st: right* premolar 2nd: left premolar
4 posterior	1st: right* premolar 2nd: right molar 3rd: left premolar 4th: left molar
7 anterior and posterior	1st: central-lateral incisors 2nd: left* canine 3rd: right canine 4th: right premolar 5th: right molar 6th: left premolar 7th: left molar
8 anterior and posterior	1st: left* canine 2nd: left central-lateral incisors 3rd: right central-lateral incisors 4th: right canine 5th: right premolar 6th: right molar 7th: left premolar 8th: left molar

*Left-handed radiographers may choose to begin the exposures on the opposite side.

Patient Preparation

To help gain patient cooperation and confidence, it is important to explain the procedure to the patient. Include specific instructions regarding the need for patient cooperation and be honest about any difficulties anticipated (see Chapter 11). Perform a cursory oral inspection and ask the patient to remove any objects from the mouth that would interfere with the procedure, such as removable dentures or orthodontic appliances, chewing gum, etc. Ask the patient to remove eyeglasses. If any metal or thick plastic parts of the eyeglasses remain in the path of the x-ray beam, they will be imaged onto the radiograph. Protect the patient with the lead apron and thyroid collar barriers.

Position the patient's head so that the occlusal plane is parallel to the floor and the midsagittal plane (midline) is perpendicular to the floor (Figure 14–15). Use the head rest to adjust the patient's position. When using a film holder with an external aiming device, the patient's head position is not as critical. However, stabilizing the patient's head against the head rest is important to prevent movement during the exposure. Place the head rest against the occipital protuberance (the back, base of the skull) for greatest stability.

Managing Exposures

All films and film-holding devices should be ready and available once the procedure begins. If not pre-tabbed, the film packets may be prepared with stick-on paper bite tabs or placed in the film-holding device. Insert the film packet into the patient's mouth and center over the area of interest (Table 14–3). The film packet should be inserted flat until the packet is completely in the patient's mouth (Figure 14–16). Then rotate the film packet until it is in a vertical position. Inserting in this manner allows the radiographer to move the tongue out of the way as the film packet is rotated. The bitetab should be held firmly against the occlusal surface of the mandibular teeth. The patient should be instructed to close so that the teeth occlude normally. Biting down correctly on the bitetab is important to obtain the proper relationship of the teeth on the radiograph. Failure to hold the tab firmly permits the film to drift lingually and distally, and increases the possibility that the tongue will move the film. This often results in a tilted or slanted occlusal plane on the radiographic image (Figure 14–17).

Practice Point

To aid in gaining the patient's understanding of what will be required, it can be helpful to perform a trial placement of the film. When using a film holder, practice the procedure by placing the holder without the film packet inserted to help the patient understand how to bite. This practice placement can also be done when using bite tabs or loops. Providing the patient with this opportunity to practice can increase the likelihood of a successful process.

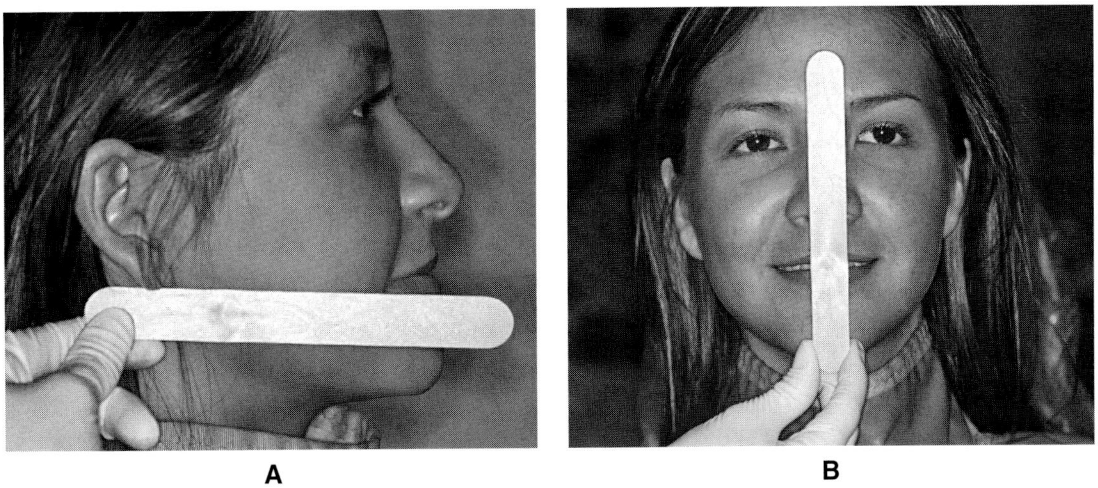

FIGURE 14-15 **Patient positioning.** The patient is positioned with the head supported against the head rest with the (**A**) occlusal plane parallel to the floor and the (**B**) midsaggital plane perpendicular to the floor.

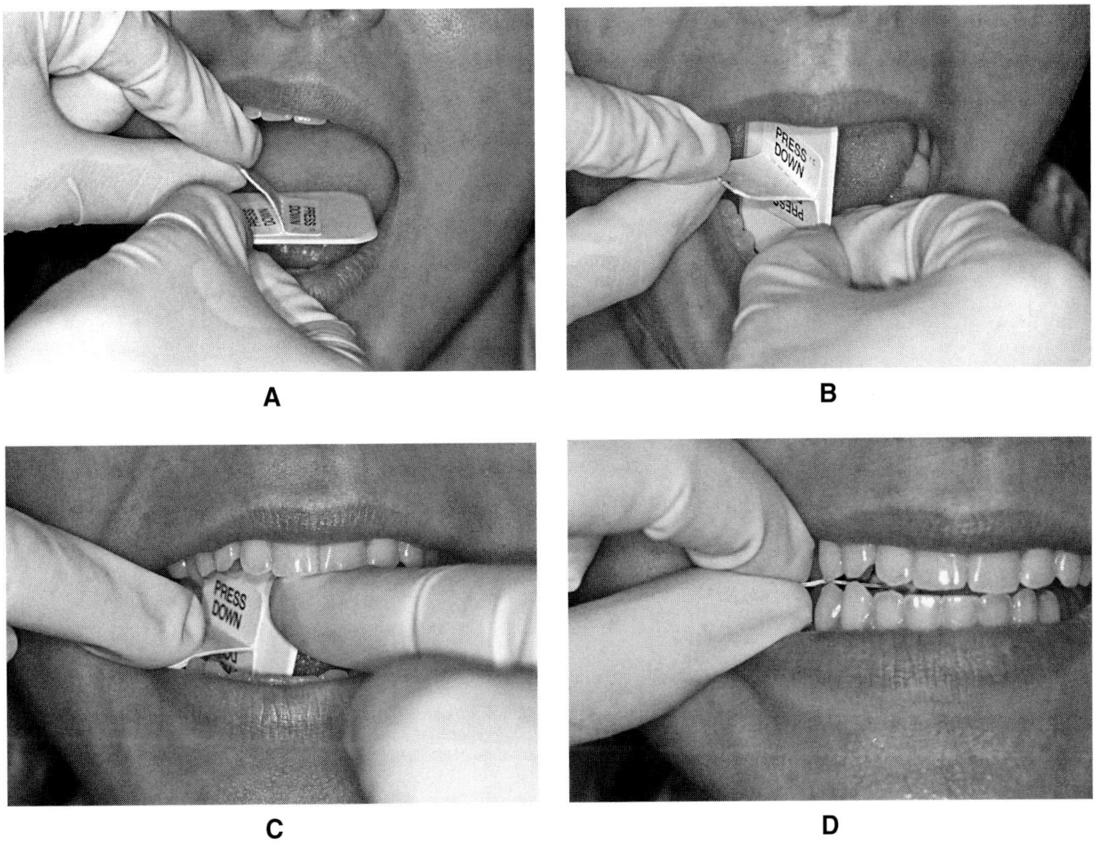

FIGURE 14-16 **Film packet placement.** (**A**) Inserting the film packet flat until the packet is completely in the patient's mouth. (**B**) Then the radiographer rotates the film packet until it is in a vertical position. Inserting in this manner allows the radiographer to move the tongue out of the way as the film packet is rotated. (**C**) The tab is held in place against the occlusal surfaces of the mandibular teeth while the top edge of the film is angled slightly toward the lingual to avoid being pushed down by the palate. (**D**) The tab is held in place until the patient closes.

TABLE 14-3 **Bitewing Radiographic Technique: A Summary**

Bitewing Radiograph	Film Packet Placement	Vertical Angulation	Horizontal Angulation	Point of Entry
Central incisors (vertical)	Center the film packet to line up behind the central and lateral incisors; if using a size #2 film, include the mesial halves of the canines.	+10	Direct the central rays perpendicularly through the left and right central incisor embrasure.	A spot on the incisal plane between the maxillary and mandibular central incisors.
Canine (vertical)	Center the film packet to line up behind the canine; include the distal half of the lateral incisor and the mesial half of the first premolar.	+10	Direct the central rays perpendicularly at the center of the canine.	A spot on the incisal plane between the maxillary and mandibular canines.
Central-lateral incisors (vertical)	Center the film packet to line up behind the central and lateral incisors; include the mesial half of central incisor on the opposite side and the mesial half of the canine.	+10	Direct the central rays perpendicularly through the central and lateral incisor embrasure.	A spot on the incisal plane between the maxillary and mandibular lateral incisors.
Premolar (horizontal or vertical)	Align the anterior edge of the film packet to line up behind the distal half of the maxillary or the mandibular canine; chose the most mesially located canine.	+10	Direct the central rays perpendicularly through the first and second premolar embrasure.	A spot on the occlusal plane between the maxillary and mandibular second premolars.
Molar (adult) (horizontal or vertical)	Align the anterior edge of the film packet to line up behind the distal half of the maxillary or the mandibular second premolar; chose the most mesially located premolar.	+10	Direct the central rays perpendicularly through the first and second molar embrasure.	A spot on the occlusal plane between the maxillary and mandibular first molars.
Molar (horizontal-child)	Align the anterior edge of the film packet to line up behind the distal half of the maxillary or the mandibular canine; chose the most mesially located canine.	+5 to +10	Direct the central rays perpendicularly through the first and second primary molar embrasure; or, if erupted, the first and second premolar embrasure.	A spot on the occlusal plane between the primary maxillary and mandibular first molars; or, if erupted, the maxillary and mandibular second premolars.
Premolar-molar (size #3)	Align the anterior edge of film packet to line up behind the distal half of the maxillary or the mandibular canine; chose the most mesially located canine.	+10	Direct the central rays perpendicularly through the second premolar and first molar embrasure.	A spot on the occlusal plane between the maxillary and mandibular second premolars.

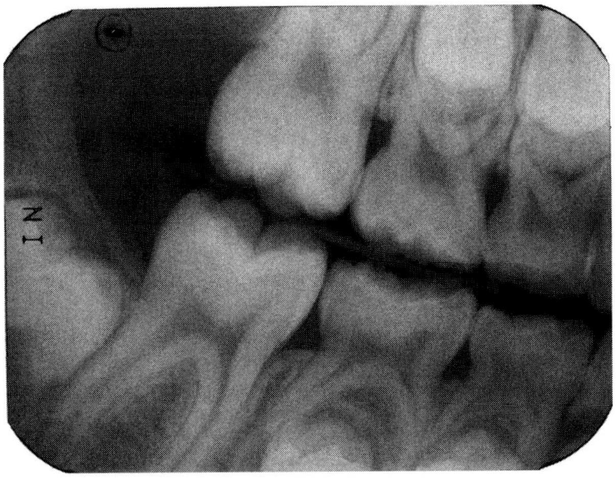

FIGURE 14–17 **Tilted film.** The slanted occlusal plane observed on this film resulted from a failure to place the film packet far enough lingually to avoid being pushed down by the palate when the patient occluded onto the bitetab.

Practice Points

Tilted Film

A sloping or slanting (tilted) occlusal plane is a frequent reason for having to retake bitewing radiographs. Probable causes include:

1. The failure of the patient to maintain a steady pressure on the bitetab.
2. The patient swallowing while the exposure is being made.
3. Anatomical obstructions such as a torus or malpositioned tooth.
4. The top edge of the film contacting the lingual gingiva or curvature of the palate.
5. Poor placement of the bitetab or film holder.

Possible corrections include:

1. Providing the patient with specific instructions about securely biting on the bitetab.
2. Cautioning the patient not to swallow or allow the teeth to separate.
3. Checking for anatomical obstructions before positioning the film packet. When obstructions such as tori are present, position the film behind the obstruction (see Chapter 25).
4. Positioning the film packet far enough away from the lingual surfaces of the teeth. This is especially important with the premolar and anterior bitewings, where the curvature of the palate will contact the anterior-superior corner of the film and cause it to be pushed down, slanting the position.
5. Exercising care in selecting and positioning the correct size film.

Altering the Number of Bitewings

There are times when additional bitewing radiographs are needed. When the patient presents with mal-aligned or crowded teeth, overlapping may occur, even when all angulations are set correctly. In this case, an additional film may have to be positioned to image the mal-aligned teeth. Managing this special need is discussed in Chapter 25.

Additionally, when the patient presents with missing teeth or edentulous areas, bitewing radiographs may not need to be exposed. Children who present with a mixed dentition of missing primary teeth and unerupted permanent teeth often allow for a visual inspection of the proximal surfaces of the erupted teeth, negating the need to expose bitewings in these areas. Managing the child patient is discussed in Chapter 23.

Avoiding Overlap

Because the interproximal surfaces of the molars are in a mesiodistal relationship to the patient's sagittal plane, conventional film placement parallel to the buccal surfaces often results in overlapping of the contact areas and closure of the embrasure spaces. In such cases, the film should be positioned perpendicularly to the embrasures to avoid distortion. Place the film slightly diagonally with the front edge of the film farther from the lingual of the teeth than the back edge (Figure 14–18). Then direct the central ray of the x-ray beam through the contact areas.

The Bitewing Techique

Figures 14–19 through 14–22 illustrate the precise film packet positions and required angulations for each of the horizontal and vertical bitewing radiographs discussed in this chapter. See Table 14–3 for a summary of the technique.

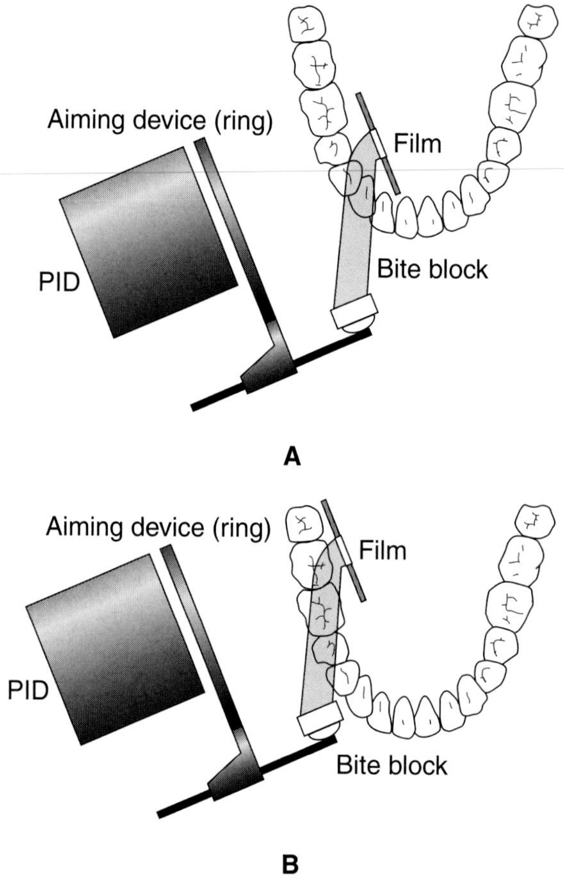

FIGURE 14–18 **Film and PID position with the Rinn bitewing instrument.** (**A**) Conventional premolar film packet placement places the film packet slightly diagonally with the front edge of the film farther from the lingual of the teeth than the back part. (**B**) Because the interproximal surfaces of the molar teeth are in a mesiodistal relationship to the sagittal plane, it is recommended that the film be positioned perpendicularly to the embrasures, resulting in a diagonal placement of the film, much like with the premolar position. (Courtesy of Dentsply Rinn)

BITEWING TECHNIQUE

Central-Lateral Bitewing Exposure

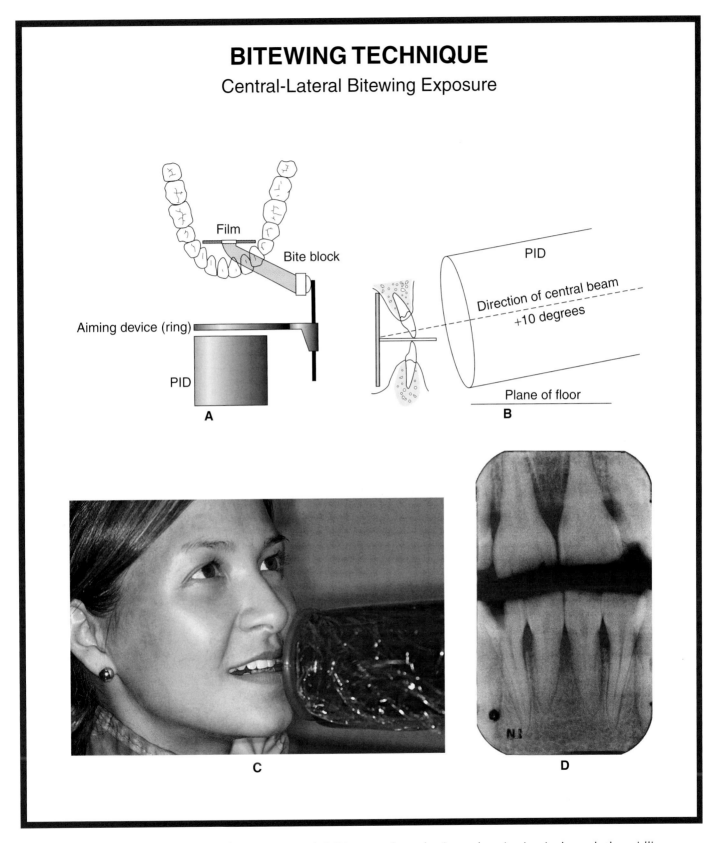

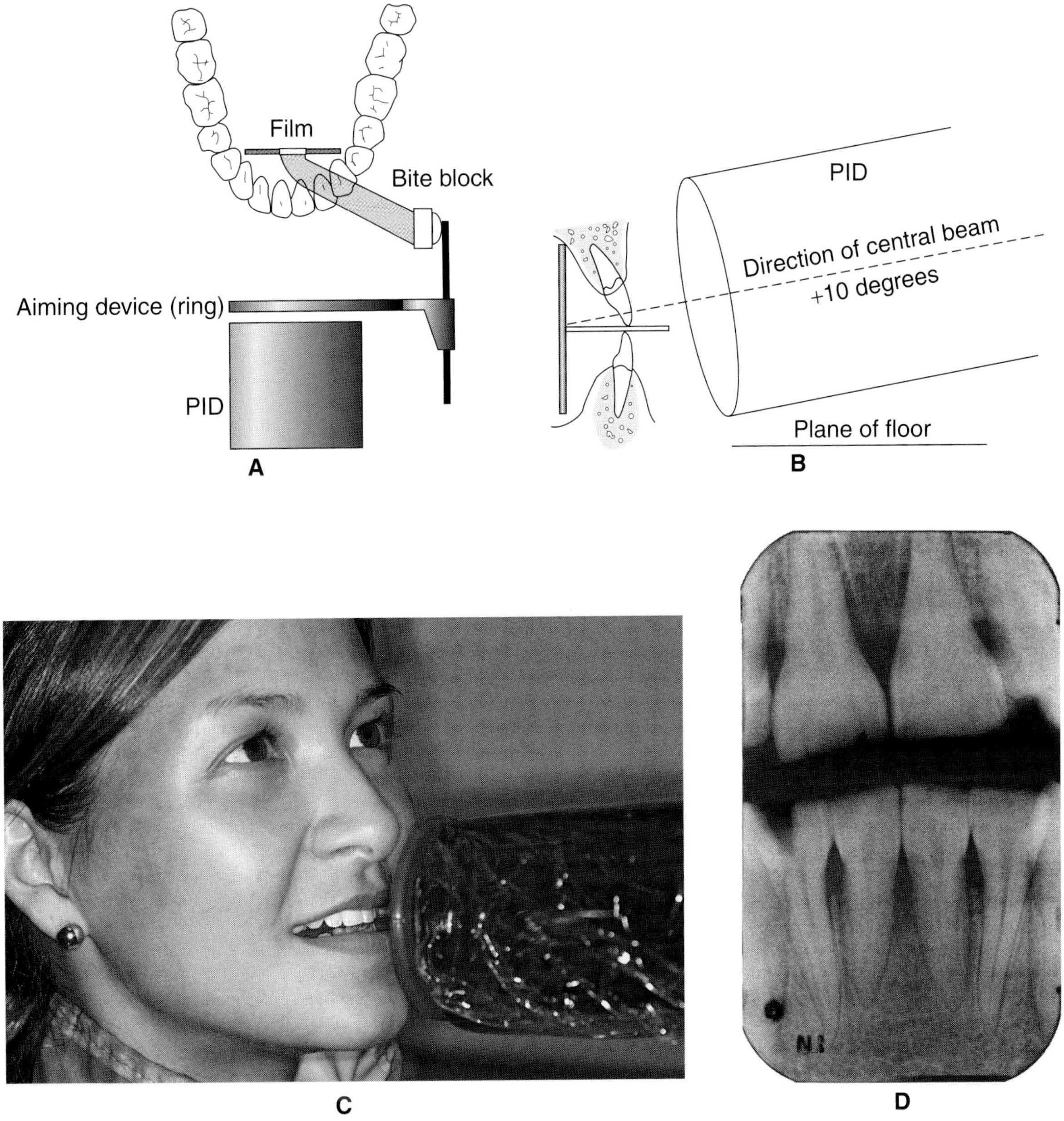

FIGURE 14–19 **Central-lateral bitewing exposure.** (**A**) Diagram shows horizontal projection is through the midline embrasure and perpendicular to the mean tangent. (**B**) Vertical projection is directed perpendicular to the film at approximately +10° with the PID tilted downward. (**C**) Position of Rinn film holder and PID. (**D**) Central-lateral bitewing radiograph.

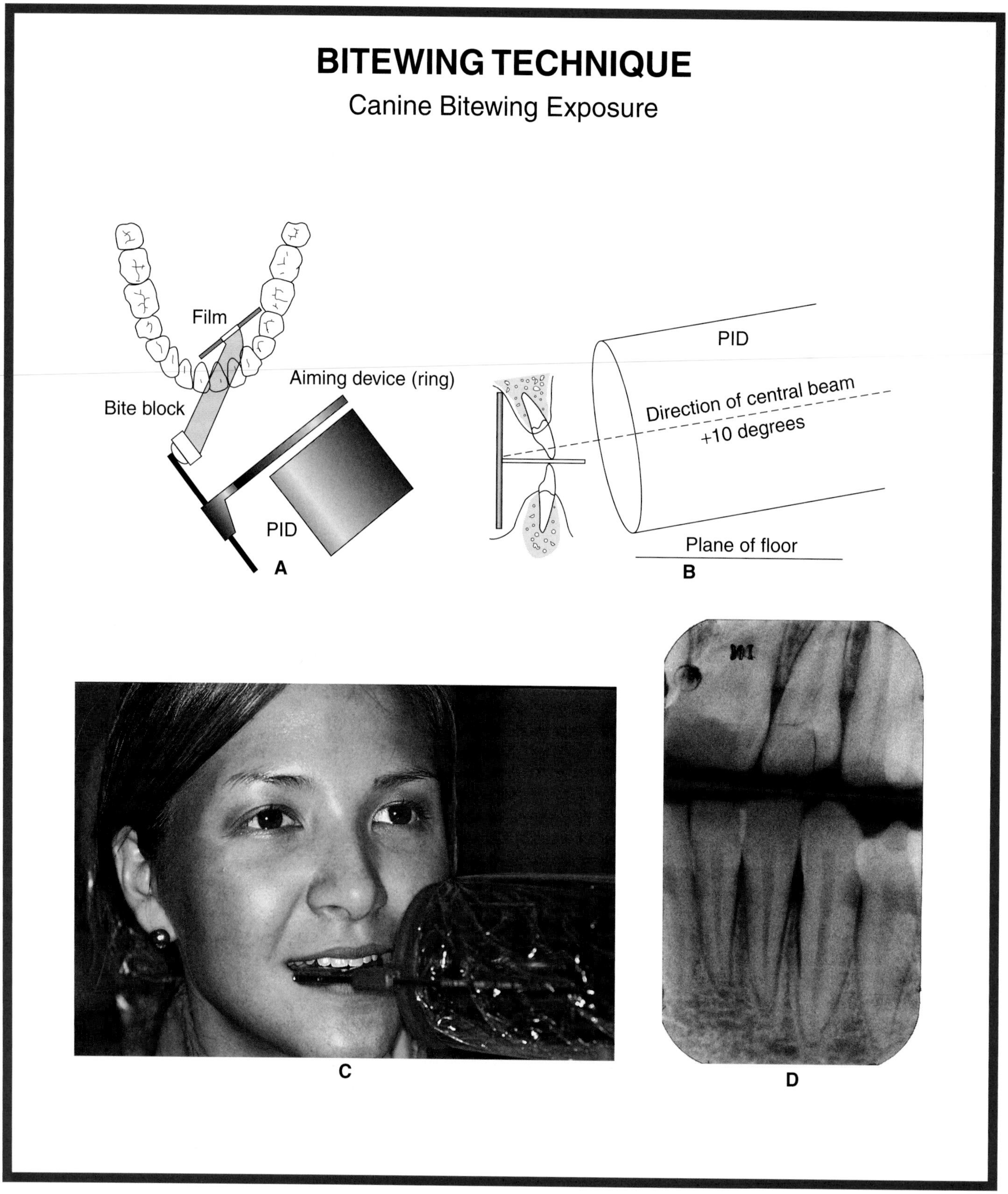

FIGURE 14–20 **Canine bitewing exposure.** (**A**) Diagram shows horizontal projection is through the canine and perpendicular to the mean tangent. (**B**) Vertical projection is directed perpendicular to the film at approximately +10° with the PID tilted downward. (**C**) Position of Rinn film holder and PID. (**D**) Canine bitewing radiograph.

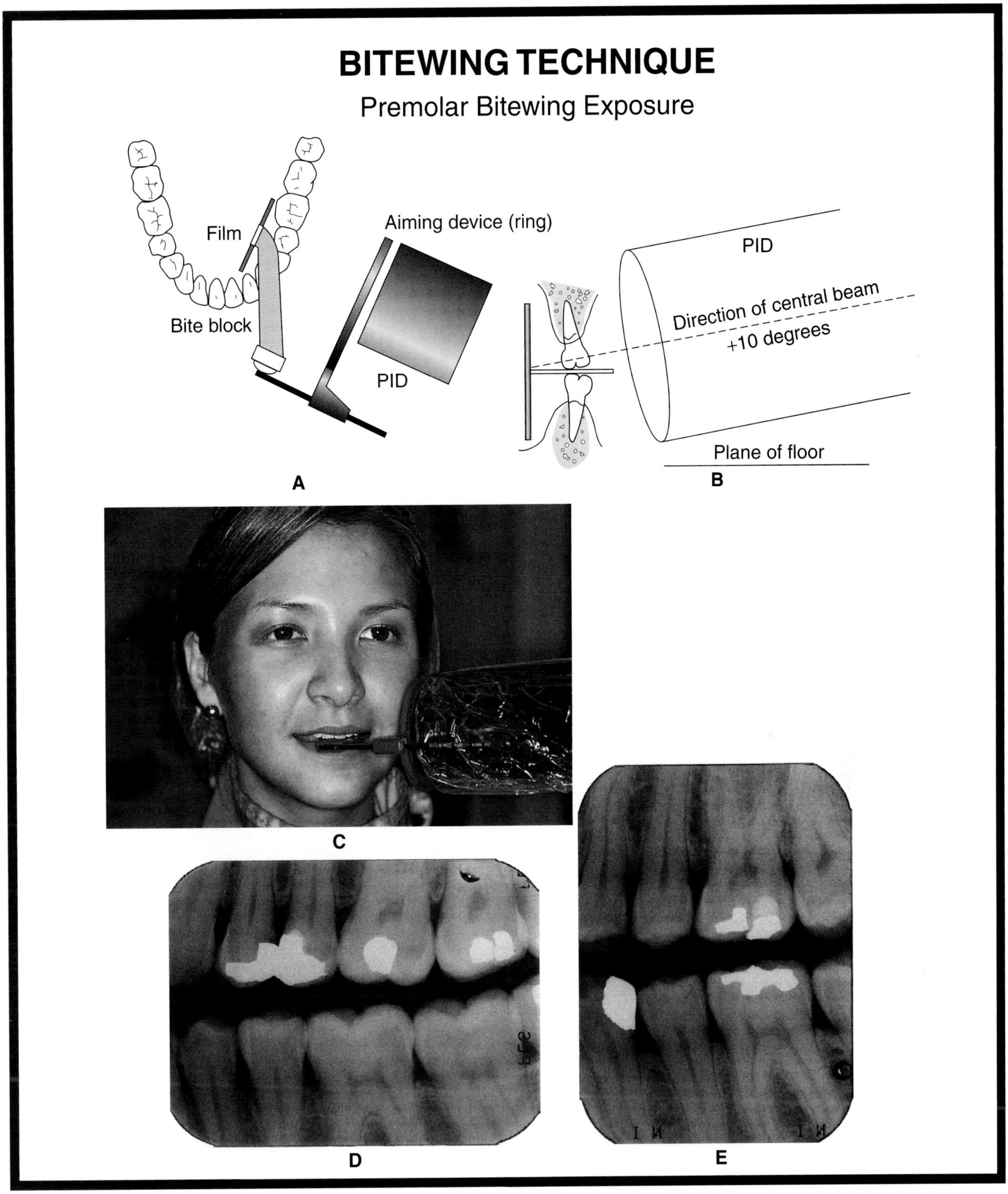

FIGURE 14–21 **Premolar bitewing exposure.** (**A**) Diagram shows horizontal projection is through the first and second premolar embrasure and perpendicular to the mean tangent. (**B**) Vertical projection is directed perpendicular to the film at approximately +10 degrees with the PID tilted downward. (**C**) Position of Rinn film holder and PID. (**D**) Horizontal premolar bitewing radiograph. (**E**) Vertical premolar bitewing radiograph.

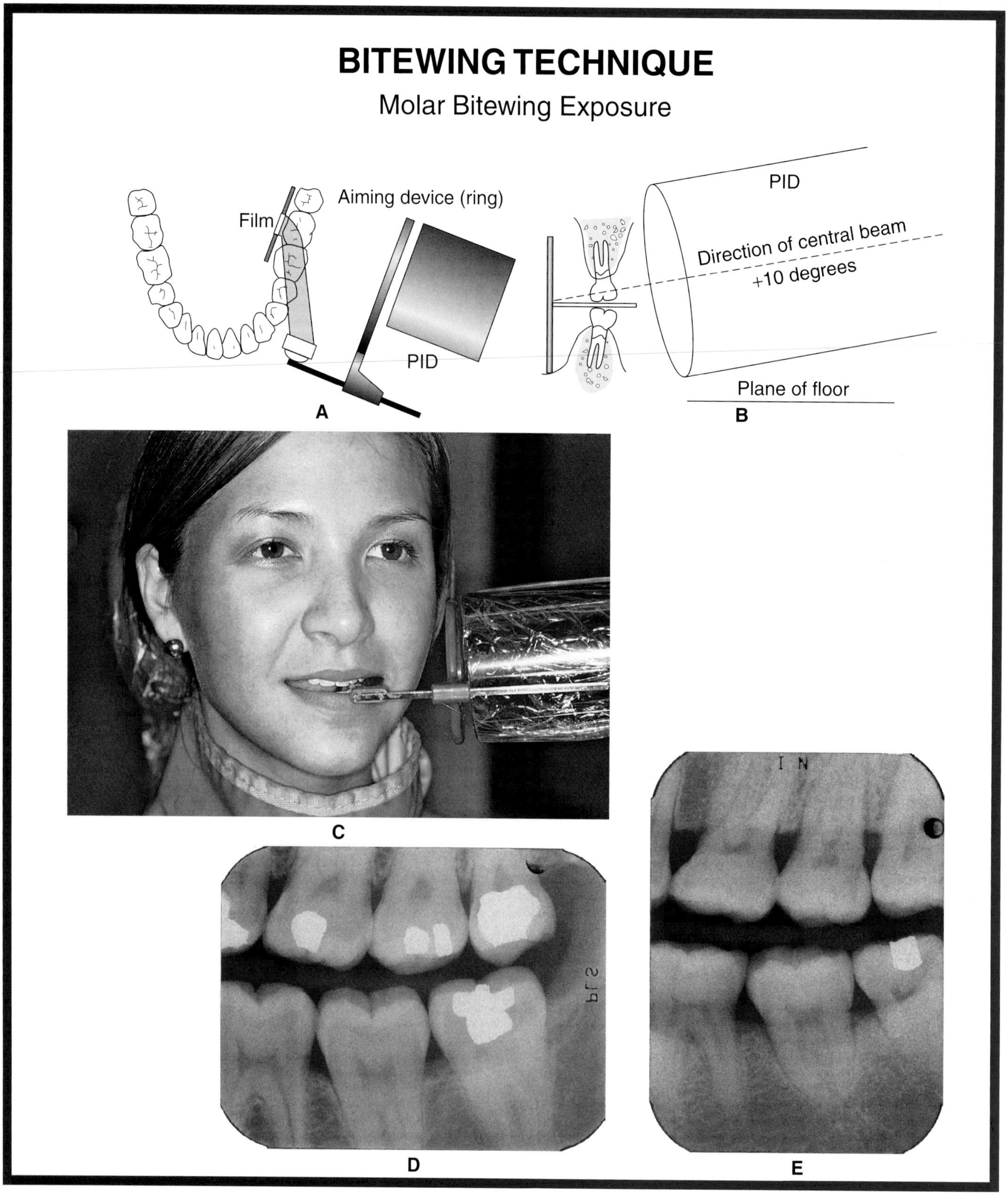

FIGURE 14–22 **Molar bitewing exposure.** (**A**) Diagram shows horizontal projection is through the first and second molar embrasure and perpendicular to the mean tangent. (**B**) Vertical projection is directed perpendicular to the film at approximately +10 degrees with the PID tilted downward. (**C**) Position of Rinn film holder and PID. (**D**) Horizontal molar bitewing radiograph. (**E**) Vertical molar bitewing radiograph.

REVIEW—Chapter Summary

Bitewing radiographs image the coronal portion of both maxillary and mandibular teeth on one film. Bitewing radiographs supplement and complete the full-mouth survey because of their improved ability to image incipient caries in the tooth contact areas and early resorptive changes in the alveolar bony crest.

The size and number of films to use to expose a bitewing radiographic series depend on the type of survey required and the size and shape of the patient's oral cavity. Care must be taken in placement of the film so that the radiograph will show the teeth of interest and image the same amount of maxillary and mandibular structures.

The vertical angulation setting for all bitewing radiographs is +10 degrees. An error in the horizontal angulation will cause overlapped images in the tooth contact areas and render the film useless for diagnostic purposes.

Some form of film retention—bitetab, film loop, or film-holder bite block—must be used. The patient prevents the film from moving by biting firmly on the bitetab or film-holder bite block in an edge-to-edge or centric relationship.

When exposing a set of bitewing radiographs, an orderly sequence should be followed. Step-by-step instructions for exposing a bitewing survey is presented.

RECALL—Study Questions

1. Which of these conditions would not be visible on a bitewing radiograph?
   a. Proximal surface caries
   b. Overhanging restoration
   c. Apical abscess
   d. Alveolar crest resorption
2. How many standard-sized #2 films are recommended for a posterior bitewing survey of an adult patient?
   a. 2
   b. 4
   c. 7
   d. 8
3. In which of the following situations would using a size #3 film be acceptable?
   a. Horizontal bitewings on a child patient
   b. Horizontal bitewings on an adult patient
   c. Horizontal bitewings on an adult patient with periodontal disease
   d. Vertical bitewings on any patient who presented with a need for them
4. Which size film is used, and how is it positioned in the anterior region of a small and narrow adult arch?
   a. Size #3 film placed vertically
   b. Size #2 film placed horizontally
   c. Size #1 film placed vertically
   d. Size #0 film placed horizontally
5. An error in which of these results in overlapping?
   a. Film packet placement
   b. Point of entry
   c. Vertical angulation
   d. Horizontal angulation
6. An error in vertical angulation will result in:
   a. Unequal distribution of the arches.
   b. Overlapping.
   c. Overexposure to the patient.
   d. Cone cut.
7. What is the approximate vertical angulation for bitewing radiographs?
   a. −10 degrees
   b. 0 degrees
   c. +10 degrees
   d. +20 degrees
8. Which of the following best fits this description: "Disposable, may be used for placing both horizontal and vertical bitewings, and provides increased imaging of the alveolar bone"?
   a. Stick-on bitetabs
   b. Pre-attached bitetabs
   c. Bite loops
   d. Rinn film holder
9. In which of the following conditions would vertical bitewing radiographs be recommended over horizontal bitewing radiographs?
   a. Child with rampant caries
   b. Adolescent with suspected third molar impactions
   c. Adult with mal-aligned teeth
   d. Adult with periodontal disease
10. When taking a set of eight vertical bitewing radiographs, which of the following should be exposed first?
    a. Left molar bitewing
    b. Left premolar bitewing
    c. Right canine bitewing
    d. Right premolar bitewing
11. The film packet placement for an adult horizontal molar bitewing is to align the film packet so that the:
    a. Central and lateral incisors are centered on the film.
    b. Canine is centered on the film.
    c. Anterior portion of the film lines up behind the distal half of the canine.
    d. Anterior portion of the film lines up behind the distal half of the second premolar.
12. The film packet placement for an adult vertical premolar bitewing is to align the film packet so that the:
    a. Central and lateral incisors are centered on the film.
    b. Canine is centered on the film.
    c. Anterior portion of the film lines up behind the distal half of the canine.
    d. Anterior portion of the film lines up behind the distal half of the second premolar.
13. Through which interproximal space should the central rays be perpendicularly directed when exposing a molar bitewing on a child with primary teeth?
    a. Between the central and lateral incisors
    b. Between the lateral incisor and canine
    c. Between the canine and first molar
    d. Between the first and second molars

14. Through which interproximal space should the central rays be perpendicularly directed when exposing a premolar bitewing on an adolescent?
    a. Between the central and lateral incisors
    b. Between the lateral incisor and canine
    c. Between the canine and first premolar
    d. Between the first and second premolars

REFLECT—Case Study

Study the dental chart and patient record below. Note the dentist's written prescription for a radiographic examination. Decide the following:

1. What type of bitewings will most likely be exposed?
2. What size film will best fit this patient?
3. How many films will be required to complete the exam?
4. Write out a detailed procedure for exposing each of the required radiographs. Include:
    a. Specific film packet placements.
    b. The vertical angulation required.
    c. How the horizontal angulation will be determined.
    d. What the point of entry will be.

RELATE—Laboratory Application

For a comprehensive three-part laboratory practice exercise on this topic, see E. M. Thomson, *Exercises in Oral Radiography Techniques: A Laboratory Manual,* 2nd ed., Upper Saddle River, NJ: Prentice Hall, 2006. Chapter 2, "Bitewing Radiographic Technique."

BIBLIOGRAPHY

Eastman Kodak. *Successful Intraoral Radiography.* Rochester, NY: Eastman Kodak, 1998.

Rinn Corporation. *Intraoral Radiography with Rinn XCP/BAI Instruments.* Elgin, IL: Dentsply/Rinn Corporation, 1989.

White, S. C. & Pharoah, M. J. *Oral Radiology Principles and Interpretation,* 5th ed. St. Louis: Elsevier, 2004.

Wilkins, E. M. *Clinical Practice of the Dental Hygienist,* 9th ed. Philadelphia: Lippincott Williams & Wilkins, 2005.

Case: New patient to your practice.
Age/Gender: 40-year-old male.
Medical History: Hypertension.
Dental History: Has had extensive dental treatment in the past as evidenced by several extractions and restored teeth.
Social History: Appears nervous of dental treatment.
Chief Complaint: Thinks he has "gum disease."
Current Oral Hygiene Status: Generalized 4–6 mm pockets; generalized moderate gingivitis.
Initial Treatment: Take a set of bitewing radiographs.

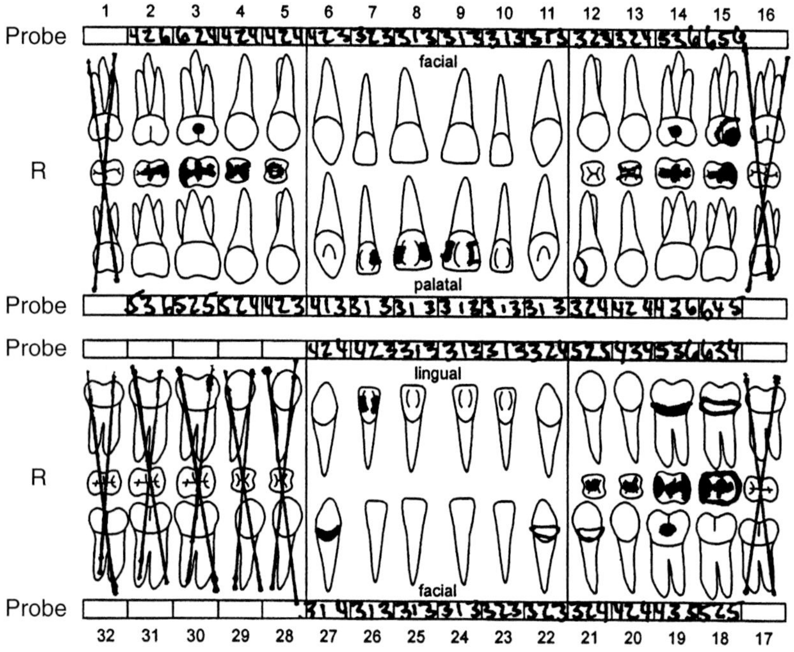

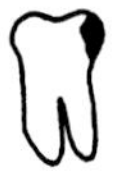
Clinically visible restoration

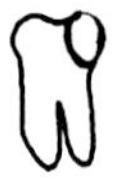
Clinically visible carious lesion

Clinically missing tooth

15

The Occlusal Examination

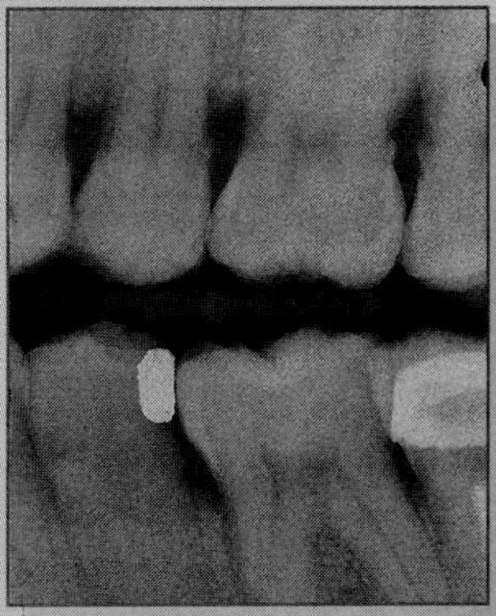

■ OBJECTIVES

Following successful completion of this chapter, you should be able to:

1. Define the key words.
2. State the purpose of the occlusal examination.
3. List the indications for occlusal radiographs.
4. Match the topographical and cross-sectional techniques with the condition to be imaged.
5. Compare the patient head positions for the topographical and the cross-sectional techniques.
6. Demonstrate the steps for the maxillary and mandibular topographical surveys.
7. Demonstrate the steps for the mandibular cross-sectional survey.

■ KEY WORDS

Cross-sectional technique
Occlusal radiographs
Topographical technique

Introduction

The purpose of the occlusal examination is to view large areas of the maxilla (upper jaw) or the mandible (lower jaw) on one radiograph. The film is placed in the mouth between the occlusal surfaces of the maxillary and mandibular teeth. The patient occludes (bites) lightly on the film to stabilize it.

The purpose of this chapter is to discuss the use and explain the procedures for the occlusal examination.

Types of Occlusal Examinations

Occlusal radiographs are either topographical or cross-sectional.

Topographical Technique

The **topographical technique** produces an image that looks like a large periapical radiograph (Figure 15–1). The topographical occlusal technique is similar to the bisecting technique used to produce periapical radiographs (see Chapter 13). Topographical occlusal radiographs may be exposed in any area of the oral cavity, the anterior and posterior regions of both the maxilla and the mandible. Topographical occlusal radiographs are best used to image conditions of the teeth and supporting structures when a larger area than that imaged by a periapical radiograph is required. Topographical occlusal surveys generally yield a greater amount of information in the alveolar crest and apical areas than periapical radiographs.

Cross-sectional Technique

The **cross-sectional technique** produces an image much like its name implies (Figure 15–1). The circular or elliptical appearance of the teeth on the radiograph and the increased coverage of the sublingual area (under the tongue) allow the cross-sectional occlusal radiograph to yield more information about the location of tori and impacted or malpositioned teeth and calcifications of soft tissues in this area.

Fundamentals of Occlusal Radiographs

The occlusal examination may be made alone or to supplement periapical or bitewing radiographs. The large size #4 occlusal film is useful for recording information that cannot be adequately recorded on the smaller periapical films. **Occlusal radiographs** are used to:

- Precisely locate supernumerary, unerupted, or impacted teeth (especially impacted canines and third molars).
- Locate retained roots of extracted teeth.
- Detect the presence, locate, and evaluate the extent of, disease and lesions (cysts, tumors, etc.).
- Locate foreign bodies in the jaws.
- Reveal the presence of salivary stones (sialoliths) in the ducts of the sublingual and submandibular glands.
- Aid in evaluating fractures of the maxilla or mandible.
- Show the size and shape of mandibular tori.

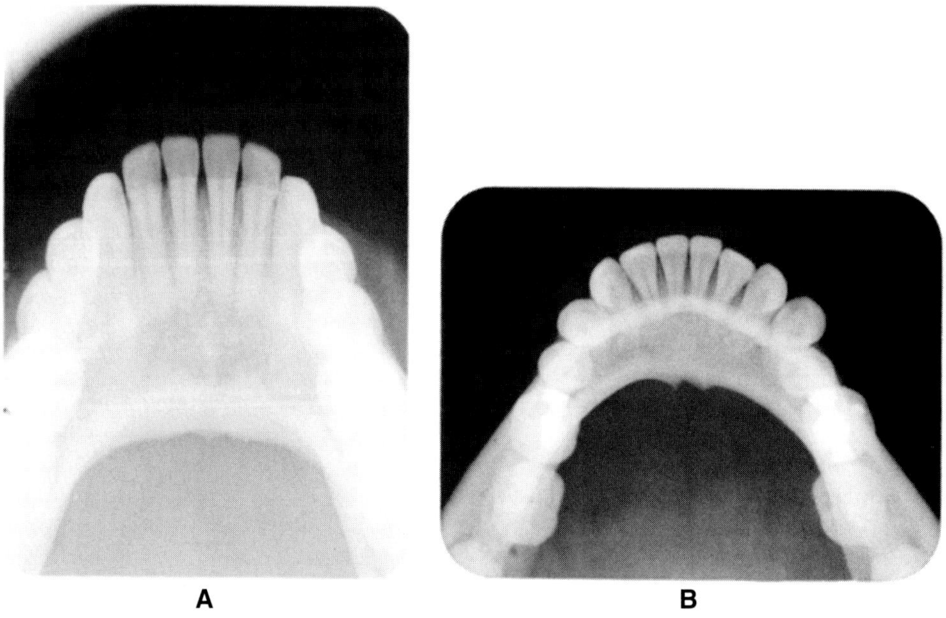

FIGURE 15–1 **A comparison of topographical and cross-sectional occlusal radiographs.** (**A**) The topographical occlusal radiograph of the anterior mandible closely resembles a periapical radiograph. Note how the large occlusal film images a larger portion of the region. (**B**) The cross-sectional occlusal radiograph of the mandibular anterior region reveals more information about the sublingual area (under the tongue) and conditions of the soft tissue than about the teeth and the supporting structures.

- Aid in examining patients with trismus who can open their mouths only a few millimeters.
- Evaluate the borders of the maxillary sinus.
- Examine cleft palate patients.
- Use as an acceptable substitute on young children who may not be able to tolerate periapical film packet placement (see Chapter 23).

Occlusal radiographs may be taken in any region of the oral cavity. This chapter focuses on five of the most common standard film packet placements:

1. Maxillary topographical (anterior)
2. Maxillary topographical (posterior)
3. Mandibular topographical (anterior)
4. Mandibular topographical (posterior)
5. Mandibular cross-sectional

Film Requirements

The large 3 × 2 1/4 in. (7.7 × 5.8 cm) #4 film is used for occlusal radiographs on most adult patients. Smaller intraoral films may also be used, depending on the area to be examined. The standard #2 periapical film is frequently used with children, either to image labiolingual or buccolingual unerupted tooth positions or in place of periapical radiographs. The #2 film may also be used on adults when the oral cavity is too small for the large occlusal film.

Orientation of the Film Packet

The film packet is positioned with the white unprinted side (front side) of the film packet against the arch of interest. If imaging the mandibular arch, the white, unprinted side of the film packet will face the mandible. If imaging the maxillary arch, the white, unprinted side of the film packet will face the maxilla. The film may be placed into the mouth with the long dimension positioned horizontally or vertically. It may be centered over one small region, such as for use in the anterior region of the arch, or over the entire right or left sides of the dental arches. The film position used will depend on the type of occlusal radiograph needed and the area to be imaged.

In the correct position, the film should be placed well back into the mouth, but with at least 1/4 in (1/2 cm) of the film packet protruding outside the mouth to avoid cutting off part of the image. Since the embossed identification dot should be positioned away from the area of interest, positioning it toward the anterior should leave it outside the mouth and therefore prevent it from interfering with the image.

Holding the Occlusal Film Packet in Position

Because pre-determined vertical angulations and points of entry are utilized in taking occlusal radiographs (just as they are for periapical radiographs using the bisecting technique), it is very important that the patient be seated with the head in the correct position for the area to be imaged. For occlusal radiographs taken on the maxilla, the patient should be seated with the occlusal plane parallel to the plane of the floor and the midsagittal plane perpendicular to the plane of the floor (see Figure 14–15). The head position for the mandibular exposures will depend on the type of occlusal radiograph to be produced. Topographical occlusal radiographs of the mandible may be taken with the head positioned the same as for maxillary exposures, the occlusal plane parallel to the floor and the midsagittal plane perpendicular to the floor. Mandibular cross-sectional occlusal radiographs are taken with the patient reclined in the chair so that the head is tipped back, positioning the occlusal plane perpendicular to the plane of the floor (Figure 15–2).

No film holders are used for occlusal radiographs. The film is held in place during the exposure by slight pressure of the teeth of the opposite jaw.

Angulation

The occlusal technique is based on the correlation of certain head positions with specific vertical angulations, making the occlusal technique similar to the bisecting technique for periapical radiographs. For this reason, occlusal radiographs will likely have some dimensional distortion and are not a substitute for periapical radiographs taken with the paralleling technique.

The vertical angulation for topographical occlusal radiographs follows the rules of the bisecting technique used for periapical radiographs, where the central rays of the x-ray beam are directed through the apices of the teeth perpendicularly toward the bisector (Figure 15–3). No film holders are used for the placement of occlusal radiographs. Instead, the patient lightly occludes on the film packet placed flat in between the arches. This film packet placement is not parallel to the long axes of the teeth being imaged. To determine the correct vertical angulation when taking a topographical occlusal radiograph, the radiographer must observe the plane of the film packet, locate the long axes of the teeth of interest and estimate the imaginary bisector of these two planes (the film packet and the long axes of teeth). If the patient's

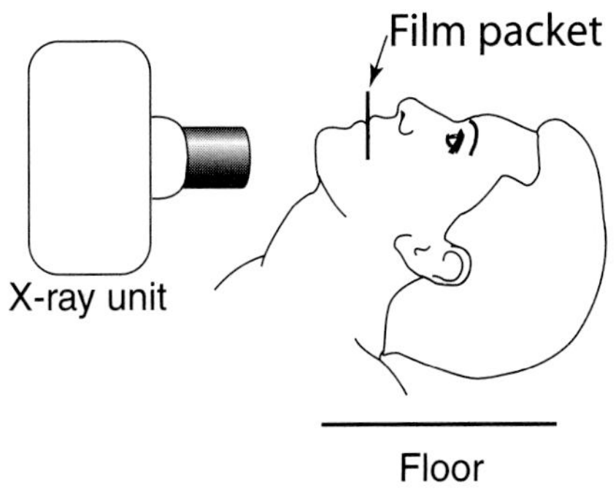

FIGURE 15–2 **Patient positioning for mandibular cross-sectional occlusal radiographs.** Patient reclined in the chair so that the head is tipped back, positioning the occlusal plane perpendicular to the plane of the floor. The central rays of the x-ray beam are directed toward the film perpendicularly.

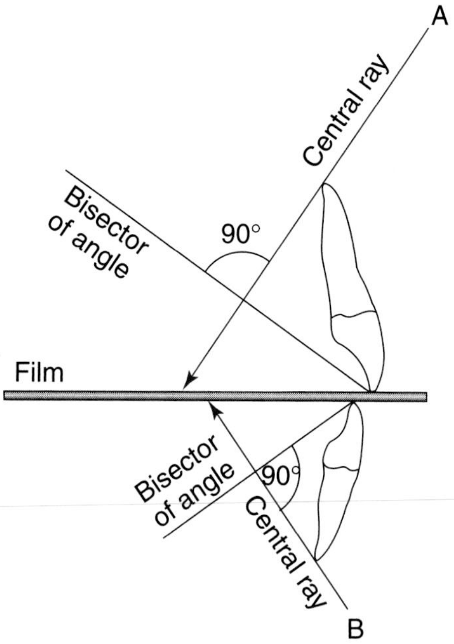

FIGURE 15-3 **Angulation theory of topographical occlusal radiographs.** The film packet placement for occlusal radiographs is clearly not parallel to the long axes of the teeth being imaged. Based on the bisecting technique, vertical angulation for (**A**) maxillary and (**B**) mandibular topographical radiographs is determined by directing the central rays of the x-ray beam perpendicular to the imaginary bisector between the film plane and the long axes of the teeth of interest.

head is in the correct position for topographical occlusal radiographs (occlusal plane parallel to the floor and the midsaggital plane perpendicular to the floor), then the radiographer can utilize pre-determined vertical angulation settings (Table 15–1).

The vertical angulation for the mandibular cross-sectional occlusal radiograph of the mandible is such that the central rays of the x-ray beam are directed toward the film perpendicularly (Figure 15–2). To achieve a perpendicular relationship between the plane of the film and the central rays of the x-ray beam, the patient's head position must be such that the occlusal plane is perpendicular to the plane of the floor. In other words, the patient should be reclined and the chin tipped upward. In this position, the vertical angulation will most likely be set at 0°, allowing the x-rays to strike the film perpendicularly.

Cross-sectional occlusal radiographs of the maxilla are sometimes needed to assess the maxillary sinus, edentulous patients, or other specific needs. However, the significant amount of bony structures located here make cross-sectional occlusal radiographs of the maxilla difficult to image with clarity. Therefore maxillary cross-sectional occlusal radiographs are exposed less frequently.

The correct horizontal angulation for all occlusal radiographs is determined by directing the central rays at the film perpendicularly. When exposing topographical occlusal radiographs, both maxillary and mandibular, the midsaggital plane may be used as a guideline. When exposing anterior topographical occlusal radiographs, direct the central rays of the x-ray beam parallel to the midsaggital plane through the anterior teeth. When exposing posterior topographical occlusal radiographs, direct the central rays of the x-ray beam perpendicular to the midsaggital plane through the posterior teeth. The horizontal angulation for the mandibular cross-sectional is also such that the central rays will intersect the film perpendicularly. Align the open end of the PID parallel to the film packet to achieve this position.

While occlusal radiographs can be made with any length position indicating device (PID), the shorter 8 in. (20.5 cm) length may be easier to position into the increased vertical angulation positions required for this technique. Additionally, because of the increased film–object distance, a longer PID length (16 in./41 cm) will likely add to the dimensional distortion of the image.

TABLE 15-1 **Recommended Vertical Angulation Settings for Occlusal Radiographs**

Occlusal Radiograph	Recommended Vertical Setting*
Maxillary topographical (anterior)	+65°
Maxillary topographical (posterior)	+45°
Mandibular topographical (anterior)	−55°
Mandibular topographical (posterior)	−45°
Mandibular cross-sectional	0°**

*The patient must be seated in the correct position, with the occlusal plane of the arch being imaged parallel to the floor and the midsaggital plane perpendicular to the floor.

**The patient must be seated in the correct position, with the occlusal plane of the mandibular perpendicular to the floor and the midsaggital plane perpendicular to the floor.

Preparation

Unit Preparation

Prior to placing the film packet intraorally, the unit should be turned on and the exposure settings selected. It is helpful to place the tube head and PID in the approximate position for the exposure to limit the time required for this step once the film packet has been placed into the patient's oral cavity.

Patient Preparation

To help gain patient cooperation and confidence, it is important to explain the procedure to the patient. Include specific instructions regarding the need for patient cooperation and be honest about any difficulties anticipated (see Chapter 11). Perform a cursory oral inspection and ask the patient to remove any objects from the mouth that would interfere with the procedure, such as removable dentures or orthodontic appliances, chewing gum, etc. Ask the patient to remove eyeglasses; if any metal or thick plastic parts of the eyeglasses remain in the path of the x-ray beam, they will be imaged onto the radiograph. Protect the patient with the lead apron and thyroid collar barriers.

Practice Point

When exposing an occlusal radiograph on the mandible, it may be necessary to modify placement of the lead barrier thyroid collar. While it is very important to use ALARA (as low as reasonably achievable) practices and utilize the lead thyroid collar to protect radiation-sensitive tissues in the head and neck region, the thyroid collar may be in the path of the primary beam during mandibular topographical and/or cross-section techniques.

You should place the lead apron and thyroid collar on the patient in the usual manner. After adjusting the patient's head position and placing the film packet, align the PID and check to be sure that the thyroid collar is not in the path of the x-ray beam. If the lead thyroid collar is in a position that will block the x-rays from reaching the film, adjust the collar position. Failure to remove the lead thyroid collar from in front of the open end of the PID will most likely result in a re-take of the radiograph.

When preparing to expose maxillary and mandibular topographical occlusal radiographs, position the patient's head so that the occlusal plane of the arch to be imaged is parallel to the floor and the midsagittal plane (midline) is perpendicular to the floor. The occlusal plane should be positioned perpendicular to the floor for the mandibular cross-sectional occlusal radiograph. The chair may be reclined and/or the head rest tipped backward to achieve the correct patient position for mandibular cross-sectional radiographs.

Managing Exposures

- The patient must bite down lightly on the film packet to hold it in place.
- The open end of the PID must be aligned as close as possibly to the patient's skin at the correct point of entry.
- Because the film will not be positioned parallel to the long axes of the teeth of interest, using a shorter target–film distance (8 in./20.5 cm PID) may help minimize distortion.
- The exposure factors (kVp, mA, and time) used for occlusal radiographs are usually the same as those settings used for periapical and bitewing radiographs in the same area.

The Occlusal Examination

Figures 15–4 through 15–8 illustrate the precise film packet positions and required angulations for each of the topographical and cross-sectional occlusal radiographs discussed in this chapter. See Table 15–2 for a summary of the technique.

PROCEDURE 15–1

PROCEDURE FOR EXPOSING OCCLUSAL RADIOGRAPHS

1. Perform infection control procedures (see Procedure Box 9–2).
2. Prepare unit. Turn on and set exposure factors.
3. Seat patient and explain the procedure.
4. Request that the patient remove objects from the mouth that can interfere with the procedure and remove eyeglasses.
5. Adjust chair to a comfortable working level.
6. Adjust the headrest to position the patient's head so that the occlusal plane is parallel to the floor and the midsagittal plane (midline) is perpendicular to the floor for maxillary and mandibular topographical occlusal radiographs, and occlusal plane and midsaggital planes both perpendicular to the floor for mandibular cross-sectional occlusal radiographs
7. Place the lead apron and thyroid collar on the patient. Check the thyroid collar to be sure that it will not block the primary beam when exposing mandibular occlusal radiographs.
8. Perform a cursory inspection of the oral cavity and determine how the film packet will be positioned. (See Table 15–2 for the film packet placements for each of the occlusal radiographs described in this chapter.)
9. Place the film packet into the oral cavity so that about 1/4 in (0.6 cm) protrudes from the patient's mouth. Position the embossed dot toward the anterior (outside the mouth.).
10. Hold the film packet against the occlusal/incisal surfaces of the teeth of the arch to be imaged while asking the patient to bite lightly. (No film holder is used.)
11. Release the film packet when the patient has closed, holding it in place.
12. Set the vertical angulation to intersect the imaginary bisector of the film plane and the long axes of the teeth perpendicularly. (See Table 15–1 for the recommended vertical angulation settings for each of the occlusal radiographs described in this chapter.)
13. Determine the correct horizontal angulation by directing the central ray of the x-ray beam perpendicular to the film in the horizontal plane. Utilize the film packet and the midsaggital plane to determine horizontal angulation. (See Table 15–2 for aid in determining the horizontal angulation for each of the occlusal radiographs described in this chapter.)
14. Center the PID over the film packet. (See Table 15–2 for point of entry recommendations for each of the occlusal radiographs described in this chapter.)
15. Make the exposure.
16. Remove the film packet from the patient's oral cavity.
17. Repeat steps 9–16 if addition films are required.
18. Remove the lead apron and thyroid collar from the patient.
19. Perform infection control procedures following the exposures (see Procedure Box 9–4).

OCCLUSAL TECHNIQUE

Maxillary Topographical Occlusal Radiograph (Anterior)

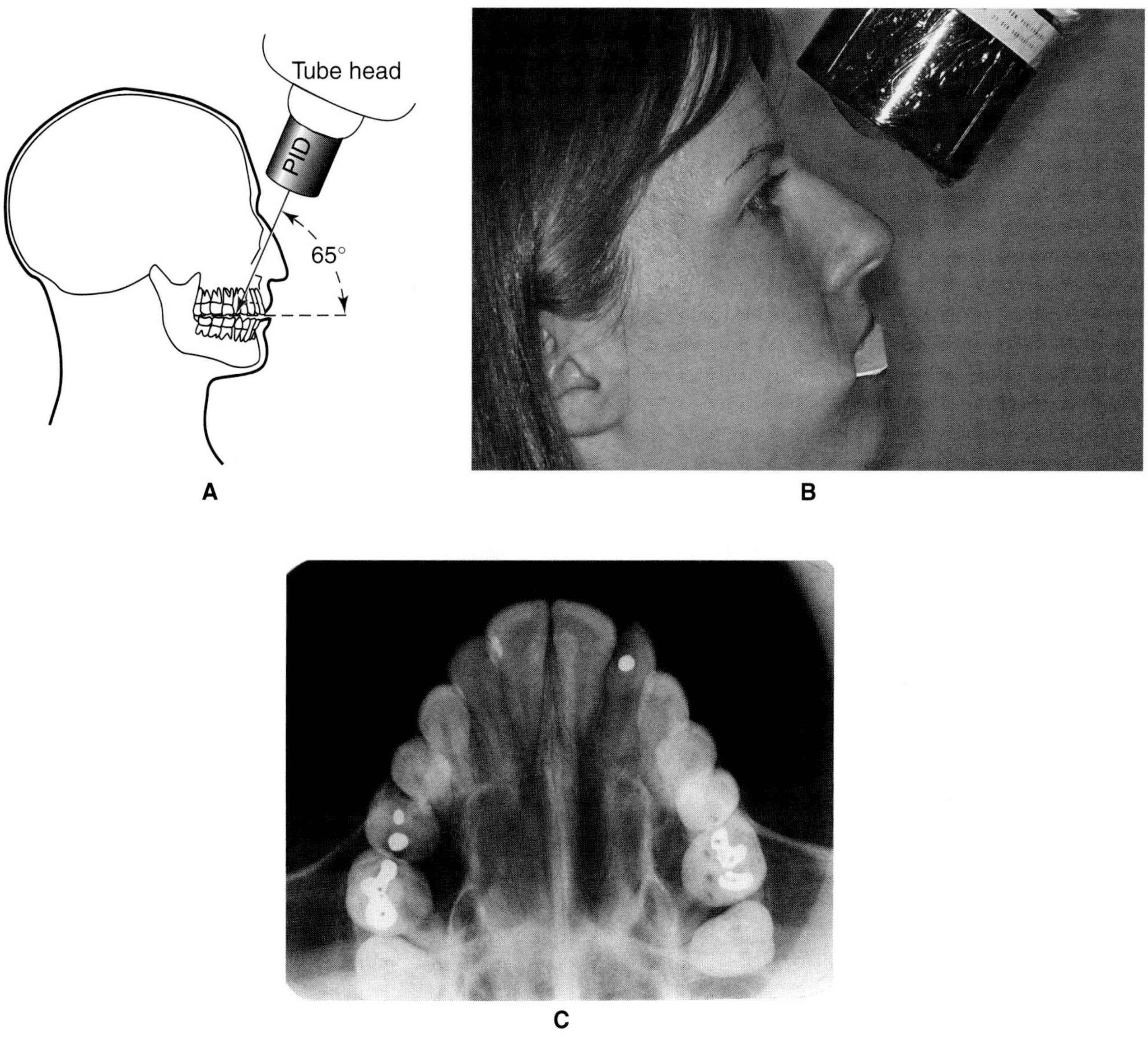

FIGURE 15–4 **Maxillary topographical occlusal radiograph (anterior).** (**A**) Diagram showing relationship of tube head and PID to occlusal film and patient. Exposure side of the film faces the maxillary arch with longer film dimension buccal-to-buccal (across the arch). The horizontal central ray is directed perpendicular to the patient's midsagittal plane, and the vertical angulation is directed approximately +65° through a point near the bridge of the nose toward the center of the film. (**B**) Patient showing position of film packet and 8 in. (20.5 cm) circular PID. (**C**) Anterior maxillary topographical occlusal radiograph.

OCCLUSAL TECHNIQUE

Maxillary Topographical Occlusal Radiograph (Posterior)

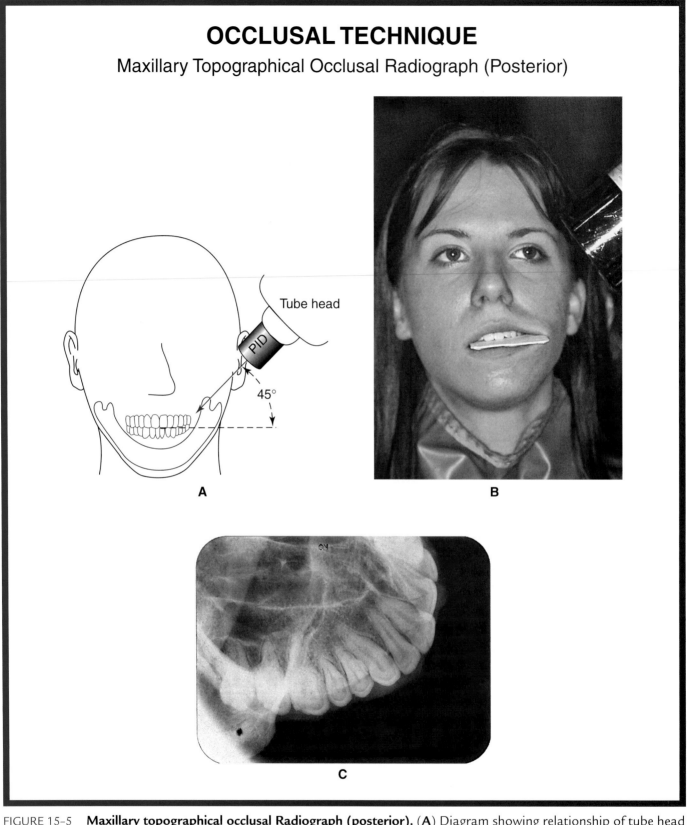

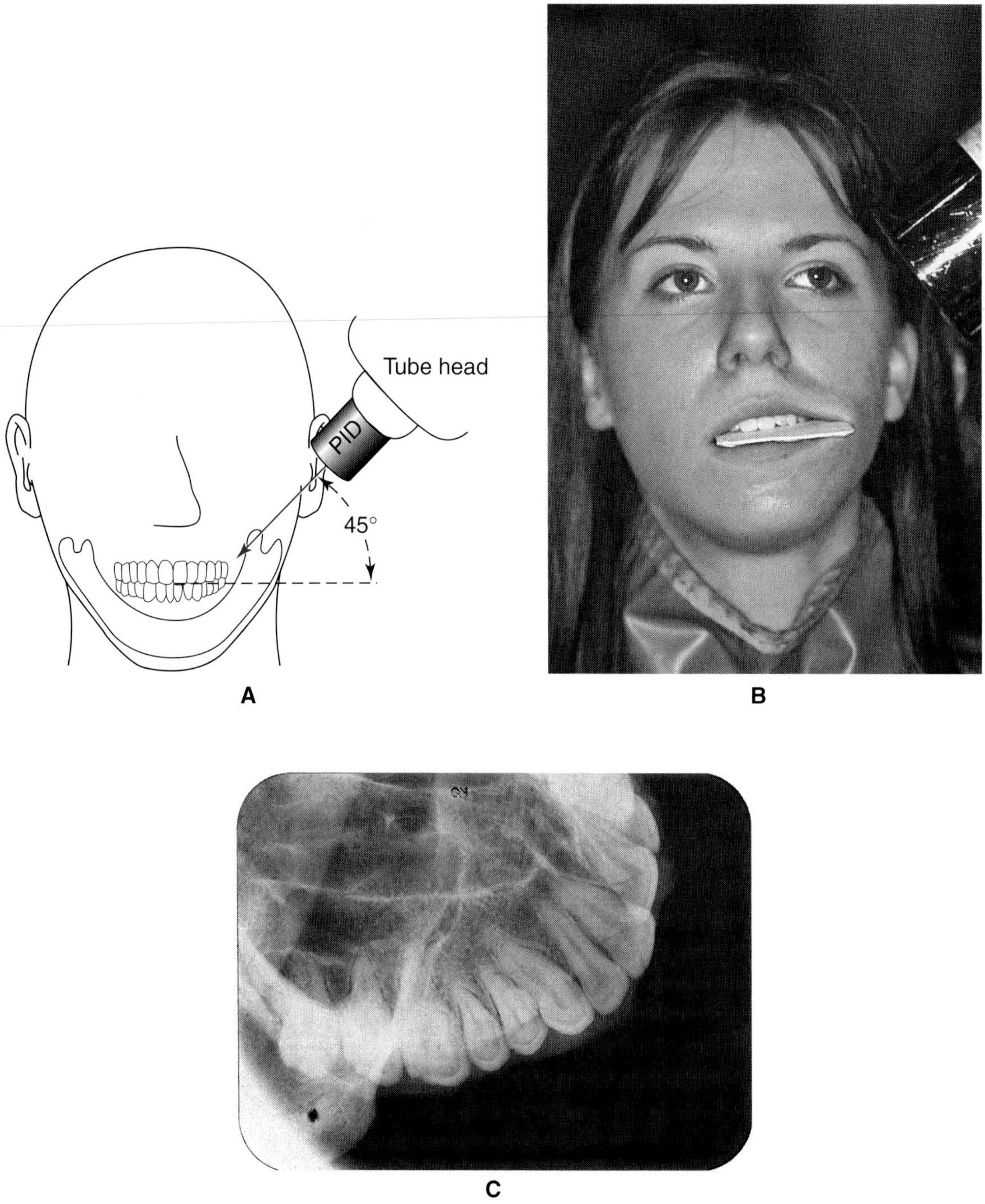

FIGURE 15-5 **Maxillary topographical occlusal Radiograph (posterior).** (**A**) Diagram showing relationship of tube head and PID to occlusal film and patient. The film packet is positioned over the left or right side, depending on the side of interest. Exposure side of the film faces the maxillary arch with longer film dimension along the midline (anterior-to-posterior). The horizontal central ray is directed perpendicular to patient's midsagittal plane, and the vertical angulation is directed approximately +45° through a point on the ala-tragus line below the outer canthus of the eye toward the center of the film. (**B**) Patient showing position of film packet and 8 in. (20.5 cm) circular PID. (**C**) Posterior maxillary topographical occlusal radiograph.

OCCLUSAL TECHNIQUE

Mandibular Topographical Occlusal Radiograph (Anterior)

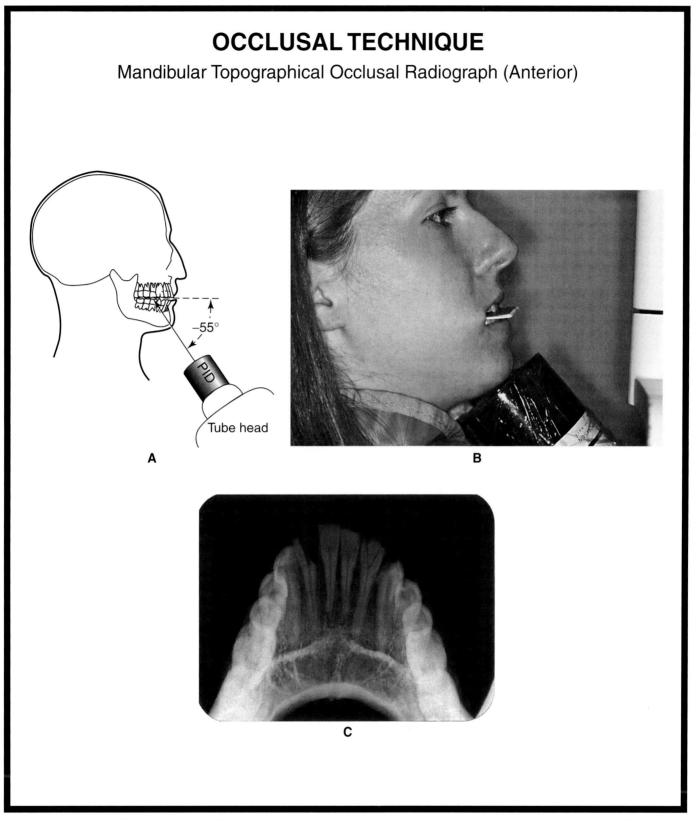

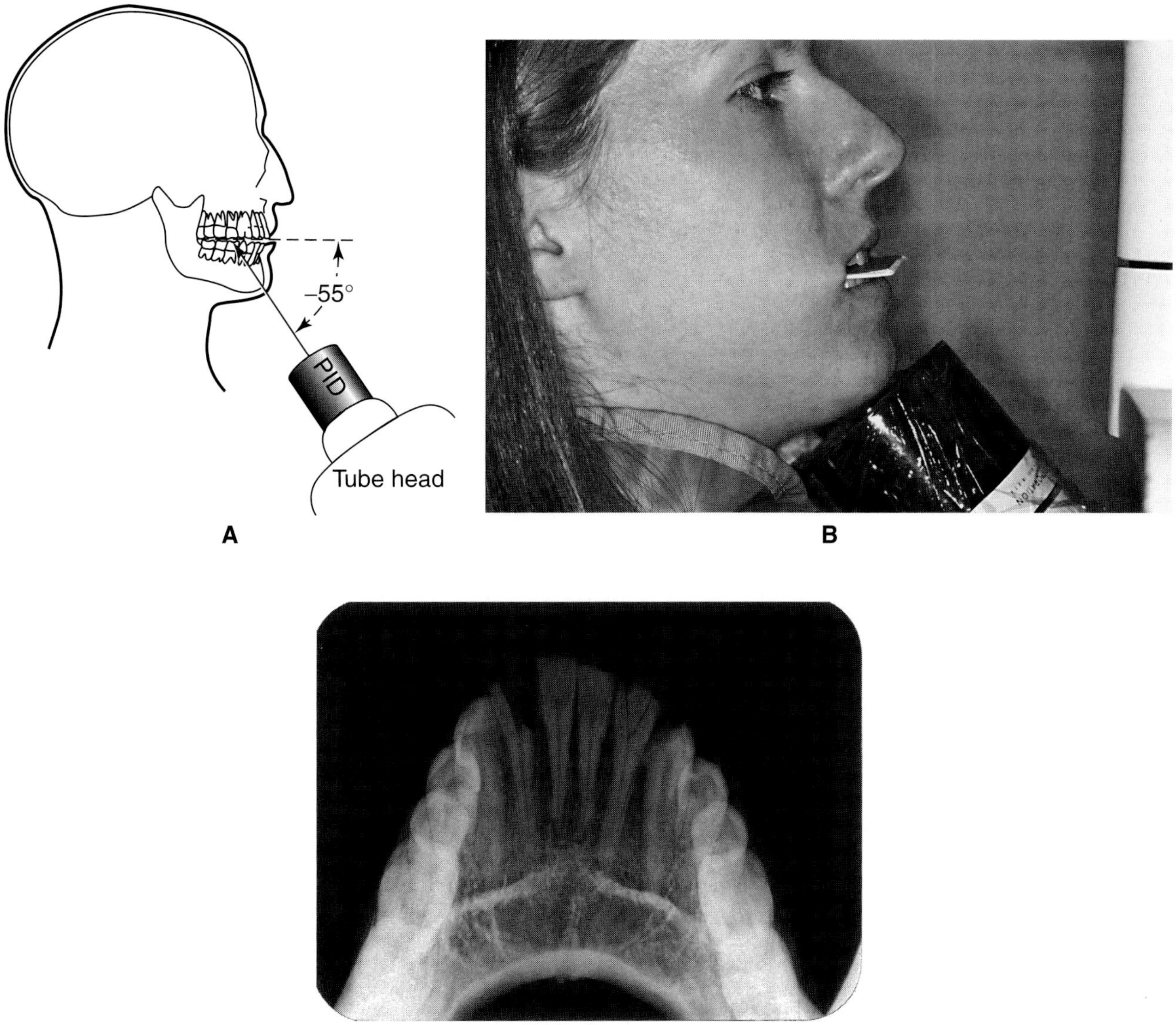

FIGURE 15-6 **Mandibular topographical occlusal radiograph (anterior).** (**A**) Diagram showing relationship of tube head and PID to occlusal film and patient. Exposure side of the film faces the mandibular arch with longer film dimension buccal-to-buccal (across the arch). The horizontal central ray is directed perpendicular to patient's midsaggittal plane, and the vertical angulation is directed approximately −55° through a point in the middle of the chin toward the center of the film. (**B**) Patient showing position of film packet and 8 in. (20.5 cm) circular PID. (**C**) Anterior mandibular topographical occlusal radiograph

OCCLUSAL TECHNIQUE

Mandibular Topographical Occlusal Radiograph (Posterior)

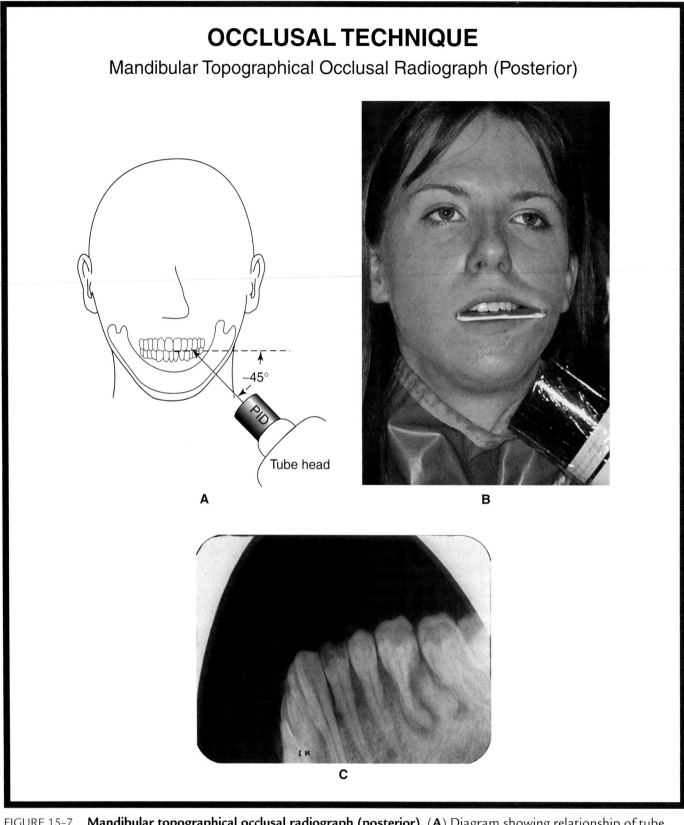

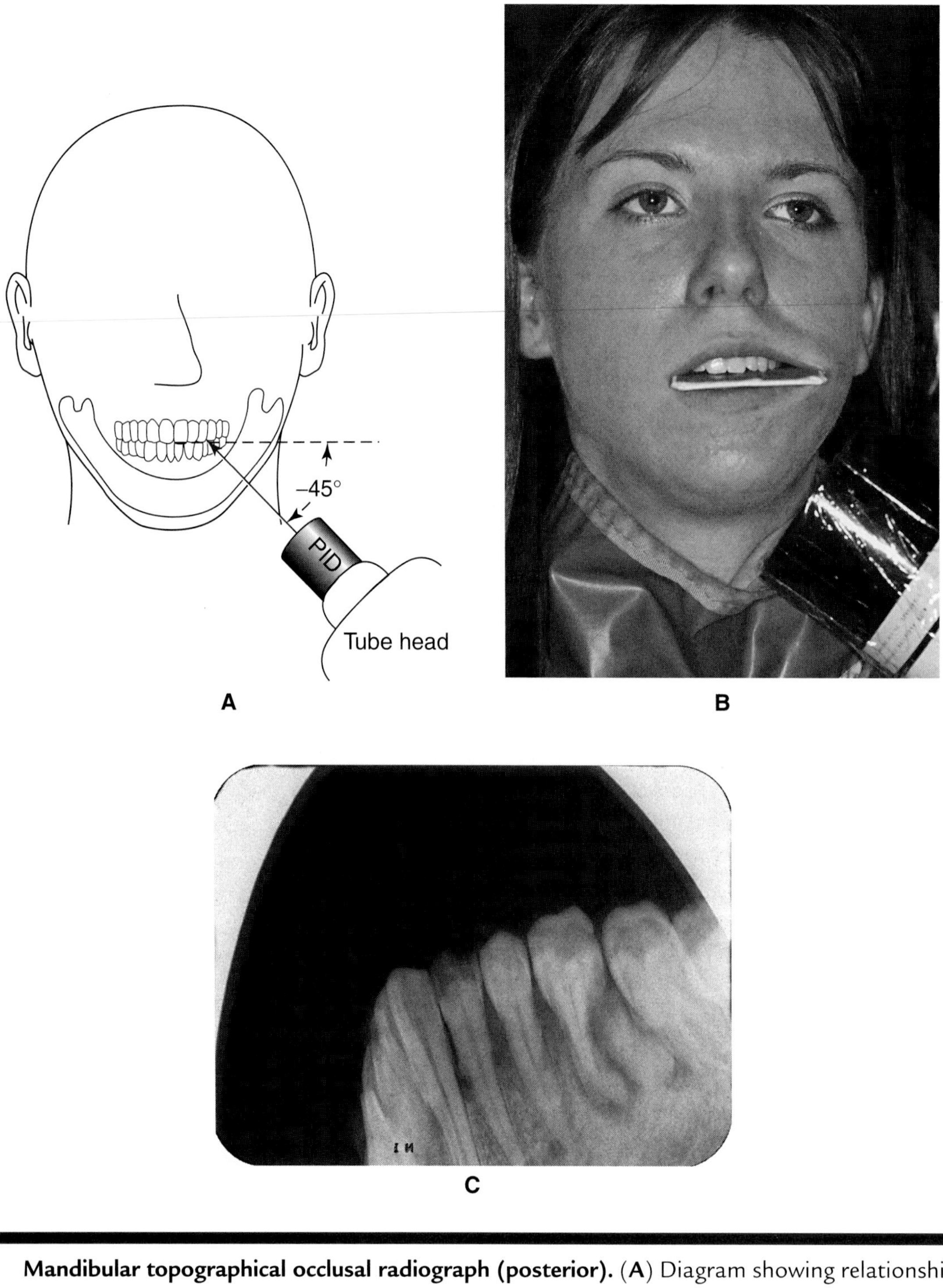

FIGURE 15-7 **Mandibular topographical occlusal radiograph (posterior).** (**A**) Diagram showing relationship of tube head and PID to occlusal film and patient. The film packet is positioned over the left or right side, depending on the side of interest. Exposure side of the film faces the mandibular arch with longer film dimension along the midline (anterior-to-posterior). The horizontal central ray is directed perpendicular to patient's midsagittal plane, and the vertical angulation is directed approximately −45° through a point on the inferior border of the mandible directly below the second mandibular premolar toward the center of the film. (**B**) Patient showing position of film packet and 8 in. (20.5 cm) circular PID. (**C**) Posterior mandibular topographical occlusal radiograph.

OCCLUSAL TECHNIQUE

Mandibular Cross-Sectional Occlusal Radiograph

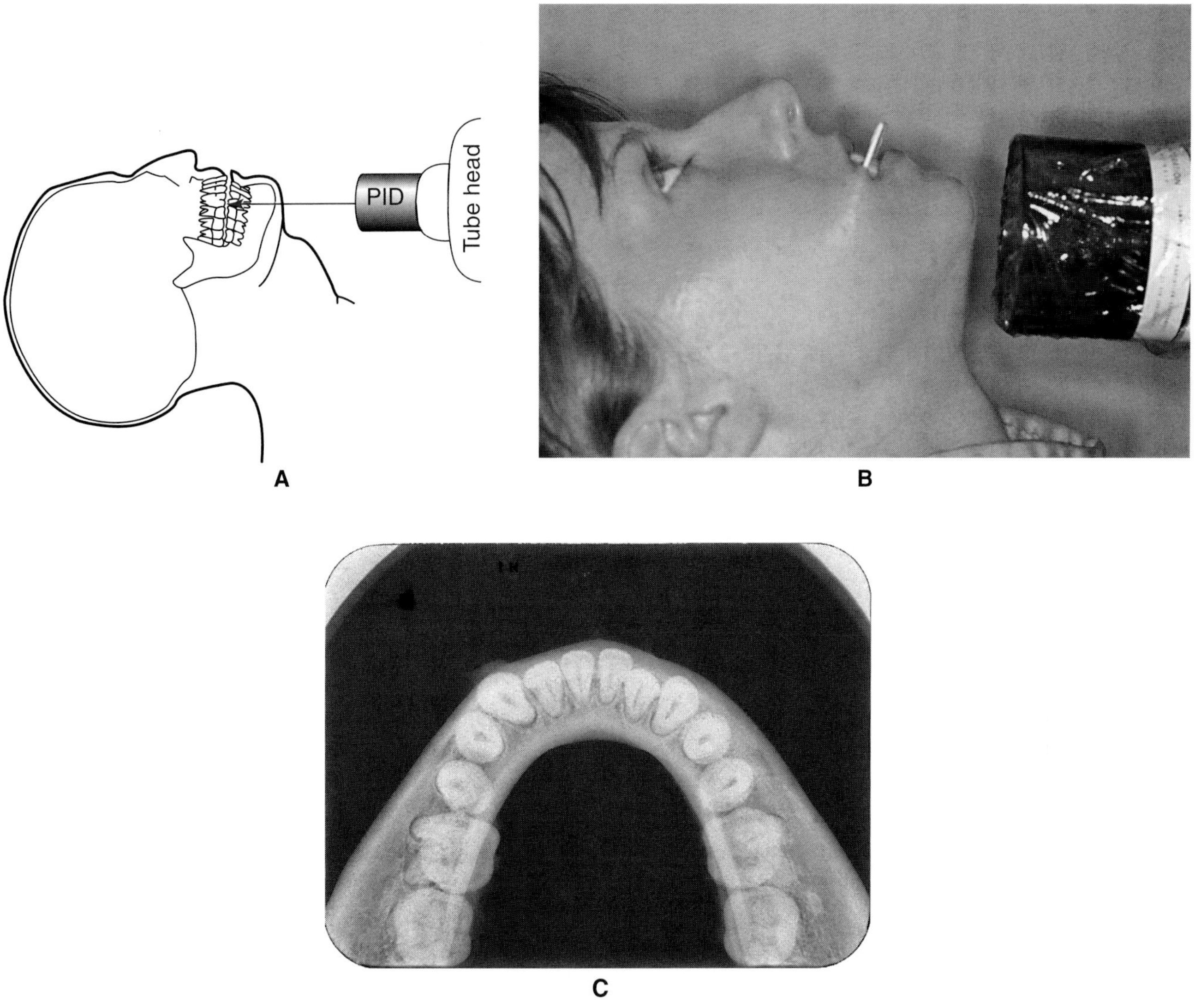

FIGURE 15-8 **Mandibular cross-sectional occlusal radiograph.** (**A**) Diagram showing relationship of tube head and PID to occlusal film and patient. The exposure side of the film faces the mandibular arch with the longer film dimension buccal-to-buccal (across the arch). The horizontal central ray is directed perpendicular to patient's midsaggittal plane, and the vertical angulation is directed approximately 0° through a point 2 in. (5 cm) back from the tip of the chin toward the center of the film. (**B**) Patient showing position of film packet and 8 in. (20.5 cm) circular PID. (**C**) Mandibular cross-sectional occlusal radiograph.

TABLE 15-2 A Summary of Occlusal Radiographic Technique

Occlusal Radiograph	Film Packet Placement	Vertical Angulation	Horizontal Angulation	Point of Entry
Maxillary topographical (anterior)	Long dimension across the mouth (buccal-to-buccal). White unprinted side toward the maxillary teeth.	Direct the central rays perpendicular to the imaginary bisector between the long axes of the teeth and the film in the vertical dimension, +65°.	Direct the central rays perpendicular to patient's midsagittal plane.	Through a point near the bridge of the nose toward the center of the film
Maxillary topographical (posterior)	Long dimension along the midline (front-to-back). White unprinted side toward the maxillary teeth.	Direct the central rays perpendicular to the imaginary bisector between the long axes of the teeth and the film in the vertical dimension, +45°.	Direct the central rays perpendicular to patient's midsagittal plane.	Through a point on the ala-tragus line below the outer cantus of the eye toward the center of the film
Mandibular topographical (anterior)	Long dimension across the mouth (buccal-to-buccal). White unprinted side toward the mandibular teeth.	Direct the central rays perpendicular to the imaginary bisector between the long axes of the teeth and the film in the vertical dimension, −55°.	Direct the central rays perpendicular to patient's midsagittal plane.	Through a point in the middle of the chin toward the center of the film
Mandibular topographical (posterior)	Long dimension along the midline (front-to-back). White unprinted side toward the mandibular teeth.	Direct the central rays perpendicular to the imaginary bisector between the long axes of the teeth and the film in the vertical dimension, −45°	Direct the central rays perpendicular to patient's midsagittal plane.	Through a point on the inferior border of the mandible directly below the second mandibular premolar toward the center of the film
Mandibular cross-sectional	Long dimension across the mouth (buccal-to-buccal). White unprinted side toward the mandibular teeth.	Direct the central rays perpendicular to the film; 0°.	Direct the central rays perpendicular to patient's midsagittal plane	Through a point 2 in. (5 cm) back from the tip of the chin toward the center of the film

REVIEW—Chapter Summary

The purpose of occlusal examinations is to image a larger area than that produced on a periapical radiograph. The topographical occlusal teachnique is based on a modification of the bisecting principle used to expose periapical radiographs. The topographical occlusal teachnique is used to view conditions of the teeth and supporting structures such as fractures and large apical lesions.

The central rays of the x-ray beam are directed at a right angle to the film to produce a cross-sectional occlusal radiograph. Cross-sectional occlusal radiographs are used to establish buccolingual dimensions and to locate impactions or erupting teeth that are out of normal alignment and to image calcifications in the soft tissue under the tongue.

No film holder is required; the patient lightly bites down on the film packet to hold it in place. Occlusal film size #4 is used for adult surveys. If indicated, a size #2 or smaller film may be used with the occlusal technique, especially for children.

The patient's head should be positioned with the occlusal plane parallel to the plane of the floor and the midsaggital plane perpendicular to the floor when exposing maxillary and mandibular topographical occlusal radiographs. The patient's head should be tipped back into a position, with both the occlusal plane and the midsaggital plane perpendicular to the plane of the floor, when exposing a mandibular cross-sectional occlusal radiograph. With the patient's head in the correct position, pre-determined vertical angulation settings may be used.

The horizontal angulation is determined in the same manner as for bitewing and periapical radiographs, where the central rays of the x-ray beam are directed perpendicularly to the film.

RECALL—Study Questions

1. All of the following are indications for exposing occlusal radiographs *except* one. Which one is this *exception?*
   a. Locate foreign bodies
   b. Examine sinus borders
   c. Reveal sialoliths
   d. Evaluate periodontal disease

2. Which of these film sizes is known as the occlusal film?
   a. #1
   b. #2
   c. #3
   d. #4
3. The ideal patient head position when exposing a maxillary topographical occlusal radiograph is to position the occlusal plane _____ to the plane of the floor and the midsaggital plane _____ to the plane of the floor.
   a. Parallel, perpendicular
   b. Perpendicular, parallel
   c. Parallel, parallel
   d. Perpendicular, perpendicular
4. The ideal patient head position when exposing a mandibular cross-sectional occlusal radiograph is to position the head rest so that the chin is tipped _____ and the occlusal plane is _____ to the plane of the floor.
   a. Down, perpendicular
   b. Up, perpendicular
   c. Down, parallel
   d. Up, parallel
5. The film should be placed with the long dimension along the midline (front to back) for which of these occlusal radiographs?
   a. Maxillary topographical anterior
   b. Maxillary topographical posterior
   c. Mandibular topographical anterior
   d. Mandibular cross-sectional
6. Assuming that the patient's head is in the correct position, which of the following is the correct vertical angulation setting for a maxillary anterior topographical occlusal radiograph?
   a. + 65 degree
   b. + 45 degree
   c. 0 degree
   d. −55 degree
7. Assuming that the patient's head is in the correct position, which of the following is the correct vertical angulation setting for a mandibular cross-sectional occlusal radiograph?
   a. +65 degree
   b. +45 degree
   c. 0 degree
   d. −55 degree
8. Where should the embossed dot be positioned when placing an occlusal film packet intraorally?
   a. Toward the apical
   b. Toward the occlusal
   c. Toward the anterior
   d. Toward the posterior
9. Which of the following will a mandibular cross-sectional occlusal radiograph best image?
   a. Cleft palate
   b. Fractured jaw
   c. Large periapical cyst
   d. Sublingual swelling

REFLECT—Case Study

Consider the following cases. After determining the radiographic assessment for each of these three cases, write out a detailed procedure chart that a radiographer can follow to obtain the needed radiographs. Begin with patient positioning. Be sure to include the steps for determining the correct film packet placement, x-ray beam angles, and landmarks for determining point of entry.

1. An adult patient presents with a sub-lingual swelling indicating the possibility of a blocked salivary gland. What type of occlusal radiograph will this patient most likely be assessed for?
2. An adult patient presents with severe pain in the mandibular left posterior region, indicating the possibility of an impacted third molar. The pain and swelling in this region is preventing the patient from opening more than a few millimeters. What type of occlusal radiograph will this patient most likely be assessed for?
3. A child patient presents with trauma to the maxillary anterior teeth after a fall off her bicycle. What type of occlusal radiograph will this patient most likely be assessed for?

RELATE—Laboratory Application

For a comprehensive laboratory practice exercise on this topic, see E. M. Thomson, *Exercises in Oral Radiography Techniques: A Laboratory Manual,* 2nd ed., Upper Saddle River, NJ: Prentice Hall, 2007. Chapter 13, "Supplemental Radiographic Techniques."

BIBLIOGRAPHY

Eastman Kodak. *Successful Intraoral Radiography.* Rochester, NY: Eastman Kodak, 1998.

Carroll, M. K. *Advanced Oral Radiographic Techniques: Part I, Occlusal and Lateral Oblique Projections* (videorecording). Jackson, MS: Health Sciences Consortium, Learning Resources, University of Mississippi Medical Center, 1993.

White, S. C & Pharoah, M. J. *Oral Radiology Principles and Interpretation,* 5th ed. St. Louis: Elsevier, 2004.

PART VI • RADIOGRAPHIC ERRORS AND QUALITY ASSURANCE

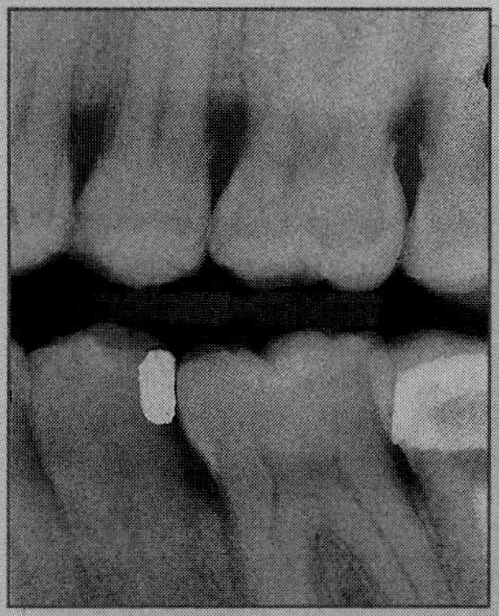

16

Identifying and Correcting Undiagnostic Radiographs

CHAPTER OUTLINE

■ OBJECTIVES

Following successful completion of this chapter, you should be able to:

1. Define the key words.
2. Recognize errors caused by incorrect radiographic techniques.
3. Apply the appropriate corrective action for technique errors.
4. Recognize errors caused by incorrect radiographic processing.
5. Apply the appropriate corrective action for processing errors.
6. Recognize errors caused by incorrect radiographic film handling.
7. Apply the appropriate corrective action for film handling errors.
8. Identify five causes of film fog.
9. Apply the appropriate corrective action for preventing film fog.

■ KEY WORDS

Artifacts
Cone cut
Distomesial projection
Double exposure
Elongation
Film fog
Foreshortening
Herringbone pattern
Mesiodistal projection
Overdevelopment
Overexposure
Overlapping
Pressure mark
Reticulation
Static electricity
Underdevelopment
Underexposure

Introduction

While radiographs play an important role in oral healthcare, it should be remembered that exposure to radiation carries a risk. The radiographer has an ethical responsibility to the patient to produce the highest diagnostic quality radiographs, in return for the patient's consent to undergo the radiographic examination. Less than ideal radiographic images diminish the usefulness of the radiograph. When the error is significant, a radiograph will have to be re-taken. In addition to increasing the patient's radiation exposure, re-take radiographs require additional patient consent and may reduce the patient's confidence in the operator and in the practice.

> **No radiograph should be retaken until a thorough investigation reveals the exact cause of the error and the appropriate corrective action is identified.**

It is important that the radiographer develop the skills needed to identify radiographic errors. Identifying common mistakes and knowing the causes will help the knowledgeable operator avoid these pitfalls. Being able to identify the cause of an undiagnostic image will allow the radiographer to apply the appropriate corrective action when re-taking the exposure.

The purpose of this chapter is to investigate common radiographic errors, identify probable causes of such errors, and to present the appropriate corrective actions.

Recognizing Radiographic Errors

In order to recognize errors that diminish the diagnostic quality of a radiograph, the radiographer must understand what a quality image looks like (Table 16–1). First and foremost, the radiograph must be an accurate representation of the teeth and the supporting structures. The image should not be magnified, elongated, foreshortened, or otherwise distorted. Film density and contrast should be correct for ease of interpretation: not too light, or too dark, or fogged. The radiograph should be free of errors.

Practice Point

All errors reduce the quality of the radiograph. However, not all errors create a need to re-expose the patient. Two examples of this are when the error does not affect the area of interest and when the error affects only one film in a series (bitewings or full mouth) where the area of interest can be viewed in an adjacent radiograph. For example, a radiograph may have a **cone cut** error, cutting off part of the image. If the cone cut error does not affect the area of interest, a re-take would not be required. Consider this situation, where a periapical radiograph is exposed to image suspected apical pathology in the posterior region. If the cone cut error occurs in the anterior portion of the film, cutting off the second premolar, but an abscess at the root apex of the first molar is adequately imaged, the film would most likely not have to be re-taken.

When exposing a set of radiographs such as a vertical bitewing or full mouth series, if an error prevents adequate imaging of a condition, adjacent films should be observed for the possibility that the condition may be adequately revealed in another radiograph. For example, if one film in a set of bitewings is overlapped, it should be determined if the adjacent films image the area adequately. If so, a re-retake film would most likely not be indicated. Determining when a retake is absolutely necessary will keep radiation exposure to a minimum.

TABLE 16–1 Characteristics of a Quality Radiograph

Bitewing Radiograph	Periapical Radiograph
Film packet placed correctly to image area of interest	Film packet placed correctly to image area of interest
Equal portion of the maxilla and mandible imaged	Entire tooth plus at least 2 mm of alveolar bone beyond the root apex imaged
Occlusal/incisal plane of the teeth is parallel to the edge of the film	Occlusal/incisal plane of the teeth is parallel with the edge of the film
Occlusal plane straight or slightly curved upward toward the posterior	A margin of 1/4 in. (6 mm) imaged beyond the incisal/occlusal edges of the crowns
Most posterior contact point imaged	Embossed dot positioned toward the incisal/occlusal edge
	In a full mouth survey, each tooth should be imaged at least once, preferably twice

Recognizing the cause of radiographic errors is important in being able to take corrective action. Errors that diminish the diagnostic quality of radiographs may be divided into three categories:

1. Technique errors
2. Processing errors
3. Film handling errors

It is important to note that errors in any of these categories may produce the same or a similar result. For example, it is possible that a dark radiographic image may have been caused by **overexposure** (a technique error) or by **overdevelopment** (a processing error), or by exposing the film to white light (a film handling error). For the purpose of defining the more common radiographic errors, we will discuss the errors according to these three categories.

Technique Errors

Technique errors include mistakes made in patient positioning or film packet placement, incorrect positioning of the PID (vertical and horizontal angulations), and setting the wrong exposure factors. Additional technical problems include movement of the patient, the film packet, or the PID.

Incorrect Positioning of the Patient or Film Packet

The most basic technique error is not imaging the correct teeth. The radiographer must know the standard film packet placements for all types of projections and must possess the skills necessary to achieve these correct placements.

Absence of Mesial Structures

- **Probable cause:** Film packet was placed too far back in the patient's oral cavity.
- **Correction:** Know what teeth must be imaged on the type of radiograph being exposed. Move the film packet mesially (toward the front of the mouth).

Absence of Distal Structures

- **Probable cause:** Film packet was placed too far forward in the patient's oral cavity.
- **Correction:** Know what teeth must be imaged on the type of radiograph being exposed. Move the film packet distally (toward the back of the mouth).

Absence of the Apical Structures (Figure 16–1)

- **Probable cause:** Film packet was not placed high enough (maxillary) or low enough (mandibular) in the patient's oral cavity to image the entire tooth, including the root tip. Ideally, there should be at least 2 mm of supporting bone imaged beyond the root apex of the tooth.

  This error is more often the result of incorrect vertical angulation, especially when utilizing the paralleling technique. Inadequate (too little) vertical angulation will result in less of the apical region being imaged onto the radiograph.
- **Correction:** In the maxillary areas, raise the film packet in the patient's oral cavity. In mandibular areas, lower the film packet in the patient's oral cavity. Ensure that the film packet is positioned correctly into the film holding device and that the patient is biting down all the way. Use the correct vertical angulation. Direct the central rays toward the film perpendicularly when utilizing the paralleling technique and direct the central rays perpendicularly toward the imaginary bisector when utilizing the bisecting technique (see Chapter 13).

Absence of Coronal Structures (Figure 16–2)

- **Probable cause:** Film packet not placed low enough (maxillary) or high enough (mandibular) in the patient's oral cavity to image the entire tooth including the crown edges. Ideally there should be a 1/4 in. (6.4 mm) margin imaged beyond the crown of the tooth.

  The use of film holders will almost always eliminate this error. When noted, the cause is most often the result of

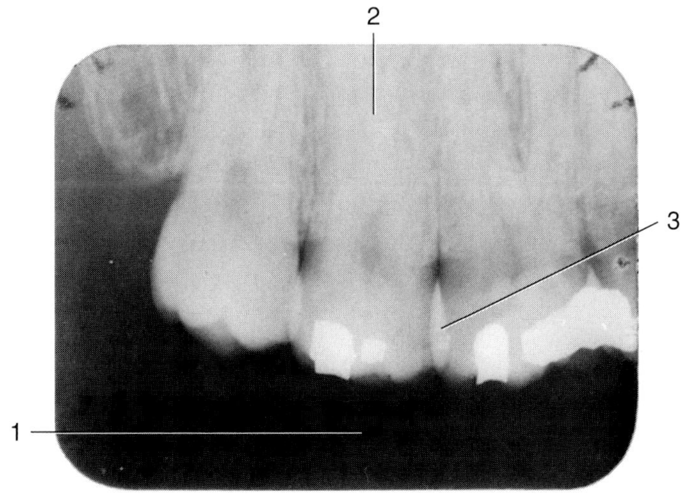

FIGURE 16–1 **Radiograph of maxillary molar area.** (**1**) Excessive occlusal margin with resultant absence of the complete apical structures is caused by film being placed too low in mouth or by inadequate vertical angulation. (**2**) Tooth structures are elongated because the vertical angulation was inadequate (not steep enough). (**3**) Overlapping results from incorrect horizontal angulation. In this example, the overlapping is more severe in the anterior (mesial) region and less severe in the posterior (distal) region, indicating distomesial projection of the x-ray beam toward the film.

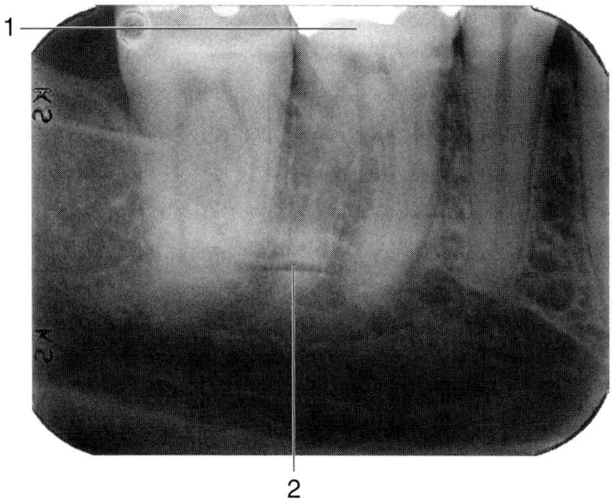

FIGURE 16–2 **Radiograph of maxillary molar area.** (**1**) Absence of occlusal margin on all coronal structures as a result of placing the film too high in mouth, or a vertical angulation that was excessive (too steep). (**2**) Note the radiolucent artifact (horizontal line) that results from bending the film packet.

incorrect vertical angulation, especially when utilizing the paralleling technique. Excessive vertical angulation will result in cutting off the occlusal/incisal edge of the teeth in the resultant image.

- **Correction:** In the maxillary areas, lower the film packet in the patient's oral cavity. In mandibular areas, raise the film packet in the patient's oral cavity. Ensure that the film packet is positioned correctly into the film-holding device and that the patient is biting down all the way. Use the correct vertical angulation. Direct the central rays toward the film perpendicularly when utilizing the paralleling technique, and direct the central rays perpendicularly toward the imaginary bisector when utilizing the bisecting technique (see Chapter 13).

Practice Point

The misuse of a cotton roll to help stabilize the film holder is often the cause of the root tips being cut off the resultant radiographic image. A cotton roll is sometimes utilized to help the patient bite down on the film-holder bite block to secure it in place (see Chapter 13). This practice is appropriate when used correctly. Correct placement of the cotton roll is on the opposite side of the bite block from where the teeth occlude. Placing the cotton roll on the same side as the teeth will prevent the film packet from being placed high enough (maxillary) or low enough (mandibular) in the mouth.

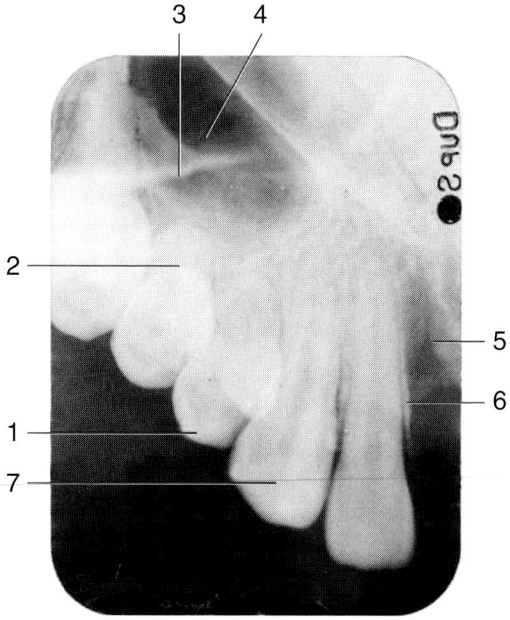

FIGURE 16–3 **Radiograph of maxillary canine area.** (**1**) Slanting or diagonal occlusal plane is caused by improper positioning of the film packet. (**2**) Foreshortened images in this example are caused by a combination of excessive vertical angulation and incorrect film position. (**3**) Distortion of image is caused by film bending. (**4**) Maxillary sinus, (**5**) recent extraction site, (**6**) lamina dura, and (**7**) canine is not properly centered on film.

Slanting or Tilted Instead of Straight Occlusal Plane (Figure 16–3)

- **Probable cause:** Edge of the film packet was not parallel with the incisal or occlusal plane of the teeth, or the film holder was not placed flush against the occlusal surfaces. This error often results from the top edge of the film packet contacting the lingual gingiva or the curvature of the palate.
- **Correction:** Straighten the film packet by positioning away from the lingual surfaces of the teeth. Place the film packet in toward the midline of the palate. Utilize this highest region of the palatal vault to stand the film up parallel to the long axes of the teeth. Ensure that the patient is biting down securely on the bite block of the film holder.

Vertical Instead of Horizontal Film Packet Placement in the Posterior Areas

- **Probable cause:** Film packet was placed with its longer dimension vertically. This is seldom desirable in posterior areas.
- **Correction:** Rotate the film packet so that the longer dimension is placed horizontally and the film edge is parallel with the occlusal plane.

Horizontal Instead of Vertical Film Packet Placement in the Anterior Areas

- **Probable cause:** Film packet was placed with its longer dimension horizontally. Such placement is undesirable and often produces dimensional distortion of the image. Furthermore, the anterior teeth are sometimes longer than the narrow dimension of the film and the root apices would most likely not be recorded on a film positioned in this manner.
- **Correction:** Rotate the film packet so that the longer dimension is placed vertically. The short edge of the film packet should be placed parallel to the incisal edges of the anterior teeth.

Herringbone or Tire-Track Pattern (Figure 16–4)

- **Probable cause:** Film packet was reversed and the back side was facing the teeth and the radiation source. The pattern represents the embossed lead foil in the back of the film packet. The image will also be significantly underexposed (too light).
- **Correction:** Pay attention to which side of the film packet is the front and which is the back. When in doubt, read the printed side of the film packet for direction. Turn the film packet so that the tube side faces toward the teeth and the radiation source.

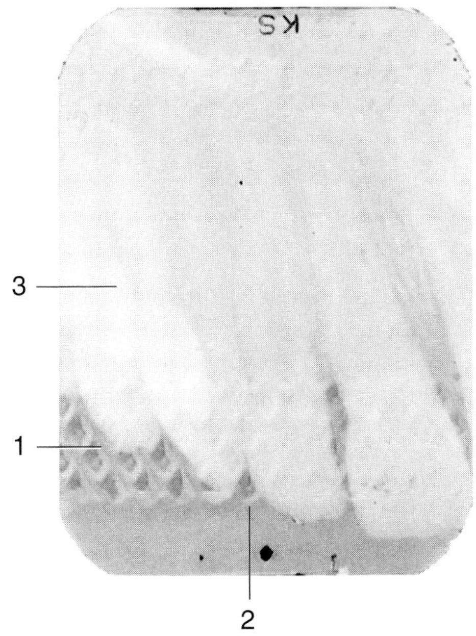

FIGURE 16-4 **Herringbone error.** (**1**) Light image and two bars of herringbone (tire-track) pattern, indicating that the film was placed backwards (reversed) in the mouth. The image is light because the lead foil absorbed some of the x-rays. (**2**) Film is not correctly centered and occlusal plane is not straight. (**3**) Foreshortening of images of the premolar and canine caused by a combination of excessive vertical angulation and incorrect film placement.

Incorrect Position of Identification Dot

- **Probable cause:** Embossed identification dot positioned in apical area.
- **Correction:** Pay attention when placing the film packet into the film holding device to position the dot in the incisal or occlusal area.

Incorrect Positioning of the Tube Head or PID

Included in this category are the errors that result from incorrect vertical and horizontal angulations and centering of the x-ray beam over the film packet. We have already discussed that incorrect vertical angulation often results in not imaging the apices or the occlusal/incisal edges of the teeth. Elongation (images that appear stretched out) or foreshortening (images that appear shorter than they are), with or without cutting off the images of the apices or the occlusal/incisal edges of the teeth, are dimensional errors that result from incorrect vertical angulation when utilizing the bisecting technique.

Elongation of the Image (Bisecting Technique Error) (Figure 16–1)

- **Probable cause:** Insufficient vertical angulation of the central beam (PID).
- **Correction:** Increase the vertical angulation. Also check the position of the film packet and the patient's head. Incorrect film packet placement and patient positioning can affect the vertical angulation.

Foreshortening of the Image (Bisecting Technique Error) (Figure 16–3)

- **Probable cause:** Excessive vertical angulation of the central beam (PID).
- **Correction:** Decrease the vertical angulation. Also check the position of the film and the patient's head. Incorrect film packet placement and patient positioning can affect the vertical angulation.

Overlapping of the Image (Figure 16–1)

- **Probable cause:** Incorrect rotation of the tube head and PID in the horizontal plane. Superimposition of the images of proximal surfaces occurs when the central beam is not directed perpendicularly toward the film through the interproximal spaces. The two common errors are mesiodistal and distomesial projections. When the angle of projection in the horizontal plane is from mesial to distal (**mesiodistal projection**), the mesiobuccal root of maxillary molars appears to be superimposed over the lingual root, and the **overlapping** contacts are more severe in the posterior part of the image. Conversely, when the angle of projection is from distal to mesial (**distomesial projection**), the distobuccal root of maxillary molars appears to be superimposed over the lingual root, and the overlapping contacts are more severe in the anterior part of the image (see Figure 14–7).
- **Correction:** Unless there is also elongation or foreshortening, maintain the vertical angulation. To compensate

for mesiodistal angulation, change the direction of the PID so that the central ray is projected more to the mesial; to compensate for distomesial angulation, change the direction of the PID so that the central ray is projected more to the distal. Ideally, the central ray of the x-ray beam should be directed perpendicular to the film through the teeth contacts.

Practice Point

Remember the phrase *"Move toward it to fix it"* when correcting mesiodistal or distomesial overlap error. If the overlapping appears more severe in the anterior (mesial) region, shift the tube head and PID toward the anterior (mesial); if the overlapping appears more severe in the posterior (distal) region, shift the tube head and PID toward the posterior (distal).

Cone Cut (Figures 16–5 and 16–6)

- **Probable cause:** The primary beam of radiation was not directed toward the center of the film and did not completely expose all parts of the film. Assembling the Rinn XCP film-holding instrument incorrectly will cause the operator to direct the central ray of the x-ray beam to the wrong place, resulting in cone cut error.
- **Correction:** Maintain horizontal and vertical angulation and move the tube head up, down, posteriorly, or anteriorly, depending on which area of the radiograph shows a clear, unexposed area. Check to see that the XCP instrument is assembled correctly, and direct the central ray of the x-ray beam to the center (middle) of the film packet.

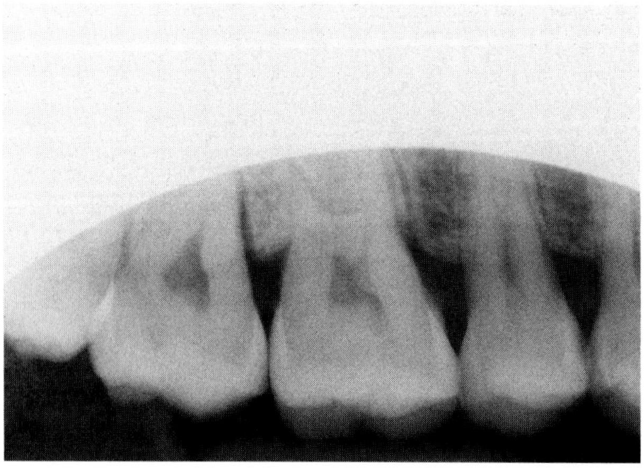

FIGURE 16-5 **Cone cut error.** Cone cut is caused by not directing the central rays toward the middle of the film. The white circular area was beyond the range of the x-ray beam, indicating no exposure. This radiograph illustrates cone cut due to posterior Rinn XCP® instrument being assembled incorrectly.

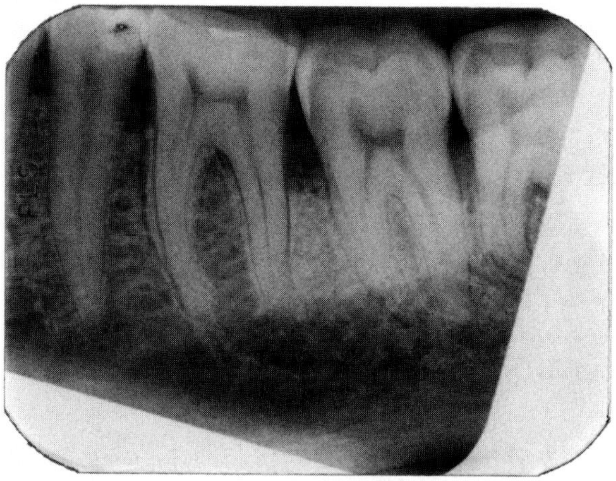

FIGURE 16-6 **Cone cut error.** Cone cut can also occur when using rectangular collimation.

Incorrect Exposure Factors

Insufficient knowledge in the use of the control panel settings and exposure button often result in less than ideal radiographic images.

Light (Thin) Image (Figures 16–4 and 16–7)

- **Probable cause: Underexposure** or insufficient exposure time in relation to milliamperage, kilovoltage, and distance selected by the operator; or as the result of timer inaccuracy or a faulty exposure switch. Light images also result when the film is placed in the oral cavity backwards. Whenever a light image results, the operator should examine it closely for the presence of a pattern that represents the embossed lead foil, indicating a backwards film packet placement. This pattern can resemble a tire-track or diamond pattern, depending on the manufacturer of the lead foils. This error is still referred to as **herringbone pattern** error, after the herringbone pattern appearance of original films. Light images that result from processing errors will be discussed below.

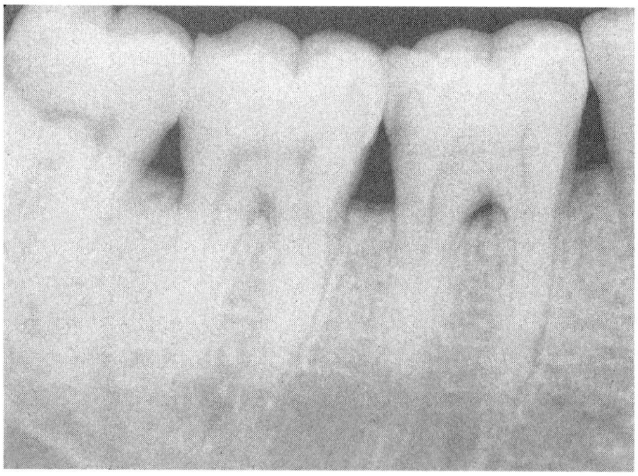

FIGURE 16-7 **Light (thin) image.** Underexposed or underdeveloped radiograph results in a light image.

- **Correction:** Increase the exposure time, the milliamperage, the kilovoltage, or a combination of these factors. The exposure button must be depressed for the full cycle. The operator must watch for the red exposure light and the audible signal to end to indicate that the exposure button may be released. If the problem persists, check the accuracy of the timer or switch for possible malfunction. Ensure that the front of the film packet faced the x-ray source.

Dark Image (Figure 16–8)

- **Probable cause:** Overexposure (excessive mA, kVp, or time). Dark images that result from processing errors will be discussed below.
- **Correction:** Decrease the exposure time, the milliamperage, the kilovoltage, or a combination of these factors.

Absence of Image

- **Probable cause:** Non-exposure to x-rays. Failure to turn on the line switch or to maintain firm pressure on the exposure button during the exposure. Alternate causes: electrical failure, malfunction of the x-ray machine or processing errors (which will be discussed below).
- **Correction:** Turn on the x-ray machine and maintain firm pressure on the exposure button during the entire exposure period. Watch for the red exposure light and listen for the audible signal indicating that the exposure has occurred.

Double Image

- **Probable cause: Double exposure** resulting from accidentally exposing the same film twice.
- **Correction:** Maintain a systematic order to exposing radiographs. Keep unexposed and exposed film packets organized.

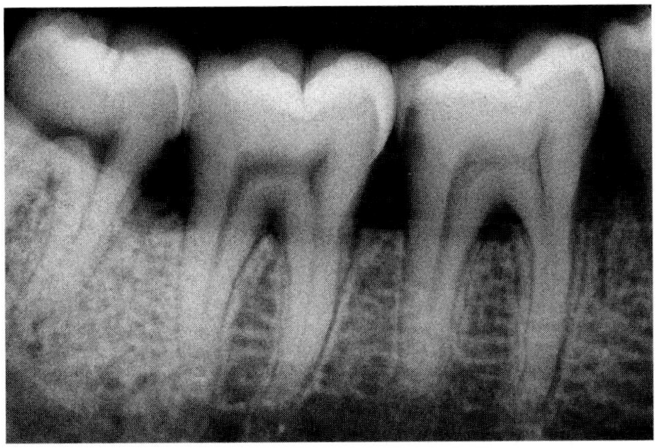

FIGURE 16–8 **Dark image.** Overexposure and overdevelopment results in a dark image.

Miscellaneous Errors in Exposure Technique

Poor Definition

- **Probable cause:** Movement during exposure. Caused by patient movement, film slippage, or vibration of the tube head.
- **Correction:** Place the patient's head into position against the head rest of the exam chair and ask him/her to hold still throughout the duration of the exposure. Explain the procedure and gain the patient's cooperation, asking him/her to maintain steady pressure on the film holder and not to move. Do not use the patient's finger to stabilize the film packet in the oral cavity. Steady the tube head before activating the exposure.

Artifacts

Artifacts are images on the film other than anatomy or pathology that do not contribute to a diagnosis of the patient's condition (Figures 16–9 and 16–10). Artifacts may be radiopaque or radiolucent.

- **Probable cause:** The presence of foreign objects in the oral cavity during exposure, e.g., appliances such as removable bridges, partial or full dentures, and space maintainers, patient glasses, facial jewelry. These will result in radiopaque artifacts.
- **Correction:** Perform a cursory examination of the oral cavity to check for the presence of appliances. Ask the patient to remove any objects that may be in the path of the primary beam. Ensure that the lead apron and thyroid collar do not block the x-rays from reaching the film.

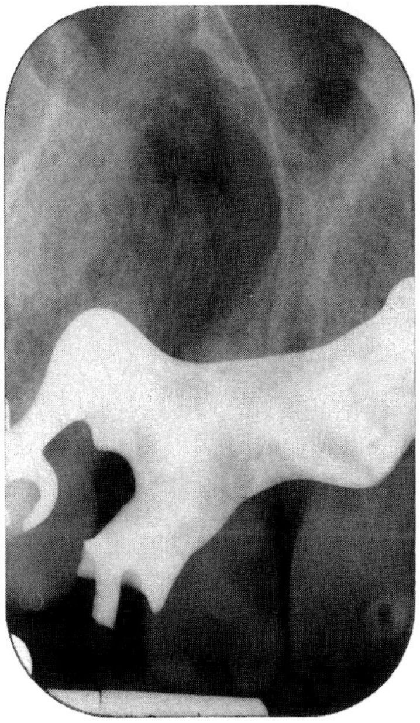

FIGURE 16–9 **Radiopaque artifacts.** Partial denture left in place during exposure, creating a radiopaque artifact on the resultant image.

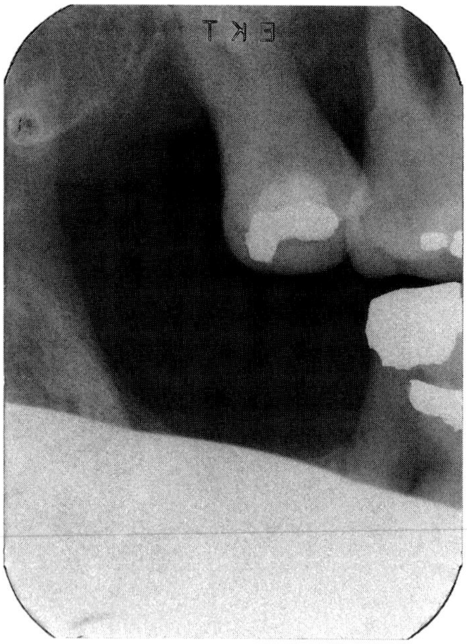

FIGURE 16-10 **Radiopaque artifacts.** Lead thyroid collar got in the way of the primary beam during exposure, creating a radiopaque artifact on the resultant image.

Processing Errors

Processing errors account for a major portion of the retake films that increase patient radiation dose, add time to a busy day's schedule, and waste money. Processing errors occur with both manual and automatic processing. Processing errors include under- and overdevelopment, incorrectly following protocols, and failure to maintain an ideal darkroom setting.

Development Error

Light Image (Figure 16–7)

- **Probable cause: Underdevelopment** results from a variety of errors. Most often the film was not left in the developer for the required time. This often occurs when the developer solution is cold. The colder the developer, the longer the time required to produce an image of ideal density. Alternate processing causes of light images include weakened, old developer or fixer contamination of the developer.
- **Correction:** When processing manually, check the temperature of the developer and consult a time–temperature chart before placing the film in the developer. Ensure that the automatic processor indicates that the solutions have warmed up and the correct timed cycle is used. If weakened or old solutions are suspected, change the solutions. Maintain good quality control to replenish solutions to keep them functioning at peak conditions.

Dark Image (Figures 16–8)

- **Probable cause: Overdevelopment** also results from a variety of errors. Usually the film is left in the developer too long. This often occurs when the developer solution is hot. The warmer the developer, the less developing time required. A dark image is also the result of using a strong developing solution (when using chemicals mixed from concentrate).
- **Correction:** When processing manually, check the temperature of the developer and consult a time–temperature chart before placing the film in the developer. Ensure that the automatic processor indicates that the solutions are maintaining the correct temperature and timed cycle. If a strong mix of chemicals is suspected, change the solutions. Maintain good quality control to replenish solutions to keep them functioning at peak conditions.

Processing and Darkroom Protocol Errors

Absence of Image

- **Probable cause:** Film was placed in the fixer before being placed in the developer, or the emulsion may have dissolved in warm rinse water. Alternate cause: Film may not have been exposed.
- **Correction:** When processing manually, the operator must have knowledge of which tank contains the developer and which tank contains the fixer. Labelling the tanks prevents confusion. Place the film in the developer solution first. To prevent the emulsion from separating from the film base, promptly remove the film at the end of the washing period.

Black Image

- **Probable cause:** Film was accidentally exposed to white light.
- **Correction:** Turn off all light in the darkroom except the proper safelight before unwrapping the film packet. Lock the door or warn others not to enter. Use an "in-use" sign. When using an automatic processor, ensure that the film has completely entered the light-protected processor before turning on the white overhead light or removing hands from the daylight loader.

Partial Image

- **Probable cause:** Level of the developer was too low to cover the entire film. This is a manual processing error.
- **Correction:** Replenish the processing solutions to the proper level or attach the films to lower clips on the film hanger to ensure that they will be submerged completely in the solution.

Green Areas on Film

- **Probable cause:** Films stuck together in the developer, preventing the solutions from reaching the sides of the film emulsion. This error occurs in manual processing when two films are attached to one clip of the film hanger through failure to separate films in double-film packets. Failing to separate double films prior to loading into an automatic processor yields the same results.

- **Correction:** The operator must be knowledgeable about the use of double film packets. When manually processing several radiographs at the same time, make certain that the films do not touch those on other hangers.

Dark Areas on Film

- **Probable cause:** Films stuck together in the fixer. The fixer was not able to remove the undeveloped silver halide crystals or to neutralize the developer in those areas, and development continues partially.
- **Correction:** During manual processing, agitate films gently when inserting into the fixer; make certain the films do not come in contact with those on other hangers. Feed films into automatic processors slowly and one at a time.

Reticulation (Figure 16–11)

- **Probable cause:** Temperature of processing solutions is too hot, or there is too great a difference between the temperature of the processing solutions and the rinse water. Temperature differences of 10°F may cause the film to become pitted and **reticulated** through the softening and melting of the emulsion.
- **Correction:** When using manual processing, maintain the processing solution temperature approximately the same as that of the rinse water. Do not begin to process the film until the circulating water has cooled or warmed the developer and fixer appropriately. In manual processing, temperatures in excess of 80°F (26.7°C) should be avoided.

Chemical Contamination

White Spots on Film

- **Probable cause:** Premature contact with fixer—drops of fixer that splash onto the work area may come in contact with the undeveloped film.
- **Correction:** Maintain a clean and orderly darkroom and work area.

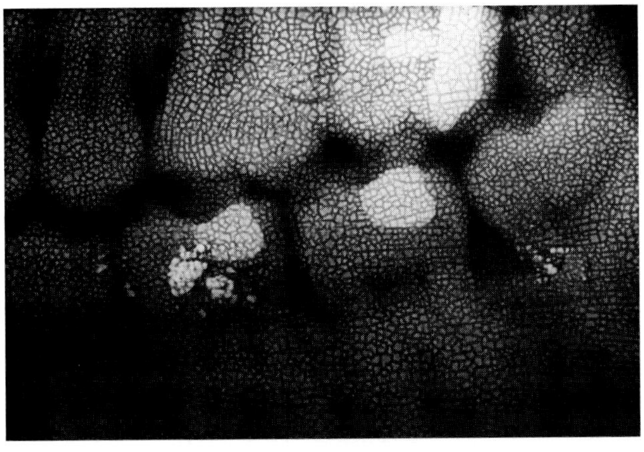

FIGURE 16–11 **Radiograph showing reticulation.**

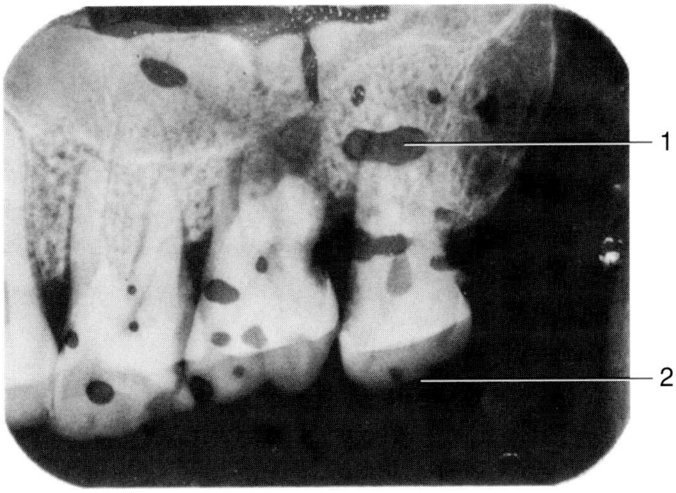

FIGURE 16–12 **Radiograph of maxillary molar area.** (**1**) Dark spots on radiograph are caused by premature contact of film surface with developer. (**2**) Uneven occlusal margin caused by incorrect film positioning.

Dark Spots on Film (Figure 16–12)

- **Probable cause:** Premature contact with developer—drops of developer that splash onto the work area may come in contact with the undeveloped film.
- **Correction:** Maintain a clean and orderly darkroom and work area.

Iridescent Stain

- **Probable cause:** Oxidation and exhaustion of developer.
- **Correction:** Maintain quality control with regular replenishment and replacing of the processing solutions.

Brownish-yellow Stains

- **Probable cause:** Insufficient or improper washing of the film. Brown stains often do not appear until several weeks after processing.
- **Correction:** When processing manually, rinse films in circulating water for at least 20 minutes, preferably 30. Always return the film that was taken out for wet-reading for completion of fixing and washing. When processing automatically, ensure that the main water supply to the unit is turned on.

Dark Brown or Gray Film

- **Probable cause:** Oxidation and exhaustion of fixer.
- **Correction:** Maintain quality control over replenishing and replacing the fixer with fresh solution.

Film Handling Errors

The manner in which film is handled contributes to its ability to record a diagnostic quality image. Bending the film produces artifacts and significantly reduces the quality of the radiographic image. Additionally, exposing the film to conditions such as static electricity and the potential for scratching the emulsion will result in undiagnostic images. These artifacts may appear radiolucent or radiopaque.

Black Pressure Marks (Bent Film) (Figures 16–2 and 16–13)

- **Probable cause:** Bending the film or excessive pressure to the film emulsion can cause the emulsion to crack. Accidentally bending the film often occurs when the radiographer is placing the film packet into a film holder. A corner of film packet is sometimes purposely bent by the radiographer to prevent discomfort to the patient.
- **Correction:** Use caution when loading the film packet into the film holding device. Films should not be bent to fit the oral cavity. Instead, use a smaller sized film, the occlusal technique (see Chapter 15), or an extraoral procedure (see Chapter 27).

White Lines or Marks (Figure 16–14)

- **Probable cause:** The film emulsion is soft and can be easily scratched by a sharp object such as a film clip or hanger. Scratching removes the emulsion from the base.
- **Correction:** Care should be used when inserting a film onto a film hanger for developing. Avoid contact with other films or hangers.

Black Paper Stuck to Film

- **Probable cause:** A tear or break in the outer protective wrapping of the film packet by rough handling enables saliva to penetrate to the emulsion. Moisture softens the emulsion, causing the black paper to stick to the film.

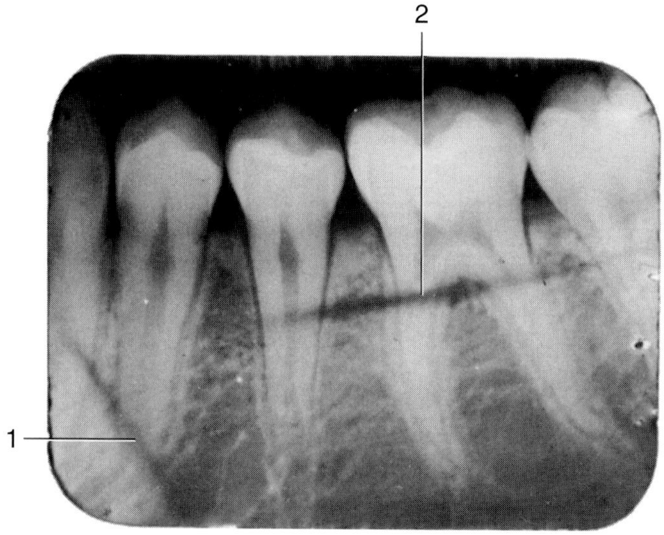

FIGURE 16-13 **Radiograph of mandibular posterior area.** (**1**) Distortion caused by bending the lower left film corner and pressure mark (thin radiolucent line). (**2**) Long radiolucent streak is a pressure mark caused by bending or by careless handling with excessive force.

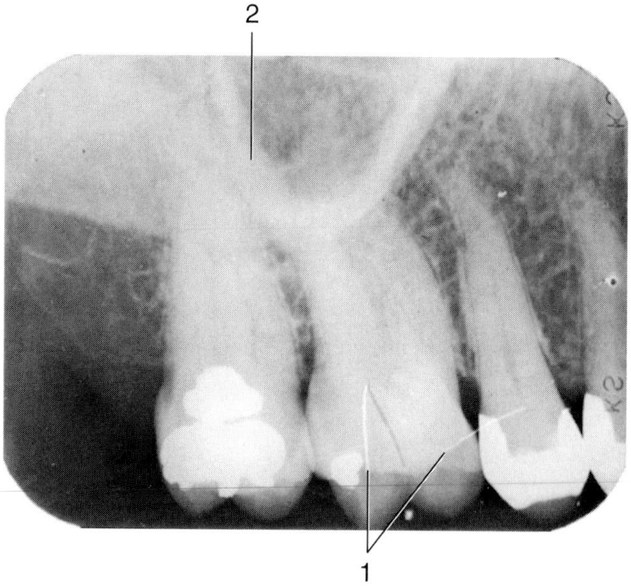

FIGURE 16-14 **Radiograph of maxillary posterior area.** (**1**) White streak marks show where the softened emulsion was scratched off the film during processing. (**2**) U-shaped radiopaque band of dense bone shows the outline of the zygoma.

- **Correction:** Careful handling prevents a break in the seal of the film packet. Always blot excess moisture from the film packet after removing it from the mouth.

Smudged Film (Figure 16–15)

- **Probable cause:** Fingermarks on the dry film or on the soft wet emulsion. Residual glove powder on the fingers will also leave black smudges.
- **Correction:** Avoid contact with the surface of the radiograph. Handle films carefully and by the edges only. Hands should be clean and free of moisture or glove powder.

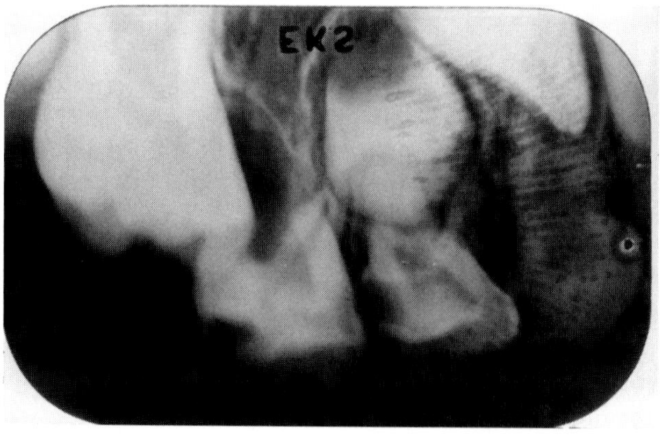

FIGURE 16-15 **Radiograph of primary molar area showing fingerprint.**

Thin Black Lines (see Figure 27–3)

- **Probable cause: Static electricity** was produced when the film was pulled out of the wrapping too fast. Static electricity creates a white light spark that exposes (blackens) the film.
- **Correction:** Pull the film out of the wrapping slowly. Reduce the occurrence of static electricity by increasing humidity in the darkroom. Use antistatic products on protective clothing to prevent the creation of static electricity.

Curled Films

- **Probable cause:** Rapid drying of the film through the use of excessive heat.
- **Correction:** Slower, more gradual drying. Avoid prolonged drying in an electric dryer.

Scratched Film

- **Probable cause:** Failure to protect the dried radiograph.
- **Correction:** Careful handling of processed radiographs. Mount the radiographs promptly and enclose in a protective envelope.

Film Fog

Still another cause of undiagnostic radiographs is the formation of a thin, cloudy layer that fogs the film surface. Fog diminishes contrast and makes it difficult and often impossible to interpret the radiograph. Fog on radiographs is produced in many ways and can occur before or after the film is exposed or during processing (Table 16–2). Most fogged radiographs have a similar appearance, making it difficult to pinpoint the cause. Careful attention to the exposure techniques and film processing method used and darkroom and film handling protocols will help reduce the occurrence of **film fog** error (Figure 16–16).

Radiation Fog

- **Probable cause:** Film is not properly protected from stray radiation before or after exposure.
- **Correction:** Store film at a safe distance from the source of x-rays or protect it by placing it in a lead-lined dispenser. Exposing a film increases its sensitivity; therefore it is very important that once a film has been exposed, it should be protected from the causes of film fog until processed.

TABLE 16–2 **Causes of Film Fog**

- Radiation
- Light
- Heat
- Humidity
- Chemical fumes
- Aging

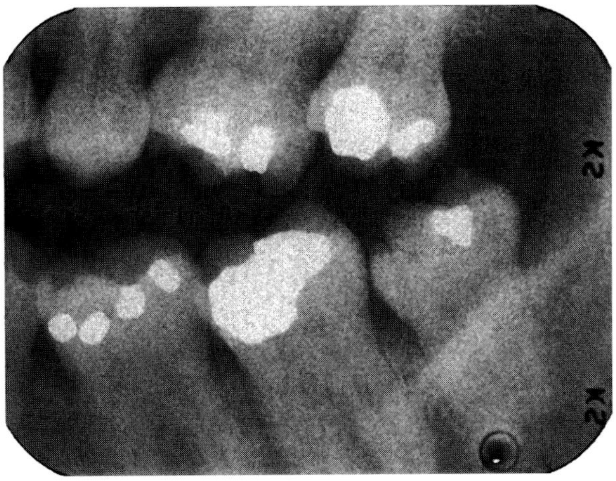

FIGURE 16–16 **Film fog.** Film fog results in lack of image contrast.

White Light Fog

- **Probable cause:** Light leak around the door of the darkroom or a minute break in the wrapping of the film.
- **Correction:** Check the darkroom for white light leaks. Handle the film packet carefully to prevent tearing the light-tight outer wrapping.

Safelight Fog

- **Probable cause:** Faulty safelighting occurs when the wattage of safelight bulb is stronger than recommended; the distance the safelight is located over the work space area is too close; the filter is the incorrect type or color for the film being used; or the filter is scratched or otherwise damaged, allowing white light through. Even when adequate, prolonged exposure to the safelight will fog film.
- **Correction:** Perform periodic quality control checks on the darkroom and safelight. Follow film manufacturer's guidelines when choosing filter color. Check the bulb wattage, the distance away from the work space and examine the filter for defects. The radiographer should develop skills necessary to open film packets aseptically within a two- to three-minute period to minimize the time films are exposed to the safelight.

Storage Fog (Heat, Humidity, and Chemical Fumes)

- **Probable cause:** Film stored in a warm, damp area or in the vicinity of fume-producing chemicals.
- **Correction:** Store in cool, dry area. Many practices store film in a refrigerator until ready to use. Film should not be stored in the darkroom unless protected from heat, humidity and fume-producing processing solutions.

Chemical Fog

- **Probable cause:** Developing films too long or at too high a temperature.
- **Correction:** Develop at recommended time–temperature cycle.

Processing Contamination Fog

- **Probable cause:** Contamination of processing chemicals.
- **Correction:** Avoid contamination of processing chemicals. Always replace the manual tank cover in the same position, with the side over the developer remaining over the developer and the side over the fixer remaining over the fixer to prevent contamination of the solutions. Thoroughly rinse films to remove developer before moving the film hanger into the fixer.

Aged Film Fog

- **Probable cause:** The film emulsion has a shelf life with an expiration date (see Figure 7–9). As film ages, it becomes increasingly fogged.
- **Correction:** Watch the date on film boxes. Rotate film stock so that the oldest film is used before newer film. Do not overstock film.

Miscellaneous Sources of Fog

Fluorescent Watch Faces and Dials

- **Probable cause:** Glowing light that reaches the film has the potential to create fog. This is especially true when processing sensitive extraoral films.
- **Correction:** Watches with fluorescent faces should not be worn, unless covered with the sleeve of the operator's gown or lab coat. Dials of equipment located in the darkroom that glow in unsafe light colors should be masked with opaque tape.

Cigarette Fog

- **Probable cause:** The glow of a cigarette is sufficient to fog the film.
- **Correction:** Smoking in an oral healthcare practice is undesirable, and in many regions, prohibited by law.

REVIEW—Chapter Summary

The dental radiographer should know what a quality diagnostic radiograph should look like and be able to identify when errors occur. No radiograph should be retaken until a thorough investigation reveals the exact cause of the error and the appropriate corrective action is identified. While radiographic errors may be classified as technique errors, processing errors and handling errors, undiagnostic radiographs are traceable to many causes. Frequently several different errors may cause similar-looking defects.

Technique errors include mistakes made in positioning the patient and the film packet, positioning of the tube head and the PID, and choosing the correct exposure factors. The film packet should not be positioned too high, low, anteriorly or posteriorly. Incorrect vertical angulation results in cutting off the occlusal/incisal edges or the apices of the teeth when utilizing the paralleling technique and elongation or foreshortening when utilizing the bisecting technique. Incorrect horizontal angulation results in overlapping.

Processing errors include development mistakes, not following protocols for processing and darkroom use, and chemical contamination. Overdevelopment causes dark images, and underdevelopment causes light images. Reticulation or a cracked emulsion appearance results when the processing solutions and water rinse temperatures are extremely different. Developer splash results in dark artifacts, and fixer splash results in light or white artifacts. Brownish-yellow stains result from improper rinsing.

Film-handling errors include bent, scratched, damaged and fogged films. Static electricity produces black lines on the resultant radiograph. Scratched emulsion will leave white or clear areas on the film. Stray radiation, light, heat, humidity, chemical fume exposure and contamination will create film fog. Film has a shelf life, and aging produces film fog.

RECALL—Study Questions

1. What is the appropriate corrective action when a film of the maxillary molar area did not image the third molar?
   a. Position the film higher in the oral cavity.
   b. Position the film lower in the oral cavity.
   c. Move the film forward in the oral cavity.
   d. Move the film back further in the oral cavity
2. What does a herringbone or tire-track pattern on the processed radiograph indicate?
   a. Embossed dot was positioned incorrectly.
   b. Lead foil was processed with the film.
   c. Film packet was placed in the oral cavity backwards.
   d. Temperatures of the processing chemicals were not equal.
3. When using the bisecting technique, which of these errors results from inadequate vertical angulation?
   a. Elongation
   b. Foreshortening
   c. Cone cut
   d. Overlapping
4. A radiograph of the maxillary molar area shows that the mesiobuccal root is superimposed over the lingual root and the overlap appears more severe in the posterior region. What correction is needed?
   a. Increase the vertical angulation.
   b. Decrease the vertical angulation.
   c. Shift the horizontal angulation toward the mesial.
   d. Shift the horizontal angulation toward the distal.
5. What error results in overlapped contacts being more severe in the second molar area than in the first premolar area?
   a. Excessive vertical angulation
   b. Inadequate vertical angulation
   c. Mesiodistal projection of horizontal angulation
   d. Distomesial projection of horizontal angulation
6. Which of these conditions results from a failure to direct the central ray toward the middle of the film packet?
   a. Overlapping
   b. Cone cut
   c. Elongation
   d. Foreshortening

7. Which of these indicates that the radiograph was overexposed?
   a. Clear image
   b. Light image
   c. Dark image
   d. Double image
8. All of the following will result in radiographs that are too light *except* one. Which one is this *exception*?
   a. Hot solutions
   b. Old film
   c. Underexposing
   d. Underdeveloping
9. All of the following will result in radiographs that are blank (clear) *except* one. Which one is this *exception*?
   a. No exposure to x-rays
   b. Placing films in the fixer first
   c. Extended time in warm water rinse
   d. Accidental white light exposure
10. Which of these conditions indicates that the level of the developer in the tank insert was too low?
   a. Herringbone effect
   b. Partial image
   c. Light image
   d. Reticulation
11. Which of these indicates that the film was not properly washed?
   a. Light image
   b. Fogging
   c. Brownish-yellow stains
   d. White spots
12. All of the following will result in black artifacts on the radiograph *except* one. Which one is this *exception*?
   a. Static electricity
   b. Bent film
   c. Glove powder
   d. Fixer splash
13. Static electricity appears radiographically as:
   a. Black lines.
   b. Scratched emulsion.
   c. White spots.
   d. Film fog.
14. All of the following are causes of film fog *except* one. Which one is this *exception*?
   a. Exposure to scatter radiation
   b. Use of old, expired film
   c. Double exposing the film
   d. Chemical-fume contamination of film

REFLECT—Case Study

You have just finished taking a full mouth series of periapical and bitewing radiographs. After processing and mounting the films, you notice the following:

1. The maxillary right molar periapical radiograph did not image the third molar.
2. The maxillary right canine periapical radiograph appears elongated and the image of the root tip is cut off.
3. The right premolar bitewing radiograph is overlapped. The overlapping appears most severe in the posterior portion of the image, and less severe in the anterior region.
4. The left molar bitewing film was bent when it was placed into the film holder.
5. The mandibular central incisors periapical radiograph appears very light, with a hint of a patterned image superimposed over the image of the teeth.
6. The film that should have been a left mandibular molar periapical radiograph is blank, with no hint of an image.
7. The left maxillary premolar periapical radiograph appears to have been double exposed.

Consider these 7 films with errors and answer the following questions:

   a. What is the most likely cause of this error? How did you arrive at this conclusion?
   b. Could there be multiple causes for this error? What other errors would produce this result?
   c. Why do you think this error occurred?
   d. What corrective action would you take when re-taking this radiograph? Be specific.
   e. What are you basing your decision to re-expose the patient on?
   f. What steps or actions would you recommend to prevent this error from occurring in the future?

RELATE—Laboratory Application

For a comprehensive laboratory practice exercise on this topic, see E. M. Thomson, *Exercises in Oral Radiography Techniques: A Laboratory Manual,* 2nd ed., Upper Saddle River, NJ: Prentice Hall, 2007. Chapter 10, "Identifying and Correcting Radiographic Errors."

BIBLIOGRAPHY

Eastman Kodak. *Exposure and Processing for Dental Radiography.* Rochester, NY: Eastman Kodak, 1998.

Eastman Kodak. *Successful Intraoral Radiography.* Rochester, NY: Eastman Kodak, 1998.

White S. C. & Pharoah, M. J. *Oral Radiology Principles and Interpretation,* 5th ed. St. Louis: Elsevier, 2004.

17

Quality Assurance in Dental Radiography

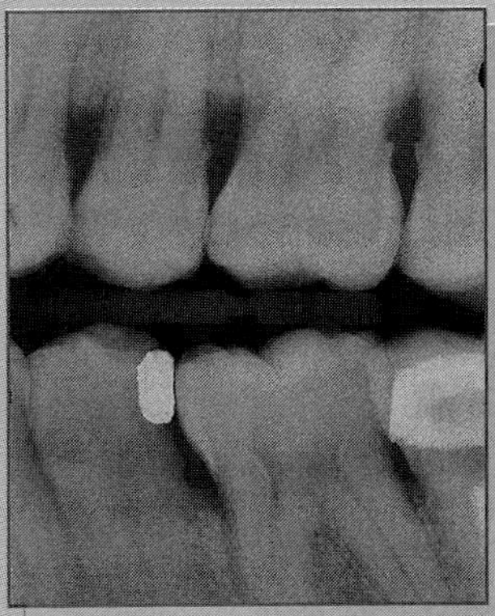

CHAPTER OUTLINE

■ OBJECTIVES

Following successful completion of this chapter, you should be able to:

1. Define the key words.
2. Explain the relationship between quality assurance and quality control.
3. List the four objectives of quality control tests.
4. Make a step wedge with cardboard and lead foil and demonstrate how to use it.
5. List two tests the radiographer can use to monitor a dental x-ray machine.
6. Explain the use of the coin test to monitor darkroom safelighting.
7. Describe how to test for light leaks in the darkroom.
8. Explain the use of a reference film to test processing chemistry.
9. Explain the use of the fresh film test to monitor the quality of a box of film.
10. List the steps of a quality assurance program.
11. Explain the role a competent radiographer plays in quality assurance.

■ KEY WORDS

Clearing time test
Coin test
Fresh film test
Light-tight
Output
Quality assurance
Quality control
Reference film
Step-wedge

Introduction

Quality assurance is defined as the planning, implementation, and evaluation of procedures used to produce high-quality radiographs with maximum diagnostic information (yield) while minimizing radiation exposure. Establishing a quality control program for radiographic procedures helps to increase the quality of radiographs produced and decrease the incidence of re-take radiographs. Quality assurance includes both quality control techniques and quality administration procedures (Table 17–1).

The purpose of this chapter is to present quality control tests that are used to monitor the dental x-ray machine; the x-ray processing system and darkroom; film storage; documentation and administrative maintenance; and operator competency.

TABLE 17–2 Quality Control Tests for Dental X-ray Machines

1. Radiation output
2. Timer accuracy
3. Milliamperage accuracy
4. Kilovoltage accuracy
5. Focal spot size
6. Filtration (beam quality)
7. Collimation
8. Beam alignment
9. Tube head stability

Quality Control

Quality control is defined as a series of tests to assure that the radiographic system is functioning properly and that the radiographs produced are of an acceptable level of quality. The objectives of quality control include:

1. Maintain a high standard of image quality.
2. Identify problems before image quality is compromised.
3. Keep patient and occupational exposures to a minimum.
4. Reduce the occurrence of re-take radiographs.

Examples of quality control measures include: tests to evaluate dental x-ray machine **output;** tests to evaluate safelighting of the darkroom; processing chemistry testing and replenishing; evaluation of film storage area; view box inspections; documentation such as records of when processing chemistry needs changing, posted technique factors near x-ray machines, and a maintenance log of re-takes to keep track of common errors and find solutions for avoiding them in the future.

Dental X-ray Machine Monitoring

Periodic comprehensive testing of the x-ray machine is essential to a quality assurance program. These tests include radiation output, timer accuracy, accuracy of milliamperage and kilovoltage settings, focal spot size, filtration (beam quality), collimation, beam alignment, and tube head stability (Table 17–2). State and local health departments may provide or require x-ray machine testing as part of their registration or licensing programs. In this case, a qualified health physicist will conduct most of these tests prior to renewing registration or license. However, the radiographer who uses the equipment on a daily basis should also play a role in monitoring the x-ray machine. Additionally, a working knowledge of the quality control tests available will help the radiographer identify when the equipment is not functioning at peak performance. Free literature on quality control tests for the oral healthcare practice entitled *Quality Assurance in Dental Film Radiology* and *Quality Control Tests for Dental Radiography* are available from Eastman Kodak Company, (*www.kodak.com/dental*, publication no. N-416).

TABLE 17–1 Quality Assurance Includes Both Quality Control and Quality Administration

Quality Control	Quality Administration
X-ray machines	Assess needs
Darkroom	Develop a written plan
Processing equipment	Assign authority and responsibility
Processing chemistry	Provide training
X-ray film and storage	Monitor maintenance schedule
X-ray viewing	Document actions and keep records/log
Operator competence	Perform periodic evaluation

Output Consistency Test (Procedure Boxes 17–1 and 17–2)

Radiation output may be monitored by the radiographer using a step wedge. A **step-wedge** is a device of layered metal steps of varying thickness used to determine film density and contrast. A step-wedge may also be used to test the strength of the processing chemicals, which will be discussed later.

A step-wedge may be obtained commercially or be made using several pieces of lead foil from intraoral film packets (Figure 17–1). To perform the radiation output test, the step-wedge is placed on a size #2 intraoral film on the counter or exam chair and the film is exposed with set exposure factors. This film is put aside, protected from stray radiation, heat and humidity, and other potential causes of film fog (see Chapter 16). The process is repeated with a new film at intervals determined by the practice. For example, the first exposure may be made in the morning, followed by a second exposure at mid-day and a third exposure at the end of the day. At the end of the desired time frame, all of the exposed films are processed at the same time and evaluated. Consistency in radiation output will produce three radiographs with images of the step wedge that are identical in densities and contrast. A failed test will produce images that are different from each other, indicating that the radiation output varied over the course of the day (Figure 17–2). A failed test

PROCEDURE 17–1

ASSEMBLING A STEP-WEDGE

1. Divide a piece of cardboard the size of a #2 x-ray film into thirds.
2. Leave the first third uncovered and cover the remaining two-thirds with two pieces of lead backing from a discarded film packet. Tape into place.
3. Cover the final third with three additional pieces of lead backing, taping them into place.

would indicate that a qualified health physicist should examine the x-ray machine.

To ensure accurate test results, film fog must be controlled. It is important that the exposed films be stored in a safe place away from stray radiation until processing. Additionally, to eliminate the possibility that the processing chemicals may change over time, it is important that all three films be processed at the same time.

Tube Head Stability

Another test the radiographer should make regularly on the dental x-ray machine is tube head stability. A drifting tube head must not be used until the support arm and yoke are properly adjusted to prevent movement of the tube head during exposure. To test for drift, the radiographer should position the tube head in various positions that will likely be needed for radiographic

PROCEDURE 17–2

PROCEDURE FOR X-RAY MACHINE OUTPUT CONSISTENCY TEST

1. Prepare a step-wedge or use a commercially made device (see Procedure Box 17–1).
2. Obtain three (or desired number) size #2 intraoral film packets from the same package.
3. Place two of the films in a safe place, protected from film fog causing elements (stray radiation, heat, humidity, chemical fumes).
4. Place one of the film packets on the counter or exam chair within reach of the x-ray tube head.
5. Place the step-wedge on top of the film packet.
6. Position the x-ray tube head over the film packet and step-wedge, and direct the central rays of the x-ray beam perpendicularly toward the film packet. Place the open end of the PID exactly 1 in. (2.5 cm) above the film packet. Use a ruler for accuracy.
7. Set the exposure factors to those utilized for an adult patient maxillary molar periapcial radiograph.
8. Make the exposure.
9. Place the exposed film in a safe place, protected from film fog causing elements (stray radiation, heat, humidity, chemical fumes).
10. Some time after the first exposure (at the desired time interval), retrieve one of the stored size #2 intraoral film packets.
11. Repeat steps 4 through 9.
12. Some time after the first two exposures (at the desired time interval), retrieve the third stored size #2 intraoral film packet.
13. Repeat steps 4 through 9.
14. When ready, process all three of the films at the same time.
15. When processing is complete, observe all three of the films for consistency in density and constrast.
16. A failed test will show a difference in density or contrast among the three images.
17. Call a qualified health physicist to examine the x-ray machine if needed.

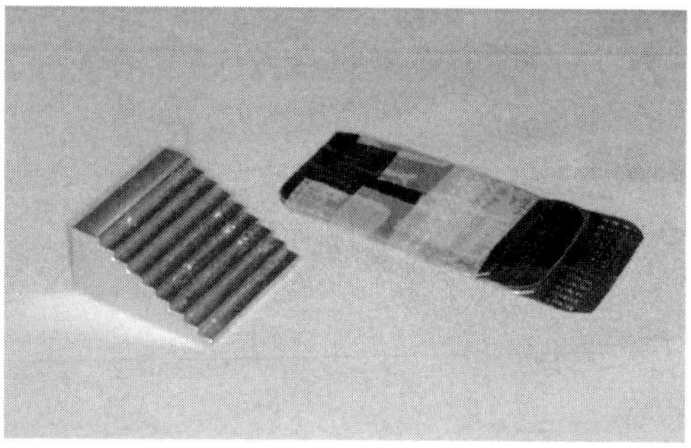

FIGURE 17-1 **Step-wedge.** (**A**) Commercially made step-wedge. (**B**) Step-wedge made from discarded sheets of lead foil from intraoral film packets.

exposures. When not in use, the support arm should be folded into a closed position with the PID pointing down to prevent weight stress from loosening the support arm and causing the drift (Figure 17–3).

Darkroom Monitoring

The darkroom should be evaluated for the presence of conditions that create film fog and compromise image quality. The darkroom should be checked to determine that it is adequately ventilated, free from chemical fumes, within the prescribed temperature and humidity range recommended by the film manufacturer, beyond the reach of stray radiation, and **light-tight.** The key to a safe darkroom is an appropriate safelight.

Safelight Test

As you will recall from Chapter 8, the safelight must have a bulb of the proper wattage, a filter color deemed safe for the film being

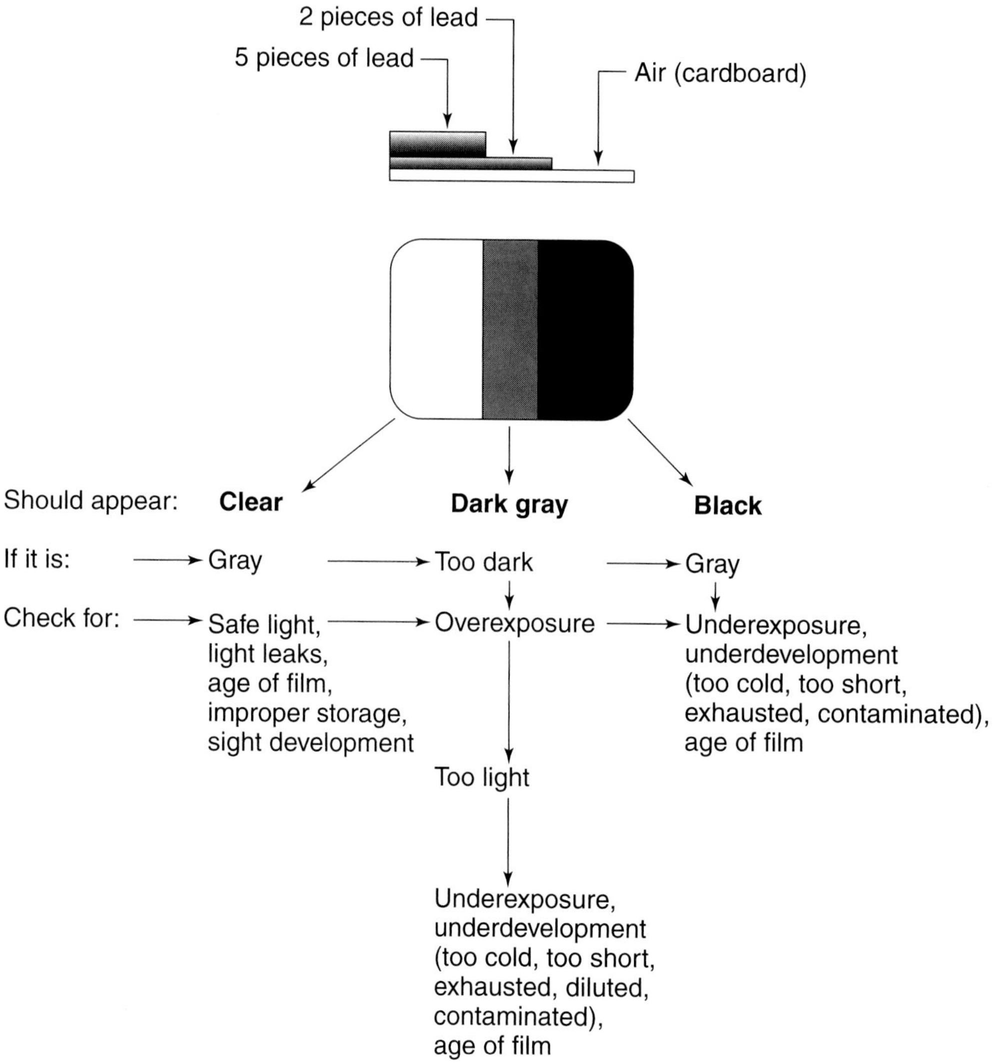

FIGURE 17-2 **Sketch of a step-wedge.** A step-wedge is useful in making visual comparisons for quality control. (Courtesy of Dr. A. Peter Fortier, Louisiana State University, School of Dentistry, and Department of Dental Diagnostic Science, School of Dentistry, University of Texas at San Antonio)

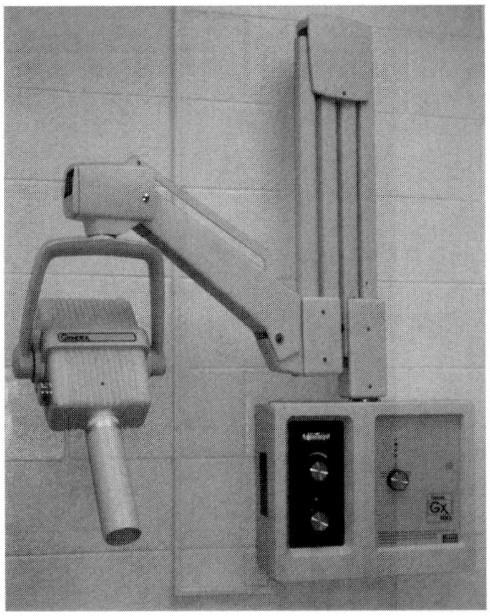

FIGURE 17-3 **Correct position of tube head when not in use.** Extension arm folded, tube head and PID aimed at the floor.

processed, and be located a safe distance from the working area where films will be unwrapped. The coin test can be used to test the safelight for adequacy.

The **coin test** uses a coin and a slightly exposed film to determine safelight adequacy (Procedure Box 17–3). Because films that have already been exposed are more sensitive to conditions that cause film fog, a true test of the safelight uses a film that is pre-exposed to a small amount of radiation. After the test film has been slightly exposed, it is unwrapped in the darkroom under safelight conditions and placed on the counter where patient films will normally be unwrapped. A coin is placed on top of the unwrapped film for two or three minutes. This period simulates the approximate time required aseptically to unwrap a full mouth series of films and load them into the processor. It is assumed that while the film is on the counter, the portion of the film that remains under the metal coin would be protected from possible light exposure, while the rest of the area would receive exposure if the light was unsafe.

When the time is up, the film is processed as usual. After processing, the film is examined. An image of the outline of the coin would indicate a failed test, suggesting that the safelight conditions in the darkroom are fogging the film. A failed test should prompt the radiographer to check to be sure that the safelight bulb wattage is correct and that the filter color is appropriate for the film used. The distance away from the working area should be checked and the safelight filter should be visually inspected for scratches or cracks in the filter that would allow white light to escape.

Test for Light Leaks

Whether the darkroom is light-tight can be determined by closing the door and turning off all lights, including the safelight. Light leaks, if present, become visible after about five minutes when the eyes become accustomed to the dark. Possible sources of light leaks include around the entry door or around the pipes leading into the darkroom. Drop ceiling tiles and ventilation screens may also allow white light to enter the darkroom. While eyes are still adjusted to the dark, white light leaks may be marked with tape or chalk to allow the radiographer to find them when the white overhead lights are turned back on. Light leaks should be sealed with tape or weather stripping.

An additional source of inappropriate light is light from illuminated dials or watch faces worn by personnel in the darkroom. Illuminated dials located in the darkroom may be masked with tape if necessary. Wristwatches with fluorescent faces should not be worn in the darkroom unless covered by the sleeve of the operator's lab coat.

Processing System Monitoring

All processing equipment, including the automatic processor, manual processing equipment, cassettes, intensifying screens, and viewbox, need to be checked on a periodic basis.

Automatic Processor

The key to peak performance of an automatic processor is maintenance. Often the unit manufacturer will recommend daily, weekly, monthly, and quarterly maintenance and cleaning procedures to ensure quality performance. A schedule of set maintenance procedures, and a log of when those procedures need to be performed, should be posted to assist those who utilize the equipment with the maintenance scheduling.

These two tests are helpful in daily monitoring of the automatic processor:

1. Begin by processing an unexposed film under safelight conditions. The film should come out of the return chute of the automatic processor clear (slightly blue tinted) and dry.
2. Then process a film that has been exposed to white light. This film should come out of the return chute of the automatic processor black and dry after processing.

A failed test should prompt the operator to check the solutions, the water supply, and film dryer. The solution levels should be checked and must be replenished and changed on a regular basis. The processor should be maintaining the correct temperature. The water supply must be turned on and the dryer operating correctly to produce a clear, dry film.

Manual Processing

Determine whether the thermometer and timer are accurate. Monitor the temperature and levels of the processing solutions and replenish and change as needed. Ensure that the work area is clean and free of dust.

Processing Solutions

As explained in Chapter 8, chemical manufacturers recommend changing processing solutions at least every four weeks with "normal" use. There are often times in practice when more or

PROCEDURE 17–3

COIN TEST FOR SAFELIGHT ADEQUACY

1. Obtain a size #2 intraoral film packet and a coin.
2. Place the film packet on the counter or exam chair within reach of the x-ray tube head.
3. Position the x-ray tube head over the film packet. Direct the central rays of the x-ray beam perpendicularly toward the film packet. Place the open end of the PID about 12 in. (30 cm) above the film packet.
4. Set the exposure factors to the lowest possible setting.
5. Make the exposure.
6. Take the slightly exposed film and a coin to the darkroom. Turn off the overhead white light and turn on the safelight.
7. Unwrap the film packet and place the film on the counter where you would normally process patient films.
8. Place the coin on top of the unwrapped film.
9. Wait approximately two or three minutes.
10. Remove the coin from the film and process the film in the usual manner.
11. When processing is complete, observe the film for any outline of the coin. (The film will have an overall appearance of darkness or slight fogging from the slight radiation exposure in step 5. However, you are looking for a distinguishable outline of the coin.)
12. A failed test will show an outline of the coin.
13. Examine the safelight for correct bulb wattage, filter color, scratches or cracks, distance away from working area. Perform additional tests to check for possible white light leaks or the presence of other light sources.

less films may be processed during any given week. Therefore it is important to monitor the strength of the processing solutions on a daily basis, before undiagnostic film images result.

The developer solution is the most critical of the processing solutions and demands careful attention. When the developer solution deteriorates and loses strength, the underdeveloped radiographic images lighten. An instrument called the Dental Radiographic Quality Control Device (Figure 17–4), available commercially (from Xray QC, *www.Xrayqc.com*) can be utilized to monitor the developer. The device has a filmstrip with several density steps for comparison to a test film. Step-by-step instructions are printed on front of the device.

The radiographer may prepare a step-wedge from discarded lead foil from intraoral film packets, discussed earlier, to monitor the developer as well (Procedure Box 17–4). Using the step-wedge, several films are exposed at the same settings, all at the same time. At the beginning of the day, immediately after fresh chemistry has been prepared, one of the exposed films is processed. This becomes the **reference film,** with the ideal image density and contrast. The remaining exposed films should be stored in a cool, dry place protected from stray radiation and other conditions that produce film fog. At the beginning of each day, one of the previously exposed films is processed and compared to the reference film. Each subsequent film should match the reference film in density and contrast. A failed test would indicate that the processing chemicals, particularly the developer, was losing strength and needed to be changed (Figure 17–2).

A **clearing time test** allows the radiographer to test the strength of the fixer solution in a manual processing tank. An unexposed film is placed in the fixer solution and timed. If the film clears in four minutes or less, the fixer solution is adequate. If the clearing time is over four minutes, the fixer should be replaced.

Cassettes and Intensifying Screens

Quality control procedures include periodically examining cassettes and intensifying screens. Extraoral cassettes should be checked for warping, light leaks, and screen–film contact. Warping and light leaks result in fogged radiographs. Poor screen contact results in an image with poor definition (fuzzy image) (see Chapter 27). Defective cassettes should be repaired or replaced.

Intensifying screens should be examined for cleanliness and scratches. Any specks of dirt, paper, or other material will absorb the light given off by the screen crystals and produce white or clear artifacts on the resultant radiographic image. Dirty screens

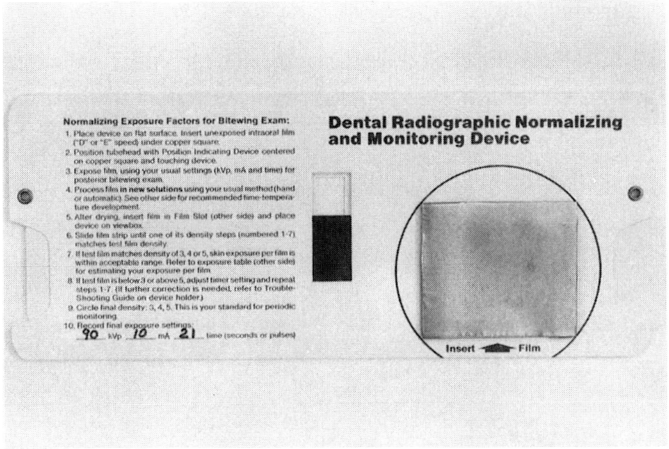

FIGURE 17-4 **Dental radiographic quality control device.** (Available from Xray QC [formerly Dental Radiographic Devices], www.xrayqc.com)

should be cleaned as needed with solutions recommended by the screen manufacturer. However, overuse of chemical cleaning should be avoided. Any scratched or damaged screen should be repaired or replaced.

Viewbox

If functioning properly the viewbox should give off a uniform, subdued light. Flickering light may indicate bulb failure. The surface of the viewbox should be wiped clean as needed. Care should be taken when using a viewbox in the darkroom. Films that are unwrapped immediately after turning off the viewbox may be fogged by the afterglow of the fluorescent light tubes. Film emulsions are sensitive to this afterglow and can be fogged.

X-ray Film Monitoring

Only fresh x-ray film should be used for exposing dental radiographs. Film manufacturers use a series of quality control tests to assure dental x-ray film quality. Film should be properly stored, protected, and used before the expiration date. Check

PROCEDURE 17-4

REFERENCE FILM TO MONITOR PROCESSING SOLUTIONS

1. Prepare a step-wedge or use a commercially made device (see Procedure Box 17–1).
2. Obtain several size #2 intraoral film packets from the same package.
3. Place one of the film packets on the counter or exam chair within reach of the x-ray tube head.
4. Place the step-wedge on top of the film packet.
5. Position the x-ray tube head over the film packet and step-wedge, and direct the central rays of the x-ray beam perpendicularly toward the film packet. Place the open end of the PID exactly 1 in. (2.5 cm) above the film packet. Use a ruler for accuracy.
6. Set the exposure factors to those utilized for an adult patient maxillary molar periapcial radiograph.
7. Make the exposure.
8. Place the exposed film in a safe place, protected from film fog causing elements (stray radiation, heat, humidity, chemical fumes).
9. Immediately repeat steps 3 through 8 with the rest of the films.
10. Following a complete solution change of the processing chemistry, process one of the exposed films. This film is the reference film.
11. Mount the reference film on the viewbox.
12. Each day immediately after replenishing the processing chemistry, retrieve one of the stored exposed films and process as usual.
13. Compare the film processed on this day to the reference film processed when the chemistry was changed. Look for similar density and contrast indicating that the processing solutions are functioning at peak levels.
14. Repeat steps 12 and 13 each day. The solutions are exhausted and need to be changed when the density and contrast of the just-processed film does not match the reference film.

the expiration date on the x-ray film box and always use the oldest film first.

The **fresh film test** can be used to monitor the quality of each box of film. When a new film box is opened for use, immediately process one of the films without exposing it. If the film is fresh, it will appear clear with a slight blue tint. If the film appears fogged, the remaining films in the box should not be used.

Quality Administration Procedures

Quality administration refers to conducting a quality assurance program in the oral healthcare practice. A quality assurance program should include an assessment of current practices, where and how the problems seem to be occurring; a written plan that identifies who is responsible and what training the personnel need to be able to carry out the quality control tests; record-keeping and periodic evaluations of the plan (Table 17–1).

Needs Assessment

This step ties in with the last evaluation step. Periodically the oral healthcare team should review patient radiographs for quality. Problems that occur should be documented and then periodically reviewed to look for areas where a change in policy, maintenance schedules, or other area is noted.

Written Plan

The oral healthcare team should develop a written plan that will guide quality control. The plan should include, but not be limited to, the purpose of the quality assurance program; assignment of authority and responsibilities; a list of equipment that requires monitoring; a list of tests that will be performed and at what time intervals (Table 17–3); a log of all quality assurance test results; a log of retake radiographs; documentation of training; and evaluation interval and report.

Careful planning and thoroughly carrying out a quality assurance program increases the likelihood of producing the highest quality radiographs while minimizing radiation exposure.

TABLE 17–3 **Suggested Time Intervals for Performing Quality Control Tests**

Quality Control Test	Suggested Time Interval
Output consistency	Annually
Tube head stability	Monthly
Darkroom safelighting	Annually
Automatic processor	Daily
Processing solutions	Daily
Cassettes and screens	Annually
Viewboxes	Monthly

Authority and Responsibilities

While the dentist is ultimately responsible for the overall quality care that his/her practice provides the patient, each oral healthcare team member can be given authority to carry out specific aspects of the quality control program. Assigning authority and clearly defining specific tasks and/or maintenance procedures helps to ensure that the procedures are being carried out. Each oral healthcare team member must be informed of how and why the tasks are to be performed and provided with training opportunities to assure compentency in performing in this capacity.

Monitoring and Maintenance Schedules

A monitoring schedule listing all the quality control tests, identification of the person responsible for each test, and the frequency of testing should be generated and posted. Check-off lists can be used to record maintenance and inspections.

Logs and Periodic Evaluation

A log should be kept of all quality control tests. Include the date, the specific test, the results, action taken if any, and the name of the person who conducted the test. Also, a log of all radiographs re-taken should be recorded to identify recurring problems.

Office personnel should meet periodically to evaluate the logs and the quality assurance program.

Competency of the Radiographer

Essential to a quality assurance program is the ability of the radiographer. Operator errors that result in undiagnostic radiographs generate the need for re-take radiographs. Re-takes result in unnecessary radiation exposure to the patient and lost time for both the patient and the practice. Not only must the radiographer be competent in exposing, processing, and mounting dental radiographs, but in identifying when errors occur. Even competent radiographers encounter situations where less than ideal radiographic images result. It is important, therefore, that the radiographer be able to recognize poor quality, identify the cause, and apply the appropriate corrective action.

Operator errors and re-takes should be recorded to identify recurring problems. Each film exposed may be recorded in a log that can be reviewed periodically to monitor for problems and the application of the appropriate corrective actions. This will also help monitor the skills of the radiographer. To aid in operator competency, educational opportunities such as continuing education courses or on-the-job-training can assist the radiographer in brushing up on skills, improving in an area of deficiency, and/or staying apprised of the newest technology and treatment recommendations.

Benefits of Quality Assurance Programs

Everyone benefits from a well organized quality assurance program. The time required to assess, plan, implement, and evaluate a quality assurance program is made up in the time saved and the benefits gained avoiding the production of poor quality radiographs and re-takes.

Periodic evaluation of the program will allow for flexibility as changes in recommended protocols or new techniques come into being. The ultimate goal of quality assurance is to produce radiographs with the greatest amount of diagnostic yield using the smallest amount of radiation exposure.

REVIEW—Chapter Summary

Quality assurance is defined as the planning, implementation, and evaluation of procedures used to produce high-quality radiographs with maximum diagnostic information (yield) while minimizing radiation exposure.

Quality control is defined as a series of tests to assure that the radiographic system is functioning properly and that the radiographs produced are of an acceptable level of quality. These tests include the monitoring of the dental x-ray machine, the darkroom, processing system, and x-ray film. A step-wedge is a valuable tool that can be used in a variety of tests.

Quality control tests for monitoring dental x-ray machines include the output consistency test and tube head stability. Quality control tests for monitoring the darkroom include the coin test for checking the safelight and for checking for light leaks. Quality control tests for monitoring the processing system include monitoring the processing solutions with the use of a reference film and the clearing time test. The fresh film test is used to monitor dental x-ray film.

Quality administration refers to conducting a quality assurance program in the oral healthcare practice. The five steps to a quality administration program are: assess needs, develop a written plan, assign authority and responsibilities, develop monitoring and maintenance schedules, and utilize a log and evaluations to check on the program.

The key to producing the highest quality diagnostic radiographs with the lowest possible radiation exposure is operator competence. Everyone, the oral healthcare team and the patients, benefits from a well organized quality assurance program.

RECALL—Study Questions

1. The goal of quality assurance is to achieve maximum diagnostic yield from each radiograph. Quality control means using tests to ensure quality.
   a. The first statement is true; the second statement is false.
   b. The first statement is false; the second statement is true.
   c. Both statements are true.
   d. Both statements are false.
2. List the four objectives of quality control.
   a. ____________________
   b. ____________________
   c. ____________________
   d. ____________________
3. The step-wedge can be used to test all of the following *except* one. Which one is this *exception?*
   a. Dental x-ray machine output consistency
   b. Processing chemistry strength
   c. Density and contrast of the image
   d. Adequacy of the safelight
4. All of the following are quality control tests for monitoring the dental x-ray machine *except* one. Which one is this *exception?*
   a. Tube head stability test
   b. Coin test
   c. Output consistency test
   d. Timer, milliamperage and kilovoltage setting accuracy test
5. The use of the coin test will monitor darkroom safelight conditions. When an image of the coin appears on the radiograph, the safelight is adequate.
   a. The first statement is true; the second statement is false.
   b. The first statement is false; the second statement is true.
   c. Both statements are true.
   d. Both statements are false.
6. A film processed under ideal conditions and used to compare subsequent radiographic images is a:
   a. Fresh film.
   b. Fogged film.
   c. Periapical film.
   d. Reference film.
7. When the automatic processor is functioning properly, an unexposed film will exit the return chute dry and:
   a. Black.
   b. Clear.
   c. Green.
   d. With the image of a coin.
8. In addition to the dentist who is responsible for planning, implementing, and evaluating a quality assurance plan?
   a. Dental assistant
   b. Dental hygienist
   c. Practice manager
   d. All of the above
9. On-the-job training and continuing education courses contribute to radiographic competence. Competent radiographers are key to a quality assurance program.
   a. The first statement is true; the second statement is false.
   b. The first statement is false; the second statement is true.
   c. Both statements are true.
   d. Both statements are false.

REFLECT—Case Study

The practice where you work needs to update their radiographic quality control plan. Currently the basic plan mentions the need to test the x-ray machine and monitor the darkroom and processing systems. Applying what you have learned in this chapter, develop a quality control plan for your practice. Include the following:

1. List of equipment you think the practice should be testing
2. The name of the test needed
3. Recommended time interval for performing the test
4. Name of the person assigned to perform the test
5. A description of what a failed test and a successful test would look like

6. The action required if a failed test results

Then prepare the following documents that your practice would use to assist the quality assurance plan:

1. A detailed, step-by-step procedure that someone could follow to perform each of the tests you have recommended
2. Forms to keep a log of the outcomes for each of the tests you recommended

RELATE—Laboratory Application

For a comprehensive laboratory practice exercise on this topic, see E. M. Thomson, *Exercises in Oral Radiography Techniques: A Laboratory Manual,* 2nd ed., Upper Saddle River, NJ: Prentice Hall, 2007. Chapter 11, "Radiographic Quality Assurance."

BIBLIOGRAPHY

American Academy of Dental Radiology Quality Assurance Committee. Recommendations for quality assurance in dental radiography. *Oral. Surg.* 55:421–426, 1983.

Eastman Kodak. *Quality Assurance in Dental Radiography.* Rochester, NY: Eastman Kodak, 1998.

Quality Assurance for Diagnostic Imaging Equipment: Recommendations of the National Council on Radiation Protection and Measurements. NCRP Report no. 99. Bethesda, MD: NCRP publications, 1988.

PART VII • MOUNTING AND VIEWING DENTAL RADIOGRAPHS

18

Mounting and Introduction to Interpretation

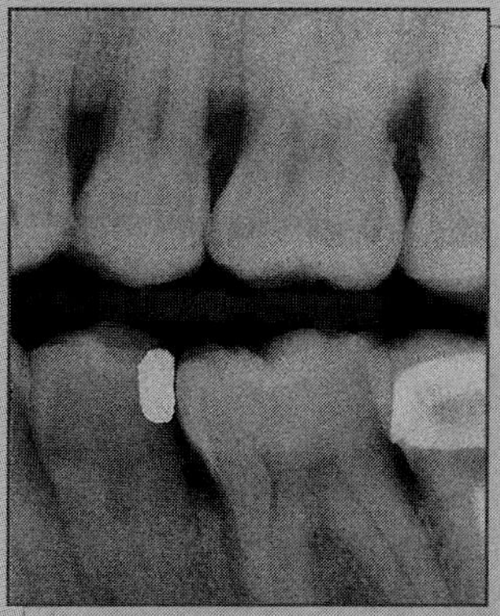

CHAPTER OUTLINE

■ OBJECTIVES

Following successful completion of this chapter, you should be able to:

1. Define the key words.
2. List at least five advantages of mounting radiographs.
3. Discuss the use and importance of the identification dot.
4. Compare labial and lingual methods of film mounting.
5. Demonstrate mounting radiographs according to the suggested steps presented.
6. List at least five anatomic generalizations that aid in mounting radiographs.
7. Compare interpretation and diagnosis.
8. Describe the roles of the film mount, viewbox, and magnification in viewing radiographs.
9. Demonstrate viewing radiographs according to the suggested steps presented.

■ KEY WORDS

Anatomical order
Diagnosis
Film mount
Film mounting
Identification dot
Interpretation
Labial mounting method
Lingual mounting method
Viewbox

Introduction

Mounting is an important step in the interpretation of dental radiographs. Dental radiographs must be mounted in the correct anatomic order to allow for a thorough and systematic interpretation. A thorough knowledge of the normal anatomy of the teeth and jaws is needed to mount radiographs correctly. Therefore, mounting and interpreting dental radiographs go hand in hand.

The purpose of this chapter is to describe the step-by-step procedures for mounting and viewing dental radiographs. To aid in this process, basic key points regarding anatomic landmarks will be discussed. Chapter 19 provides the detailed radiographic interpretation of normal radiographic anatomy.

Mounting Radiographs

Film mounting is the placement of radiographs in a holder arranged in **anatomical order** (Figure 18–1). The advantages of film mounting are:

- Intraoral radiographs are easier to view and interpret in the correct anatomical position.
- Mounting decreases the chance of error caused by confusing the patient's right and left sides.
- Viewing films side by side allows for easy comparison between different views.
- Less handling of individual radiographs results in fewer scratches and fingerprint marks.
- Film mounts can mask out distracting side light, making radiographs easier to view and interpret.
- Film mounts provide a means for labeling the radiographs with patient's name, date of exposure, name of the practice, etc.
- Mounted films are easy to store.
- Patient education and consultations are enhanced when films are mounted.
- When mounted labially, radiographic findings can be easily transferred to the patient's dental chart.

Film mounting generally refers only to intraoral films. Large extraoral radiographs must be labeled with lead letters or tape that identify the right and left sides and are often placed in an envelope so that the patent's name and the date of the exposure can be written on the outside.

Occasionally, single intraoral radiographs are not mounted, but are placed into a coin envelope and attached to the patient record. However, it is better to mount even a single or a small group of radiographs; a full-mouth series should always be mounted for accurate viewing. Additionally, the film mount provides a place to record the patient's name, date and other pertinent information.

Film Mounts

Film mounts are celluloid, cardboard, or plastic holders with frames or windows for the radiographs (Figure 18–2). Attaching the radiographs to the film mounts is called film mounting. Film mounts are available in many sizes and with numerous combinations of windows or frames to fit films of different sizes. Mounts may be large enough to accommodate a full-mouth series of radiographs, or hold only a few or even a single radiograph. Standard commercially made mounts are available, or companies will make custom mounts to suit special needs. Black plastic or gray cardboard mounts are often preferred over clear plastic mounts because these can block out extraneous light from the viewbox, enhancing viewing and interpretation.

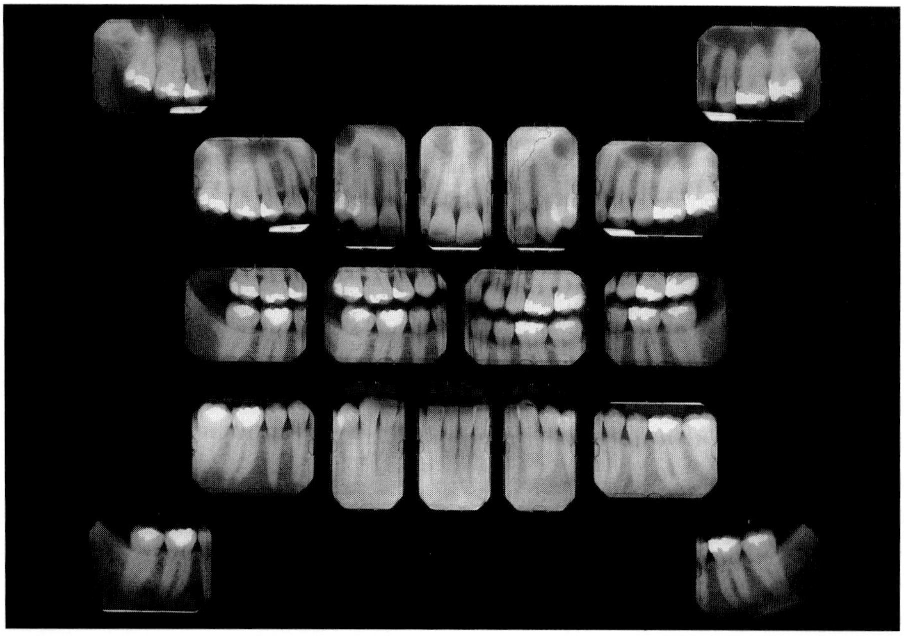

FIGURE 18–1 **Full-mouth series mounted in an opaque mount.**

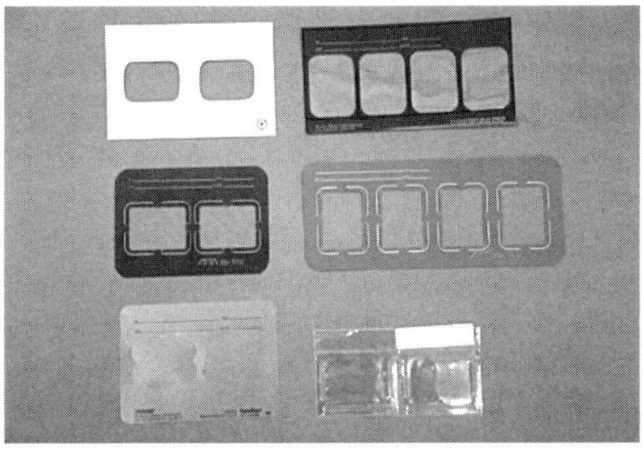

FIGURE 18-2 **Examples of various film mounts.** Film mounts are available in a variety of sizes and film combinations.

Identification Dot

An embossed **identification dot** near the edge of the film appears convex or concave, depending on the side from which the film is viewed. If the film packet was placed in the patient's oral cavity correctly, the raised portion of the identification dot (the convexity) automatically faces the x-ray tube and the source of radiation. Therefore, when the radiograph is viewed later, the identification dot may be relied on to determine which is the patient's left and right sides. Since the radiograph may be viewed from either side, it is important that the radiographer understand the role the identification dot plays in film orientation.

Film Mounting Methods

Since the radiograph may be viewed from either side, two methods of film mounting have been used. The first method, now obsolete but still used by some dentists, is the lingual method. With the **lingual mounting method,** the radiographs are mounted so that the embossed dot is concave. In this position, the viewer is reading the radiograph as if standing behind the patient (Figure 18–3). Therefore, what the viewer observes on the right side of the radiograph would correspond to the patient's right as well. Essentially, the viewer's right is the patient's right.

The second method, recommended by the American Dental Association and the American Academy of Oral and Maxillofacial Radiology, is the **labial mounting method.** With the labial method of film mounting, the radiographs are mounted so that the embossed dot is convex. In this position, the viewer is reading the radiographic as if standing in front of, and facing, the patient (Figure 18–4). Therefore, what the viewer observes on the right side of the radiograph would correspond to the patient's left side. Essentially, the viewer's right is the patient's left. This also corresponds to the order in which teeth and anatomical structures are drawn on most dental and periodontal charts.

Film Mounting Procedure

Radiographs should be mounted immediately after processing. Handle films by the edges to avoid smudging or scratching them, and label the radiographs to prevent loss or mixing them up with

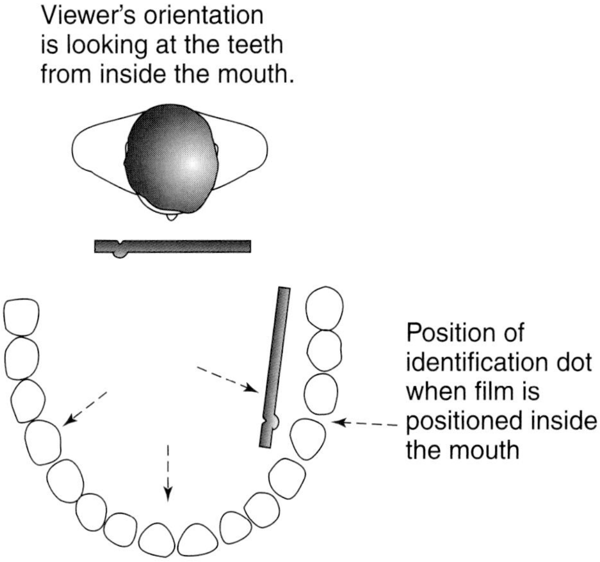
Viewer's orientation is looking at the teeth from inside the mouth.
Position of identification dot when film is positioned inside the mouth

FIGURE 18-3 **Lingual method of film mounting.** When the identification dot is viewed in the concave position, the viewer's orientation is from behind the patient. The patient's left is the viewer's left.

other patient films. An orderly sequence to the mounting procedure is suggested (Procedure Box 18–1). This is especially true for the beginner. While the sequence for mounting is often a matter of preference, the first step in mounting all radiographs should be to orient the embossed dot the same way for all the films. When mounting using the labial method, orient all the films so that the embossed dot is convex.

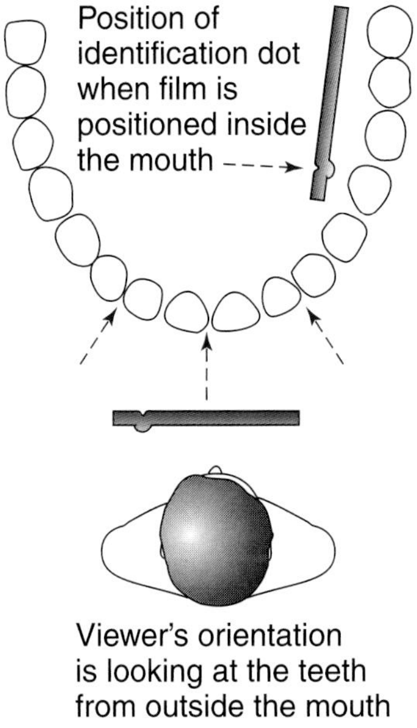
Position of identification dot when film is positioned inside the mouth
Viewer's orientation is looking at the teeth from outside the mouth

FIGURE 18-4 **Labial method of film mounting.** When the identification dot is viewed in the convex position, the viewer's orientation is in front of and facing the patient. The patient's left is the viewer's right.

PROCEDURE 18–1

SUGGESTED SEQUENCE FOR MOUNTING A FULL MOUTH SERIES OF RADIOGRAPHS

1. Place the films on a clean white or light-colored paper towel or tray cover on the counter in front of a viewbox.
2. Wash hands to prevent smudging the films.
3. Orient the embossed dots all the same way.
4. Separate the bitewing from the periapical radiographs.
5. Separate the anterior periapicals from the posterior periapicals.
6. Separate the maxillary from the mandible periapical radiographs.
7. Orient the periapical radiographs so that the roots are pointing up for the maxilla and down for the mandible.
8. Orient the bitewing radiographs so that the occlusal plane slants upward in the posterior, producing a slight "smile" appearance.
9. Place the anterior periapical radiographs into the appropriate frame on the left or right side of the film mount.
10. Place the posterior periapical radiographs into the appropriate frame on the left or right side of the film mount.
11. Place the bitewing radiographs into the appropriate frame on the left or right side of the film mount.
12. Label the film mount with the patient's name, date of exposure, facility name, and other pertinent information.
13. Check the mounted films to be sure they are secured in the mount and are mounted appropriately. (Embossed dots all facing the same direction, no films upside down.)
14. Place the mounted radiographs on the viewbox for use during the patient appointment and for interpretation.

When mounting a full mouth series of periapical and bitewing radiographs, it is helpful to use the film sizes and orientation in the oral cavity to help with the mounting process. Size #1 film is often used to radiograph the anterior region. Additionally, anterior periapical radiographs are placed in the oral cavity with the long dimension of the film packet positioned vertically, whereas posterior periapical radiographs are placed in the oral cavity with the long dimension of the film packet positioned horizontally. These clues may be utilized to help the radiographer determine where to position the films in the mount.

To mount correctly, the radiographer must have a base knowledge in radiographic anatomy. Chapter 19 covers radiographic anatomy observed on intraoral radiographs and Chapter 28 covers radiographic anatomy observed on panoramic radiographs in detail (Table 18–1). However, to aid in the mounting procedure, the following generalizations are offered:

- Roots and crowns of the maxillary anterior teeth are larger and longer than those of the mandibular teeth.
- Canine teeth generally have the longest roots when compared to adjacent teeth.
- Maxillary molars generally have three roots. The presence of the palatal root makes it difficult to visual three distinct roots.
- Mandibular molars generally have two divergent roots that are distinctly observed. Bone is visible in between the two roots.
- Most roots curve toward the distal.
- Large radiolucent areas denoting the nasal fossa or the maxillary sinus indicate that the radiograph is of a maxillary area.
- The body of the mandible has a distinct upward curve toward the ramus in the molar area. The film should be oriented so that a slight "smile" appearance is detected.

After the last radiograph has been mounted, the entire film mount should be carefully checked to see that:

- Identification dots all face the same direction.
- All radiographs are arranged in proper anatomical order.
- No radiographs were reversed or mounted upside down.

TABLE 18–1 **Anatomical Landmarks Distinguishing Maxillary Radiographs from Mandibular Radiographs**

Area	Maxillary Anatomical Landmarks	Mandibular Anatomical Landmarks
Incisor	Incisive foramen Median palatine suture Nasal fossa Nasal septum Anterior nasal spine	Lingual foramen Genial tubercles Nutrient canals Mental ridge Mental fossa
Canine	Inverted Y Lateral fossa	
Premolar	Maxillary sinus	Mental foramen
Molar	Maxillary sinus Zygomatic process of maxilla Zygoma Maxillary tuberosity Hamulus Coronoid process of mandible	Mandibular canal Oblique ridge Mylohyoid ridge Submandibular fossa

- The radiographs are firmly attached to the mount.
- The patient's name and date have been recorded on the mount.

Viewing the Radiographs

Proper viewing is essential for the interpretation of dental radiographs. One must be familiar with and understand optimal viewing conditions and the proper sequence of viewing the radiographs.

Interpretation versus Diagnosis

Dental radiographs are viewed by any trained professional (dentist, dental hygienist, or dental assistant) with a knowledge of normal anatomic landmarks of the maxilla, mandible, and related structures. Radiographs may be interpreted by all members of the oral healthcare team, but the dentist is responsible for the final interpretation and diagnosis. **Interpretation** is explanatory, and may be defined as reading the radiograph and explaining what is observed in terms the patient understands. Items that a dental hygienist or dental assistant may interpret are radiographic errors such as overlapped contacts or elongated images; artifacts that may have appeared on the radiograph such as the image of a film holder; normal radiographic anatomy such as the absence of a developing permanent tooth under a primary tooth or the presence radiographically of unerupted third molars. **Diagnosis** is defined as the determination of the nature, and the identification of an abnormal condition or disease. An example of interpretation would be showing the patient the image of the developing third molar on the radiograph, whereas diagnosis would be the dentist determining that the third molar is impacted. Referring a patient to the dentist for evaluation of a radiolucent finding on the proximal surface of a tooth that appears on a bitewing is interpretation. Dental hygienists and dental assistants are trained to identify this deviation from normal-appearing enamel and can point out these deviations for further evaluation by the dentist. Telling the patient that the radiolucency is caries and requires treatment is diagnosis, a responsibility of the dentist.

The dental hygienist and dental assistant play a valuable role in the preliminary diagnosis, by interpreting deviations from normal radiographic anatomy and calling these to the attention of the dentist. The more pairs of eyes evaluating the radiographs, the more benefit to the patient.

Viewing Equipment

A **viewbox** and a magnifying glass are required for optimal film viewing (Figure 18–5). Holding radiographs up to the overhead room light will not provide adequate conditions in which to observe detailed, subtle changes often revealed by radiographs.

- **Viewbox.** Many types of viewboxes are available. The ideal type for the oral healthcare practice has a dark non-reflective frame, a frosted glass panel, and a rheostat to vary the intensity of the light. The viewbox lighting must be of uniform intensity and be evenly diffused. The viewing surface should be large enough to accommodate a full set of intraoral radiographs as well as typical dental extraoral radiographs, i.e., panoramic radiographs. The film mount or a cardboard template should be used to mask out distracting light around the mount. Blocking out excess sidelight reduces glare and facilitates viewing. The use of gray or black cardboard or frosted plastic film mounts helps to reduce glare and enhances the detail of the images. Always use subdued room lighting to allow the eyes to adapt to the light level of the radiographs.

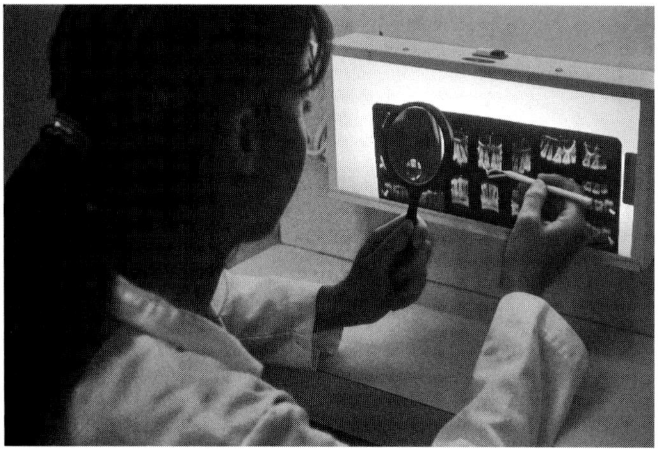

FIGURE 18-5 **Radiographer viewing radiographs.** Radiographs should be viewed in subdued room lighting, using a viewbox and a magnifying glass. Note the black film mount that blocks distracting light around the films.

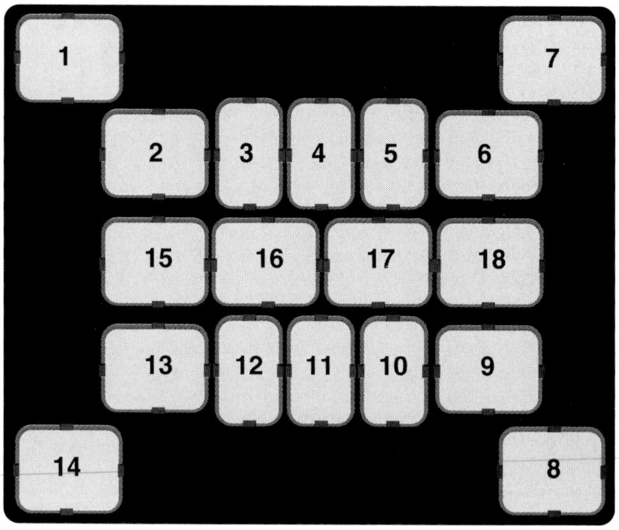

FIGURE 18-7 **Proper sequence for viewing radiographs.** The radiographer should view the radiographs in the sequence illustrated. Start with number 1 and proceed clockwise through number 18.

- **Magnifying glass.** Some viewers are equipped with a magnifying device (Figure 18–6). Otherwise, a hand-held magnifying glass should be used to aid the viewer.

Depending on the radiographer's training and responsibility, the individual may now proceed to make a preliminary interpretation and discuss it with the dentist who will make the final diagnosis regarding any findings. A thorough examination is best accomplished when a specific sequence of analysis is used (Procedure Box 18–2 and Figure 18–7). The mounted radiographs must be viewed in a systematic order to prevent errors in interpretation. All available radiographs should be examined for a specific condition, and then the examination process should be repeated for the next condition. For example, the radiographs may be examined first for the presence or absence of teeth and other development anomalies. A second examination could concentrate on detecting caries, and the third examination would look for periodontal conditions. Interpreting these conditions is discussed in Chapters 20, 21, and 22.

When interpreting more than one radiograph, such as a set of bitewings or a full mouth series, the teeth and the supporting structures are often imaged more than once. While maintaining a systematic order of interpretation, it is helpful to compare each area in all of the views. For example, a suspected periodontal condition may be observed on a maxillary periapical radiograph, while the bitewing radiograph may possibly image the level of bone with more detail. Comparing adjacent films will add to a thorough interpretation.

All radiographic findings must be noted in the patient's record after confirmation by the dentist. Although all professionals may record findings, the final interpretation and diagnosis is the responsibility of the dentist.

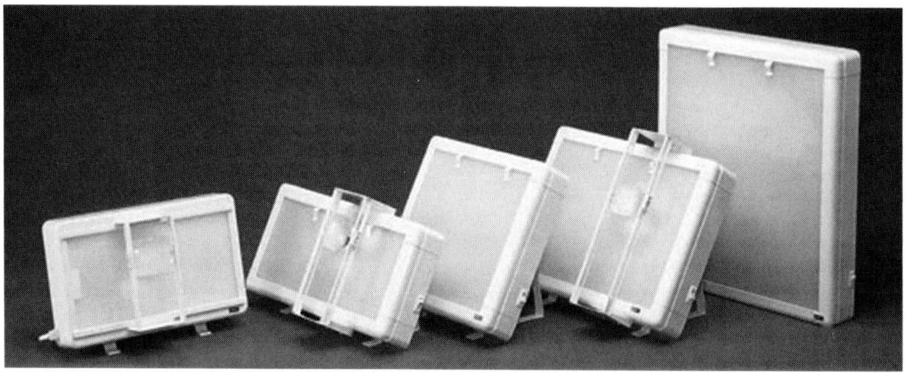

FIGURE 18-6 **Viewboxes come in many varieties.** Note the attached magnifying device on three of these viewboxes. (Courtesy of Dentsply Rinn)

PROCEDURE 18–2

SUGGESTED SEQUENCE FOR VIEWING A FULL MOUTH SERIES OF RADIOGRAPHS

1. Place the mounted radiographs on the viewbox.
2. Dim the overhead lights and turn on the viewbox light.
3. Using a magnifying glass, begin the examination in the patient's maxillary right posterior region (Figure 18–7).
4. Proceed horizontally to the anterior region and continue to the patient's maxillary left posterior region.
5. Next, move down to the patient's mandibular left posterior region.
6. Proceed horizontally to the anterior region and continue to the patient's mandibular right posterior region.
7. Next, move up to the bitewing radiographs, starting with the right molar bitewing radiograph on the left side of the film mount. Proceed horizontally, examining each bitewing radiograph until you finish with the left molar bitewing radiograph on the right side of the film mount.
8. Repeat steps 3 through 7 for the following conditions:
   a. Presence or absence of teeth
   b. Tooth morphology and eruption patterns
   c. Deviations from normal and/or suspected pathology
   d. Presence, type, and condition of dental materials
   e. Caries
   f. Periodontal conditions and risk factors
9. Document all findings on a preliminary radiographic interpretative form.
10. Collaborate with the dentist regarding findings.
11. After confirmation and diagnosis of findings by the dentist, record findings on the patient's permanent record.
12. Assist the dentist in explaining findings and treatment plan to the patient using the radiographs.

Using Mounted Radiographs

Radiographs should be developed and mounted as soon as possible and placed on the viewbox during the patient's appointment for easy reference during treatment. At each subsequent appointment the latest radiographs should be placed on the viewbox, where they can be easily accessed as needed.

After the appointment, all radiographs should be thoroughly interpreted during time set aside for this purpose. Unless only one or two radiographs were taken, there may not have been enough time during the patient's appointment to thoroughly review each film for all possible conditions. Once the interpretation is complete, the radiographs should be filed appropriately and kept indefinitely as part of the patient's permanent record. The need for an orderly filing system cannot be overstressed. Misplaced radiographs can result in inappropriate treatment being rendered, risk management problems, and may have legal implications. All radiographs should be handled with care to prevent smudging or scratching. Radiographs should be protected from heat damage by storage in cool, well ventilated areas.

Although radiographs will lose value after more than six months or one year because oral conditions change constantly in most patients, they are valuable for comparing present with previous conditions. Sometimes radiographs are needed in a court of law. Therefore, radiographs should be preserved until the statute of limitations has expired. Since laws vary from state to state, and may not always apply under certain conditions, radiographs should be kept indefinitely (see Chapter 10).

REVIEW—Chapter Summary

A thorough knowledge of normal radiographic anatomical landmarks is needed for mounting and interpreting radiographs. Mounting films is recommended for its many advantages. Film mounts vary in size and number of frames, but all have space for documenting information such as the patient's name and date of exposure. Each film has an embossed identification dot used to determine the patient's left and right sides. Lingual mounting places the identification dot in a concave position, so that the patient's left side is the viewer's left side.

Labial mounting places the identification dot in a convex position, so that the patient's left side is the viewer's right side. Labial mounting method is the recommended method.

To aid in fast and accurate mounting of radiographs, a systematic procedure should be followed. The first step in film mounting is to orient the embossed identification dot the same way (convex) for all radiographs. There are several generalizations regarding the teeth and oral cavity anatomy that can be used to aid in mounting radiographs correctly.

Interpretation is explanatory, as is the reading of radiographs. Diagnosis uses radiographs to determine the nature and identification of the disease or abnormality. Dental radiographs may be interpreted by the dentist, dental hygienist, or dental assistant. The dentist is responsible for the final diagnosis.

Viewing radiographs is facilitated with the use of a viewbox and magnification. Mounted radiographs must be viewed in a systematic order to prevent errors in interpretation.

Radiographs should be interpreted thoroughly during or after the patient's appointment. Radiographs should be accurately labeled and filed and kept indefinitely.

RECALL—Study Questions

1. List four advantages of mounting intraoral radiographs:
   a. ____________________
   b. ____________________
   c. ____________________
   d. ____________________
2. Which of these helps to determine whether the radiograph is the patient's left or right side?
   a. Slight "smile" appearance
   b. Distally curved roots
   c. Large crowns
   d. Identification dot
3. A desirable film mount should be:
   a. Made of cardboard.
   b. Made of plastic.
   c. Translucent, to allow light to reach the film.
   d. Black, to block out light transmission and prevent glare.
4. Labial method film mounting positions the identification dot concave. The labial method is the recommended film mounting method.
   a. The first statement is true; the second statement is false.
   b. The first statement is false; the second statement is true.
   c. Both statements are true.
   d. Both statements are false.
5. Lingual method film mounting positions the identification dot convex. When utilizing the lingual method, the viewer's right is the patient's left.
   a. The first statement is true; the second statement is false.
   b. The first statement is false; the second statement is true.
   c. Both statements are true.
   d. Both statements are false.
6. Mounting is the placement of radiographs in a holder arranged in anatomical order. All radiographs should be handled with care to prevent smudging or scratching.
   a. The first statement is true; the second statement is false.
   b. The first statement is false; the second statement is true.
   c. Both statements are true.
   d. Both statements are false.
7. Which of the following should be done first when mounting radiographs?
   a. Orient the identification dot the same way
   b. Separate bitewing from periapical films
   c. Separate the anterior from the posterior films
   d. Orient the teeth roots to point in the correct direction
8. All of the following will aid the radiographer in correctly mounting radiographs *except* one. Which one is this *exception?*
   a. Anterior films were positioned with the long dimension vertically.
   b. Canine teeth generally have the longest roots.
   c. Maxillary molars usually have three roots.
   d. Roots and crowns of mandibular teeth are usually larger than maxillary teeth.
9. Reading and explaining radiographic images is:
   a. Diagnosing.
   b. Interpreting.
   c. Viewing.
   d. Mounting.
10. The final responsibility to diagnose the radiograph rests with the:
    a. Dental assistant.
    b. Dental hygienist.
    c. Dentist.
    d. Patient.
11. Mounted radiographs must be viewed in a systematic sequence to prevent errors in interpretation. Mounted radiographs may be adequately viewed by holding the mount up to room light.
    a. The first statement is true; the second statement is false.
    b. The first statement is false; the second statement is true.
    c. Both statements are true.
    d. Both statements are false.
12. In which region is it best to begin the interpretation process when viewing radiographs mounted using the labial method?
    a. Maxillary left posterior
    b. Maxillary right posterior
    c. Mandibular left posterior
    d. Mandibular right posterior
13. Following diagnosis by the dentist, the radiographic findings must be recorded on the patient's record by the:
    a. Dental assistant.
    b. Dental hygienist.
    c. Dentist.
    d. Any of the above.

REFLECT—Case Study

These four radiographs have just exited the automatic processor. Based on what you learned in this chapter, correctly "mount" each of these four radiographs by writing the corresponding number in the correct frame of the film mount. Assuming the identification dots are all positioned convex, label the film mount indicating the left and right sides. Then address the following:

1. Describe how you determined which side was the left and which side was the right.
2. List the steps you followed to mount these radiographs correctly.
3. List three generalizations you used to mount these films.
4. List three final checks you would make to double-check your mounting procedure.

RELATE—Laboratory Application

For a comprehensive laboratory practice exercise on this topic, see E. M. Thomson, *Exercises in Oral Radiography Techniques: A Laboratory Manual,* 2nd ed., Upper Saddle River, NJ: Prentice Hall, 2007. Chapter 8, "Film Mounting and Radiographic Landmarks."

BIBLIOGRAPHY

Langland, O. E. & Langlais, R. P. *Principles of Dental Imaging,* 2nd ed. Philadelphia: Lippincott Williams & Wilkins, 2002.

White, S. C. & Pharoah, M. J. *Oral Radiology Principles and Interpretation,* 5th ed. St. Louis: Elsevier, 2004.

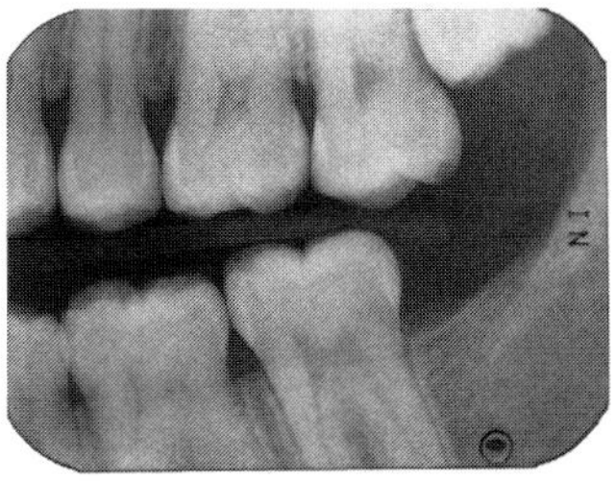
1

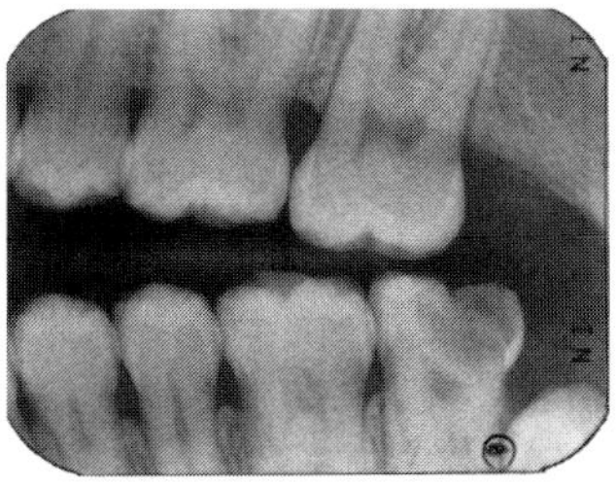
2

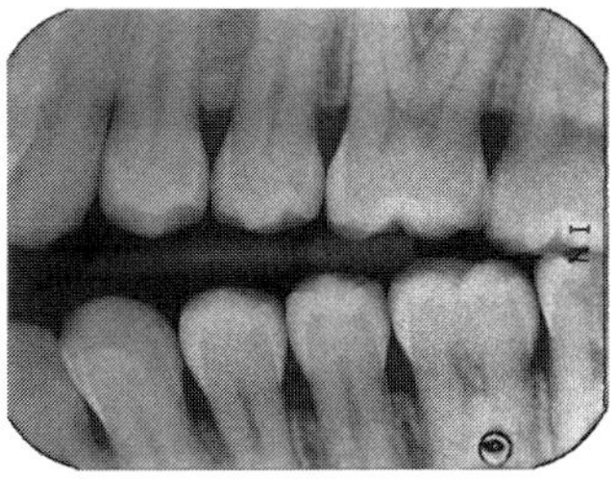
3

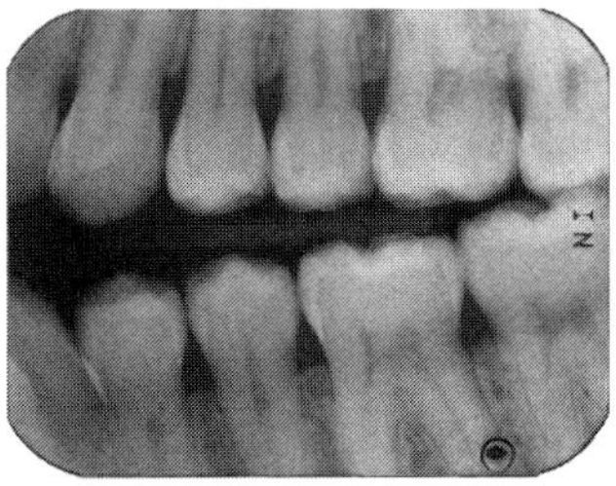
4

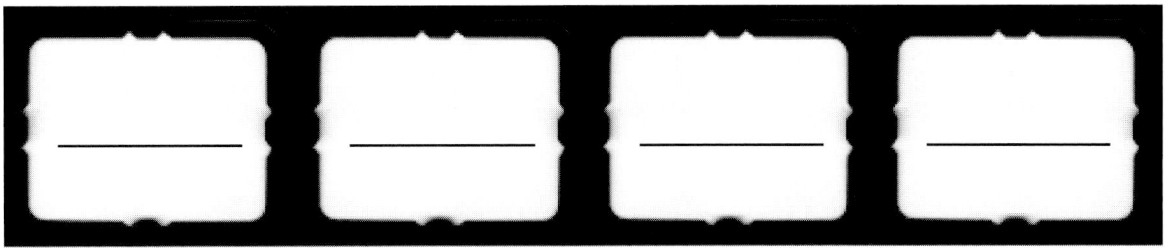

19

Recognizing Normal Radiographic Anatomy

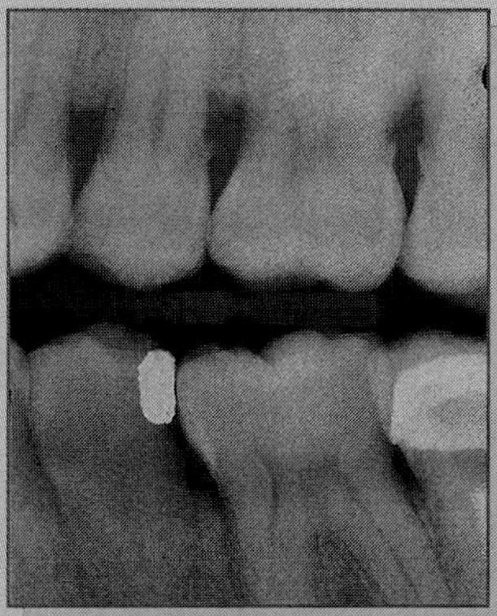

CHAPTER OUTLINE

■ OBJECTIVES

Following successful completion of this chapter, you should be able to:

1. Define the key words.
2. Provide three rationales for why it is important to recognize and identify normal anatomical landmarks of the face and head.
3. Describe and identify the facial and cranial bones.
4. Differentiate between the lamina dura and the periodontal ligament space.
5. Describe and identify the radiographic appearance of all structures of the teeth.
6. Name all of the anatomical landmarks of the maxilla and mandible.
7. Name and identify all landmarks or features normally seen on intraoral radiographs of the maxilla and mandible.

■ KEY WORDS

Alveolar bone
Alveolar process
Alveolus
Angle of mandible
Anodontia
Anterior nasal spine
Apical foramen
Cancellous bone
Cementum
Condyle
Coronoid process of the mandible
Cortical bone
Dentin
Dentition
Enamel
Exfoliation
External auditory meatus (foramen)
Floor (border) of the maxillary sinus
Foramen
Frontal bone
Genial tubercles
Hamulus
Impacted teeth
Incisive (anterior palatine) foramen
Inferior border of mandible
Inverted Y
Lamina dura
Lateral fossa
Lingual foramen
Mandible
Mandibular canal
Mandibular foramen
Mastoid process
Maxilla
Maxillary sinus
Maxillary tuberosity
Median palatine suture
Mental foramen

Mental fossa	Ramus
Mental ridge	Septum
Mylohyoid ridge	Sigmoid (mandibular) notch
Nasal bones	Sinus (maxillary)
Nasal conchae	Sphenoid bone
Nasal fossa (cavity)	Styloid process
Nasal septum	Submandibular fossa
Nasal spine	Supernumerary teeth
Nutrient canal	Suture
Nutrient foramen	Symphysis
Oblique ridge	Temporal bone
Occipital bone	Torus mandibularis (lingual torus)
Periodontal ligament (PDL)	Trabecular bone
Permanent teeth	Tubercle
Primary teeth	Tuberosity (maxillary)
Process	Zygoma
Pterygoid plates	Zygomatic arch
Pulp chamber (cavity)	Zygomatic process

Introduction

As you learned in Chapter 18, knowledge of normal radiographic anatomy is required for mounting and interpreting dental radiographs. Before the radiographer can identify a deviation from the normal, a solid base knowledge of what is normal is required. The beginning radiographer first learns to identify facial landmarks that assist in aligning the correct angles and direction of the PID for proper technique (see Figure 12–9). But it is while learning to read radiographic images and to recognize normal radiographic anatomy that the radiographer begins to develop an appreciation for precise film packet placement and accurate techniques. The importance of learning to identify normal radiographic anatomy may be summarized as follows:

1. To evaluate a film for correct positioning so that the areas of interest and anatomical structures are clearly visible, enhancing the diagnostic value of the radiograph.
2. To assist in determining into which frame of the x-ray mount each radiograph is to be mounted.
3. To assist in interpreting radiographs and recognizing a deviation from the normal that would require referral to the dentist for evaluation.

The purpose of this chapter is to review the anatomy of the head and neck region and to describe these anatomical structures as they often appear on dental radiographs.

Significant Normal Anatomical Landmarks

Although most anatomical landmarks observed on intraoral radiographs are located on the maxilla or the mandible, the radiographer should also be able to recognize and identify the major bones and anatomical structures of the cranium and face. Such knowledge is particularly useful when reading cephalometric, temporomandibular joint, or panoramic exposures.

Some of the other cranial and facial bones that may be imaged onto dental radiographs are illustrated in Figures 19–1 and 19–2. These include the: **frontal bone,** the right and left parietal bones, the **occipital bone,** the right and left **temporal bones,** the right and left **zygomas** (zygomatic bone, also called malar bone or cheekbone), the **zygomatic arch,** which is made up of the temporal process of the zygoma and the zygomatic process of the temporal bone, the **sphenoid bone,** the right and left **nasal bones,** the **external auditory meatus (foramen),** the **styloid process,** the **mastoid process** of the temporal bone, the right and left **maxilla,** and the **mandible.**

The teeth are located within the alveolar processes of the maxillae and the mandible; thus most dental radiographs include portions of these bones. The maxillae are actually two bones, a right and left maxilla, whereas the mandible is a single bone. Generally, but not always, the same landmarks appear on both right and left sides.

It is helpful to consider the overall location of these features prior to learning how and where each will appear on an intraoral radiograph. Figure 19–3 shows the **nasal septum** and the **nasal spine.** Figure 19–4 illustrates the location of the **median palatine suture, maxillary tuberosity** area, and the **incisive (anterior palatine) foramen.** The **maxillary sinus** is an empty space within the maxilla. Figures 19–5 and 19–6 illustrate the structures of the mandible: body, **ramus, inferior border, alveolar process, angle of the mandible, condyle, coronoid process, sigmoid (mandibular) notch, mandibular foramen, mental foramen, mandibular canal** which is located within the

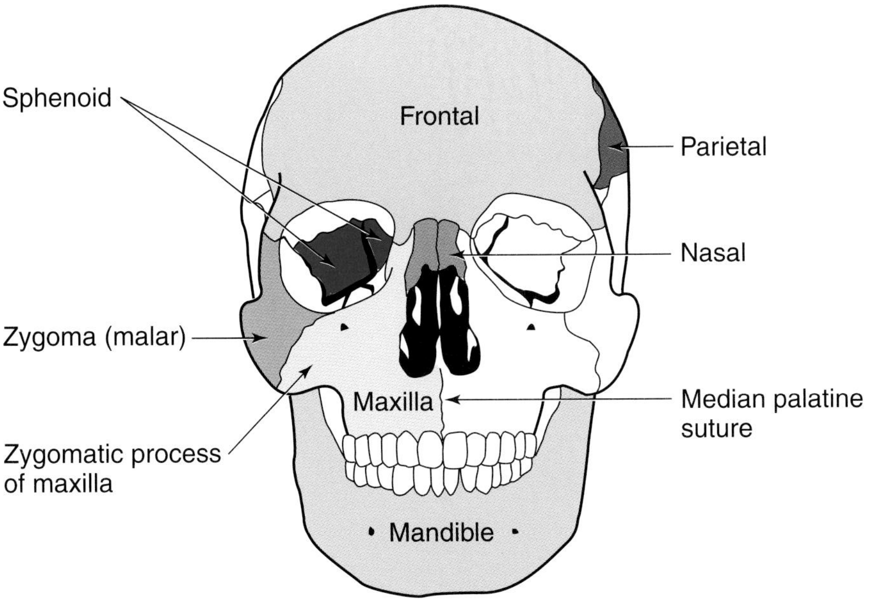

FIGURE 19–1 **Frontal view of the skull.**

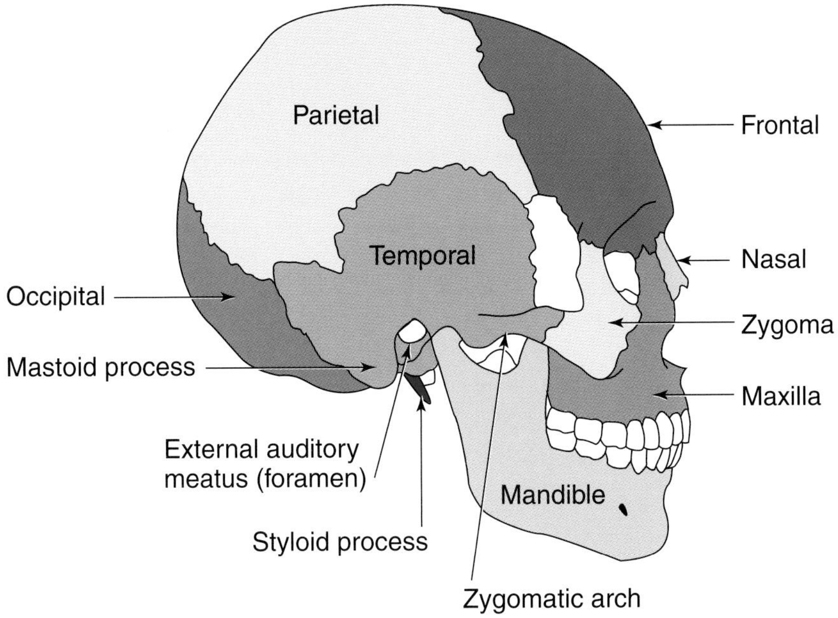

FIGURE 19–2 **Lateral view of the skull.**

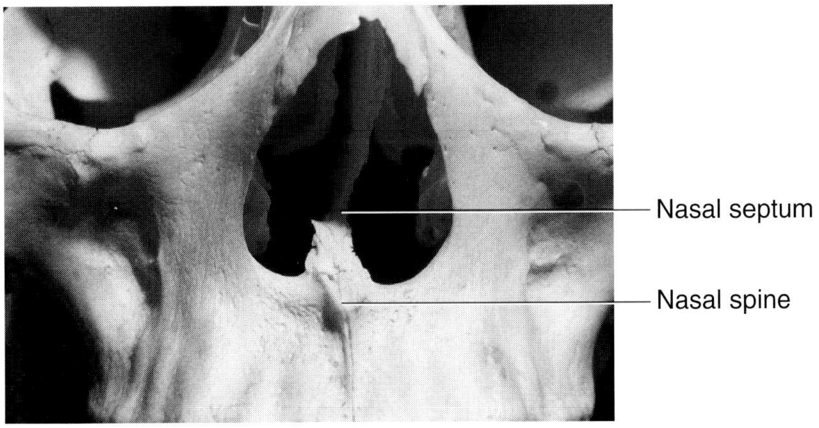

FIGURE 19–3 **Frontal view of the nose.**

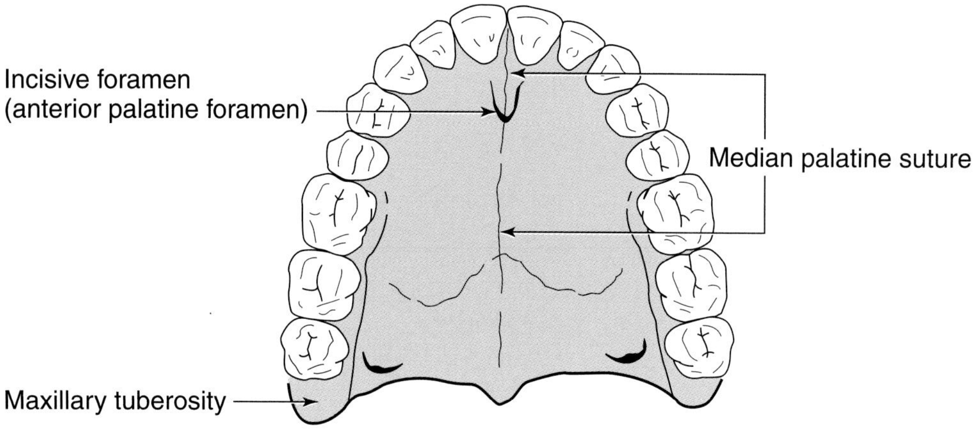

FIGURE 19-4 **Palatal view of maxilla.**

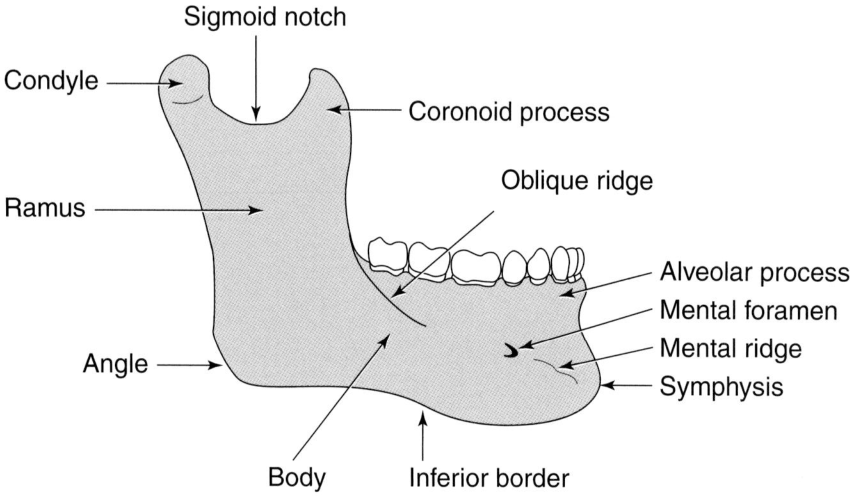

FIGURE 19-5 **Lateral view of detached mandible.**

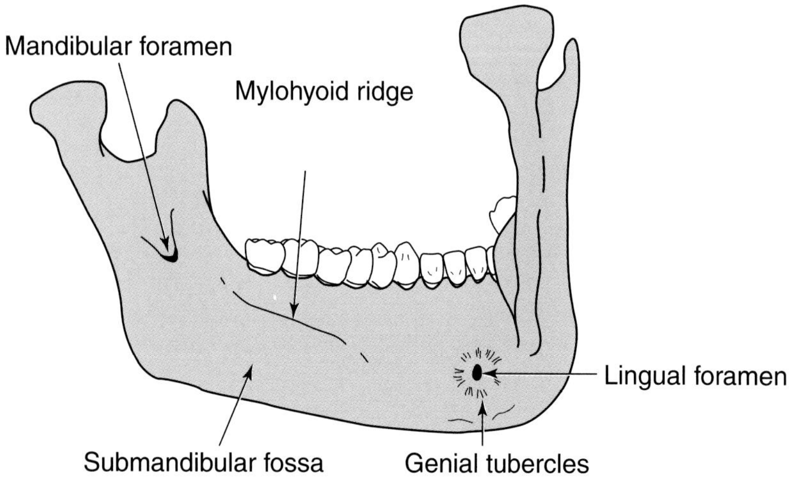

FIGURE 19-6 **Lingual view of detached mandible.**

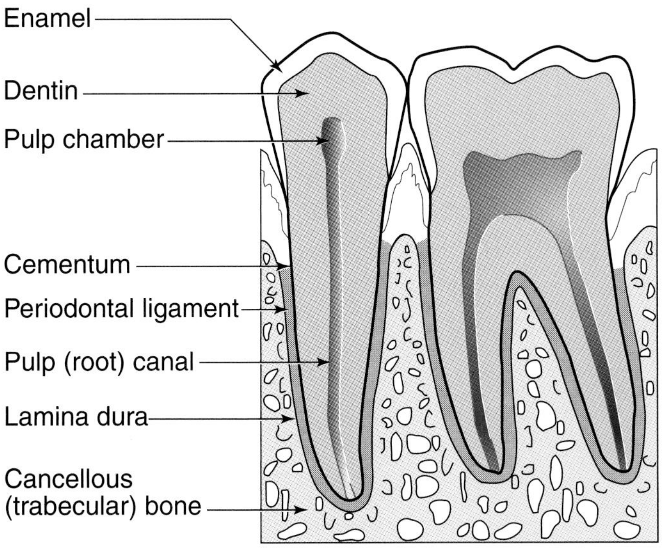

FIGURE 19–7 **Drawing of mandibular premolar–molar area.**

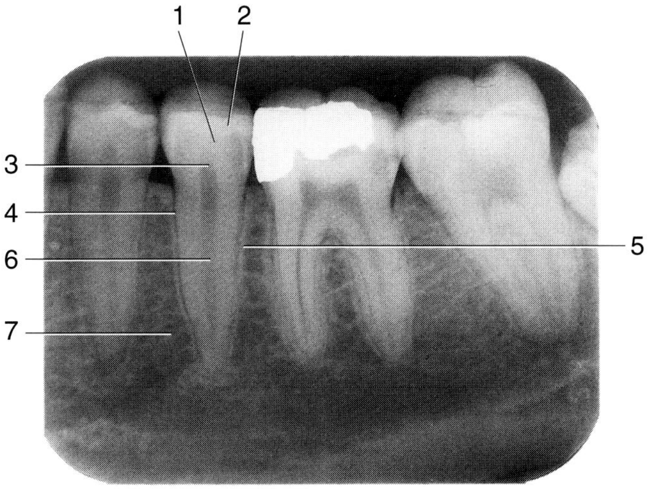

FIGURE 19–8 **Radiograph of mandibular premolar area.** This radiograph shows (**1**) dentin, (**2**) enamel, (**3**) pulp chamber, (**4**) periodontal ligament space, (**5**) lamina dura, (**6**) pulp (root) canal, and (**7**) cancellous (trabecular) bone. Note that because only a very thin layer of cementum covers the root, it is radiographically indistinguishable from the underlying dentin.

mandible between the mandibular foramen and the mental foramen, **mental ridge, symphysis, lingual foramen, genial tubercles, oblique ridge, mylohyoid ridge,** and the **submandibular fossa.**

Some of these landmarks are visible only on larger occlusal and extraoral radiographs. Depending on the film packet placement, patient positioning and the angle of the x-ray beam, certain landmarks may or may not be imaged. Furthermore, the angle of the x-ray beam may distort the appearance of the structure so that it may not always appear exactly as illustrated in this textbook. However, a working knowledge of what structures are likely to be imaged will further assist the radiographer in achieving competence in this skill.

Radiographic Appearance of the Alveolar Bone and Tooth Area

Before considering the appearance of these specific bones and their features on a full mouth series of radiographs, it is important to recognize and identify the normal appearance of **alveolar bone** and the structures of the teeth. Compare the drawing in Figure 19–7 with a radiograph of the same area shown in Figure 19–8.

Bone

Although bones appear solid, they are solid only on the outside and are honeycombed within. Bone is classified as **cortical bone,** a compact or dense form of bone, such as that which lines the outside layers of the maxillae and the mandible, and **cancellous** or spongy **bone,** which forms the bulk of the inner bone.

Small, interconnected **trabeculae** (bars or plates of bone) form a multitude of various-sized compartments that account for the honeycomb appearance. These trabecular spaces are usually filled with fat, blood, or bone cells, which accounts for the difference in the radiographic appearance of bone.

All bone tissues appear radiopaque. The compact or cortical outside layer appears extremely radiopaque (white), whereas the cancellous bone varies in radiopacity (shades of gray) according to the size and number of the trabecular spaces. The area may even appear almost radiolucent (black) if these spaces are very large or if the bone is thin, as is the case in the area of the submandibular fossa.

By definition, the **alveolar process** is that portion of the maxilla or mandible that surrounds and supports the teeth. It is composed of the **lamina dura** and the supporting bone.

Lamina Dura

The lamina dura is the hard, cortical bone that lines the **alveolus** (the tooth socket). On radiographs, the lamina dura appears as a thin radiopaque (white) border that outlines the shape of the alveolus (the root of the tooth). The supporting bone is cancellous and varies in density in the different parts of the alveolar process.

Periodontal Ligament Space

The teeth are attached to the lamina dura by the fibers of the **periodontal ligament (PDL).** The PDL itself is made up of soft tissues and therefore will not be imaged on a radiograph. However, the space in which the PDL lies is often visible as a thin radiolucent (dark) border between the lamina dura and the roots of the teeth.

Nutrient Canals

Nutrient canals are thin radiolucent lines of fairly uniform width that sometimes exhibit radiopaque borders. They contain blood vessels and nerves that supply the teeth, bone, and gingivae. Nutrient canals are most often visualized in the anterior of the mandible and in edentulous areas. Sometimes a **nutrient foramen** will be imaged as a tiny radiolucent dot.

Teeth

The tooth structures are enamel, dentin, cementum, and pulp. **Enamel,** the hardest body structure, covers the crown and is very radiopaque. The underlying **dentin** is not as dense and appears less radiopaque. The **cementum** that covers the roots is even less dense. Because only a thin layer of cementum covers the root, it is generally indistinguishable radiographically from the underlying dentin (Figure 19–8). Although all three highly calcified tooth structures vary in radiopacity in direct proportion to the thickness of each structure in the path of the x-ray beam, for descriptive purposes enamel, dentin, and cementum are considered radiopaque.

The tooth pulp that occupies the **pulp chamber** and the root canals is the only noncalcified tooth tissue. As this soft tissue offers only minimal resistance to the passage of x-rays, it appears radiolucent. The end of the root canal is called the **apical foramen.** This foramen permits the passage of nerves and blood vessels that nourish the tooth structures.

Dentition

To correctly identify and interpret radiographs, one needs to understand the **dentition.** Young children have 20 **primary teeth** that are gradually lost as they grow older. During the transition years a mixed dentition—that is, both primary and permanent teeth—may be present. A radiograph may show the primary teeth with partially resorbed roots, which are in a process of **exfoliation,** as well as permanent teeth whose roots are not yet fully formed, which are in the process of eruption. This is a normal phenomenon and is often observed in radiographs of children 10 to 12 years old and younger (Figure 19–9). There are 32 **permanent teeth,** including all four of the third molars (wisdom teeth).

Occasionally, teeth form but are unable to erupt: These are described as **impacted teeth.** Some people have one or more extra teeth; these are called **supernumerary teeth.** Another deviation is the congenital absence of certain teeth, described as **anodontia.** These conditions occur so frequently that, although not normal, they are not considered pathologic.

Anatomy Basics, Intraoral Radiographs

Learning to identify anatomical structures and their specific landmarks takes practice. Radiographs provide a two-dimensional image of three-dimensional structures. When imaging the head and neck region, multiple structures may be be imaged superimposed on top of each other, adding to the difficulty of correctly identifying these structures. The first step in becoming competent at this skill is to understand what basic anatomy may be in the path of the x-ray beam and hence, end up being imaged on the radiograph (Figure 19–10).

Additionally, it is helpful to be aware of which structures appear radiopaque and radiolucent. As you will recall from Chapter 4, structures that are dense and absorb or resist the passage of x-rays will appear light or white on the radiograph. Struc-

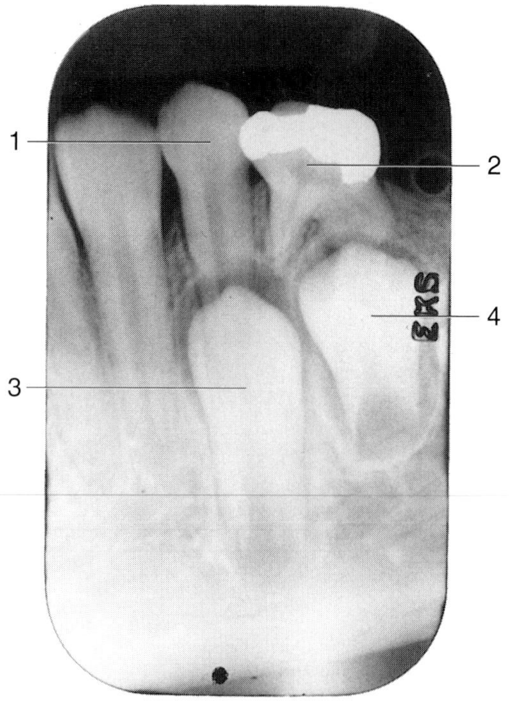

FIGURE 19-9 **Radiograph of mixed dentition in mandibular canine area.** This radiograph shows (**1**) primary canine, (**2**) primary first molar with partially resorbed roots, (**3**) permanent canine, and (**4**) permanent first premolar with incomplete root formation.

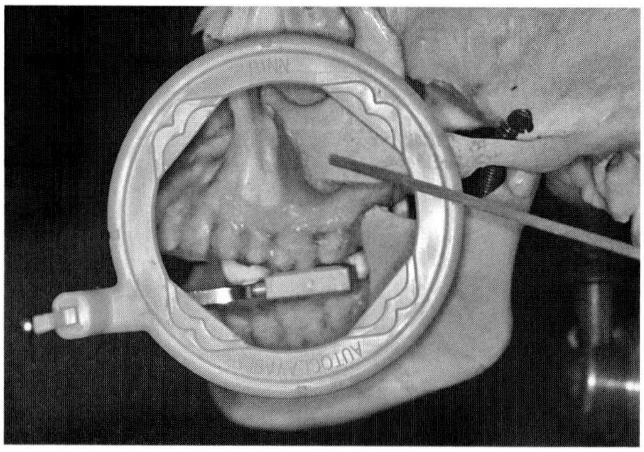

FIGURE 19-10 **Facial bones imaged on radiographs.** Note the position of the PID when exposing a maxillary posterior periapical radiograph. The zygomatic arch will most likely be imaged on this radiograph.

TABLE 19–1 **Radiopaque and Radiolucent Features**

Radiopaque	Radiolucent
Bone	Canal
Border (wall)	Foramen
Process	Fossa
Ridge	Meatus
Spine	Sinus
Tubercles	Space (PDL)
Tuberosity	Suture

tures that permit the passage of x-rays with little or no resistance will appear dark or black. Bone and its dense features such as a ridge, spine, or tubercle will appear radiopaque, while less dense features such as a foramen, canal, or suture will appear radiolucent. To aid the radiographer in learning the radiographic appearance of anatomy, it is helpful to remember that a landmark called the oblique *ridge* will be a radiopaque structure and a landmark called the mental *foramen* will appear radiolucent (Table 19–1).

Just as it is helpful to follow a systematic order when mounting and interpreting films, the radiographer will benefit from organizing the identification of anatomical landmarks into specific steps. Because memorizing the structures that make up the head and neck region can be a overwhelming task, the following system is offered to assist the beginning radiographer in learning to identify structures commonly imaged on intraoral radiographs (Figure 19–11).

As illustrated by the flow chart in Figure 19–11, differentiating among which structures will most likely be imaged on intraoral radiographs of the maxilla and which structures will be imaged on intraoral radiographs of the mandible will help the radiographer organize the anatomy terms and narrow the possible choices. When beginning the interpretation process, first determine if the intraoral radiograph you are looking at is a maxillary view or a mandibular view. See Chapter 18 for generalizations that aid in determining whether or not a radiograph is of the maxilla or the mandible. Once it has been determined which arch is imaged, determine if the view is of the anterior or the posterior region. As you will recall, anterior film packets are usually positioned with the long dimension vertically, whereas posterior film packets are placed with the long dimension positioned horizontally (see Chapter 18). Certain anatomical structures are more likely to be visible on radiographs of the anterior region, while others are more likely to be visible in the posterior region. Furthermore, prior to deciding which anatomical structure is being observed, the radiographer should determine whether or not the structure is radiopaque or radiolucent. A radiopaque appearance indicates a structure that is dense, hence eliminating labeling that structure as a foramen or fossa or other feature that would not present as radiopaque. Likewise, a radiolucent appearance indicates a structure that is less dense, so the terms process or ridge would not apply to radiolucent observations.

Organizing the interpretation of normal radiographic anatomy in this manner (Figure 19–11) will assist the beginning radiographer by providing a framework upon which to learn the terms associated with head and neck radiography, and will continue to be a basis for building on these basic interpretative skills. A working knowledge of the radiographic appearance of normal anatomy must be mastered in order to develop the skills needed to recognize deviations from the normal such as periodontal disease, caries and growth and development anomalies.

In keeping with the system laid out in Figure 19–11, anatomical landmarks in this chapter are separated into anatomy that is most likely to be observed on intraoral radiographs of the:

1. Maxillary anterior region.
2. Maxillary posterior region.
3. Mandibular anterior region.
4. Mandibular posterior region.

Depending on the manner in which the film was positioned, and the angle at which the exposure was made, the expected anatomical landmark may or may not be visible. Sometimes the landmark is visible on only the right or only the left side. Keeping this in mind, the following descriptions offer guidance for learning these structures.

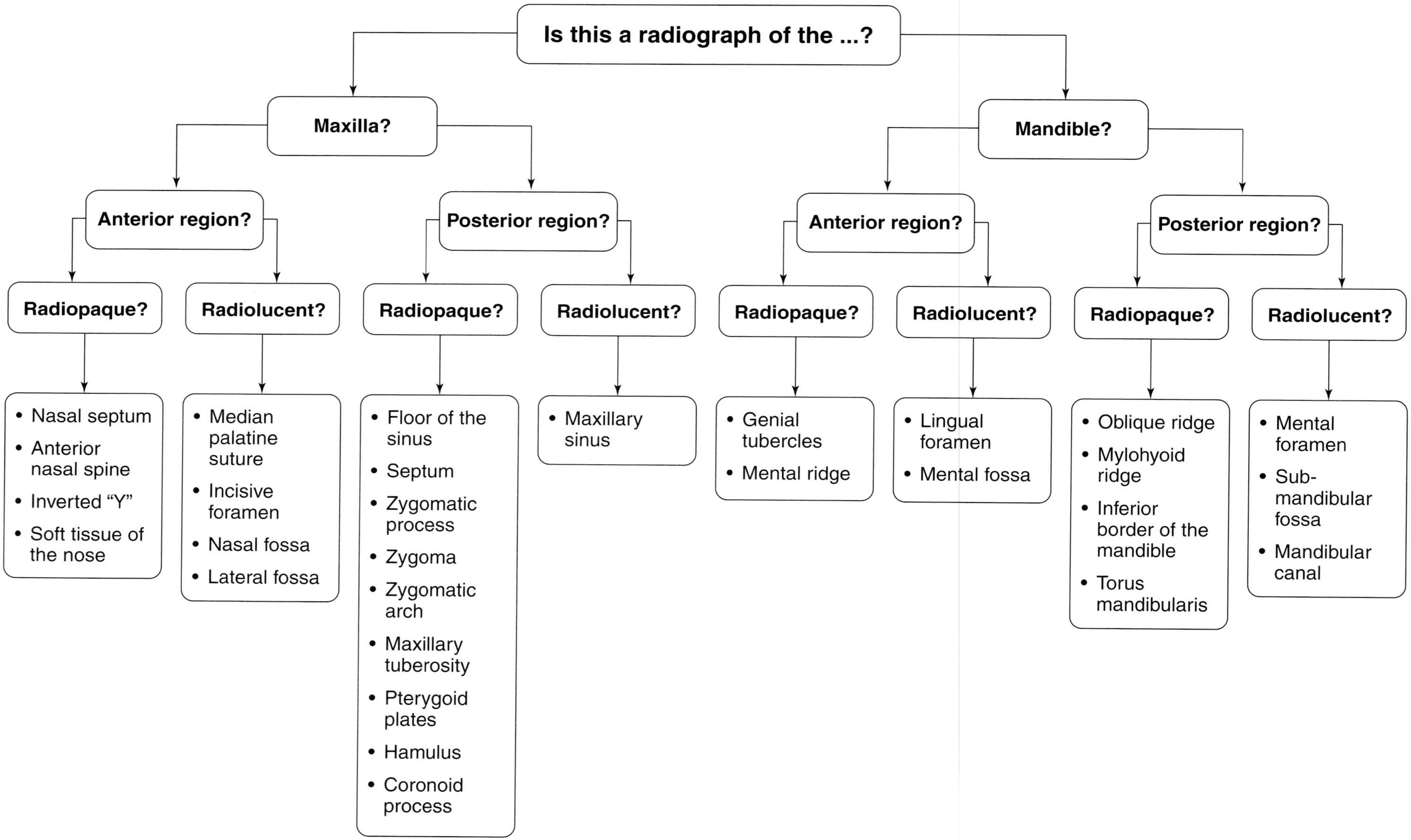

FIGURE 19–11 **Sequence for interpreting normal radiographic anatomy.**

Maxillary Anterior Region (Figures 19–12 through 19–15)

Radiopaque Features

1. **Nasal septum.** A dense cartilage structure that separates the right nasal fossa from the left. Usually appears as a vertical radiopaque line separating the paired radiolucencies of the nasal cavity.
2. **Anterior nasal spine.** A V-shaped projection from the floor of the nasal fossa in the midline. Usually appears as a triangle-shaped radiopacity.
3. **Inverted Y.** An important landmark seen in the canine–premolar area, made up of the lateral wall of the nasal fossa and the anterior-medial wall of the maxillary sinus. The intersection of these two radiopaque lines often criss-cross each other in the form of the letter Y. This Y shape often appears upside down or turned on its side.
4. **Soft tissue of the nose.** Sometimes an outline of the soft tissue of the nose may be shadowed onto anterior intraoral radiographs (Figures 19–16 and 19–17).

Radiolucent Features

1. **Median palatine suture.** A radiolucent thin line that delineates the midline of the palate and the junction of the right and left maxilla. Frequently seen between the central incisors, this structure should not be mistaken for a fracture.
2. **Incisive foramen (anterior palatine foramen).** A round or pear-shaped radiolucent opening that varies greatly in size serves for the passage of nerves and blood vessels. It is often visible near or between the apices of the central incisors. (This foramen should not be mistaken for an abscess, cyst, or other pathological condition.)
3. **Nasal fossa (cavity).** A large air space divided into two paired radiolucencies by the radiopaque nasal septum, often visible above the roots of the incisors. The radiolucency of the nasal cavities will vary in dark appearance, depending on the angle of the x-ray beam. At times, the x-ray beam may have to penetrate the **nasal conchae,** thin bony extensions of the nasal wall, and result in a less radiolucent appearance of the nasal fossa itself.
4. **Lateral fossa.** A radiolucency between the maxillary lateral incisor and the maxillary canine representing the decreased thickness in bone in this area.

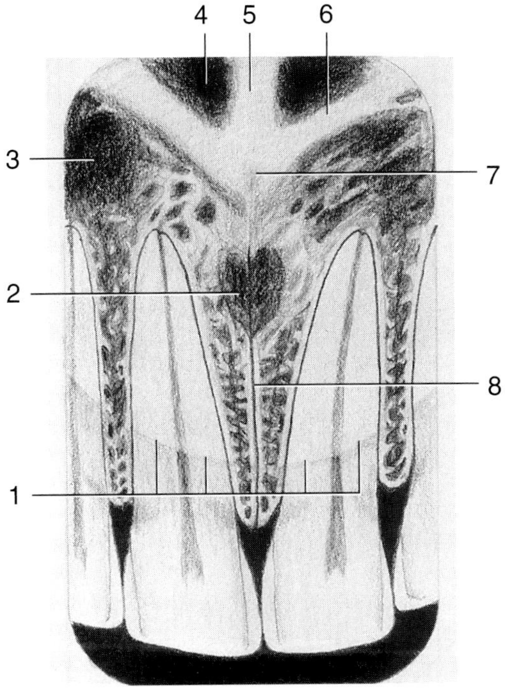

FIGURE 19–12 **Drawing of maxillary midline area.** Shown are the (**1**) outline of nose, (**2**) incisive foramen (anterior palatine foramen), (**3**) lateral fossa, (**4**) nasal fossa, (**5**) nasal septum, (**6**) border of nasal fossa, (**7**) anterior nasal spine, and (**8**) median palatine suture.

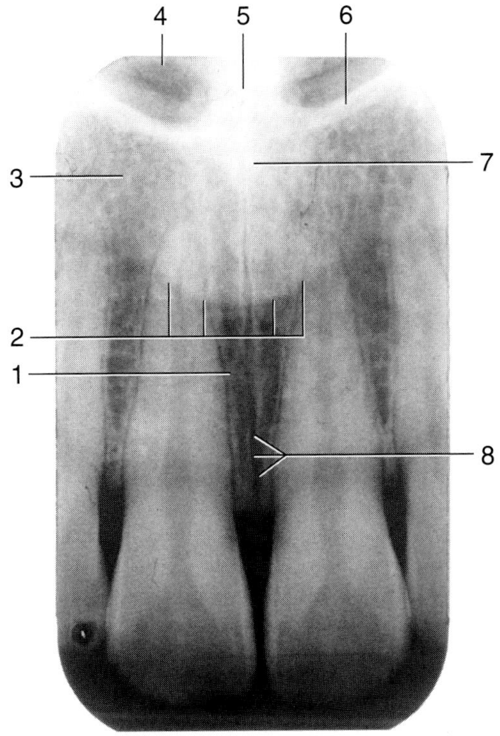

FIGURE 19–13 **Radiograph of maxillary midline area.** This radiograph shows the (**1**) incisive (anterior palatine) foramen, indicated by an irregularly shaped, rounded radiolucent area. Also seen are the (**2**) outline of the nose, (**3**) lateral fossa, (**4**) nasal fossa (radiolucent), (**5**) nasal septum (radiopaque), (**6**) border of nasal fossa, (**7**) anterior nasal spine, and (**8**) median palatine suture.

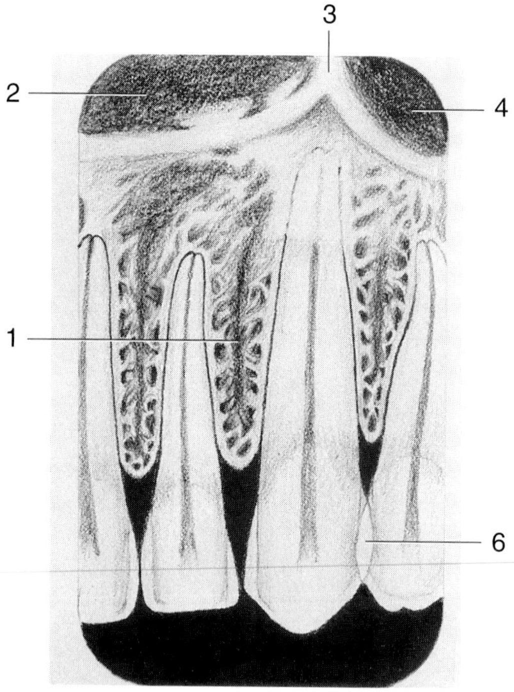

FIGURE 19-14 **Drawing of maxillary canine area.** The drawing shows the (**1**) lateral fossa, (**2**) nasal fossa, (**3**) inverted Y (intersection of the borders of nasal fossa and maxillary sinus), and (**4**) maxillary sinus. (**5**) Note the dense radiopaque area caused by overlapping of the mesial surface of the first premolar over the distal surface of the canine. This overlapping is common in this region of the oral cavity because of the curvature of the arch.

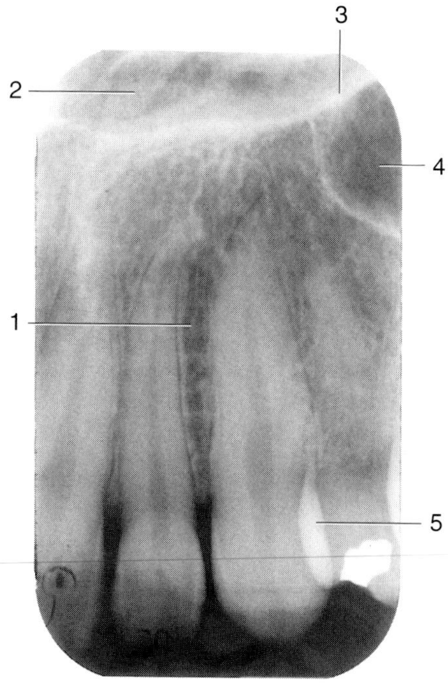

FIGURE 19-15 **Radiograph of maxillary canine area.** Shown are the (**1**) lateral fossa, (**2**) nasal fossa, (**3**) inverted Y (intersection of the borders of the nasal fossa and maxillary sinus), (**4**) maxillary sinus, and (**5**) dense radiopaque area caused by overlapping of the mesial surface of the first premolar over the distal surface of the canine. This overlapping is common in this region of the oral cavity because of the curvature of the arch.

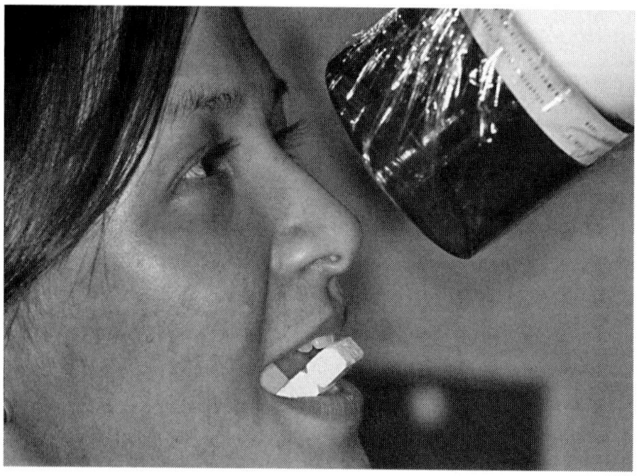

FIGURE 19-16 **Soft tissue of the nose in the path of the x-ray beam.** Note that the soft tissue of the nose will be in the path of the x-ray beam in this exposure. The resultant radiograph will most likely show an image of the soft tissue, outlining the tip of the nose.

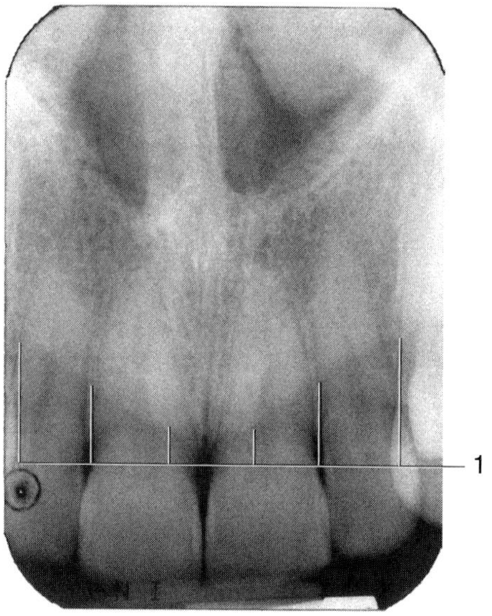

FIGURE 19-17 **Soft tissue image of the nose.** (**1**) The resultant image of the soft tissue of the nose is often magnified to a large size. According to the rules of shadow casting (see Chapter 4), the further an object is from the film packet, the more likely that object will appear magnified. The tip of the nose is at an increased distance from the intraoral film packet, resulting in a magnification of the size of the nose.

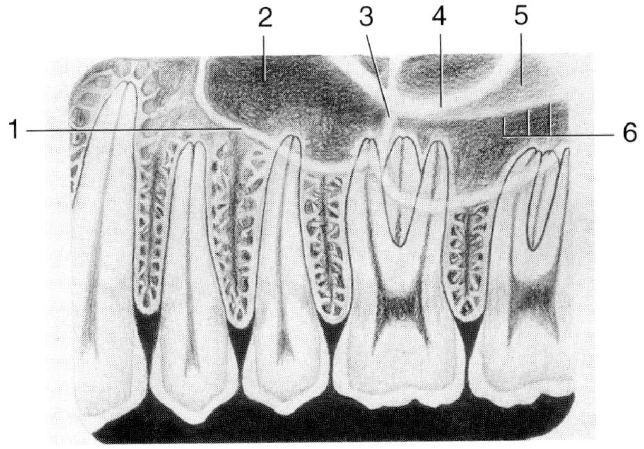

FIGURE 19-18 **Drawing of maxillary premolar area.** Drawing shows the (**1**) border (floor) of maxillary sinus, (**2**) maxillary sinus, (**3**) septum in maxillary sinus dividing the sinus into two compartments, (**4**) zygomatic process of maxilla, (**5**) zygoma, and (**6**) lower border of zygomatic arch.

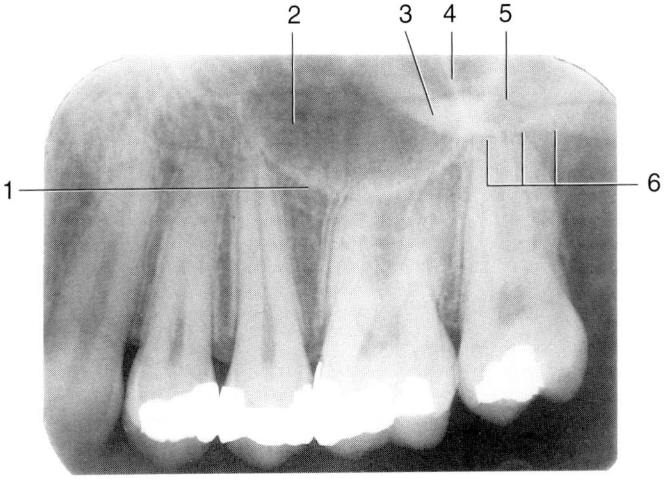

FIGURE 19-19 **Radiograph of maxillary premolar area.** This radiograph shows the (**1**) border (floor) of maxillary sinus, (**2**) maxillary sinus, (**3**) zygomatic process of maxilla, (**4**) septum in maxillary sinus dividing the sinus into two compartments, (**5**) zygoma, and (**6**) inferior border of the zygomatic arch.

Maxillary Posterior Region (Figures 19-18 through 19-22)

Radiopaque Features

1. **Floor** or **inferior border** of the sinuses. A thin, dense bone indicating the walls of the maxillary sinuses, whereas the sinus cavities themselves are referred to as radiolucent. The term radiopaque is used when referring to the sinus walls. The anterior extent of the maxillary sinus is often visible on an intraoral radiograph of the canine region as well.
2. **Septum.** A radiopaque wall (or partition) may be seen separating the maxillary sinus into two or more compartments. Septa are not always visible on all patients.
3. **Zygomatic process** of the maxilla. Appearing as a broad U-shaped band often seen above or superimposed over the roots of the first and second molars.
4. **Zygoma** (malar or cheekbone). Extends laterally and distally from the zygomatic process of the maxilla.

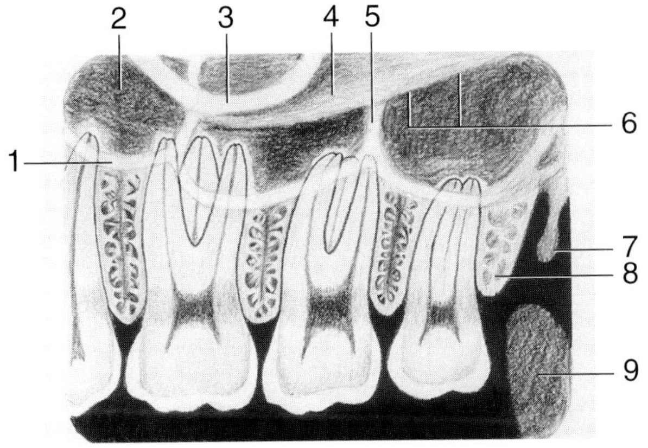

FIGURE 19-20 **Drawing of maxillary molar area.** Illustrated in the drawing are the (**1**) border (floor) of maxillary sinus, (**2**) maxillary sinus, (**3**) zygomatic process of maxilla, (**4**) zygoma, (**5**) septum in maxillary sinus, (**6**) lower border of zygomatic arch, (**7**) hamulus (hamular process), (**8**) maxillary tuberosity, and (**9**) coronoid process (mandible).

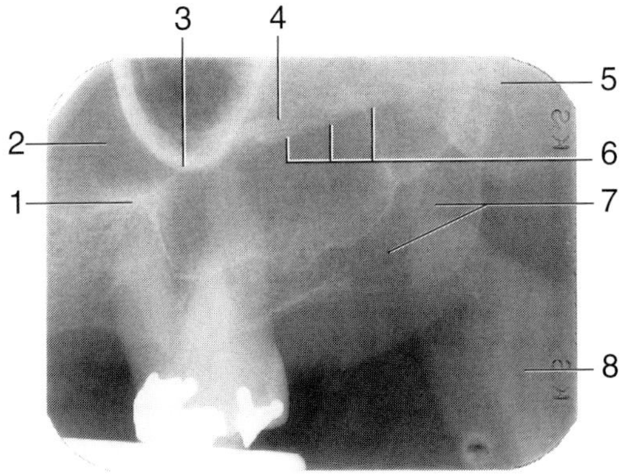

FIGURE 19-21 **Radiograph of maxillary molar area.** This radiograph shows (**1**) border (floor) of maxillary sinus, (**2**) maxillary sinus, (**3**) zygomatic process of maxilla, (**4**) zygoma, (**5**) lateral pterygoid plate, (**6**) lower border of zygomatic arch, (**7**) maxillary tuberosity, and (**8**) coronoid process of the mandible.

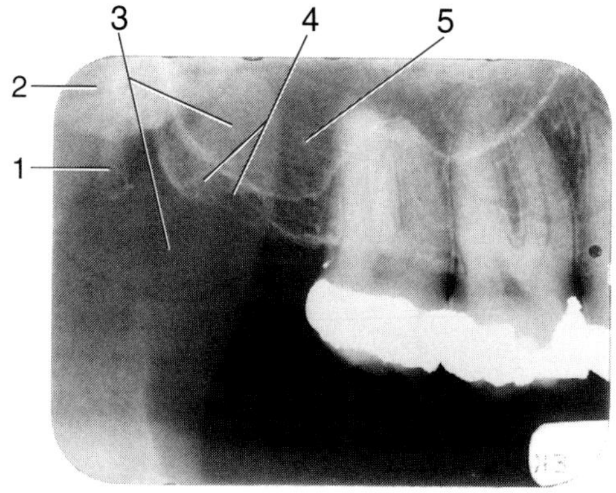

FIGURE 19–22 **Radiograph of maxillary molar area.** This radiograph shows (**1**) hamulus (hamular process), which is a downward projection of the medial pterygoid plate, (**2**) lateral pterygoid plate, (**3**) coronoid process of the mandible, (**4**) maxillary tuberosity, and (**5**) maxillary sinus.

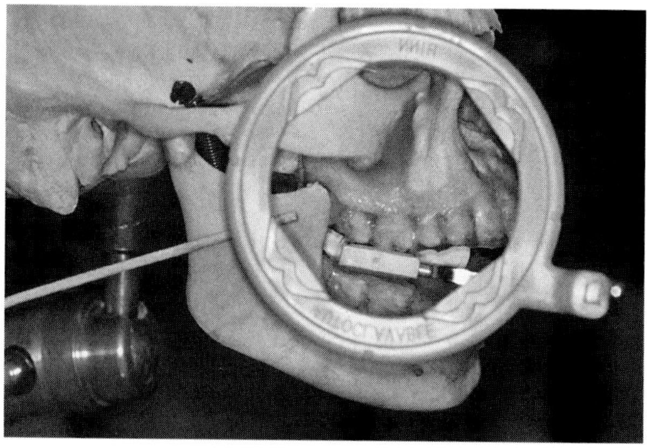

FIGURE 19–23 **Coronoid process of the mandible may be imaged on intraoral radiographs of the maxillary posterior region.** Note the position of the film holder when exposing a maxillary posterior periapical radiograph. The coronoid process of the mandible will most likely be imaged on this radiograph.

5. **Zygomatic arch.** Is continuous with the zygoma and extends distally. Because radiographs are a two-dimensional picture of three-dimensional structures, it is difficult to distinguish radiographically where the zygomatic process, zygoma, and zygomatic arch end and begin.
6. **Maxillary tuberosity.** The extension of the alveolar bone behind the molars marking the posterior limits of the maxillary arch. The maxillary tuberosity is usually referred to as radiopaque; however, depending on the size of the trabeculae located here, the radiopacity will vary.
7. **Pterygoid plates** of the sphenoid will usually appear only on the most posterior intraoral radiograph. To distinguish this structure from the maxilla, look for the posterior outline of the maxilla, distal to the maxillary tuberosity. A radiolucent suture may be detected separating the lateral ptyergoid plate from the maxilla, or the pterygoid plate may appear to overlap onto the maxilla.
8. **Hamulus** (hamular process). A downward projection of the medial pterygoid plate. It appears as a radiopaque pointed, sometimes hooklike, structure that serves as a muscle attachment. The hamulus is usually observed on only the most posterior intraoral radiographs.
9. **Coronoid process** of the mandible is sometimes seen as a triangle or large pointed radiopacity superimposed over the maxillary tuberosity. While this structure is technically a feature of the mandible, it is often in the path of the x-ray beam when positioning the PID for images of the maxillary posterior region (Figure 19–23).

Radiolucent Features

1. **Maxillary sinus.** This large air chamber inside the maxilla is visible in almost all periapical radiographs from the region of the canines posterior to the molars. The thin, radiopaque sinus wall can be observed outlining the radiolucent sinus.

Mandibular Anterior Region (Figures 19–24 through 19–27)

Radiopaque Features

1. **Genial tubercles.** Are made up of four small, bony crests on the lingual surface of the mandible that serve for muscle attachments. Generally visible as a round radiopaque "doughnut" at the midline below the apices of the central incisors.
2. **Mental ridge.** Located on the lateral surface of the mandible, the mental ridge appears as a horizontal radiopaque line extending from the premolar region to the symphysis (the midline of the mandible where the left and right sides of bone are fused together).

Radiolucent Features

1. **Lingual foramen.** A very small circular radiolucency in the middle of the radiopaque genial tubercles. Becuase it is so small, the lingual foramen often goes unnoticed.
2. **Mental fossa.** A depression on the labial aspect of the mandibular incisor area. Some consider the mental fossa to be an accentuated thinness of the mandible in the incisor area. On a mandibular incisor radiograph, the mental fossa appears as a generalized radiolucent area around the incisor apices.

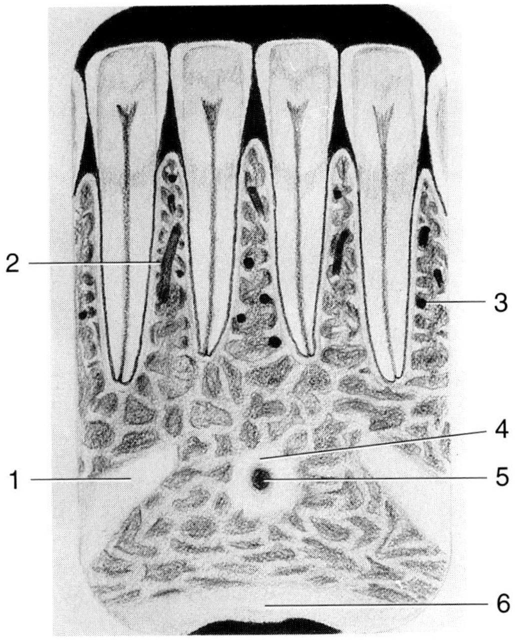

FIGURE 19-24 **Drawing of mandibular midline area.** The illustration shows (**1**) mental ridge, (**2**) nutrient canal, (**3**) nutrient foramen, (**4**) genial tubercles, (**5**) lingual foramen, and (**6**) inferior border of mandible.

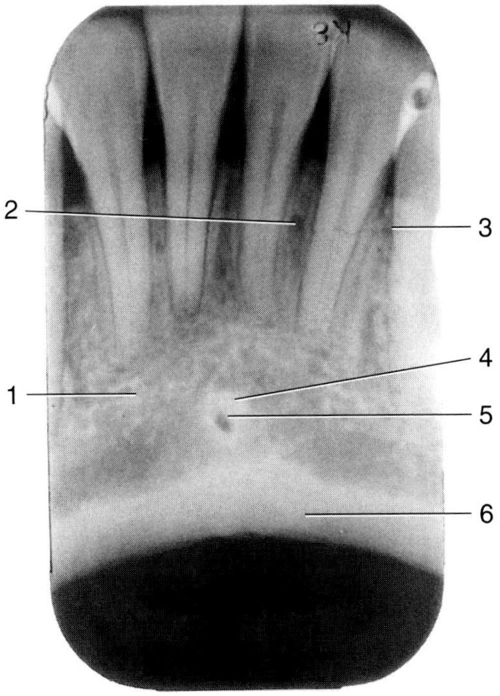

FIGURE 19-25 **Radiograph of the mandibular midline area.** This radiograph shows the (**1**) mental ridge, (**2**) nutrient canal, (**3**) nutrient foramen, (**4**) genial tubercles surrounding the (**5**) lingual foramen, and (**6**) inferior (lower) border of the mandible (radiopaque band of dense cortical bone).

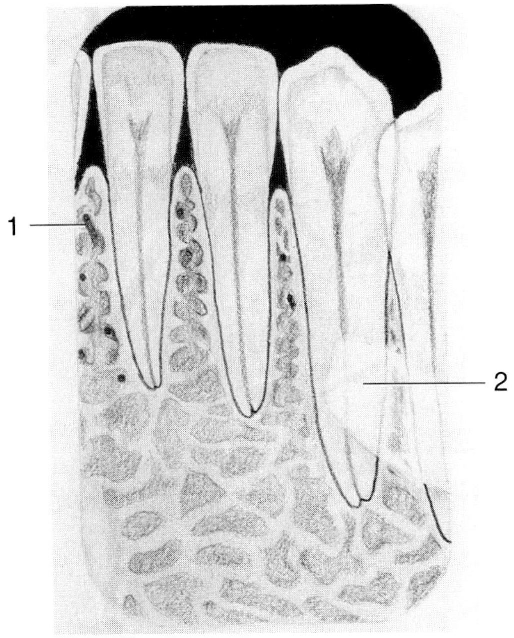

FIGURE 19-26 **Drawing of mandibular canine area.** Illustrated in the drawing are a (**1**) nutrient canal, and (**2**) torus mandibularis (lingual torus).

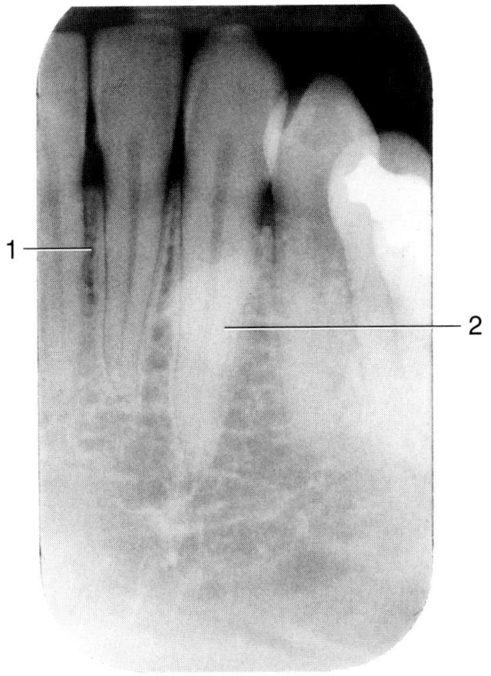

FIGURE 19-27 **Radiograph of mandibular canine area.** A (**1**) nutrient canal, and (**2**) torus mandibularis (lingual torus) are seen in this radiograph.

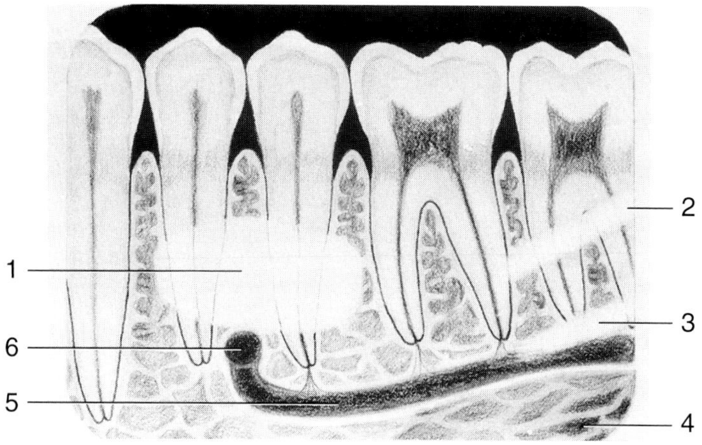

FIGURE 19-28 **Drawing of mandibular premolar area.** This drawing shows a (**1**) torus mandibularis, (**2**) oblique ridge, (**3**) mylohyoid ridge, (**4**) submandibular fossa, (**5**) mandibular canal, and (**6**) mental foramen.

Mandibular Posterior Region (Figures 19-28 through 19-33)

Radiopaque Features

1. **Oblique ridge.** A continuation of the anterior border of the ramus that extends downward and forward on the lateral surface of the mandible. The oblique ridge (sometimes called the external oblique ridge) appears as a radiopaque horizontal line of varied width superimposed across the molar roots.
2. **Mylohyoid ridge** is an irregular crest of bone for muscle attachments on the lingual surface of the mandible in the molar region. The mylohyoid ridge appears as a horizontal radiopaque line parallel and always inferior to (below) the oblique ridge. The mylohyoid ridge will most likely be imaged apcial to (below) the teeth roots.
3. **Inferior border of the mandible** is a heavy layer of cortical bone that is imaged only if the radiograph is deeply depressed in the floor of the mouth or the vertical angle of the x-ray beam is excessive. The inferior border of the mandible will appear as a distinct, thick radiopaque border.
4. **Torus mandibularis (lingual torus).** This bony growth extending out from the lingual surface of the mandible is normal, but not present on all patients. Depending on the size of the torus, the increased thickness in the bone will appear as a radiopaque fuzzy cotton ball imaged over or apical to the roots of posterior teeth.

Radiolucent Features

1. **Mental foramen.** A small opening on the lateral side of the body of the mandible, often seen near the apices of the premolars. This foramen should not be mistaken for an abscess, cyst, or other pathological condition.
2. **Submandibular fossa.** A large irregular-shaped area below the mylohyoid ridge and the roots of the mandibular molars, where the bone is thin, allowing more x-rays to

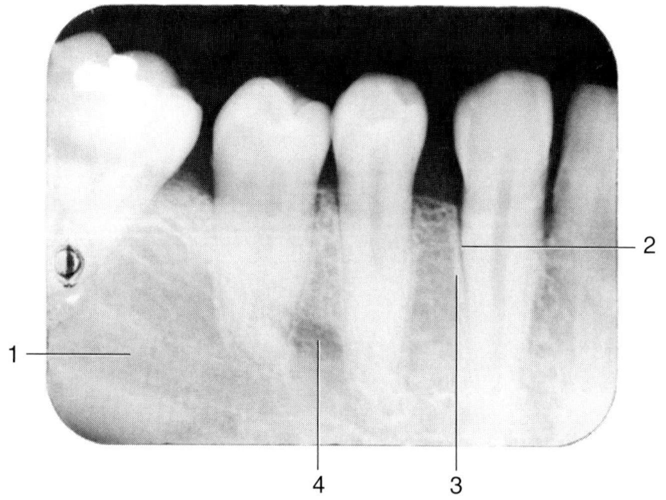

FIGURE 19-29 **Radiograph of mandibular premolar area.** Radiograph shows the (**1**) submandibular fossa, (**2**) a thin radiolucent line indicating the periodontal ligament space, (**3**) thin radiopaque line representing the lamina dura, and (**4**) the mental foramen.

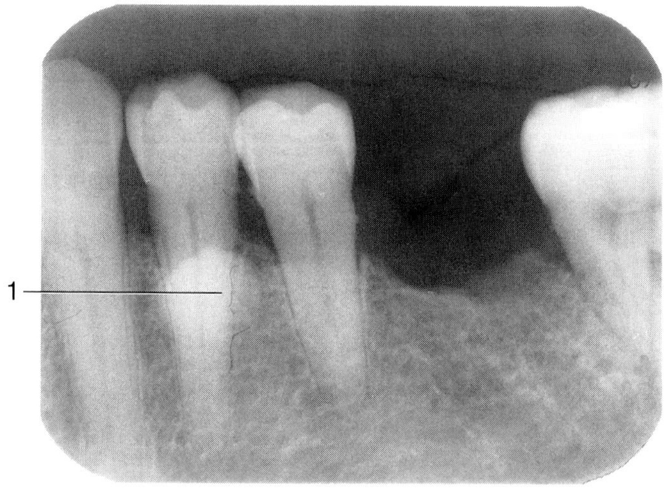

FIGURE 19-30 **Radiograph of mandibular premolar area.** Shows a small (**1**) torus mandibularis (lingual torus).

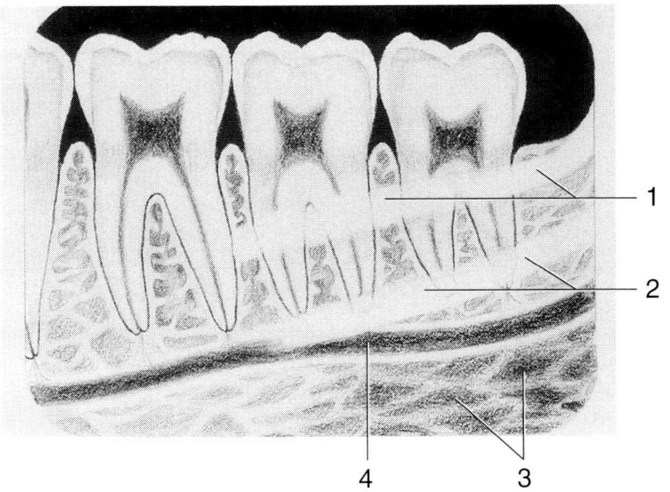

FIGURE 19-31 **Drawing of mandibular molar area.** Drawing illustrates the (**1**) oblique ridge, (**2**) mylohyoid ridge, (**3**) submandibular fossa, and (**4**) mandibular canal, a wide diagonal radiolucent area outlined above and below by thin parallel radiopaque lines representing the bony walls of the canal.

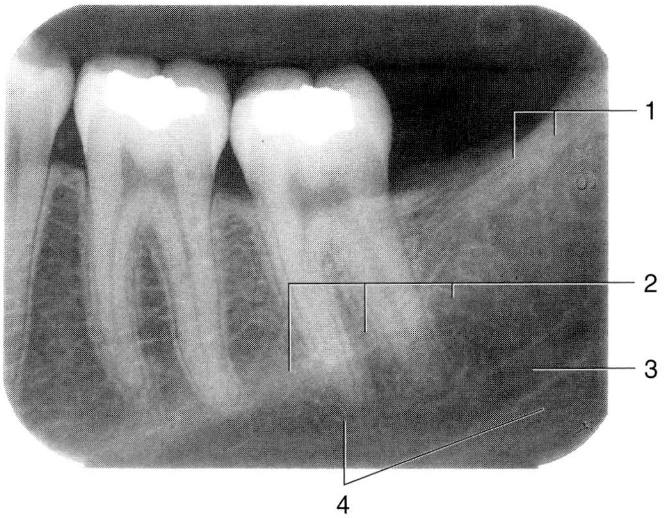

FIGURE 19-32 **Radiograph of mandibular molar area.** Shown are the (**1**) oblique ridge, (**2**) mylohyoid ridge, (**3**) mandibular canal, and (**4**) submandibular fossa.

penentrate this area and reach the film. The submandibular fossa should not be mistaken for pathology.

3. **Mandibular canal.** A canal for the passage of the mandibular nerve and blood vessels, it is outlined by two paired, thin, barely visible, parallel radiopaque lines which represent thin layers of cortical bone. The mandibular canal is often imaged in the premolar–molar areas below the apices of the teeth.

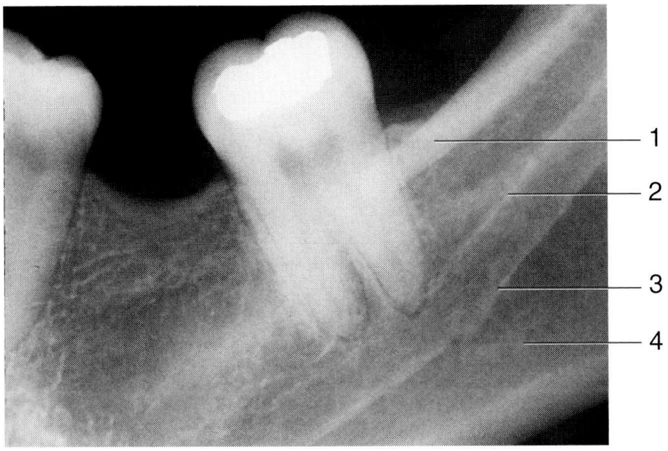

FIGURE 19-33 **Radiograph of mandibular molar area.** Shown are the (**1**) oblique ridge, (**2**) mylohyoid ridge, (**3**) mandibular canal, a wide diagonal radiolucent area outlined above and below by thin parallel radiopaque lines representing the bony walls of the canal, and (**4**) submandibular fossa.

REVIEW—Chapter Summary

Knowledge of the anatomical landmarks of the face and skull is needed to properly position the film packet, to clearly image the area of interest; to assist in mounting intraoral radiographs; and to develop the ability to interpret radiographs and recognize deviations from normal.

The radiographer should be able to identify cranial and facial bones as well as the specific landmarks and features of the maxilla and mandible. The radiographic appearance of the alveolar bone and the structures of the teeth was presented.

For the purpose of organizing anatomical structures for learning, landmarks are divided into the following categories depending on where they would be most likely to appear: maxillary anterior region, maxillary posterior region, mandibular anterior region, and mandibular posterior region. Anatomical landmarks are also separated into radiopaque images or radiolucent images. A systematic procedure is helpful to the beginning radiographer in learning to identify normal radiographic anatomy.

RECALL—Study Questions

1. A competent dental hygienist and dental assistant must be able to identify which of the following radiographically?
   a. Caries
   b. Periodontal abcess
   c. Normal anatomy
   d. Periapical pathology
2. Which of the following facial bones would most likely appear on a periapical radiograph?
   a. Occipital
   b. Parietal
   c. Frontal
   d. Zygoma

3. Bone sometimes has a mixed radiopaque-radiolucent appearance due to the nature of the:
   a. Cortical plates.
   b. Trabeculae patterns.
   c. Alveolar process.
   d. Genial tubercles.
4. Which of the following will most likely appear as a radiopacity outlining the tooth root?
   a. PDL space
   b. Lamina dura
   c. Nutrient canal
   d. Cementum
5. When nutrient canals open at the surface of the bone, they often appear radiographically as:
   a. Small radiolucent dots.
   b. Large radiopaque lines.
   c. Small radiolucent lines.
   d. Small radiopaque dots.
6. Which of these structures appears radiolucent?
   a. Enamel
   b. Cementum
   c. Dentin
   d. Pulp
7. A periapical radiograph of a 10-year-old will most likely reveal developing permenant dentition. Evidence of a congenitally missing permanent tooth is called an impaction.
   a. The first statement is true; the second statement is false.
   b. The first statement is false; the second statement is true.
   c. Both statements are true.
   d. Both statements are false
8. On a periapical radiograph of the maxillary molars, which of the following structures may be imaged superimposed onto the roots of the teeth?
   a. Mastoid process
   b. Maxillary tuberosity
   c. Zygomatic process
   d. Mylohyoid ridge
9. All of these features will appear radiolucent *except* one. Which one is this *exception?*
   a. Foramen
   b. Suture
   c. Canal
   d. Spine
10. All of these features will appear radiopaque *except* one. Which one is this *exception?*
    a. Ridge
    b. Sinus
    c. Tubercles
    d. Process
11. Which of the following is the best recommended sequence for learning to identify normal radiographic anatomy?
    a. 1. Determine if radiograph is of the maxilla or mandible.
       2. Determine if radiograph is of the anterior or posterior region.
       3. Determine if the structure is radiopaque or radiolucent.
    b. 1. Determine if radiograph is of the anterior or posterior region.
       2. Determine if the structure is radiopaque or radiolucent.
       3. Determine if radiograph is of the maxilla or mandible.
    c. 1. Determine if the structure is radiopaque or radiolucent.
       2. Determine if radiograph is of the maxilla or mandible.
       3. Determine if radiograph is of the anterior or posterior region.
    d. 1. Determine if radiograph is of the maxilla or mandible.
       2. Determine if the structure is radiopaque or radiolucent.
       3. Determine if radiograph is of the anterior or posterior region.
12. All of the following may appear on a periapical radiograph of the maxillary anterior region *except* one. Which one is this *exception?*
    a. Nasal septum
    b. Median palatine suture
    c. Maxillary tuberosity
    d. Inverted Y
13. All of the following may appear on a periapical radiograph of the maxillary posterior region *except* one. Which one is this *exception?*
    a. Maxillary sinus
    b. Incisive foramen
    c. Zygomatic arch
    d. Hamulus
14. A mandible landmark feature that may be imaged on a periapical radiograph of the maxillary posterior region is the:
    a. Mandibular canal.
    b. Submandibular fossa.
    c. Inferior border of the mandible.
    d. Coronoid process.
15. All of the following may appear on a periapical radiograph of the mandibular anterior region *except* one. Which one is this *exception?*
    a. Genial tubercles
    b. Mental ridge
    c. Coronoid process
    d. Lingual foramen
16. All of the following may appear on a periapical radiograph of the mandibular posterior region *except* one. Which one is this *exception?*
    a. Mental foramen
    b. Pterygoid plate
    c. Mandibular canal
    d. Mylohyoid ridge
17. The inverted Y landmark is composed of the intersection of which two structures?
    a. Lateral wall of the nasal cavity and anterior border of the maxillary sinus
    b. Anterior border of the maxillary sinus and inferior border of the mandible
    c. Lateral wall of the nasal cavity and soft tissue shadow of the nose
    d. Inferior border of the zygomatic process and the anterior nasal spine

REFLECT—Case Study

Your colleague is viewing a full mouth series of radiographs that he just finished mounting. As he is describing the following features, see if you can tell him the name of the anatomic landmark.

1. A dense, vertical radiopacity separating two paired oval radiolucencies observed in the maxillary anterior region
2. Large, paired oval radiolucencies separated by a dense, vertical radiopacity observed in the maxillary anterior region
3. A thin radiolucent line resembling a fracture observed between the maxillary central incisors
4. A round or pear-shaped radiolucency observed between the maxillary central incisors
5. A broad, U-shaped radiopacity observed superimposed over the maxillary posterior teeth roots
6. A radiopaque downward projection of bone that appears pointed or hook-like observed in the far posterior region of the maxilla
7. A large triangular shaped radiopacity observed superimposed over the maxillary tuberosity region
8. A large radiolucency outlined by a thin radiopaque border that is observed in almost all the periapical radiographs of the maxilla, from the canine posteriorly
9. A very small, round radiolucency observed in the midline apical (below) the mandibular incisors
10. A horizontal radiopaque line extending from the premolar region to the symphysis
11. A round radiolucency that resembles an abscess observed near the apex of the mandibular second premolar
12. A horizontal radiopaque line observed in the mandibular posterior region, superimposed across the molar roots
13. Another horizontal radiopaque line observed in the mandibular posterior region, but inferior to (below) the line described in 12 above. This line is observed inferior to the molar roots.
14. A large, irregularly shaped radiolucency observed below the line described in 13 above

RELATE—Laboratory Application

Developing the ability to recognize, identify, and describe radiographic anatomy of the head and neck region takes practice. Using the illustrations in this chapter, compare the appearance of the structures labeled with how they appear on a dry skull. Looking at a skull, point out each of the landmarks in the figures. To make it easier to locate these bones or structures, turn the skull so that it is oriented in the same direction as the illustration at which you are looking. Many structures can be seen readily; others may only be seen from one specific direction.

BIBLIOGRAPHY

Farman A. G., Nortje C. J., & Wood R. E. *Oral and Maxillofacial Diagnostic Imaging.* St Louis: C. V. Mosby, 1993.

White S. C. & Pharoah M. J. *Oral Radiology Principles and Interpretation,* 5th ed. St. Louis: Elsevier, 2004.

20

Recognizing Deviations from Normal Radiographic Anatomy

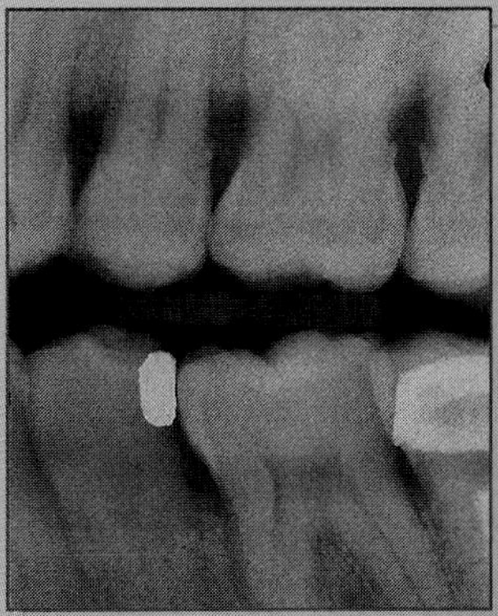

CHAPTER OUTLINE

■ OBJECTIVES

Following successful completion of this chapter, you should be able to:

1. Define the key words.
2. Identify the radiographic appearance of dental materials.
3. Identify the radiographic appearance of developmental anomalies.
4. Identify the radiographic appearance of periapical abscess, cyst, and granuloma.
5. Identify the radiographic appearance of external and internal tooth resorption.
6. Identify the radiographic appearance of calcifications and ossifications.
7. Identify the radiographic appearance of odontogenic tumors.
8. Identify the radiographic appearance of nonodontogenic tumors
9. Identify the radiographic appearance of fractures.

■ KEY WORDS

Abscess
Amalgam
Amalgam tattoo
Ameloblastoma
Amelogenesis imperfecta
Anodontia
Anomaly
Base material
Benign
Carcinoma
Cementoma
Composite
Concrescence
Condensing osteitis
Crown
Cyst
Dens in dente
Dentigerous cyst
Dentinogenesis imperfecta
Dilaceration
Exostosis
External resorption
Follicular (eruptive) cyst
Foreign body
Fracture line
Fusion
Gemination
Globulomaxillary cyst
Granuloma
Gutta percha
Hypercementosis
Idiopathic resorption
Incisive canal cyst
Internal resorption

Malignant
Mesiodens
Nonodontogenic cyst
Odontogenic cyst
Odontoma
Ossification
Osteosclerosis
Overhang
Phleboliths
Post and core
Pulp stone
Radicular cyst
Residual cyst
Resorption
Retained root
Retention pin
Rhinoliths
Sarcoma
Sclerotic bone
Sialolith
Silver point
Supernumerary tooth
Taurodontia
Torus
Tumor

Introduction

The most important skill in interpreting radiographs that a dental hygienist and dental assistant can possess is the ability to recognize deviations from normal radiographic anatomy. While the dentist is responsible for the final diagnosis and treatment of dental disease, all members of the oral health care team should be able to recognize radiographic deviations from the normal. Patient care is enhanced when the entire team views and interprets the radiographs.

Interpretation is a skill that requires a great deal of practice. The beginning radiology student is often frustrated by not being able to "see" what the expert easily identifies. To help develop this skill, a solid working knowledge of normal radiographic anatomy is needed. The radiographer should first identify normal radiographic anatomy, then systematically progress through a sequence of evaluation, naming each radiopaque and radiolucent structure observed.

Practice Point

The rule follows that when viewing radiographs you should *give everything you see a name*. Every radiopaque and radiolucent object observed on the radiograph should be identified as an anatomical landmark. Is the observation in question the mental foramen, the submandibular fossa, or the periodontal ligament space? When you have exhausted all possibilities of what a finding could be, it then becomes a deviation from the normal, requiring the attention of the dentist.

The purpose of this chapter is to help the student build on the skills acquired in Chapter 19 and to begin to identify common radiographic features that patients often present with (Procedure Box 20–1). These include the radiographic appearance of restorative materials, developmental anomalies, periapical pathology and other common pathological conditions of the teeth and the jaws, and the effects of trauma.

Prior to the discussion of the radiographic appearance of these materials and conditions, it should be noted that interpretation of radiographic findings is enhanced when the patient is present, allowing the practitioner to compare the radiographic findings with the clinical examination of the patient. Attempting to determine what a particular finding is from the radiograph alone may sometimes be difficult; for example, a radiolucency observed in the otherwise radiopaque enamel of a maxillary central incisor may give the appearance of caries. However, a clinical examination of this tooth may reveal the presence of a composite restoration, which can sometimes mimic decay radiographically. Additionally, the dentist will always use radiographs in conjunction with the patient's clinical examination, medical and dental histories, and physical signs and symptoms, together with other necessary diagnostic tests to make a final diagnosis.

Radiographic Appearance of Dental Restorative Material

It is important to observe restorative materials radiographically for the presence of recurrent decay, defective margins that contribute to periodontal disease, and for other potential problems. Restorative materials may appear radiopaque or radiolucent and some can be differentiated by their relative degree of radiopacity or radiolucency (Table 20–1). Others are better identified by their size and contour or by their probable location on the tooth. However, because radiographs are a two-dimensional image of three-dimensional objects, the image of a restoration on one surface may be superimposed on the image of another large restoration on the same tooth, thus giving the appearance of only one restoration instead of two, or even more. Often, there is more than one type of material superimposed. For example, the appear-

PROCEDURE 20–1

SEQUENCE FOR INTERPRETING A FULL MOUTH SERIES FOR DEVIATIONS FROM NORMAL RADIOGRAPHIC ANATOMY

1. See Procedure Box 18–2, Suggested Sequence for Viewing a Full Mouth Series of Radiographs.
2. Examine one anatomic structure at a time. Compare each finding with its appearance in adjacent films.
3. First, examine the supporting structures (the bones of the head and neck):
   a. Identify each landmark (see Chapter 19)
   b. Determine if the landmark is in the appropriate region
   c. And of accurate size and shape
   d. Examine the trabecular spaces and cortical plate of the bones
4. Second, examine the teeth.
   a. Determine if each tooth is present or absent
   b. Examine the shape and morphology of the crowns and roots
   c. Look for developmental stages and/or abnormalities
   d. Examine the pulp chamber and root canals
5. Third, observe any dental restorations and the presence of dental materials:
   a. Check for shape and contour
   b. And appropriate placement
   c. Look for radiolucencies that suggest recurrent decay (see Chapter 21)
6. Fourth, examine the teeth for possible carious lesions (see Chapter 21).
7. Fifth, examine the supporting alveolar bone and the periodontal ligament space for evidence of periodontal disease (see Chapter 22).
8. Present a preliminary interpretation for the dentist's review.
9. Following confirmation by the dentist, document all findings on the patient's permanent record.

ance of a base material may be observed apical to a metallic restoration, or the presence of metallic retention pins may be detected apical to a crown. Additionally, it is not always possible to determine on which tooth surface the restoration is located. A restoration looks the same whether it is on the facial (buccal) or lingual surface of the tooth.

Metallic Restorations

The images of all metallic restorations of approximately equal density appear extremely radiopaque. Thus it is impossible to determine whether the material is gold, silver, or a base metal alloy. Only by looking at the size and contour of the restoration is it possible to make an educated guess based on what materials are generally used in such circumstances. For example, metal crowns will most often appear to have smooth margins while amalgam restorations have irregular margins (Figure 20–1).

Non-metallic Restorations

Aesthetic materials, such as **composites,** porcelain, silicate, and acrylic resins (plastics) may appear radiopaque or radiolucent,

TABLE 20–1 **Metallic and Non-metallic Restorations**

Metallic Dental Materials	Non-metallic Dental Materials	
Radiopaque	Less Radiopaque	Sometimes Radiolucent
Amalgam	Composite	Composite
Gold	Porcelain	Acrylic resins
Stainless steel	Acrylic resins	Silicate
Retention pins	Silicate	
Post and core	Base	
Silver points	Cement	
Orthodontic appliances	Temporary filling	
	Gutta percha	
Implants	Sealants	

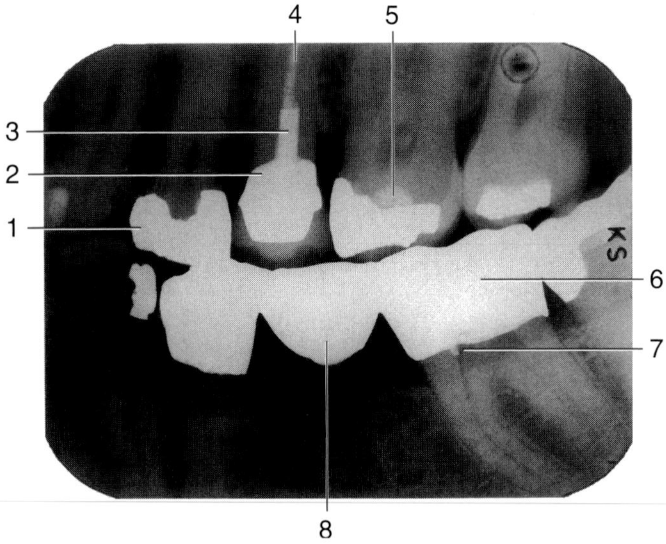

FIGURE 20–1 **Dental materials.** This radiograph shows several metallic and non-metallic dental materials. Since all of the metal restorations are equally radiopaque, their size and shape is observed to determine the type of material. The materials present in this radiograph are: (**1**) amalgam; (**2**) porcelain-fused-to-metal crown; (**3**) post and core; (**4**) gutta percha; (**5**) base material; (**6**) full metal crown, which is the posterior abutment of a three-unit bridge; (**7**) retention pin; and (**8**) metal pontic (part of the three-unit bridge).

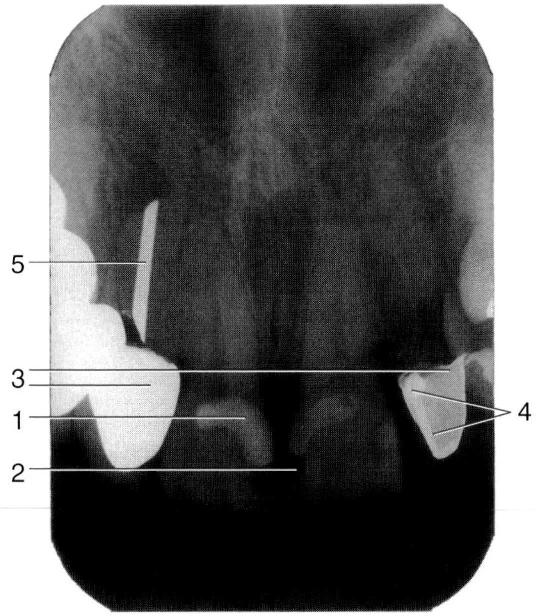

FIGURE 20–2 **Comparision of radiopaque and radiolucent appearance of composite.** This radiograph shows the appearance of (**1**) radiopaque and (**2**) radiolucent restorative materials (composites, acrylic resins or silicates) on the central incisors. (**3**) Note the appearance of the porcelain-fused-to-metal crowns on the lateral incisors. The overexposure (darkness) of this radiograph makes it especially difficult to view the porcelain on the patient's left lateral incisor. (**4**) However, the overexposure made it possible to image the cement under this crown. (**5**) Note the silver point endodontic filler.

and may be barely visible or not detected at all. Radiolucent dental materials have a tendency to mimic decay radiographically, so some manufacturers add radiopaque particles to their product so that the viewer will not mistake it for caries (Figure 20–2).

Other restorative materials such as **base material** (calcium hydroxide pastes) (Figure 20–1) and cements (Figure 20–2) exhibit about the same degree of radiopacity as dentin. Sealants will also appear very slightly radiopaque, or not at all.

Identification of Common Restorative Materials

- **Amalgam.** The most common restorative material; appears radiopaque with irregular margins and varies in size and shape. The amalgam radiopacity observed will most likely not cover the entire crown of the teeth; the less radiopaque enamel cusps are often still visible. Radiographs help to image the contours of amalgam restorations and can reveal poorly contoured margins called **overhangs** (Figure 20–3).

  Radiographs sometime reveal particles of amalgam in the soft tissue. Often found in edentutous areas of the mandible, amalgam that fractures during an extraction and falls into the root socket or under the gingival tissue may impart a bluish-purple color to the tissue called an **amalgam tattoo** (Figure 20–4).
- **Composite.** Varies in appearance from radiopaque to radiolucent. When radiolucent, composite may mimic caries

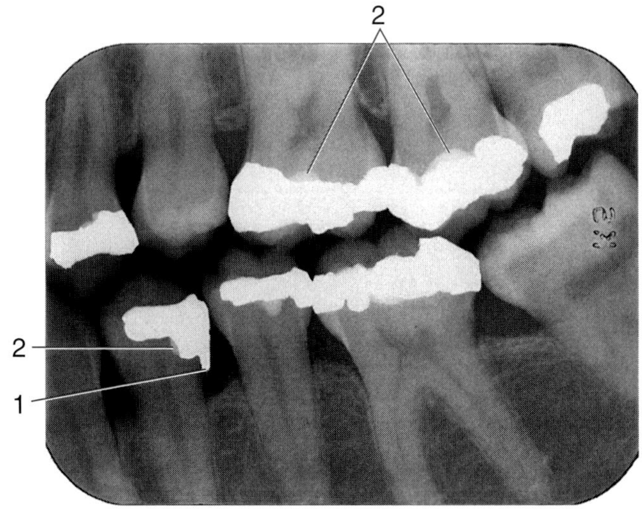

FIGURE 20–3 **Overhang.** (**1**) This bitewing radiograph reveals an amalgam overhang on the mandibular first premolar. (**2**) Base material. Note the many shapes and sizes of the amalgam restorations in this radiograph.

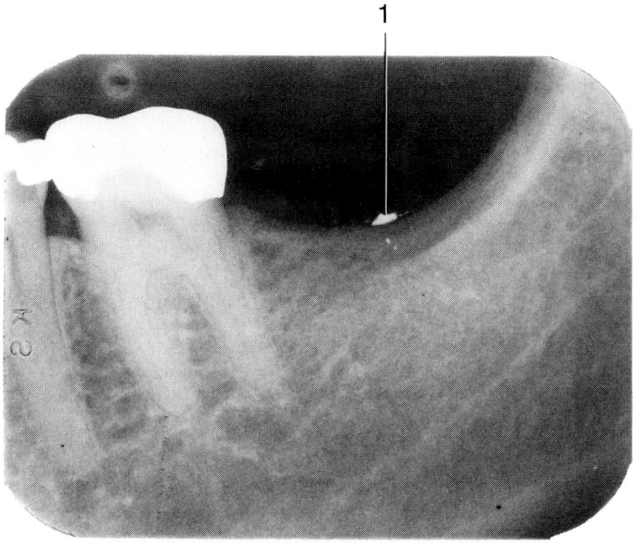

FIGURE 20–4 **Fragments of amalgam (1), seen under the soft tissue, probably left after an extraction.** Clinically, the gingiva appears bluish-purple. This is called an amalgam tattoo.

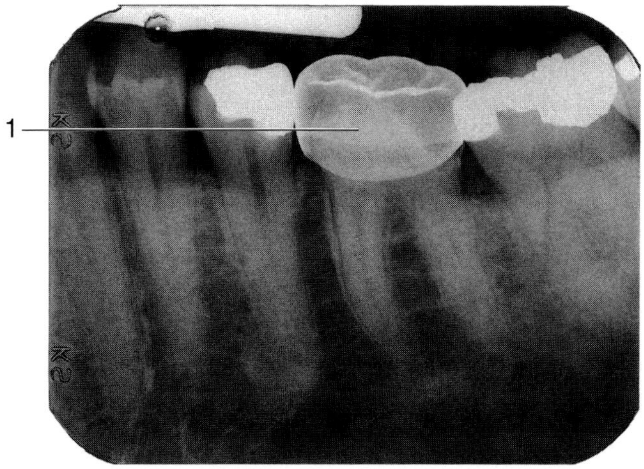

FIGURE 20–5 **Stainless steel crown (1).** Note the "see-through" appearance.

(Figure 20–2). To help distinguish composite from caries, look for the the restoration to appear to have straight margins and a prepared looked, whereas the radiolucency of caries appears more diffuse (see Figure 21–17). A clinical examination may be needed to determine definitively whether caries or composite is present.

- **Crown (full metal).** Appears radiopaque and is distinguished from amalgam by its smooth margins. Full metal **crowns** usually cover the entire crown of the tooth and will be contoured to resemble the correct shape of the cusps of the tooth (Figure 20–1).
- **Crown (porcelain fused to metal).** The metal core of the crown appears radiopaque, whereas the porcelain appears less radiopaque. The radiopaque shape of the metal core will be more rounded than a full metal crown and is not contoured to resemble the correct shape of the cusps of the tooth. Instead, the porcelain will take the shape of the cusps (Figure 20–1).
- **Crown (porcelain jacket).** Appears less radiopaque than a full metal crown because no metal is present. The porcelain material will appear to be about the same radiopacity as dentin.
- **Crown (stainless steel).** As a temporary restoration, this metal is less dense and will allow the passage of more x-rays, giving the material a "see-through" appearence. These crowns are pre-fabricated and do not appear to fit the tooth very well (Figure 20–5).
- **Retention pin.** A metal pin used to support a restoration. **Retention pins** appear radiopaque in a very easy-to-identify shape (Figures 20–1 and 20–6). Since another restorative material such as an amalgam or crown will be placed over the retention pin, it may not be imaged on the radiograph. It should be noted that retention pins will only be located in the dentin and will not be observed penetrating the pulp. A retention pin should not be confused with a post and core restoration, which penetrates the pulp chamber and must be observed in conjunction with an endodontic filling material (Figures 20–1 and 20–7). These materials are described below.

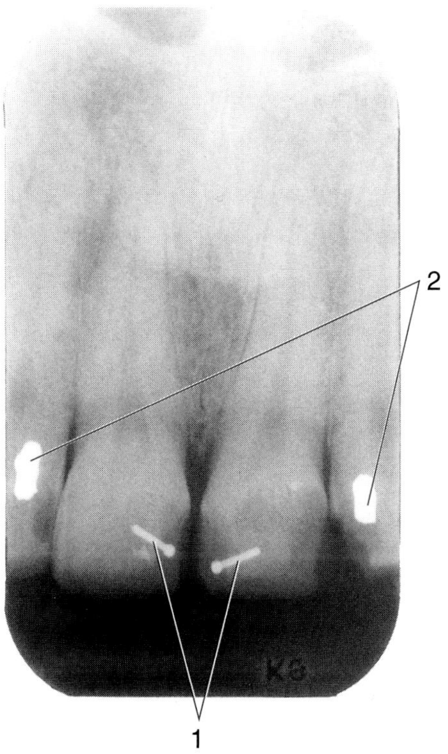

FIGURE 20–6 **Retention pins.** (**1**) Radiopaque pins help retain the radiolucent composite restorations. (**2**) Small radiopaque amalgam restorations.

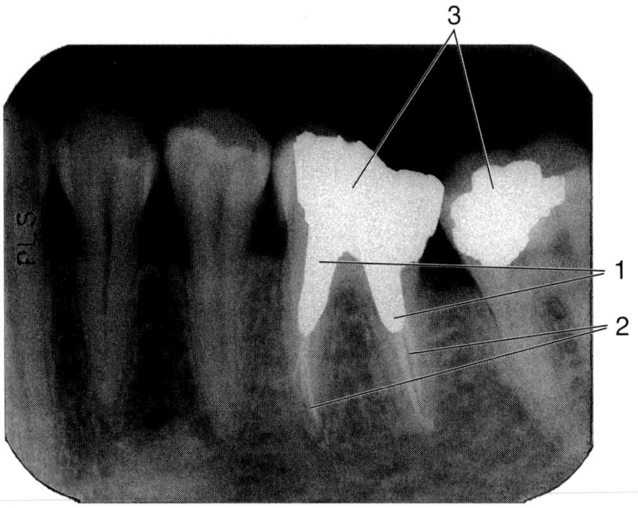

FIGURE 20-7 **Post and core.** (**1**) Large radiopacities within the root canal. (**2**) Endodontic filling material will also be present when a post and core restoration is observed. (**3**) Amalgam restorations.

- **Base material (calcium hydroxide pastes).** Base materials are used to line the cavity preparation to protect the tooth's pulp. Since another restorative material such as an amalgam will be placed over the base, it may not be observed on the radiograph. When observed, the base material will appear very slightly radiopaque (Figure 20–1).
- **Endodontic fillers.** Radiopacities observed within the pulp chamber may be either **silver points** (Figure 20–2), a very radiopaque metal root canal filling, or **gutta percha,** a less radiopaque filling (Figures 20–1 and 20–7).
- **Post and core.** A metal restoration that builds up a tooth to that it can support a crown; appears radiopaque. The core section penetrates the pulp chamber, so the presence of endodotic filler will be obeserved along with a post and core. It should be noted that in addition to location, a post and core restoration can be distinguished from a retention pin by its significantly larger size (Figure 20–7).
- **Implant.** Appears as a distinct radiopacity. The implant is located in an area of a missing tooth (Figure 20–8).
- **Orthodontic and surgical materials.** Metal orthodontic bands, wires and brackets and surgical wires, pins, and screws all appear as distinct radiopacities (Figures 20–9 and 20–10).

Radiographic Appearance of Developmental Anomalies

An **anomaly** is defined as any deviation from normal. Dental anomalies are numerous, so it is important that the dental hygienist and the dental assistant be skilled at identifying the more common of these. Such anomalies include:

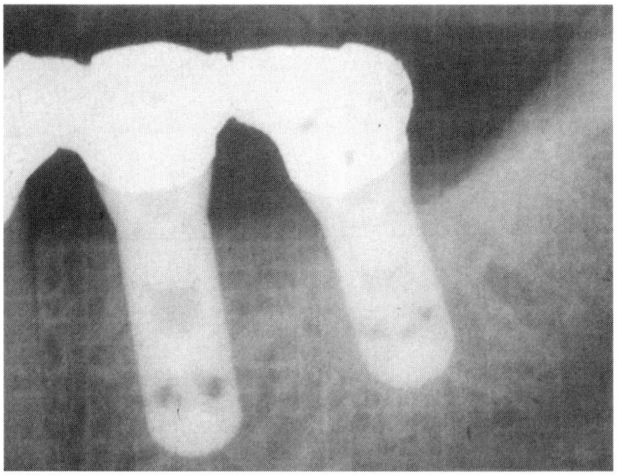

FIGURE 20-8 **Implants.** Integral implants take the shape of the missing teeth roots.

- **Anodontia.** Absence of the teeth (may be complete or partial). The third molars are the most common congenitally missing teeth, followed by the premolars (Figure 20–11) and the maxillary lateral incisors. It is important when viewing radiographs of children that the presence of the developing permanent teeth be noted.

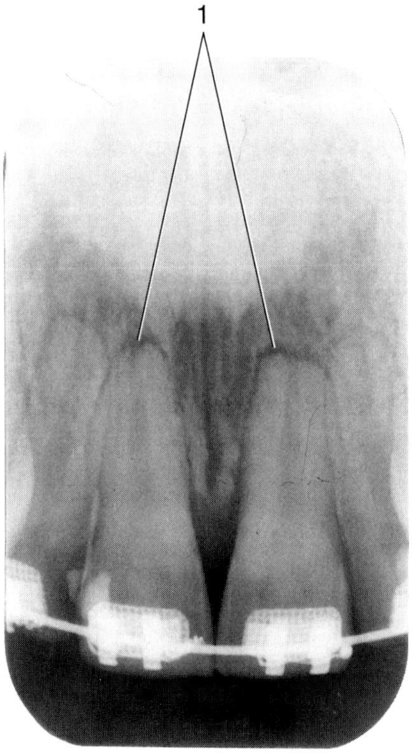

FIGURE 20-9 **Orthodontic appliance.** (**1**) Note the root-end external resorption caused by trauma of orthodontic treatment.

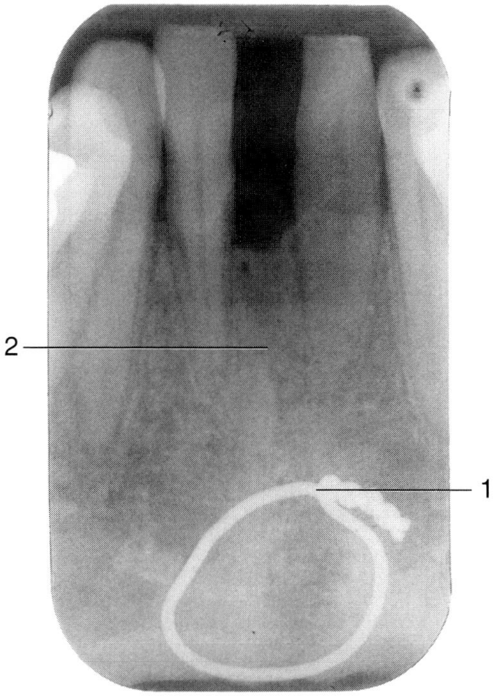

FIGURE 20-10 **Surgical wire (1) used to reduce a fracture (2) (radiolucent line).**

- **Supernumerary teeth (extra teeth).** It is equally important that the presence of **supernumerary teeth** be detected. Often there is not a space for these extra teeth to erupt into, or the radiopacities may be deformed and not resemble normal tooth form (Figure 20–12). Complications caused by supernumerary teeth include the possibility of

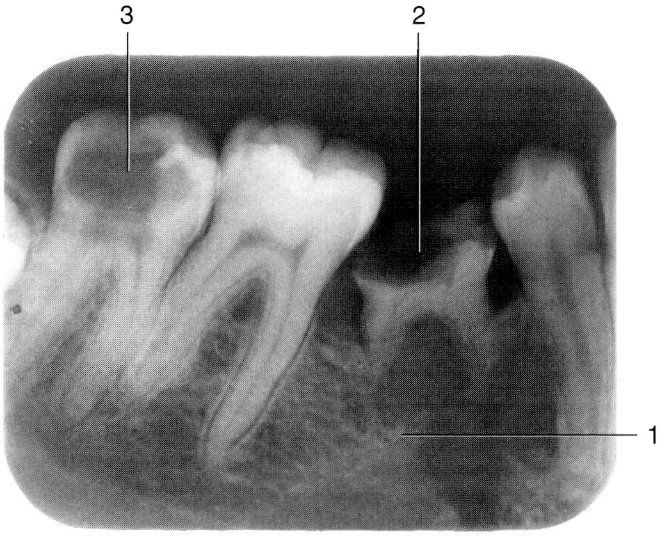

FIGURE 20-11 **Congenitally missing second premolar** (**1**). Note the extensive caries (**2**) in the second primary molar and (**3**) the second permanent molar.

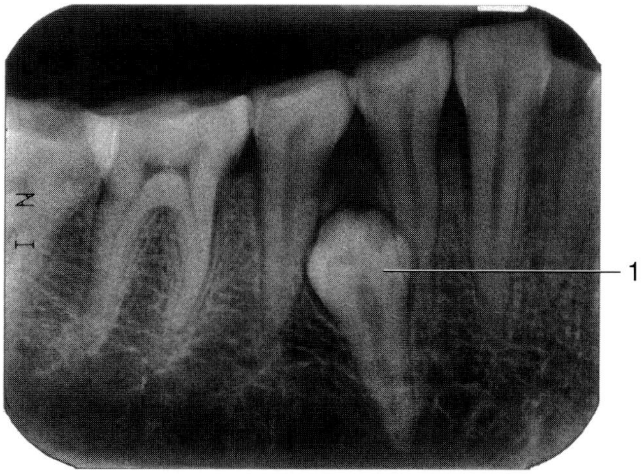

FIGURE 20-12 **Supernumerary premolar (1).**

cyst formation and the malposition, noneruption, or both of the normal teeth.

- **Mesiodens.** A supernumerary tooth located in the maxillary midline (Figure 20–13).
- **Dens in dente** (dens invaginatus). Literally, a tooth within a tooth, an invagination of the enamel within the body of the tooth. This anomaly occurs most frequently in the maxillary lateral incisor (Figure 20–14).
- **Hypercementosis.** Usually appears radiopaque and is caused by excessive cementum formation. The excessive cemen-

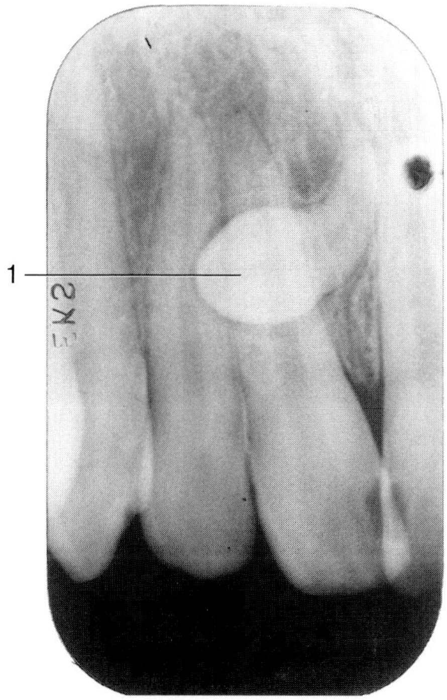

FIGURE 20-13 **Mesiodens.** (**1**) A small supernumerary tooth, located in the midline between the central incisors.

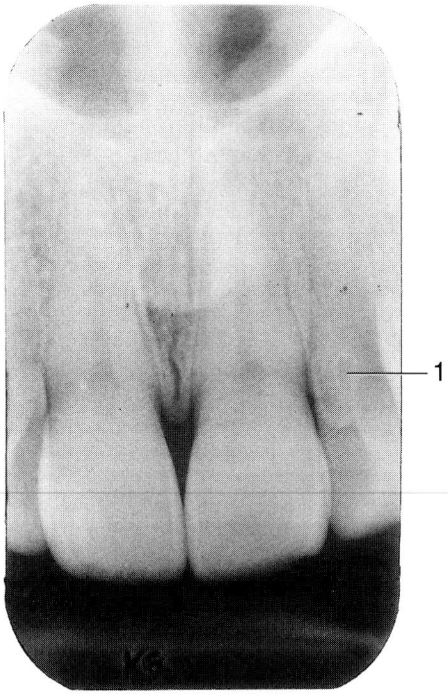

FIGURE 20–14 **Dens in dente.** (**1**) An invagination of the enamel within the body of the lateral incisor.

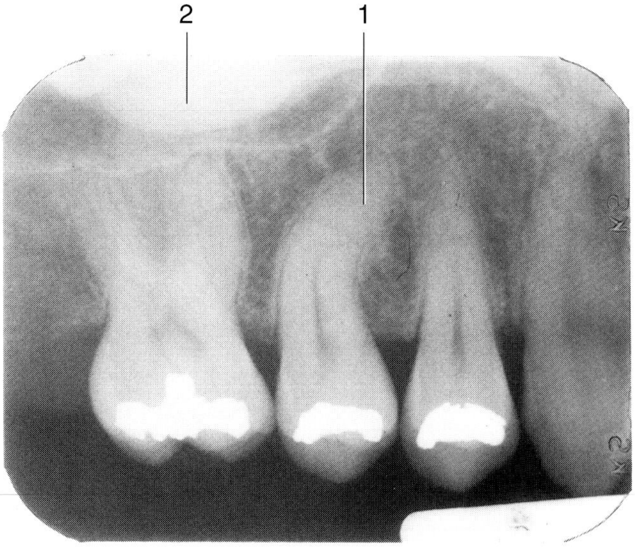

FIGURE 20–16 **Dilaceration** (**1**). A sharp bend in the root of the tooth. Note the (**2**) torus palatinus, a radiopaque overgrowth of bone on the midline of the palate.

tum on the roots often causes a bulbous enlargement along the root surface, with the area near the apex appearing most bulbous (Figure 20–15). **Hypercementosis** is distinguished from other radiopacities that appear in the bone by the outline of the periodontal ligament (PDL) space. When observing hypercementosis, the PDL contains the radiopacity and separates it from the bone. This distinction will help to avoid mistaking hypercementosis for sclerotic bone, explained later.

- **Dilaceration.** Refers to a tooth with a sharp bend in the root (Figure 20–16). **Dilaceration** usually develops as a result of trauma during root formation.

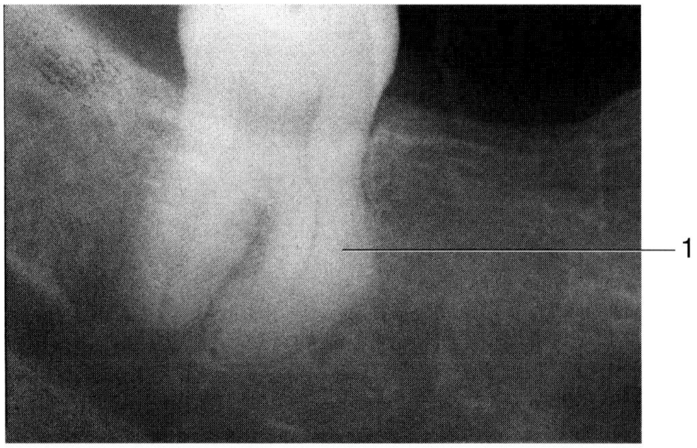

FIGURE 20–15 **Hypercementosis (1) on the roots of the molar.**

- **Taurodontia.** Characterized by very large pulp chambers and very short roots.
- **Gemination (twinning).** A single tooth bud that divides and forms two teeth. The presence of adjacent teeth help to distinguish this condition from fusion.
- **Fusion.** A condition where the dentin and one other dental tissue of adjacent teeth are united (Figure 20–17). In this case, two adjacent teeth will be involved, distinguishing fusion from gemination.
- **Concrescence.** A condition where the cementum of adjacent teeth is united. This condition is often difficult to distinguish radiographically because the angle of the x-ray

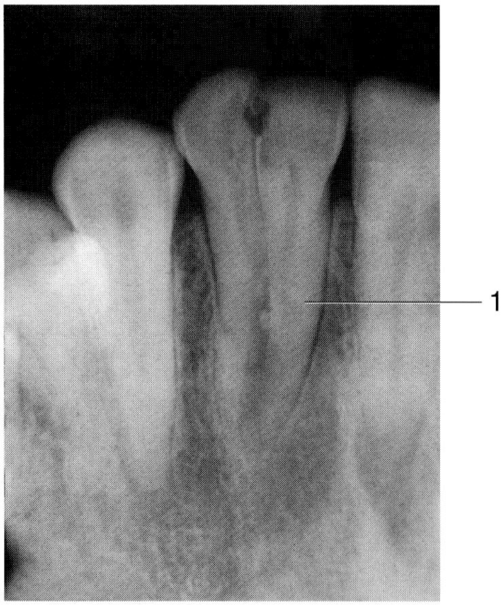

FIGURE 20–17 **Fusion (1) of two adjacent incisors.**

beam may superimpose the images of adjacent teeth, giving them a joined appearance when, in fact, concrescence is not present.

Other less frequently encountered anomalies include the following:

- **Dentinogenesis imperfecta** (hereditary opalescent dentin). Characterized by imperfectly formed dentin that has an opalescent or amber color. Radiographs reveal small underdeveloped roots and obliterated pulp chambers.
- **Amelogenesis imperfecta.** Characterized by teeth with scant or totally missing enamel.

Radiographic Appearance of Apical Disease

Radiolucencies surrounding the apices or root tips of the teeth indicate pathological changes in the hard (bony) tissues. These radiolucenies can not usually be distinguished from each other based on the radiographic image alone. The appearance of apical pathology on a radiograph must be carefully correlated with other diagostic information before a diagnosis can be made. The three most common periapical lesions observed on radiographs are **abscess, granuloma,** and **cyst** (Figure 20–18).

- **Periapical abscess.** Periapical infections usually result from pulpal inflammation. Bacteria from caries infect the pulp and gain access to the periapical bone by way of the root canals. As a rule, an acute abscess (early stage of pulpal or periapical infection) is barely discernible radiographically, becoming more radiolucent as it becomes chronic. In fact, in the very early acute stage there may be no radiographic evidence at all. The earliest sign may be a break, or loss of radiopacity, in the lamina dura. A chronic abscess may appear as a circular radiolucency around the root apices and eventual turn into a granuloma.
- **Granuloma.** A mass of granulation tissue usually surrounded by a fibrous sac continuous with the periodontal ligament space that appears attached to the root apices. Under certain conditions, epithelial elements may proliferate to form a cyst.
- **Cyst.** Epithelium-lined sac filled with fluid or semi-solid material. The periapical cyst (also known as a **radicular cyst**) is a cyst around the end of the tooth root. Unless the cyst is completely removed at the time of the extraction or surgery, it will remain, and is then called a **residual cyst.** Because of osmotic imbalance within a cyst, pressure is exerted in all directions; therefore, cysts tend to be spherical unless unequal resistance is encountered. Although usually unilocular (made up of one compartment), cysts may also be multilocular (made up of several compartments). Radiographically, a cyst may appear as a fairly uniform radiolucent cavity within the bone and surrounded by a well defined radiopaque border that resembles the lamina dura.

Another type of cyst frequently observed on radiographs of young patients is the **dentigerous cyst** (Figure 20–19). A dentigerous cyst occurs frequently with impacted teeth—

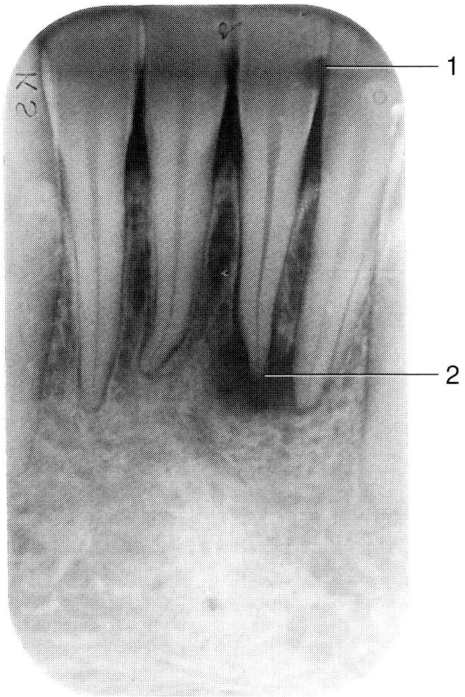

FIGURE 20-18 **Periapical pathology.** This radiograph shows (**1**) caries on the distal surface of the left central incisor, and (**2**) a round radiolucent lesion that may be a periapical abscess, a granuloma, or a cyst.

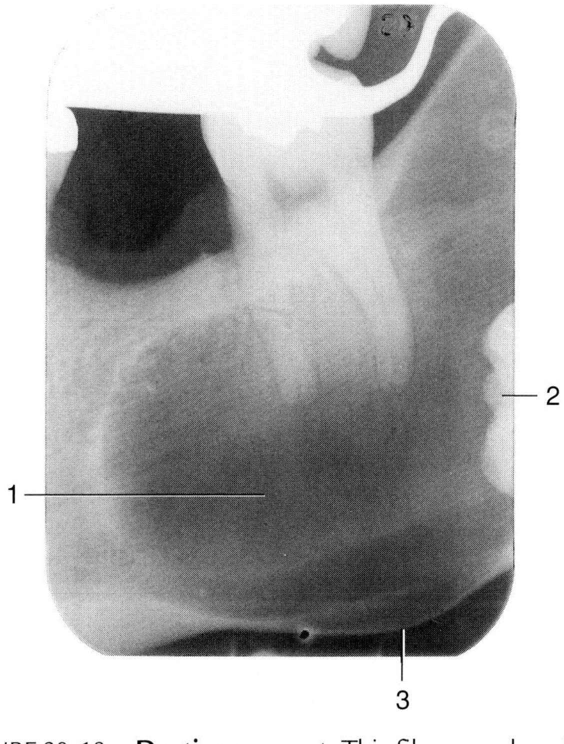

FIGURE 20-19 **Dentigerous cyst.** This film was placed in a vertical position instead of the usual horizontal position to show (**1**) a dentigerous cyst involving (**2**) the impacted third molar, and (**3**) expansion and thinning of the cortical bone of the mandible.

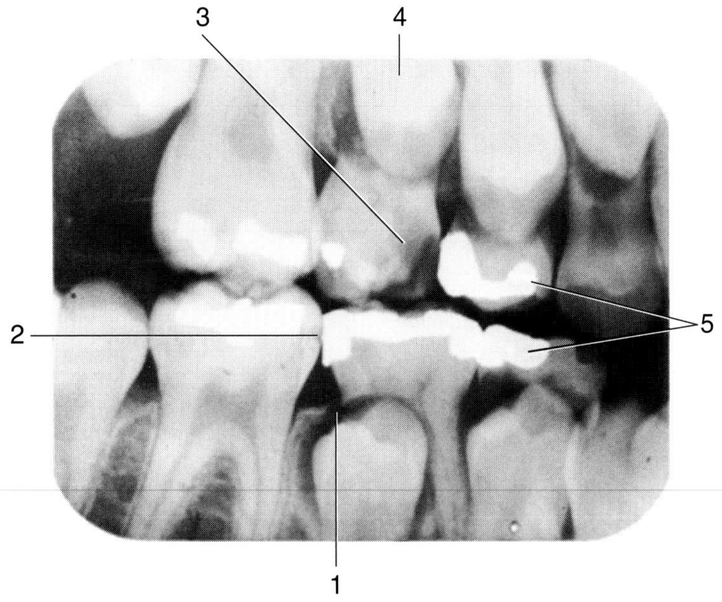

FIGURE 20-20 **Follicular (eruptive) cyst (1) around the crown of the second mandibular premolar.** Note the (**2**) incipient caries on the permanent molar, (**3**) advanced caries on the primary second molar, (**4**) erupting second maxillary premolar, (**5**) primary first molars about to be exfoliated. Note the physiologic external resorption of the primary roots.

most often third molars and supernumerary teeth—and is always associated with the crown only of the involved tooth. If the tooth causing the cyst continues to develop and is able to erupt, the cyst is often destroyed by natural means. Hence it is also known as a **follicular (eruptive) cyst** (Figure 20–20).

Periapical, residual, and dentigerous cysts are categorized as **odontogenic cysts,** which means of tooth origin. **Nonodontogenic cysts** arise from epithelium other than that associated with tooth formation. Two types of nonodontogenic cysts are the **incisive canal** (nasopalatine) **cyst** (Figure 20–21), located within the incisive canal, and the rare **globulomaxillary cyst** (Figure 20–22), which arises between the maxillary lateral incisor and the canine.

Radiographic Appearance of Tooth Resorption

Evidence of tooth **resorption** is a common finding on dental radiographs. Natural physiologic resorption, such as when the roots of primary teeth resorb in response to the erupting permanent teeth is considered normal (Figure 20–20). Other resorptive processes, however, are the result of infection, trauma, or some unusual condition. Tooth resorption may be external or internal. **External resorption** is most often characterized by root-end resorption, where the roots of the teeth appear shorter than normal (Figure 20–23). External resorption is not limited to the root end, but can occur anywhere along the tooth root. Other examples of external resorption include the resorption caused by pressure from an adjacent impacted or unerupted tooth; resorption caused by slowly growing tumors; or trauma, such as when teeth

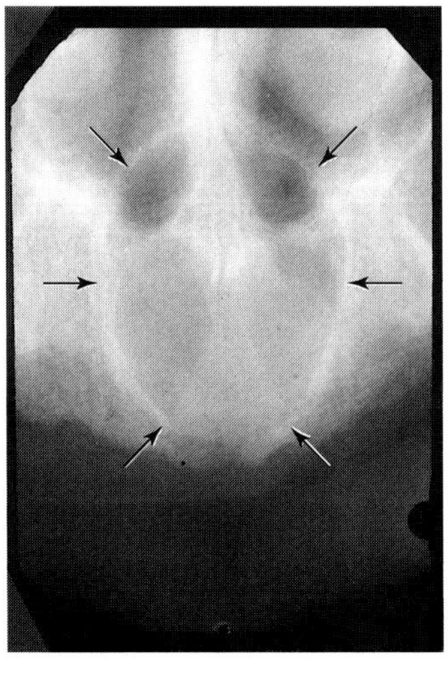

FIGURE 20-21 **Incisive canal cyst.** Arrows outline an incisive canal (nasopalatine) cyst in an edentulous maxilla.

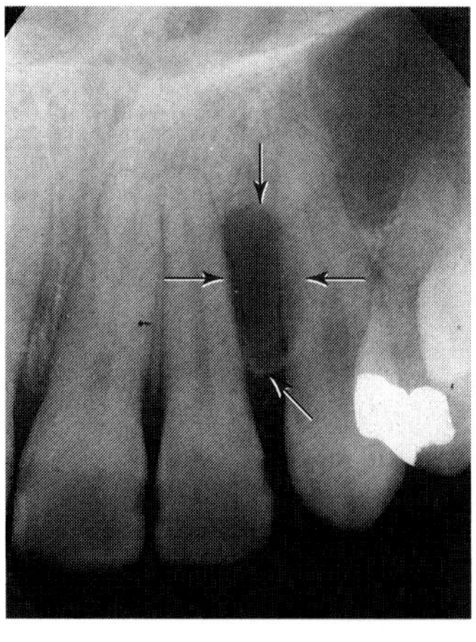

FIGURE 20-22 **Globulomaxillary cyst.** Arrows outline a globulomaxillary cyst that arises between the maxillary lateral incisor and the canine.

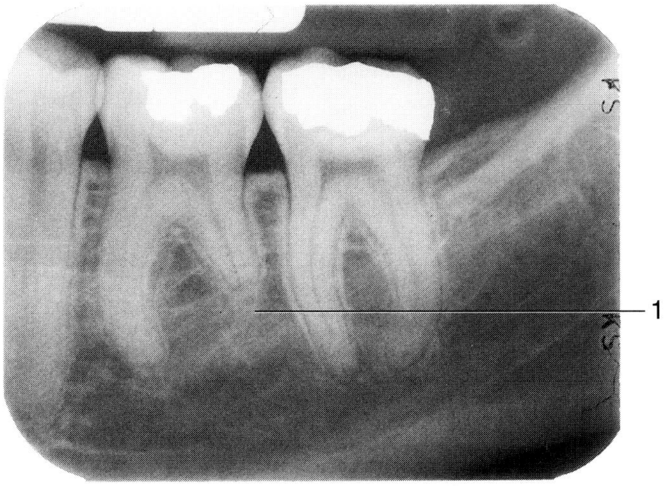

FIGURE 20–23 **External resorption.** (**1**) Idiopathic resorption of the distal root of the first molar.

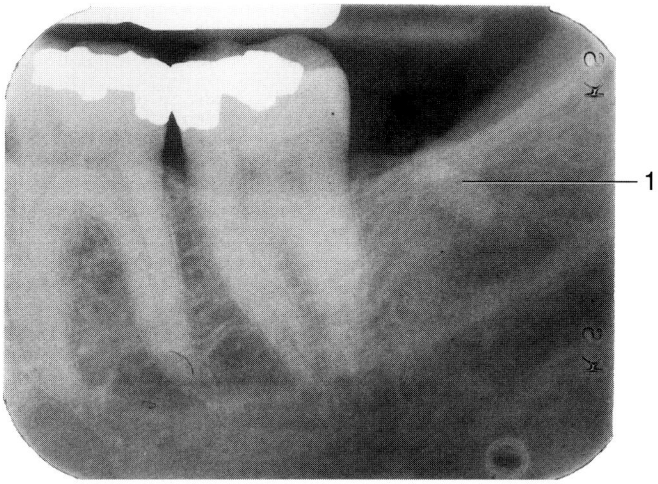

FIGURE 20–25 **Retained root (1) fragment in an extraction site.**

are moved too rapidly during orthodontic treatment (Figure 20–9). When the resorption cause is unknown, it is called **idiopathic resorption.**

Internal resorption typically appears as a radiolucent widening of the root canal, representing the resorption process taking place from the inside out (Figure 20–24).

Although not classified as resorption, the appearance of **retained root** fragments may be observed on radiographs of an edentulous area (Figure 20–25). These structures may have broken off the tooth and were left behind following extraction, or remain as the result of severe decay or trauma which broke off the crown of the tooth, leaving behind the root. The patient did not seek dental tratment for the condition and the root tip remained. Retained root tips may be clearly visible radiographically, or less so depending on their size and degree of resorption.

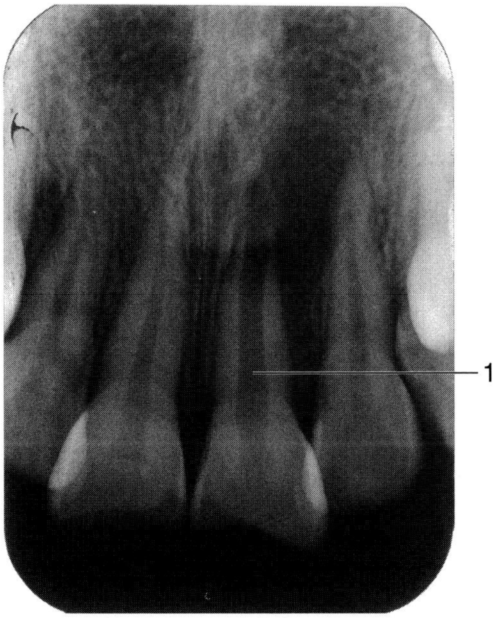

FIGURE 20–24 **Internal resorption.** (**1**) Idiopathic resorption of the tooth. Note the widening of the pulp chamber.

Radiographic Appearance of Calcifications and Ossifications

Calcifications in the dental pulp occur in the form of small nodules called **pulp stones** (Figure 20–26). These appear as radiopaque ovoid structures of varied size. Pulp stones are very common but of little significance, unless root canal therapy is needed on the affected tooth.

Other less frequently encountered calcifications are **sialoliths,** depositions of calcium salts in the salivary glands and ducts (Figure 20–27); **rhinoliths,** stones within the maxillary sinuses; and **phleboliths** or calcified thrombi, calcified masses that are observed as round or oval bodies in the soft tissues of the cheeks.

Two forms of **ossification** (the conversion of structures into hardened bone) are often imaged on radiographs. **Condensing**

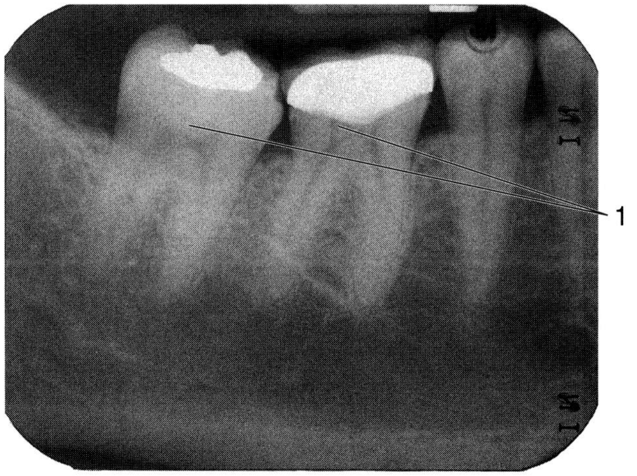

FIGURE 20–26 **Pulp stones.** (**1**) Ovoid radiopaque calcifications observed in the pulp chambers.

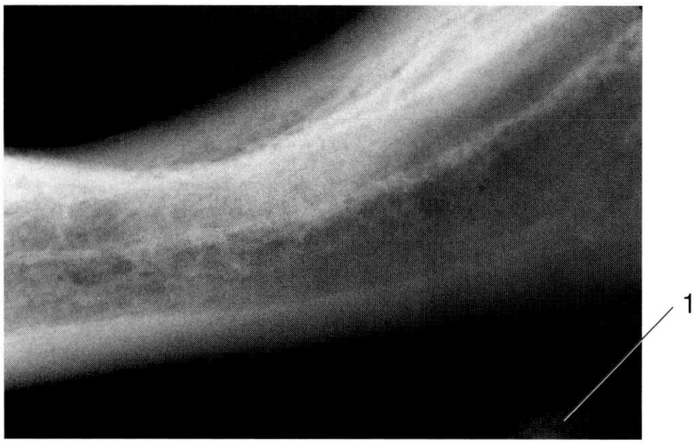

FIGURE 20-27 **Sialolith in a salivary gland.** (**1**) Note that this radiograph is of an edentulous mandible.

osteitis occurs when **sclerotic** (hardened) **bone** is formed as a result of infection (Figure 20–28). The increased radiopacity of the bone is often accompanied by a increased widening (radiolucency) of the periodontal ligament space. **Osteosclerosis** occurs when regions of abnormally dense bone form, but not as a direct result of infection (Figure 20–29). Although the cause is unknown, osteosclerosis commonly occurs in the interseptal premolar area and may be associated with fragments of retained primary roots.

Radiographic Appearance of Odontogenic Tumors

Odontogenic tumors result from abnormal proliferation of cells and tissues involved in odontogenesis (the formation of the teeth). The three types occasionally seen on radiographs are **ameloblastomas, odontomas,** and **cementomas.** Ameloblastomas have the greatest potential for serious implications for the patient. These appear as large radiolucencies of enamel origin. Radiographically, ameloblastomas may be monolocular (one compartment) or multilocular (many compartments). The monolocular form closely resembles a dentigerous cyst (Figure 20–30). The multilocular form has a characteristic "soap bubble" appearance.

Odontomas are the most common ondontogenic tumors (Figure 20–31). These are tumors of small misshaped teeth whose number in each odontoma varies widely. These toothlike structures appear radiopaque and are located within a radiolucent fibrous capsule that often resembles a cyst.

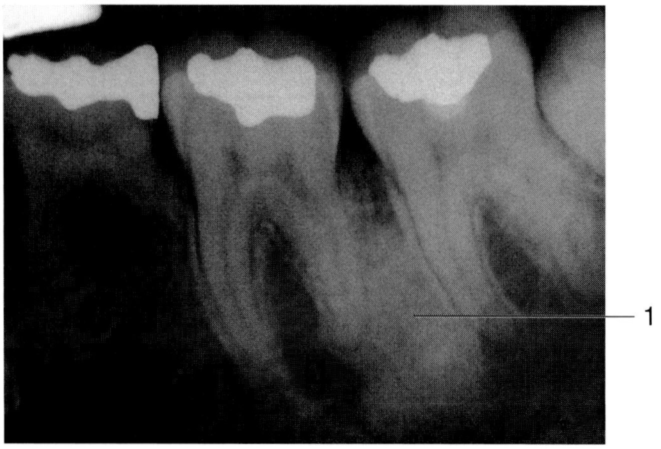

FIGURE 20-28 **Condensing osteitis.** (**1**) Radiopaque, sclerotic (hardening of) bone.

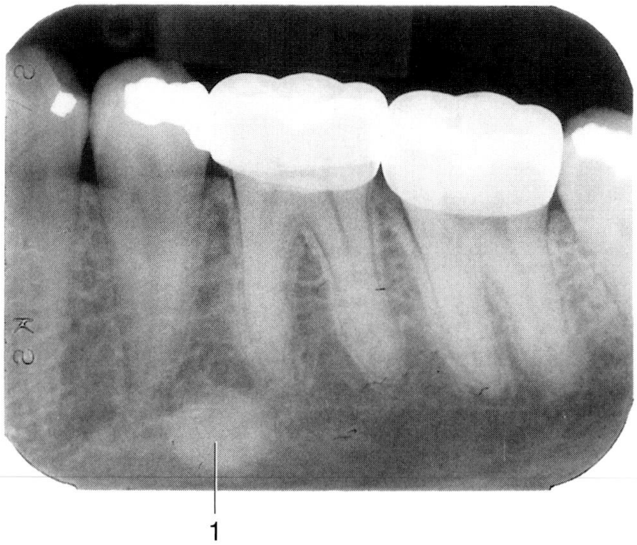

FIGURE 20-29 **Osteosclerosis.** (**1**) Diffuse idiopathic osteosclerosis.

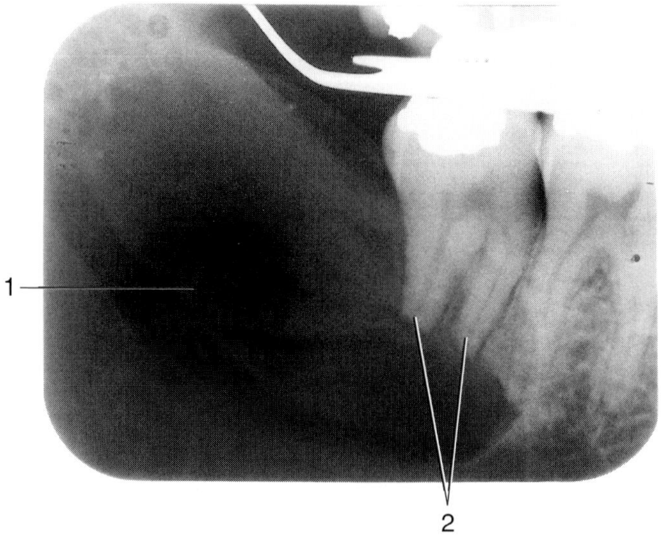

FIGURE 20-30 **Ameloblastoma.** (**1**) Large radiolucency. (**2**) Note the resorption of the molar roots caused by pressure of the tumor.

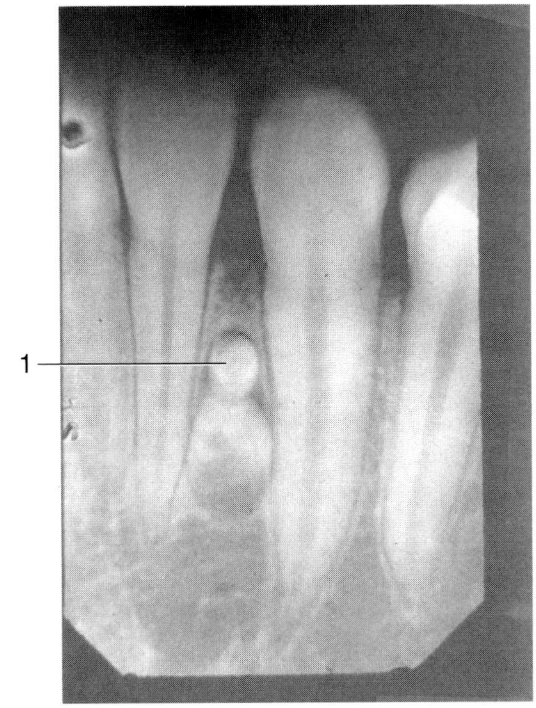

FIGURE 20-31 **Odontoma.** (**1**) Consisting of small, misshaped teeth located within a radiolucent fibrous capsule.

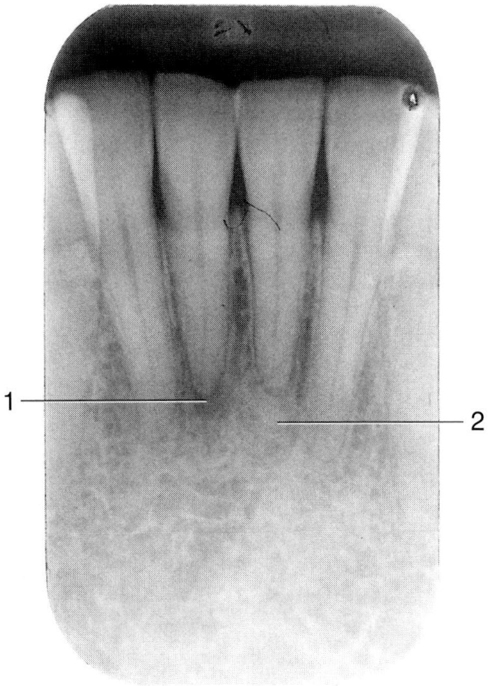

FIGURE 20-32 **Cementoma.** (**1**) Early cementoma (radiolucent), and (**2**) cementoma in late stage of development (radiopaque). The teeth are vital.

Cementomas, also called cementifying fibromas, are derived from the periodontal ligaments of fully developed and erupted teeth. Early cementomas are radiolucent and appear identical to radicular cysts. In the later stages of development, cementomas appear as radiopaque masses surrounded by a radiolucent line (Figure 20–32). Cementomas occur most frequently in the mandibular incisor region of women. The teeth are vital and the cementomas need no treatment.

Radiographic Appearance of Nonodontogenic Tumors

The majority of tumors found in the head and neck region do not have a characteristic radiographic appearance that enables a diagnosis from the radiograph alone. In fact, a diagnosis of a **tumor** cannot be made until the dentist, the pathologist, and the radiologist have combined their findings. However, the oral health care professional may be the first to detect the presence of a lesion and make the appropriate referral.

Tumors are classed as **benign** (doing little or no harm) and **malignant** (very dangerous or life threatening). Fortunately, most tumors detected in the oral health care practice are benign. Careful examination of the radiograph can often help to differentiate benign from malignant lesions.

Benign tumors may be either radiolucent or radiopaque, with well defined margins. Malignant tumors tend to have irregular margins and are less distinct, blending into the adjacent bone.

Exostoses and tori are the most frequently encountered forms of benign tumors. An **exostosis** is a localized overgrowth of bone. The term **torus** (plural tori) is often used to describe an exostosis that occurs near the midline of the palate (torus palatinus) (Figure 20–16) and on the lingual surface of the mandible (torus mandibularis) (see Figures 19–26 and 19–27). Radiographically, both appear as an area of increased radiographic density (radiopaque).

The two main types of oral malignancies are **carcinoma** and **sarcoma.** Both grow rapidly and spread into adjacent tissues. Carcinomas are malignant tumors of epithelial origin, and sarcomas are malignant tumors of connective tissue origin. The radiographic appearance of these tumors is radiolucent, with irregular and poorly defined borders. Sarcomas often have a "patchy" appearance with no demarcation from normal surrounding bone. Radiographs are vitally important in early detection because sarcomas produce changes in bone early in their development.

Radiographic Appearance of Trauma

The two most common injuries observed on dental radiographs are fractures of facial bones and teeth. **Fracture lines** are thin radiolucent lines that demarcate the region of bone or tooth separation (Figure 20–10). Fractures may on occasion have a similar appearance to the nutrient canals described in Chapter 19.

Radiographs will sometimes reveal the presence of **foreign bodies.** Note the broken dental instrument imaged in Figure 20–33.

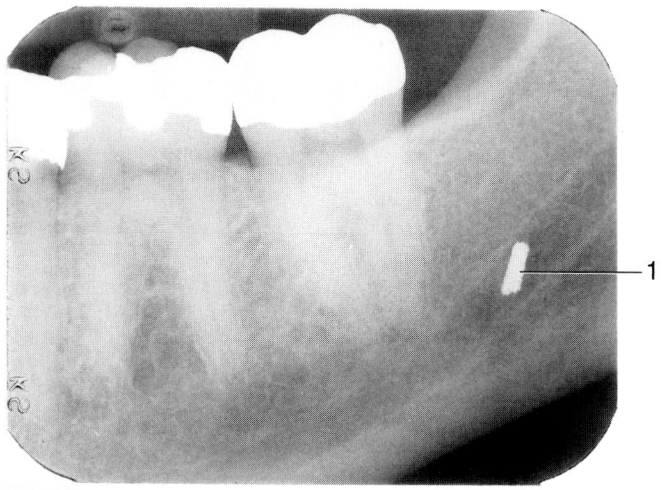

FIGURE 20-33 **Foreign object imaged on radiograph of mandibular molar region.** This radiograph shows (**1**) a broken burr, which probably lodged there when the third molar was removed.

REVIEW—Chapter Summary

The dental hygienist and dental assistant should possess the ability to recognize deviations from the normal. Developing this skill requires practice. While identifying deviations from the normal radiographically is important, a diagnosis can not be made from the radiograph alone. Common radiographic observations that the dental hygienist and dental assistant should be able to identify radiographically include the appearance of restorative materials, developmental anomalies, periapical pathology and other pathological conditions, and the effect of trauma.

Metallic restorative materials such as amlagam, metal crowns, retention pins, post and core and silver points appear radiopaque and are distinguished from each other by their size and shape. Non-metallic restorative materials such as composite, porcelain, base material, and gutta percha appear less radiopaque than metal. Some composites, may appear slightly radiopaque or radiolucent.

Developmental anomalies that may be imaged on radiographs include anodontia, supernumerary teeth, hypercementosis, dilaceration, gemination, fusion, concrescence, dentinogenesis imperfecta, and amelogenesis imperfecta.

Periapical abscess, granuloma, and cyst all appear radiolucent and can not be distinguished from each other radiographically.

Radiographs may image external and internal tooth resorption. Radiographic evidence of calcifications and ossifications include pulp stones, sialoliths, rhinoliths, phleboliths, condensing osteitis and osteosclerosis.

Although tumors may not be diagnosed from radiographs alone, the presence of ameloblastomas, odontomas, cementomas and benign and malignant tumors may be detected radiographically.

Fractures of the tooth and bone and foreign objects may be imaged radiographically.

RECALL—Study Questions

1. Amalgam and a full metal crown can be distinguished from each other radiographically by their:
   a. Degree of radiopacity.
   b. Shape and margins.
   c. Location in the mouth.
   d. Use of retention pins.
2. Which of these dental restorative materials appears most radiopaque?
   a. Amalgam
   b. Porcelain
   c. Silicate
   d. Acrylic resin
3. Which of these dental restorative materials is most likely to mimic decay radiographically?
   a. Gold
   b. Stainless steel
   c. Amalgam
   d. Composite
4. Dens in dente appears radiographically as:
   a. A tiny tooth.
   b. A large tooth.
   c. Twin teeth.
   d. A tooth within a tooth.
5. A tooth with a sharp bend in the root is called:
   a. Taurodontia.
   b. Hypercementosis.
   c. Dilaceration.
   d. Concresence.
6. Radiographically, it is not possible to accurately differentiate between a periapical abscess, a granuloma, and a cyst. Radiographically, it is not possible to accurately differentiate between carcinoma and sarcoma.
   a. The first statement is true; the second statement is false.
   b. The first statement is false; the second statement is true.
   c. Both statements are true.
   d. Both statements are false.
7. Which of these appears radiolucent on a radiograph?
   a. Sialolith
   b. Abscess
   c. Torus
   d. Odontoma
8. A large radiolucency surrounding the crown only of an unerupted tooth is most likely what type of cyst?
   a. Dentigerous
   b. Radicular
   c. Residual
   d. Periapical
9. The evidence of resorption that appears to shorten the tooth root is called:
   a. Internal resorption.
   b. External resorption.
   c. Primary resorption.
   d. Secondary resorption.

10. The radiographic appearance of a small ovoid radiopacity within the pulp chamber of the tooth is called a:
    a. Rhinolith.
    b. Phlebolith.
    c. Pulp stone.
    d. Pulp cap.
11. Which of the following appears radiolucent in its early stages and as a radiopaque mass in later stages?
    a. Condensing osteitis
    b. Periapical granuloma
    c. Osteosclerosis
    d. Cementoma
12. Which of the following tumors appears radiolucent radiographically?
    a. Torus palatinus
    b. Odontoma
    c. Sarcoma
13. Radiographic evidence of a bone fracture appears as a radiolucent line that may resemble a:
    a. Nutrient canal.
    b. Cyst.
    c. Tumor.
    d. Retained root tip.

REFLECT—Case Study

You have just accepted a position in a large oral health care clinic at a university-based dental school where your primary role will be to process, mount, and prepare a preliminary interpretation of full mouth series of radiographs taken on incoming patients. You know how valuable it is to follow a systematic order when mounting films, so you decide to apply an orderly system to interpreting the radiographs as well.

Design a form that will guide you and other radiographers through the interpretive process. Your form should include the following:

1. A place to record basic information (the patient's name, date the radiographs were taken, name of the person interpreting the radiographs, date of interpretation, etc.).
2. A step-by-step guide to where to begin and end the interpretive process.
3. A list of common conditions or deviations from normal that you will be looking for. (Organize the conditions you will be interpreting logically.)
4. Organize the conditions according to what you will examine the radiographs for first, second, third, etc.
5. Prepare columns, rows of boxes, or whatever your design requires as a place to record or list the condition.
6. Label the columns, rows of boxes, or whatever your design uses, with the appropriate headings.
7. Prepare a place to document that the condition needs a referral to the dentist.
8. Prepare your form in such a manner that other professionals may be able to utilize the form. Prepare written instructions for utilizing the form as needed.

RELATE—Laboratory Application

For a comprehensive laboratory practice exercise on this topic, see E. M. Thomson, *Exercises in Oral Radiography Techniques: A Laboratory Manual,* 2nd ed., Upper Saddle River, NJ: Prentice Hall, 2006. Chapter 12, "Radiographic Interpretation."

BIBLIOGRAPHY

Farman, A. G., Nortje, C. J., & Wood, R. E. *Oral and Maxillofacial Diagnostic Imaging.* St. Louis: C. V. Mosby, 1993.

Farman, A. G., Ruprecht, A., Gibbs, S. J., & Scarfe, W. C. (eds.). *IADMFR/CMI '97: Advances in Maxillofacial Imaging.* Amsterdam: Elsevier, 1997.

Langlais, R. P. & Kasle, M. J. *Exercises in Oral Radiographic Interpretation,* 3rd ed. Philadelphia: W. B. Saunders, 1992.

Langlais, R. P., Langland, O. E., & Nortje, C. J. *Diagnostic Imaging of the Jaw.* Philadelphia: Williams & Wilkins, 1995.

White, S. C. & Pharoah, M. J. *Oral Radiology Principles and Interpretation,* 5th ed. St. Louis: Elsevier, 2004.

21

The Use of Radiographs in the Detection of Dental Caries

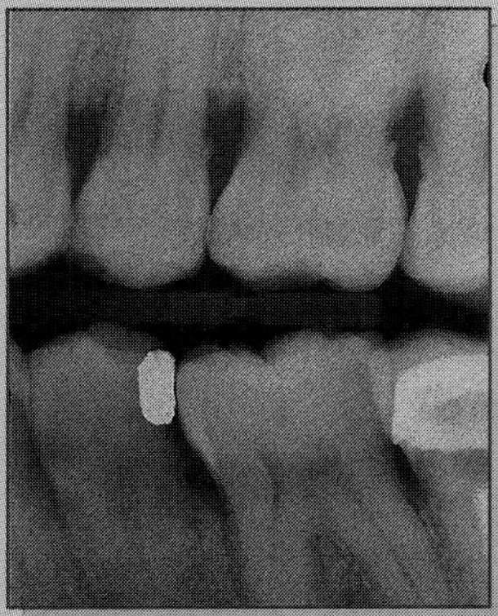

CHAPTER OUTLINE

■ OBJECTIVES

Following successful completion of this chapter, you should be able to:

1. Define the key words.
2. Explain why caries appear radiolucent on radiographs.
3. Define the role radiographs play in detecting caries.
4. Identify the ideal type of projection, technique and exposure factors that enhance a radiograph's ability to image caries.
5. List and describe the four categories of the caries depth grading system.
6. List the four locations of dental caries and identify their radiographic appearance.
7. Define and identify the radiographic appearance of recurrent dental caries.
8. List three conditions that resemble dental caries radiographically and discuss how to distinguish these from caries.

■ KEY WORDS

Advanced caries
Arrested caries
Buccal caries
Caries
Cemental (root) caries
Cementoenamel junction (CEJ)
Cervical burnout
Dentinoenamel junction (DEJ)
Incipient (enamel) caries
Interproximal
Interproximal caries
Lingual caries
Mach band effect
Moderate caries
Non-metalic restoration
Occlusal caries
Proximal caries
Rampant caries
Recurrent (secondary) caries
Severe caries

Introduction

The detection of caries (tooth decay) is probably the most common reason for exposing dental radiographs. The dental hygienist and dental assistant who is skilled in identifying normal radiographic anatomy should be able to differentiate between the appearance of normal tooth structures and dental caries on a radiograph.

The purpose of this chapter is to describe the radiographic appearance of dental caries, identify a caries depth grading system, and to offer some tips that may influence caries interpretation (Procedure Box 21–1).

Dental Caries

Description

Dental caries, or tooth decay, is a pathological process consisting of localized destruction of dental hard tissues by organic acids produced by microorganisms. The caries process is one of demineralization of tooth structure (enamel, dentin, cementum). This demineralization of tooth density allows more x-rays to pass through the tooth and darken the film. Therefore, **caries** appear radiolucent on the radiograph (Figure 21–1).

Detection

Radiographs reveal carious lesions that may go undetected clinically, especially caries on the proximal surfaces (in between the teeth) (Table 21–1). To be a useful diagnostic aid, the radiographs must be precisely exposed and meticulously processed. Improper angulation can render a radiograph worthless for caries detection. Incorrect vertical angulation obliterates viewing carious lesions on a radiograph (Figure 21–2). The horizontal angulation is particularly important. Overlapping of the contact areas between the teeth will make it impossible to detect lesions in these areas (Figure 21–3).

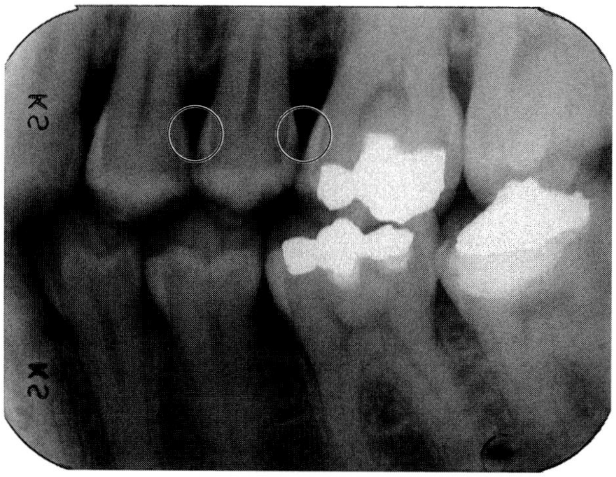

FIGURE 21–1 **Carious lesions.** Radiograph showing multiple carious lesions. Note interproximal caries are found just apical to the contact area between two adjacent teeth.

PROCEDURE 21–1

RADIOGRAPHIC INTERPRETATION FOR CARIES

1. See Procedure Box 18–2, Suggested Sequence for Viewing a Full Mouth Series of Radiographs.
2. View all surfaces of each tooth.
3. Examine the contact points and just apical to the gingival margin for radiolucencies indicating proximal caries.
4. Examine the dentin just apical to the occlusal enamel for radiolucencies indicating occlusal caries.
5. Examine the dentin in the middle of the tooth for a round radiolucency indicating buccal or lingual caries.
6. If there is bone loss and evidence that cementum is exposed in the oral cavity, examine the cervical region of the tooth for an ill-defined, radiolucent saucer-shaped area below the cementoenamel junction (CEJ) indicating cemental (root) caries.
7. Examine existing restorations for recurent decay.
8. Confirm findings and/or clarify uncertain interpretations with a clinical exam of the patient.
9. Consult the patient's chart for confirmation or clarification of findings as needed.
10. Present a preliminary interpretation for the dentist's review.
11. Following confirmation by the dentist, document all findings on the patient's permanent record.

TABLE 21-1 Radiographic Appearance of Caries

Grade	Severity	Proximal	Occlusal	Buccal/lingual	Cemental
C-1	Incipient	Radiolucent notch in the enamel only. Radiolucency is less than half-way through the enamel.	Not evident radiographically.	Not evident radiographically.	Not applicable because enamel is not involved in this type of caries.
C-2	Moderate	Radiolucent triangle with the apex pointing toward the DEJ. Radiolucency is more than half-way through the enamel, but does not invade the DEJ.	Not evident radiographically.	Not evident radiographically.	Not applicable because enamel is not involved in this type of caries.
C-3	Advanced	Radiolucency takes on a double triangle shape, first through the enamel with the apex pointing toward the DEJ and a second triangle base spreading along the DEJ with the apex pointing toward the pulp. Radiolucency is less than half-way through the dentin toward the pulp.	Flat radiolucent line, often with no or little change detected in the enamel. Radiolucency is less than half-way through the dentin toward the pulp.	Not possible to distinguish advanced from severe. Both appear as a round radiolucency in the middle of the tooth with well defined borders.	Although enamel is not involved in this type of caries, at this stage an ill-defined, radiolucent, saucer-shaped area below the cementoenamel junction (CEJ) may be observed. Bone loss must be evident.
C-4	Severe	Radiolucency may retain a double triangle shape, or be so severe as to appear as a large diffuse radiolucency. Radiolucency is more than half-way through the dentin toward the pulp.	Large radiolucency detected in the dentin below the occlusal enamel. Depending on the extent of destruction, radiolucent breaks in the occlusal enamel may be imaged. Radiolucency is more than half-way through the dentin toward the pulp.	Not possible to distinguish advanced from severe. Both appear as a round radiolucency in the middle of the tooth with well defined borders.	Although enamel is not involved in this type of caries, at this stage an ill-defined, radiolucent, saucer-shaped area below the cementoenamel junction (CEJ) may be observed. Bone loss must be evident.

The bitewing radiograph, described in Chapter 14, is the radiograph of choice for the evaluation of caries due to the precise parallelism established between the tooth and the film plane. However, a precisely placed periapical radiograph exposed using the paralleling technique will adequately image dental caries as well as bitewing radiographs (Figure 21–4).

While the exposure factors (mA, kVp and impulses) used will depend on the patient and the area to be exposed, generally, practitioners prefer to use a lower kVp to best image caries. A lower setting, such as 70 kVp, will result in an image that has a high contrast: black and white with few shades of gray in between. Since caries appear radiolucent against a radiopaque enamel (or lesser radiopaque dentin), a high contrast image is often preferred by the practitioner for imaging carious lesions.

Interpreting Dental Caries

Dental caries is a process of decalcification and requires 40 to 50 percent loss of calcium and phosphorus before the decreased density can be seen on a radiograph. For this reason, the depth of penetration of a carious lesion is deeper clinically than it appears on the radiograph. Also, because the proximal surfaces of posterior teeth are broad, the loss of small amounts of mineral from incipient lesions may be difficult to see on the radiograph (Figure 21–5).

Caries Depth Grading System

Several systems are used to grade the depth of penetration of caries. This text will use a grading system suggested by Haugejorden and Slack, 1977 (Figure 21–6). The advantage of this system is that it allows one to accurately grade the penetration of caries (establish a baseline) and to track the progression of the carious lesions at future appointments. These grades may also be called incipient, moderate, advanced, or severe.

- **C-1: Enamel caries,** also called **incipient caries** (incipient means the first stage of existence), penetrate less than halfway through the enamel of the tooth toward the **dentinoenamel junction (DEJ)** (Figure 21–6, 1).

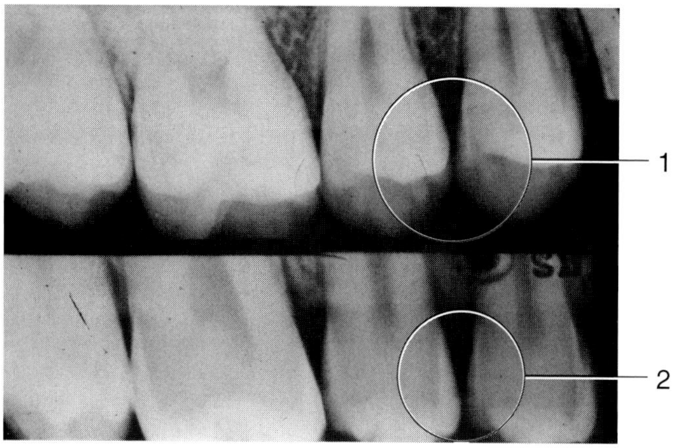

FIGURE 21-2 **Vertical angulation.** (**1**) Improper vertical angulation (excessive) obliterates viewing this proximal surface carious lesion. (**2**) Proper vertical angulation shows interproximal caries.

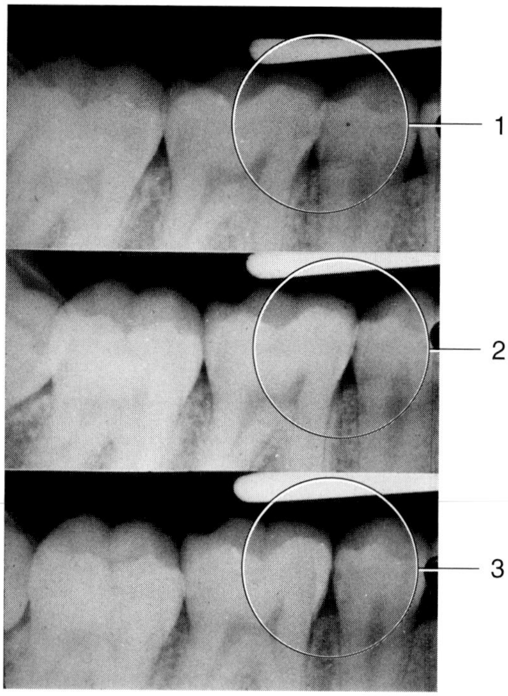

FIGURE 21-3 **Horizontal angulation.** (**1**) Improper horizontal angulation prevents viewing interproximal caries. (**2**) Improved horizontal angulation, but caries difficult to view. (**3**) Proper horizontal angulation shows interproximal caries.

- **C-2: Moderate caries,** penetrating over halfway through the enamel toward the dentinoenamel junction (DEJ), but not reaching the DEJ. Moderate caries are only seen in the enamel (Figure 21–6, 2).
- **C-3: Advanced caries** are caries of enamel and dentin definitely at or through the dentinoenamel junction (DEJ), but less than halfway through the dentin toward the pulp (Figure 21–6, 3). Advanced caries are seen in both the enamel and dentin.
- **C-4: Severe caries** are caries of enamel and dentin penetrating over halfway through the dentin toward the pulp (Figure 21–6, 4). Severe caries are seen in both the enamel and the dentin.

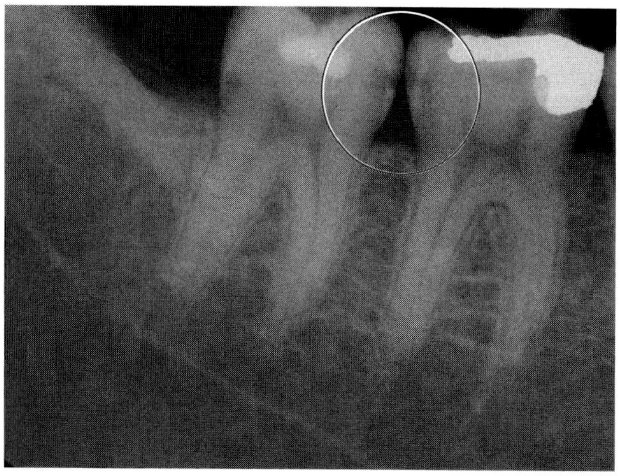

FIGURE 21-4 **Periapical radiograph showing interproximal caries.**

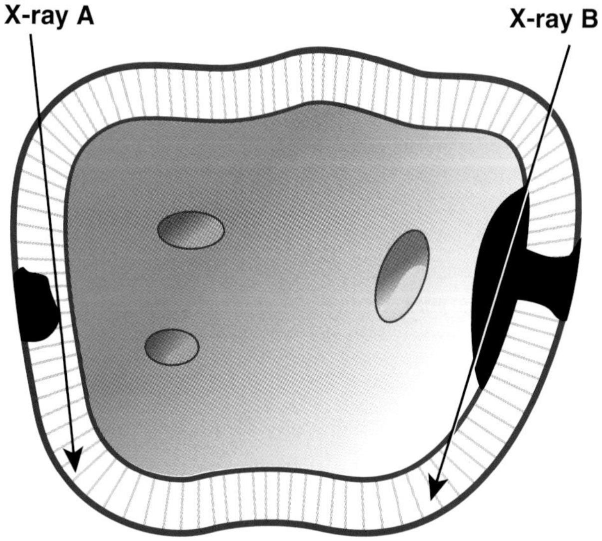

FIGURE 21-5 **Drawing showing ratio of caries to enamel.** This drawing shows **x-ray A** passing through a small ratio of caries to enamel, resulting in the caries being difficult to view and **x-ray B** passing through a large ratio of caries to enamel, resulting in the caries being easier to view.

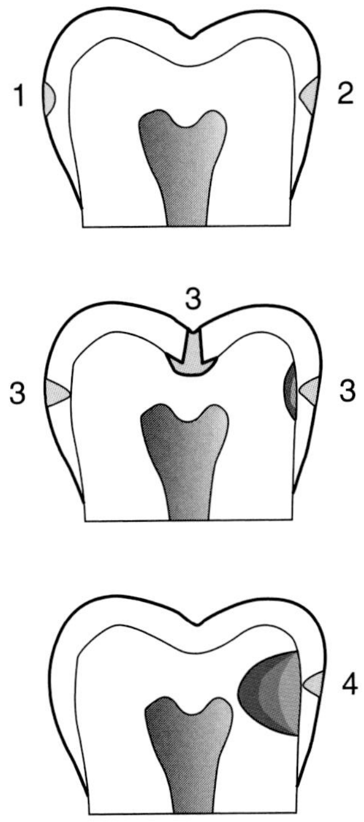

FIGURE 21-6 **Diagram of classification of dental caries recommended by Haugejorden and Slack.** (1) **C-1 caries.** Enamel caries less than halfway through the enamel (incipient caries). (2) **C-2 caries.** Enamel caries penetrated over halfway through the enamel (moderate caries). (3) **C-3 caries.** Caries definitely at or through the dentino-enamel junction (DEJ), but less than halfway through the dentin toward the pulp (advanced caries). (4) **C-4 caries.** Caries that has penetrated over halfway through the dentin toward the pulp (severe caries).

Classification of the Radiographic Appearance of Caries

The radiographic appearance of dental caries may be classified according to their location on the tooth.

There are four locations of caries:

1. Proximal
2. Occlusal
3. Buccal/lingual
4. Cemental (root surface)

Caries may be categorized as recurrent, rampant, or arrested.

Radiographs are often prescribed to detect proximal surface caries. Occlusal, buccal/lingual, and cemental caries are more readily detected clinically than with radiographs. In fact, early (incipient and moderate) occlusal, buccal/lingual and cemental caries often do not show up on radiographs even though these may be detected clinically. However, moderate and severe occlusal, buccal/lingual, and cemental caries will appear radiographically, so it is important that the radiographer recognize these.

Proximal Caries

Interproximal means between two adjacent surfaces. On dental radiographs, **proximal** surface **caries** often referred to as **interproximal caries** are located on the tooth surface that contacts the adjacent tooth. The interproximal is an area that is almost impossible to examine clinically, making the use of radiographs vitally important in caries detection. The tooth surface should be examined for caries at the point of contact, and just apical to this point of contact, to the gingival margin (Figure 21–7). The location of the height of the gingival margin, which is soft tissue, is not imaged on the radiograph. So the gingival margin location is estimated based on where the alveolar bone crest height is imaged. Assume that the gingival margin will be located at least 1 mm above the level of bone imaged on the radiograph.

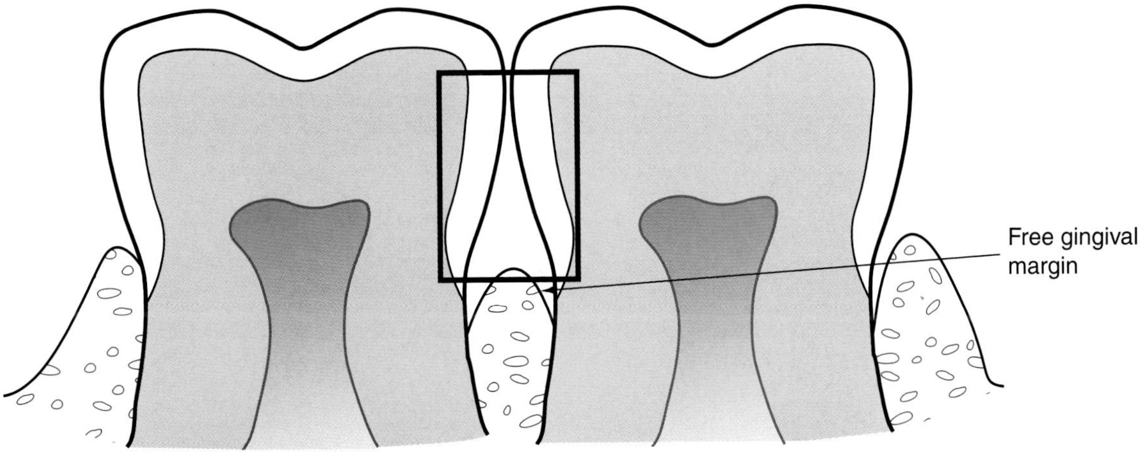

FIGURE 21-7 **Drawing indicating the area to examine for interproximal caries.** To best detect proximal surface caries, view the area where two adjacent teeth contact, apical down to the area where the gingival margin would most likely be (boxed area). Cervical burnout is most likely to be imaged apical to the gingival margin.

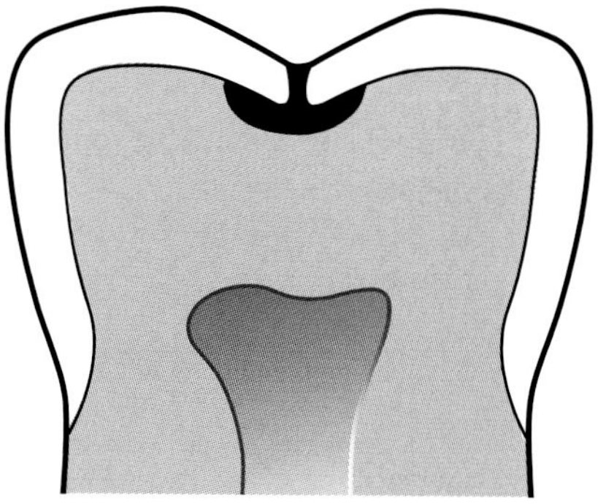

FIGURE 21-8 **Drawing of occlusal caries, early stage.** Early occlusal caries (C-1 and C-2) extend along the dentinoenamel junction (DEJ) and may not be seen on the radiograph even though the lesion may be detected clinically.

The shape of proximal caries begins as a radiolucent notch on the enamel (C-1) (Figure 21–6, 1). As the carious lesion progresses, it takes on a triangular shape (like a pyramid) with the apex pointing toward the dentinoenamel junction (DEJ) and the base toward the outer surface of the tooth (C-2) (Figure 21–6, 2). At the DEJ the caries spreads, undermining normal enamel, and again takes on a triangular shape as it penetrates toward the pulp (C-3) (Figure 21–6, 3). The base of this second triangle is along the DEJ and the apex points toward the pulp (C-4) (Figure 21–6, 4).

Occlusal Caries

Occlusal caries are carious lesions located on the chewing surface of the posterior teeth. Because of the superimposition of the buccal and lingual cusps, occlusal caries in early stages (incipient and moderate) may not be imaged on a radiograph (Figure 21–6, 3, and Figure 21–8) even though a clinical examination does detect incipient or moderate occlusal caries.

After occlusal caries has reached the DEJ (advanced caries), it may be imaged on the radiograph (Figures 21–9 and 21–10).

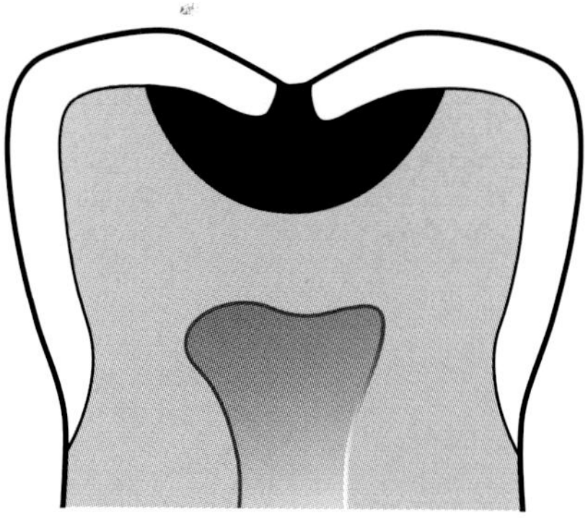

FIGURE 21-9 **Drawing of advanced occlusal caries.** Advanced (up to half-way toward the pulp) or severe occlusal caries (more than half-way toward the pulp) will most likely be imaged radiographically.

At the DEJ occlusal caries will appear as a flat radiolucent line. Often no or little change is detected in the enamel radiographically at this stage. As the carious lesion progresses, the size of the radiolucency increases. It is important to note that when examining radiographs for occlusal caries, the area of interest is below the occlusal enamel, in the area of the dentin, and not from the top of the tooth. The irregularity of the cusps and occlusal surface pits and fissures do not usually indicate the presence of caries. Changes (radiolucencies) in the dentin below the occlusal enamel are indicative of occlusal caries. As advanced caries progress to a severe stage, changes in the occlusal enamel are more likely to be imaged.

Buccal and Lingual Caries

Buccal caries involves the buccal surface of a tooth and **lingual caries** involves the lingual surface (Figure 21–11). Buccal and lingual caries are best detected clinically. Early buccal and lingual carious lesions are almost impossible to detect radiographically. This is due to the superimposition of the normal tooth structures over the caries. As the lesion becomes severe, it will appear as a radiolucency characterized by its well defined borders. This has been characterized as looking into a hole on the radiograph (Figure 21–12). However, because the radiograph is a two-dimensional image of three-dimensional structures, it is impossible to tell the depth of buccal or lingual caries or the relationship to the pulpal tissue.

Cemental (Root) Caries

Cemental caries (also known as **root caries**) develop between the enamel border and the free margin of the gingiva on the cemental surface (Figure 21–13). Bone loss and recession of the gingival tissue are necessary for the caries' process to start on the root surfaces. Cemental caries may appear on the buccal, lingual, mesial, or distal surface of the tooth.

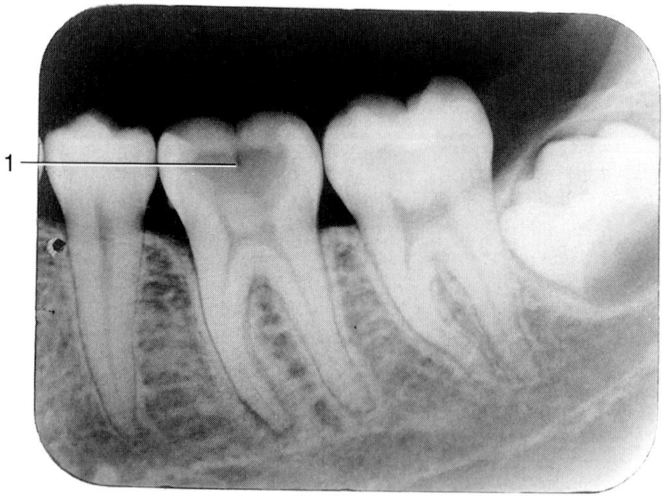

FIGURE 21-10 **Radiograph of occlusal caries.** This radiograph shows (**1**) severe occlusal caries, which appears as a large radiolucent lesion in the first molar.

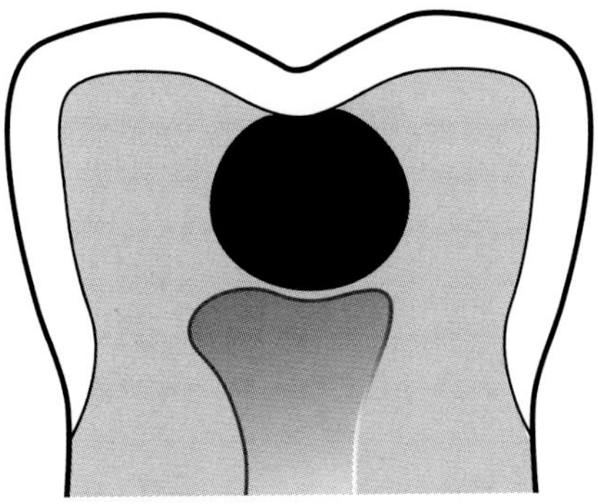

FIGURE 21-11 **Drawing of buccal or lingual caries.** Advanced buccal or lingual caries have well defined borders.

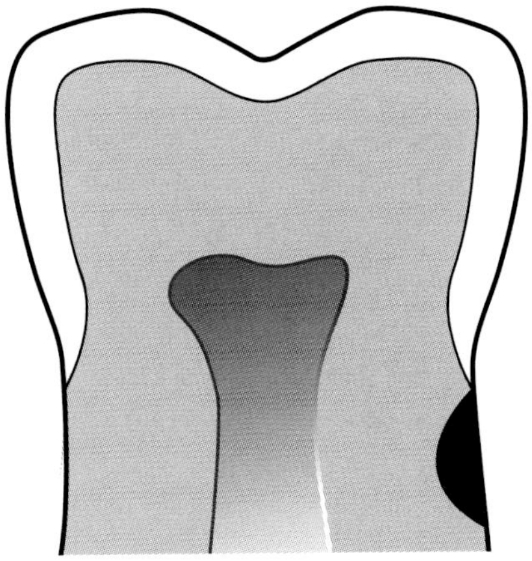

FIGURE 21-13 **Drawing of cemental (root) caries.** Cemental caries involves only the roots of teeth. Gingival recession and bone loss precede the caries' process to expose the root surfaces.

Radiographically, cemental caries appear as an ill defined, radiolucent, saucer-shaped area just below the **cementoenamel junction (CEJ)** (Figure 21–14). Cemental caries may at times be misinterpreted as cervical burnout, an optical illusion of the radiographic image. (Cervical burnout is discussed later in this chapter.) Cemental caries are more easily detected clinically than radiographically.

Recurrent (Secondary) Caries

Recurrent or **secondary caries** is decay that occurs under a restoration or around its margins. Recurrent caries occur because of poor cavity preparation, defective margins of the restoration, or incomplete removal of the caries prior to the placement of the restoration. Recurrent caries appears on a radiograph as a radiolucent area beneath a restoration or apical to the interproximal margin of a restoration (Figure 21–15).

Rampant Caries

The term rampant means growing rapidly or spreading unchecked. **Rampant caries** are severe, unchecked caries that affect multiple teeth (Figure 21–16).

Arrested Caries

The term arrested means stopped or inactive. **Arrested caries** are caries that are no longer active. Carious lesions may become arrested if there is a significant shift in the oral environment from factors that cause caries to those that slow down the caries' process. Incipient enamel caries (C-1) can remain dormant for long periods of time. Some carious lesions may even be reversed

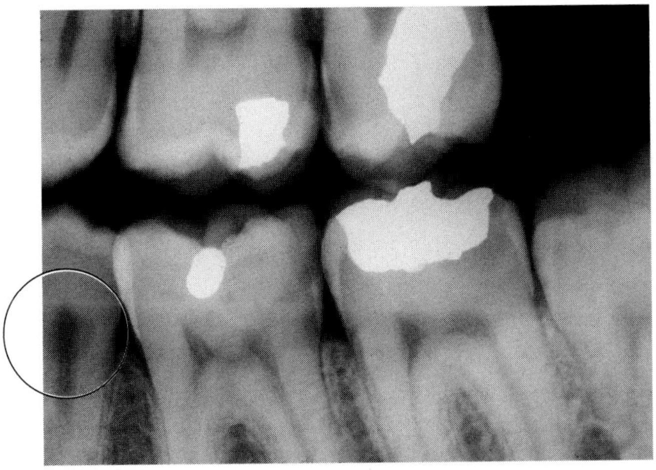

FIGURE 21-12 **Radiograph of buccal or lingual caries.** Buccal or lingual caries on this mandibular second premolar appears as a round radiolucency (superimposed over the pulp chamber).

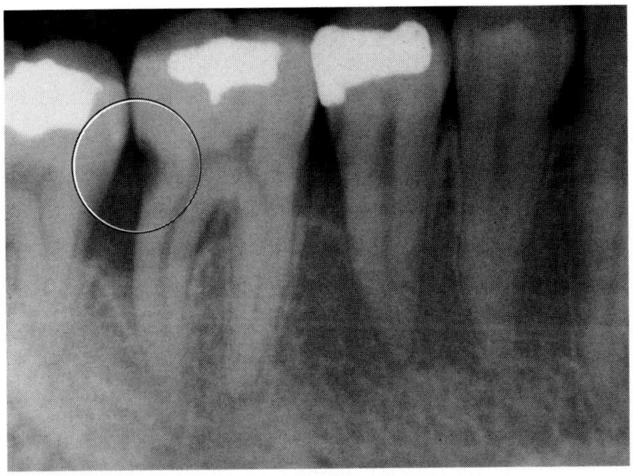

FIGURE 21-14 **Radiograph of cemental (root) caries.** The large radiolucency on the distal surface of the distal root of the first mandibular molar is cemental caries. Note the bone loss exposing the root surface.

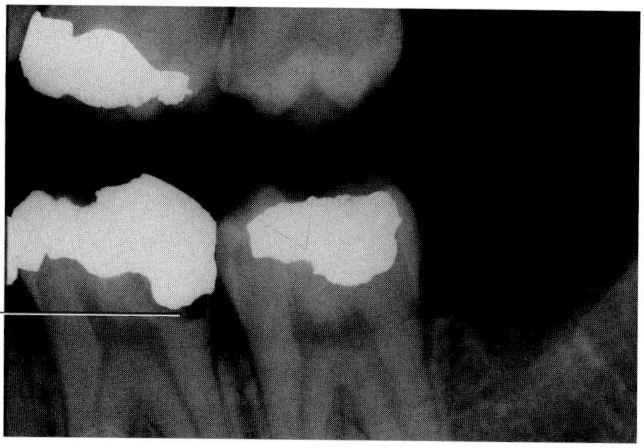

FIGURE 21–15 **Radiograph of recurrent caries.** This radiograph shows (**1**) radiolucent caries under the metallic restoration.

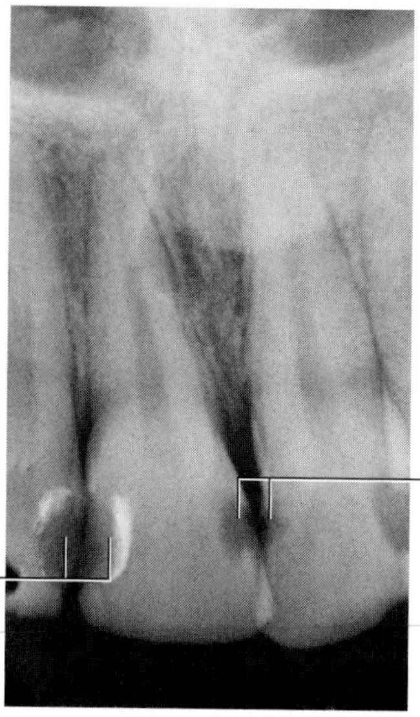

FIGURE 21–17 **Radiograph of nonmetalic restorations and carious lesions in anterior teeth.** This radiograph shows (**1**) radiolucent non-metallic restorations on the mesial surface of the lateral incisor and distal surface of the central incisor. Note that under both restorations is a base of radiopaque material. (**2**) The radiolucencies on the mesial surfaces of both central incisors are carious lesions.

by remineralization. It is important that radiographic exams continue to monitor arrested caries.

Conditions Resembling Caries

Three conditions that resemble caries are **non-metallic restorations, cervical burnout,** and **mach band effect.**

Non-metallic Restorations

Non-metallic esthetic restorations in anterior teeth may mimic decay radiographically (Figure 21–17). Non-metallic restorations such as composite, silicate, and acrylic resin discussed in Chapter 20 may mimic decay when they appear radiolucent. To aid in distinguishing a restoration from caries, look for the restoration to have straight borders, or a prepared look, with an overall even radiolucency. A radiopaque base material may also be present under the radiolucent non-metallic restoration. Caries tend to have more diffuse borders and an uneven radiolucency that takes on a triangular shape, with the apex pointing toward the DEJ or pulp. A clinical examination may be required to make a final determination.

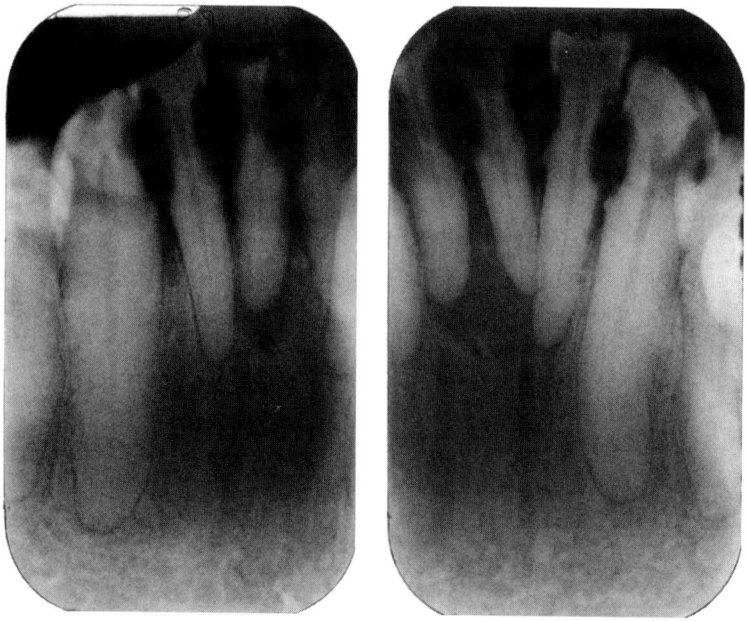

FIGURE 21–16 **Radiograph of rampant caries.** This radiograph shows multiple teeth affected.

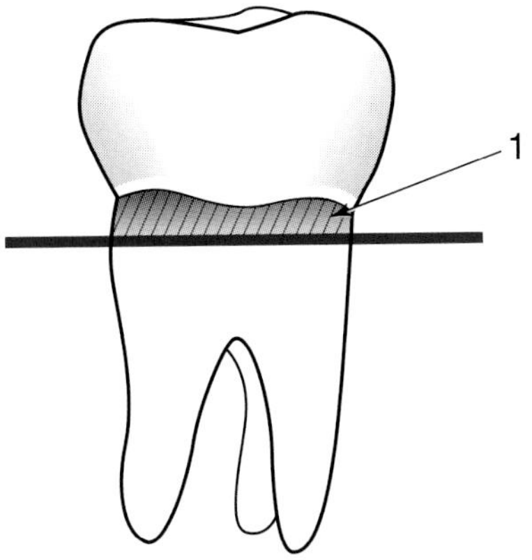

FIGURE 21-18 **Drawing of cervical burnout.** This drawing shows (**1**) cervical root surface between crown and alveolar crest of bone. The thin root surface allows more x-rays to pass than the dense enamel crown and alveolar bone, and therefore is radiolucent.

Cervical Burnout

Cervical burnout is an optical illusion created when the eye must distinguish between a very light (white) area and a very dark (black) area on the radiograph. The area of the tooth most likely to produce this optical illusion is the cervical root, or neck of the tooth. In this region, the concavity of the root surfaces allow greater penetration by the x-rays (Figure 21–18). This region will appear especially dark next to radiopaque structures. When the radiopaque enamel on one side and the radiopaque lamina dura on the other side sandwich the radiolucent cervical of the tooth in between, the effect is an increased darkness called cervical burnout. Cervical burnout often appears as an irregularly shaped radiolucent area with a fuzzy outline seen on the mesial and/or the distal surfaces of the tooth along the cervical line (Figure 21–19). To assist in distinguishing cervical burnout from caries, remember to focus caries detection only in the area of the contact point of adjacent teeth and apical to the gingival margin (Figure 21–7). Cervical burnout appears more apical, apparently under the gingival margin.

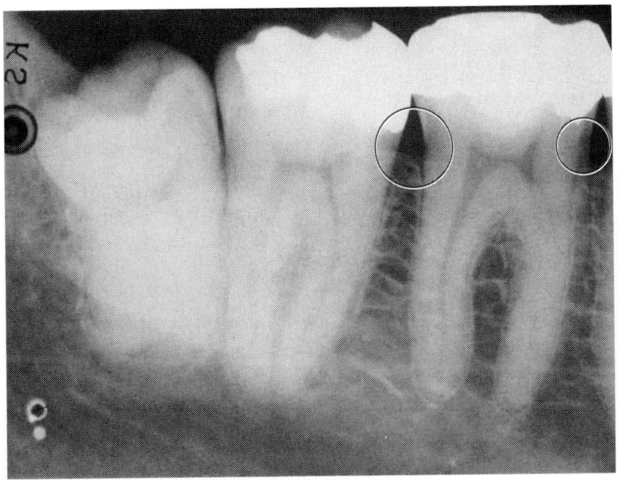

FIGURE 21-19 **Radiograph demonstrating cervical burnout.** This radiograph shows the radiolucent optical illusion of cervical burnout on the mesials and distals between the enamel and restorations and the alveolar crest of bone.

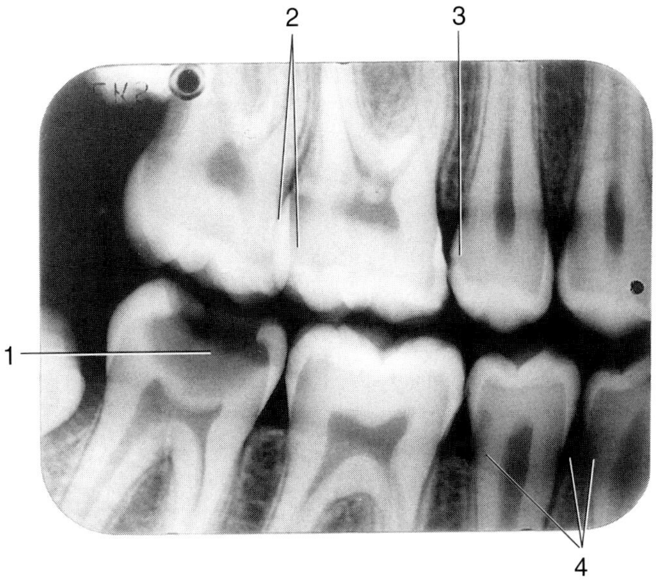

FIGURE 21-20 **Bitewing radiograph.** This radiograph shows (**1**) large occlusal caries, (**2**) radiolucent lines or mach band effect (an optical illusion caused by overlapped enamel), (**3**) interproximal caries, and (**4**) cervical burnout.

Mach Band Effect

Another optical illusion is a radiolucency caused by overlapping images of the teeth. When two proximal surfaces overlap (caused either by natural overlap of misaligned teeth or by improper horizontal angulation of the x-ray beam), the result is a dense radiopaque area surrounded by radiolucent lines. These radiolucent lines represent an optical illusion called the mach band effect resulting from the high contrast between the normal enamel and the dense overlapped enamel (Figure 21–20). The ability of these overlapped structures to produce this optical illusion illustrates how important it is to produce radiographs that do not have angulation errors.

REVIEW—Chapter Summary

The detection of caries is probably the most common reason for taking dental radiographs. Caries appear radiolucent because the demineralization of the tooth allows more x-rays to pass through to darken the film. Only precisely exposed and meticulously processed radiographs are useful in detecting caries.

Bitewing radiographs and carefully positioned periapical radiographs, exposed for a high contrast image (low kVp), are best at imaging caries. Radiographs detect more proximal surface caries than a clinical exam alone. A clinical exam is better at detecting early occlusal, buccal/lingual, and cemental caries. The depth of the caries penetration is deeper clinically than it appears on the radiograph.

An example of a caries depth grading system is presented. These grades may also be referred to as incipient caries, moderate caries, advanced caries, and severe caries.

The radiographic appearance of dental caries may be classified according to their location on the tooth: proximal, occlusal, buccal/lingual, and cemental (root surface). Three conditions that resemble caries are non-metallic restorations, cervical burnout, and mach band effect.

RECALL—Study Questions

1. Caries appear radiopaque, *because* more radiation is passing through the caries than the surrounding tissues.
   a. The first part of the statement is true, but the second part of the statement is false.
   b. The first part of the statement is false, but the second part of the statement is true.
   c. Both parts of the statement are true.
   d. Both parts of the statement are false.
2. All of the following will produce an ideal radiographic image for detecting caries *except* one. Which one is this *exception?*
   a. Bitewings
   b. Low kVp
   c. No overlapping
   d. Excessive vertical angulation
3. Caries in the earliest stage is called:
   a. Incipient.
   b. Moderate.
   c. Advanced.
   d. Severe.
4. Radiographs are best at detecting incipient caries of which of these locations on the tooth?
   a. Occlusal
   b. Proximal
   c. Buccal/lingual
   d. Cemental
5. The key to successfully interpretating radiographs for proximal surface caries is to examine the contact point between adjacent teeth and just apical to the:
   a. DEJ.
   b. CEJ.
   c. Gingival margin.
   d. Alveolar bone crest.
6. Proximal surface carious lesions appear:
   a. Triangular
   b. Square
   c. Round
   d. Saucer-like
7. Which of the following appears radiographically as a radiolucent notch that is less than half-way through the enamel?
   a. Incipient proximal caries
   b. Moderate proximal caries
   c. Advanced proximal caries
   d. Severe proximal caries
8. Which of the following appears radiographically as a radiolucent double triangle that is less than half-way through the dentin toward the pulp?
   a. Incipient proximal caries.
   b. Moderate proximal caries.
   c. Advanced proximal caries.
   d. Severe proximal caries.
9. The key to successfully interpretating radiographs for occlusal caries is to examine:
   a. The occlusal surface for changes in the pits and fissures.
   b. Under the occlusal surface for changes in the dentin.
   c. The contact point between adjacent teeth for changes in the enamel.
   d. Just apical to the contact point for changes in the DEJ.
10. Which of the following appears radiographically as a round radiolucency in the middle of the tooth with well defined borders?
   a. Proximal caries
   b. Occlusal caries
   c. Cemental caries
   d. Buccal/lingual caries
11. Which of the following appears radiographically as an ill-defined saucer-shaped radiolucency below the CEJ?
   a. Proximal caries
   b. Occlusal caries
   c. Cemental caries
   d. Buccal/lingual caries
12. Caries that occur under a restoration or around its margins are called:
   a. Recurrent caries.
   b. Cemental caries.
   c. Root caries.
   d. Buccal caries.
13. All of the following may mimic caries radiographically *except* one. Which one is this *exception?*
   a. Composite restorations
   b. Stainless stain crowns
   c. Cervical burnout
   d. Mach banding
14. An optical illusion created by an increased radiolucency observed at the cervical area of the tooth is called mach banding. Mach banding effect increases when overlap error occurs.
   a. The first statement is true; the second statement is false.
   b. The first statement is false; the second statement is true.
   c. Both statements are true.
   d. Both statements are false.

REFLECT—Case Study

You are interpreting a full mouth series of radiographs on a patient who had dental hygiene services at your facility this morning. The completed patient's dental examination chart is available, but the patient has been dismissed. As you examine the radiographs, you notice the following:

1. Incipient proximal caries on the distal of the maxillary right first molar.
   a. Describe the radiographic appearance of this lesion.
   b. Indicate why you classified this lesion as incipient.
2. Moderate proximal caries on the mesial of the maxillary left first premolar.
   a. Describe the radiographic appearance of this lesion.
   b. Indicate why you classified this lesion as moderate.
3. Advanced proximal caries on the mesial of the mandibular left second premolar.
   a. Describe the radiographic appearance of this lesion.
   b. Indicate why you classified this lesion as advanced.
4. Severe proximal caries on the distal of the mandibular right first molar.
   a. Describe the radiographic appearance of this lesion.
   b. Indicate why you classified this lesion as severe.
5. Advanced occlusal caries on the maxillary right second molar.
   a. Describe the radiographic appearance of this lesion.
   b. Indicate why you classified this lesion as advanced.
6. Cemental caries on the mesial of the mandibular right first premolar.
   a. Describe the radiographic appearance of this lesion.
   b. Indicate why you classified this lesion as cemental.
7. The patient's chart indicates incipient occlusal caries detected clinically on the maxillary left first and second molars. However, these do not seem to be evident radiographically.
   a. Explain why these caries are not observed on the radiographs.
8. The patient's chart indicates incipient buccal caries detected clinically on the mandibular left first molar. However, this lesion does not seem to be evident radiographically.
   a. Explain why the buccal caries is not observed on the radiographs.
9. The radiographs reveal two radiolucencies resembling cemental (root) caries around the cervical of the mandibular right first and second premolars. However, the patient's chart does not indicate that cemental caries were detected clinically.
   a. Explain the possible cause of these radiolucencies.
10. The periapical radiograph of the maxillary left molar region is overlapped between the maxillary first and second molars.
    a. Explain why detecting caries in this area will be compromised.
    b. What optical illusion will most likely present in this area?
    c. Describe the appearance of this optical illusion.

RELATE—Laboratory Application

For a comprehensive laboratory practice exercise on this topic, see E. M. Thomson, *Exercises in Oral Radiography Techniques: A Laboratory Manual,* 2nd ed., Upper Saddle River, NJ: Prentice Hall, 2006. Chapter 12, "Radiographic Interpretation."

BIBLIOGRAPHY

Berry, H. Cervical burnout and mach band: Two shadows of doubt in radiologic interpretation of carious lesions. *J. Am. Dent. Assoc.* 106: 622, 1983.

Langlais, R. P., & Kasle, M. J. *Exercises in Oral Radiographic Interpretation,* 3rd ed. Philadelphia: Saunders, 1992.

Langlais, R. P., Langland, O. E., & Nortje, C. J. *Diagnostic Imaging of the Jaws.* Philadelphia: Williams & Wilkins, 1995.

Langland, O. E. & Langlais, R. P. *Principles of Dental Imaging.* Philadelphia: Williams & Wilkins, 1997.

White, S. C. & Pharoah M. J. *Oral Radiology Principles and Interpretation,* 5th ed. St. Louis: Elsevier, 2004.

White, S. C. & Yoon, D. C. Comparative performance of digital and conventional images for detecting proximal surface caries. *Dentomaxillofac. Radiol.* 26:32, 1997.

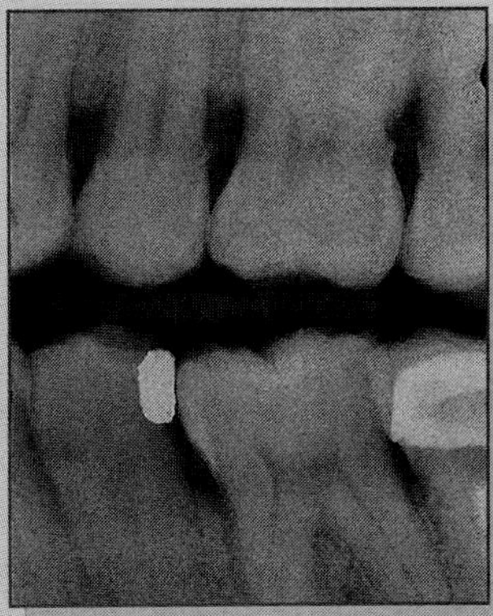

22

The Use of Radiographs in the Evaluation of Periodontal Diseases

CHAPTER OUTLINE

■ OBJECTIVES

Following successful completion of this chapter, you should be able to:

1. Define the key words.
2. List the uses of radiographs in the assessment of periodontal diseases.
3. Differentiate between horizontal and vertical bone loss.
4. Recognize the role vertical and horizontal angulations play in imaging periodontal diseases.
5. Identify three predisposing factors for periodontal disease that radiographs can help locate.
6. Explain how imaging anatomical configurations aids in the prognosis of periodontally involved teeth.
7. List the limitations of radiographs in the assessment of periodontal diseases.
8. Utilize the appropriate radiographic techniques to best detect and evaluate periodontal diseases.
9. Describe the radiographic appearance of the normal periodontium.
10. List four American Academy of Periodontology disease classification case types and describe their radiographic appearance.

■ KEY WORDS

Alveolar (crestal) bone
Calculus
Cementoenamel junction (CEJ)
Furcation involvement
Generalized bone loss
Gingivitis
Horizontal bone loss
Interdental septa
Lamina dura
Localized bone loss
Occlusal trauma
Periodontal diseases
Periodontal ligament space
Periodontitis
Periodontium
Predisposing factors
Triangulation
Vertical bone loss (angular bone loss)
Vertical bitewing series

Introduction

Dental radiographs play a key role in the diagnosis, prognosis, management and evaluation of periodontal diseases. Properly exposed and meticulously processed radiographs are invaluable aids in the diagnosis of periodontal diseases. To get the most diagnostic information from radiographs taken to image periodontal status, radiographers should have an extensive knowledge of the radiographic techniques that will produce quality films. The purpose of this chapter is to introduce the dental radiographer to the radiographic appearance of periodontal diseases; to outline the radiographic examinations and techniques best suited to produce quality radiographs for the purpose of evaluating periodontal diseases; and to describe predisposing factors for the disease that radiographs help to identify.

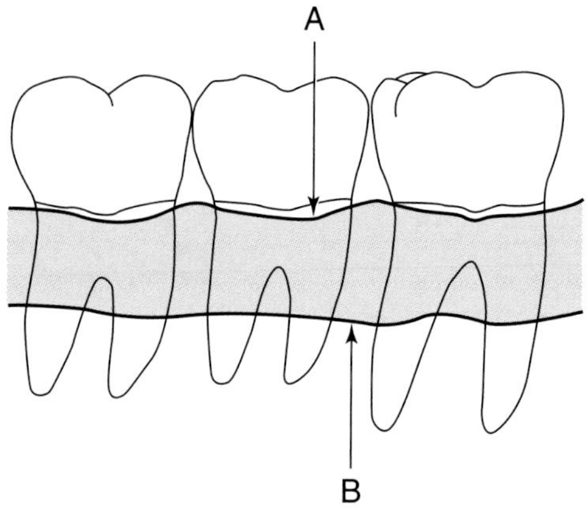

FIGURE 22–1 **Drawing showing horizontal bone loss.** (**A**) Normal (physiologic) level of bone (alveolar bone parallel to the cementoenamel junction) and (**B**) Bone level of patient with periodontal disease. Horizontal bone loss is the difference between (**A**) and (**B**) (shaded area).

Radiographic Appearance of Periodontal Diseases

Periodontal diseases are diseases that affect both soft tissues (gingiva) and bone around the teeth. The severity of periodontal disease may range from a simple inflammation of the gingiva to the destruction of supporting bone and the periodontal ligament. The most common periodontal diseases are gingivitis and periodontitis. **Gingivitis** is inflammation of the gingiva and limited to the soft tissue (gingiva). **Periodontitis** is also the result of infection, but includes loss of **alveolar bone.**

The proper diagnosis and evaluation of periodontal diseases must be made with a combination of radiographic and clinical examinations.

Radiographic Examination

Uses (Table 22–1)

Radiographs, along with a thorough clinical examination, allow the dentist and dental hygienist to evaluate and document periodontal diseases. The uses of radiographs in the assessment of periodontal diseases include:

1. **Imaging the supporting bone.** Radiographs allow the practitioner to evaluate crestal bone irregularities and **interdental septa** changes (alveolar bone changes between the teeth). Radiographs document the amount of bone remaining rather than the amount lost. The amount of bone loss is estimated as the difference between the physiologic bone level and the height of the remaining bone (Figure 22–1).

   Radiographs also allow the practitioner to determine the pattern of bone loss; horizontal or vertical. **Horizontal bone loss** describes height loss around adjacent teeth in a region. In horizontal bone loss, both buccal and lingual plates have been resorbed as well as the intervening interdental bone. Horizontal bone loss occurs in a plane parallel to the **cementoenamel junctions (CEJ)** of adjacent teeth (Figure 22–2). **Vertical bone loss,** sometimes called **angular bone loss,** occurs in a vertical direction where the resorption of one tooth root sharing the interdental septum

TABLE 22–1 **Periodontal Bone Changes Imaged by Radiographs**

- Crestal irregularities
- Interdental alveolar bone changes
- Pattern of bone loss (horizontal/vertical)
- Distribution of bone loss (localized/generalized)
- Severity of bone loss (slight, moderate, advanced)
- Furcation involvement

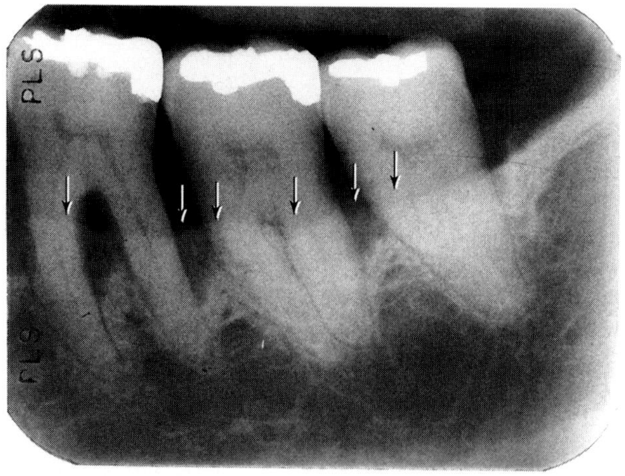

FIGURE 22–2 **Horizontal bone loss.** Arrows show bone level of patient with periodontal disease. Note that the level of bone loss is parallel to an imaginary line drawn between the cementoenamel junctions of the adjacent teeth.

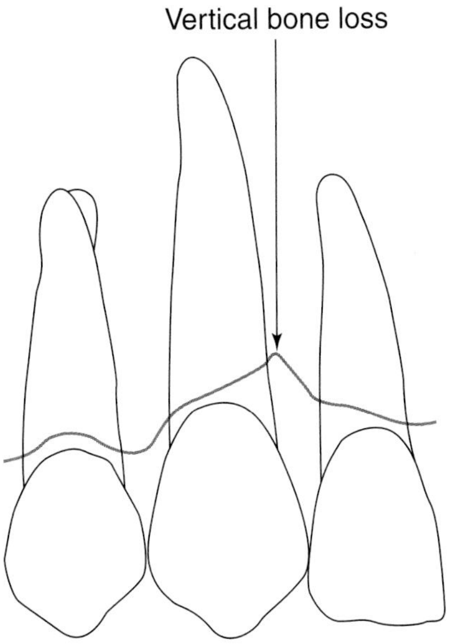

FIGURE 22-3 **Drawing showing vertical bone loss.** Vertical bone loss appears angular where the resorption is greater on the side of one tooth than on the side of the other tooth.

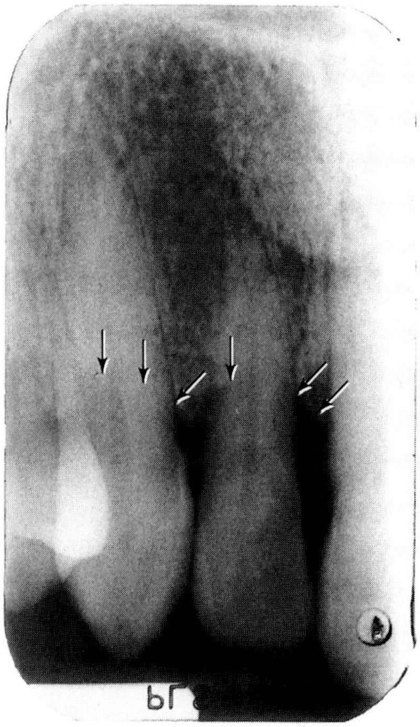

FIGURE 22-4 **Vertical bone loss.** Arrows show bone level of patient with periodontal disease.

(bone between the teeth) is greater than the other tooth (Figures 22–3, 22–4, and 22–5).

Radiographs can help the practitioner determine the distribution of bone loss; localized or generalized. **Localized bone loss** occurs in local areas and involves one or only a few teeth. (Figures 22–6 and 22–7). **Generalized bone loss** occurs throughout the entire dental arches (Figure 22–8).

Radiographs can reveal the severity of bone loss; slight, moderate, or advanced; and **furcation involvement** (bone loss between the roots) of multi-rooted teeth (Figure 22–9).

2. **Locating predisposing factors.** Radiographs can detect amalgam overhangs (see Chapter 20), poorly contoured crown margins, and **calculus** deposits that act as food traps and lead to the build-up of bacterial deposits that cause periodontal diseases (Figures 22–10 and 22–11). Calculus, hardened plaque, appears slightly radiopaque (about the radiopacity of dentin) and must be significantly calcified in order to be imaged on radiographs. Depending on the density and the amount of the deposit, calculus may appear as pointed or irregular projections on the proximal root surfaces, or as a ring-like radiopacity around the cervical neck of a tooth.

   Radiographs often reveal the effects of traumatic occlusion. **Occlusal trauma** does not cause periodontal disease, but has been shown to hinder the body's response to the disease. The effects of excessive occlusal forces show up on radiographs as a widening of the periodontal ligament space

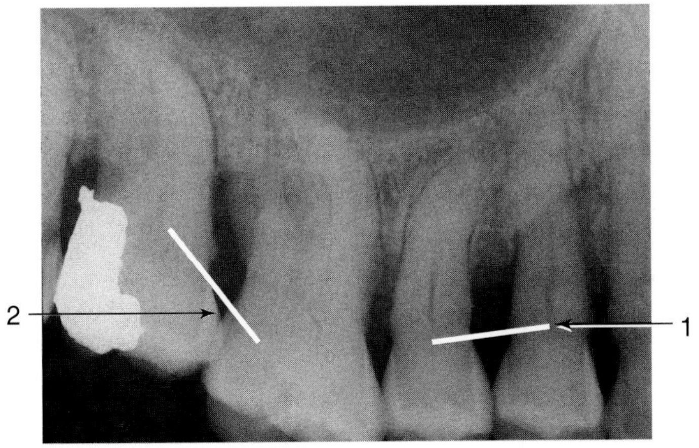

FIGURE 22-5 **Comparison of horizontal and verical bone loss.** Using the CEJ of adjacent teeth as a guideline; (**1**) horizontal bone loss and (**2**) vertical bone loss are evident on this radiograph.

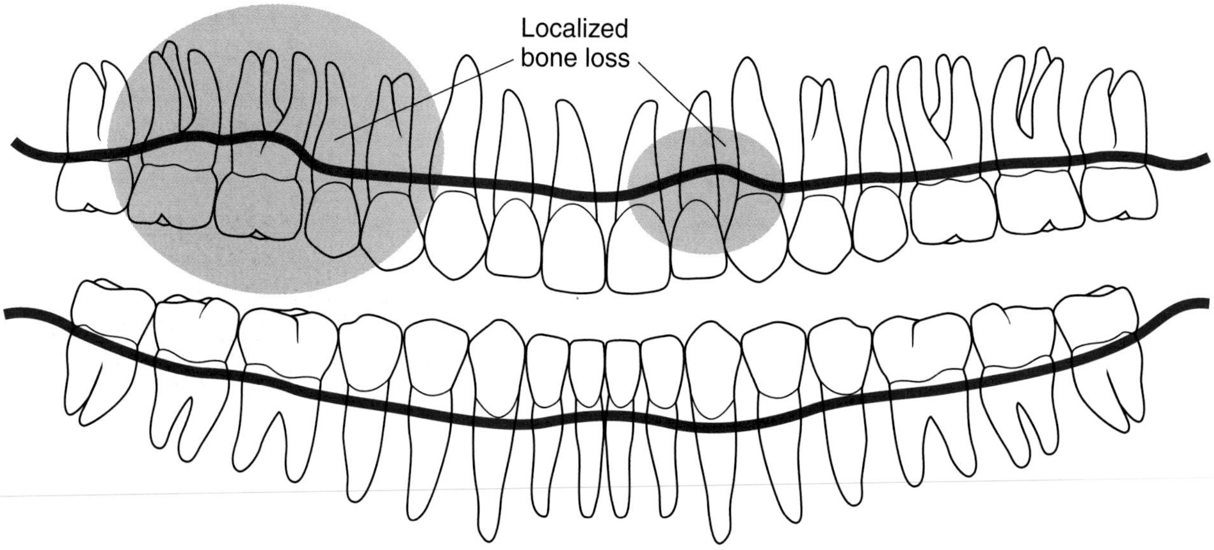

FIGURE 22-6 **Drawing showing localized bone loss.**

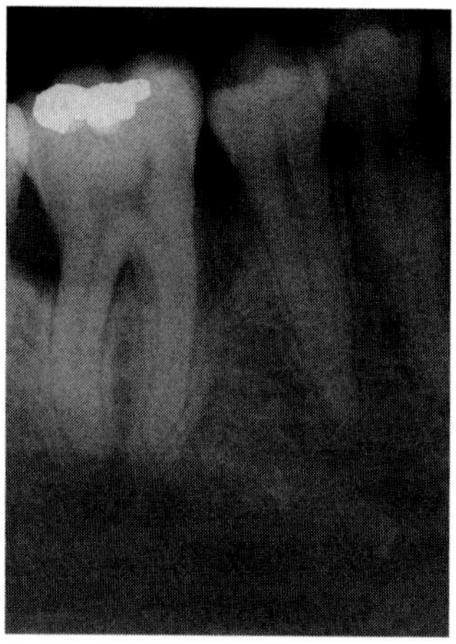

FIGURE 22-7 **Radiograph showing localized bone loss.**

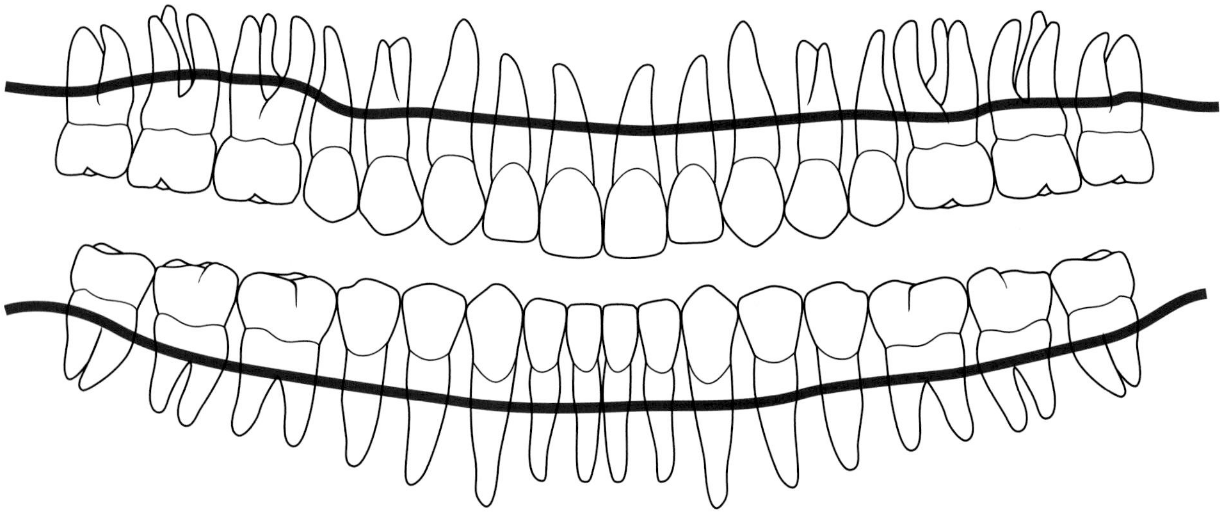

FIGURE 22-8 **Drawing showing generalized bone loss.**

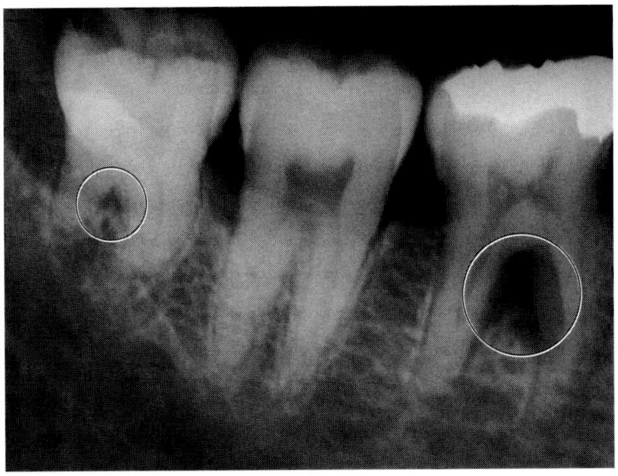

FIGURE 22-9 **Radiograph showing furcation involvement of the molars.** Note the radiolucency in between the roots of these multi-rooted teeth.

(Figure 22–12), often accompanied by an increased radiopacity in the bone (osteosclerosis; see Chapter 20) and/or an overgrowth of cementum (hypercementosis; see Chapter 20). **Triangulation** is bordered by the lamina dura, the root surface of the tooth, and its base is toward the tooth crown.

3. **Imaging anatomical configurations.** Radiographs can reveal information about root morphology, such as root length and the presence of dilacerations (see Chapter 20); root shape and width, such as multi-rooted teeth with ample supporting bone in between the roots or narrow, close or fused roots, all of which can help determine the treatment and treatment outcomes. For example, a tooth with a shortened root as a result of external resorption (see Chapter 20) will have a poor prognosis, while a tooth with a normal or long root may have a better prognosis (Figure 22–13). Additionally, teeth that have ample bone surrounding widely spaced roots will be more likely to have a better prognosis because of the amount of bone support.

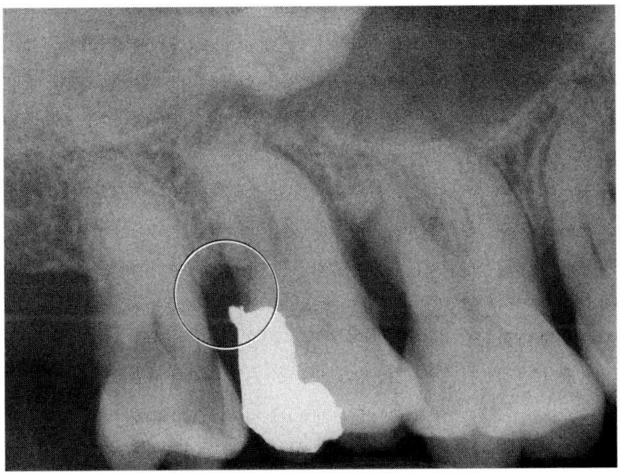

FIGURE 22-10 **Radiograph showing amalgam overhang on the maxillary second molar.** This predisposing factor will collect bacterial plaque that can contribute to the progression of periodontal diseases.

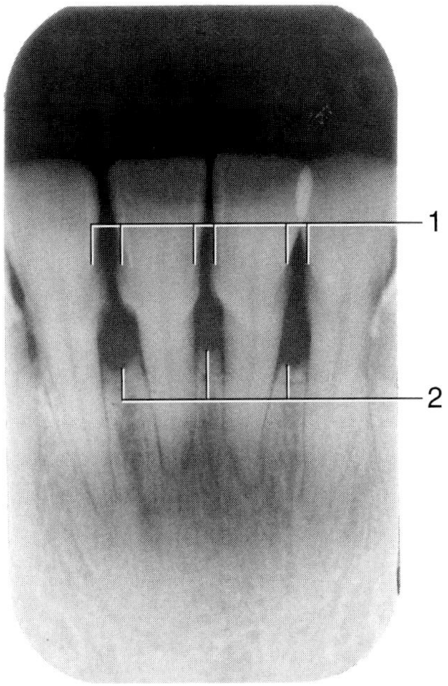

FIGURE 22-11 **Radiograph of mandibular incisor region.** This radiograph shows (**1**) large deposits of calculus around the necks of the teeth and (**2**) radiolucent areas indicating bone loss that is typical of periodontal disease.

4. **Evaluating the prognosis and treatment intervention needs.** By providing information on the tooth root-to-crown ratio, and adjacent tooth proximity, radiographs help the practitioner plan treatment and predict outcomes.
5. **Serving as a baseline and as a means for evaluating the results of treatment.** Radiographs provide documentation on the progression of disease and provide a permanent record of the condition of the bone throughout the course of the disease.

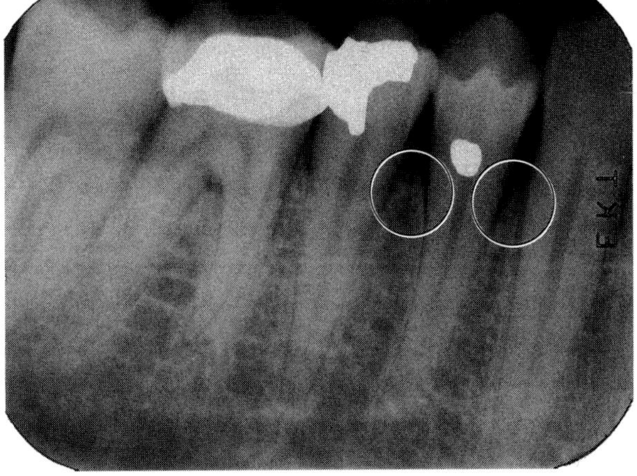

FIGURE 22-12 **Triangulation.** Widening of the periodontal ligament space indicative of occlusal trauma.

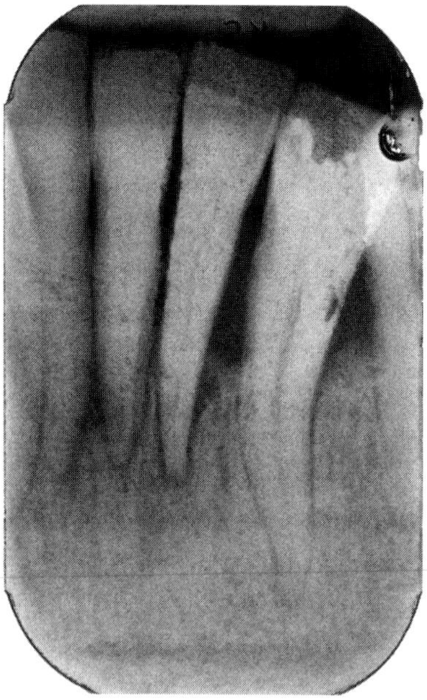

FIGURE 22-13 **Root length and root-to-crown ratio.** While the bone loss observed on this radiograph is significant, the radiograph reveals a longer than normal, dilacerated root that improves the prognosis for the canine.

Limitations

1. **Radiographs are a two-dimensional image of three-dimensional objects.** Radiographs lack the third dimension of depth, which results in bone and tooth structures being superimposed over each other. This will often hide bone loss on the buccal and lingual surfaces and furcation involvement, especially in the posterior region of the oral cavity.
2. **Changes in soft tissue not imaged.** Because soft tissue is not imaged on radiographs, gingivitis can not be detected radiographically. Radiographs do not add any information regarding the location and/or depth of periodontal pockets.
3. **Cannot distinguish treated versus untreated disease.** Radiographs do not indicate the presence or absence of active disease.
4. **Actual destruction more advanced clinically.** Radiographs can not detect early signs of periodontal diseases. A significant loss of bone density must occur before radiographic changes are detected.

Radiographic Techniques

Bitewings, especially the **vertical bitewing series,** described in Chapter 14, are most useful for examining the **periodontium** (Figure 22–14). The precise parallelism established between the tooth and the film plane when taking bitewing radiographs makes it possible to image the alveolar crestal bone accurately. To achieve this same degree of accuracy when using periapical radiographs to image the periodontium, the paralleling technique

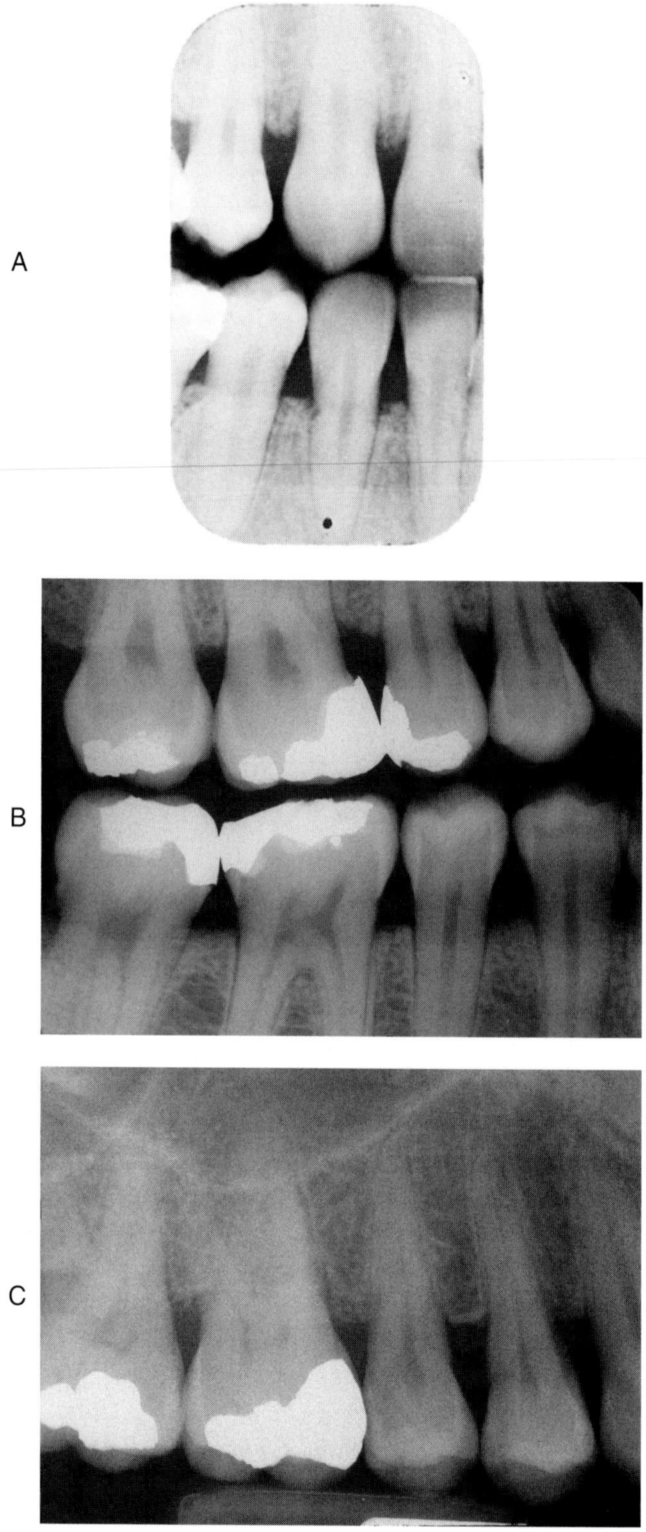

FIGURE 22-14 **Comparsion of bitewing and periapcial radiographs imaging the periodontium.** (**A**) vertical bitewing, (**B**) horizontal bitewing, and (**C**) periapical.

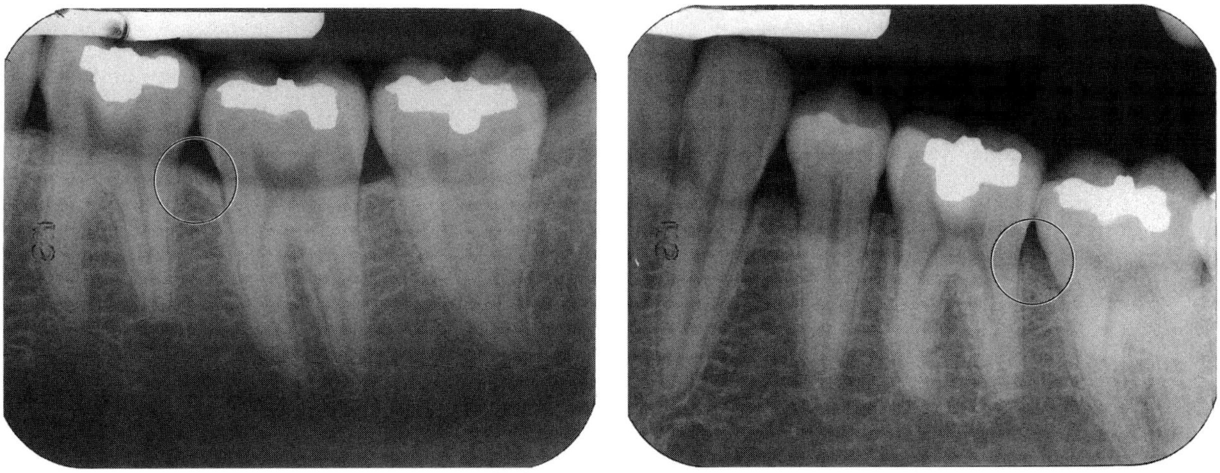

A B

FIGURE 22-15 **Example of incorrect vertical angulation.** (**A**) This radiograph has been correctly exposed. Note the appearance of the crestal bone between the mandibular first and second molars, indicating no bone loss. (**B**) This radiograph was exposed using incorrect vertical angulation. Note the same mandibular first and second molars. There is a false radiolucent, cupping-out appearance of the lamina dura. (Reprinted from *Journal of Practical Hygiene,* vol. 3, no. 2, E. M. Thomson & S. L. Tolle, "A Practical Guide for Using Radiographs in the Assessment of Periodontal Diseases. Part 2: Interpretation and Future Advances," p. 12, copyright 1994, with permission from Montage Media.)

must be utilized. The film packet must be placed parallel to the long axis of the teeth to ensure that the images of the bone and teeth on the radiograph are not distorted.

To be a useful diagnostic aid, the radiographs must be precisely exposed and meticulously processed. Improper angulation can render a radiograph worthless for evaluating periodontal disease. Excessive vertical angulation may not reveal bone loss, while inadequate vertical angulation may result in a radiographic image that falsely indicates bone loss when there is none (Figures 22–15 and 22–16). Accurate horizontal angulation is also important in evaluating periodontal disease. Faulty horizontal angulation results in overlapping of the contact areas between the teeth, making it impossible to determine the condition of interdental bone (bone in between the teeth). Second, varying

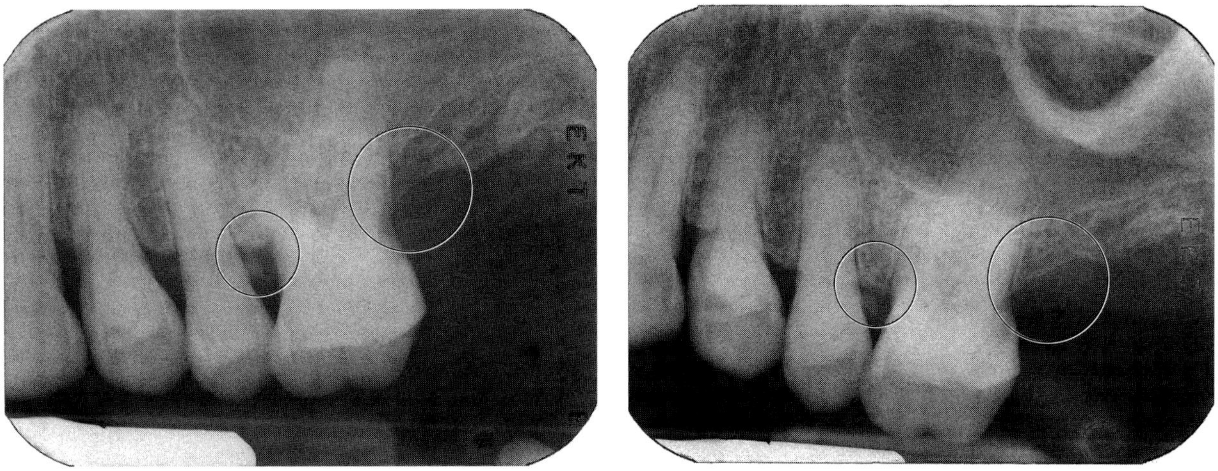

A B

FIGURE 22-16 **Example of incorrect vertical angulation.** (**A**) This radiograph has been correctly exposed. Note the level of the crestal bone mesial and distal to the maxillary first molar, indicating bone loss. (**B**) This radiograph was exposed using incorrect vertical angulation. Note the same areas, mesial and distal to the maxillary first molar. There is a false appearance to the level of bone. (Reprinted from *Journal of Practical Hygiene,* vol. 3, no. 2, E. M. Thomson & S. L. Tolle, "A Practical Guide for Using Radiographs in the Assessment of Periodontal Diseases. Part 2: Interpretation and Future Advances," p. 12, copyright 1994, with permission from Montage Media.)

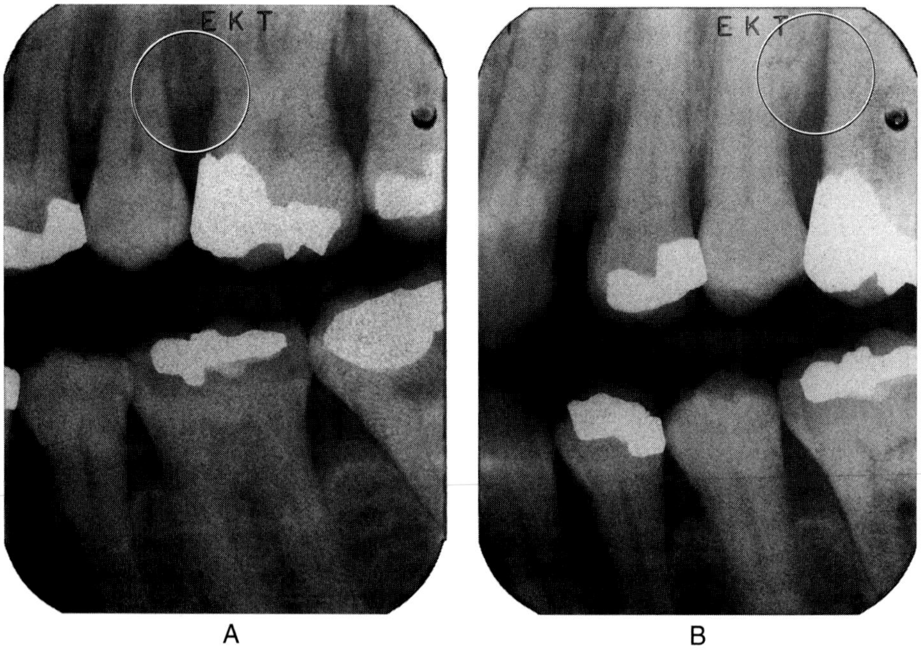

FIGURE 22–17 **Example of varying horizontal angulation.** (**A**) This radiograph, although adequately exposed at the correct horizontal angulation, does not reveal the vertical (angular) defect on the mesial of the maxillary first molar that is evident in the radiograph labeled (**B**). These two radiographs varied the horizontal angulation slightly to reveal more information. (Reprinted from *Journal of Practical Hygiene,* vol. 3, no. 2, E. M. Thomson & S. L. Tolle, "A Practical Guide for Using Radiographs in the Assessment of Periodontal Diseases. Part 2: Interpretation and Future Advances," p. 13, copyright 1994, with permission from Montage Media.)

the horizontal angulation slightly may actually increase the chances of imaging interdental defects and furcation involvement. For example, a bitewing series of seven films (discussed in Chapter 14) and a full mouth series of multiple periapical and bitewing radiographs (discussed in Chapter 13) will contain images that were produced with different horizontal angles. The varying angulations used allow for multiple views of the condition of the periodontium (Figure 22–17).

While the exposure factors (mA, kVp and impulses) used will depend on the patient and the area to be exposed, generally, practitioners prefer to use a higher kVp to best image subtle bone changes. A higher setting, such as 90 kVp, will result in an image that has a low constrast: black and white with many shades of gray in between. Since bone changes that accompany periodontal diseases appear as a radiolucency within the radiopaque bone, a low-contrast image is often preferred by the practitioner for

PROCEDURE 22–1

RADIOGRAPHIC INTERPRETATION FOR PERIODONTAL DISEASE

1. See Procedure Box 18–2, Suggested Sequence for Viewing a Full Mouth Series of Radiographs.
2. View all surfaces of each tooth.
3. Note the alveolar bone height. Use the CEJ as a reference point. Measure with a probe as needed (see Figure 18–5).
4. Examine the periodontal ligament space, following it around the entire tooth. Note widening, triangulation.
5. Examine the furcation area of multi-rooted teeth.
6. Identify local predisposing factors such as restoration overhangs and calculus.
7. Confirm findings and/or clarify uncertain interpretations with a clinical exam of the patient.
8. Consult the patient's chart for confirmation or clarification of findings as needed.
9. Present a preliminary interpretation for the dentist's review.
10. Following confirmation by the dentist, document all findings on the patient's permanent record.

TABLE 22-2 **American Academy of Periodontal Disease Classification**

Classification	Radiographic Appearance[a]
Case Type I: Gingivitis	*Alveolar crest:* Unbroken, radiopaque at a level 1.5–2.0 mm below and parallel to the CEJ
	Anterior: Pointed *Posterior:* Flat, smooth
Case Type II: Slight Chronic Periodontitis	*Alveolar crest:* Loss of density with slight radiolucencies evident; triangulation observed
	Anterior: Blunted *Posterior:* Fuzzy, cupping-out appearance
Case Type III: Moderate Chronic or Aggressive Periodontitis	*Alveolar crest:* Level greater than 2.0 mm below the CEJ indicating 30–50 percent bone loss
	Anterior and posterior: Horizontal and/or vertical patterns of bone loss observed
	Posterior: Furcation radiolucencies evident
Case Type VI: Advanced Chronic or Aggressive Periodontitis	*Alveolar crest:* Easily identified with level of bone loss greater than 50 percent
	Anterior and Posterior: Evidence of tooth position changes, drifting

[a]Modified from Perry, D. A., Beemsterboer, P., & Taggart, E. J. *Periodontology for the Dental Hygienist,* 2nd ed. W. B. Saunders, 2001.

imaging these early signs of bone destruction. A low kVp, such as 70kVp, results in a high contrast image, which is preferred for imaging caries.

Radiographic Interpretation of Periodontal Diseases

The dental radiographer should be familiar with the radiographic appearance of the normal periodontium to be able to identify deviations from normal that may indicate possible periodontal diseases (Procedure Box 22–1). The American Academy of Periodontology classifies periodontal disease based on etiologic factors of the disease and tissue response to treatment. Four classifications of periodontal disease are described based on changes in the periodontium as seen on radiographs (Table 22–2).

Case Type I: Gingivitis

Radiographs do not image soft tissue and thus, the radiographic appearance of the periodontium in all types and severities of gingivitis appears the same as normal bone. The **lamina dura** (dense cortical plate of the bony tooth socket) appears as an unbroken, dense radiopaque line around the roots of the teeth. The alveolar crest is located 1.5 to 2.0 mm apical to the cementoenamel junctions (CEJ) of the teeth (Figure 22–18). In the anterior region of the oral cavity, the alveolar crest appears pointed and sharp (Figure 22–19). In

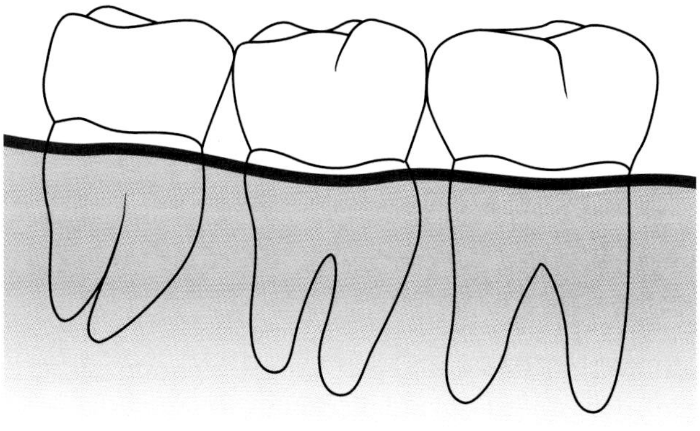

FIGURE 22-18 **Drawing showing normal bone level.** The alveolar crest located 1.5 to 2.0 mm apical to the cementoenamel junctions (CEJ) of the teeth.

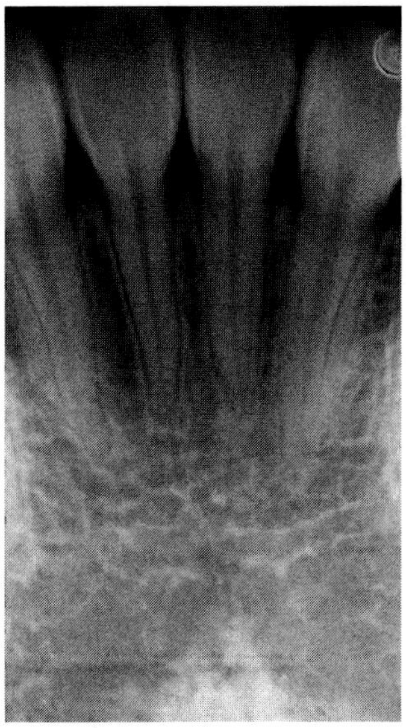

FIGURE 22-19 **Radiograph showing normal periodontium or Case Type I: Gingivitis.** Note the normal pointed radiopaque appearance of the lamina dura and thin radiolucent line of the periodontal ligament space.

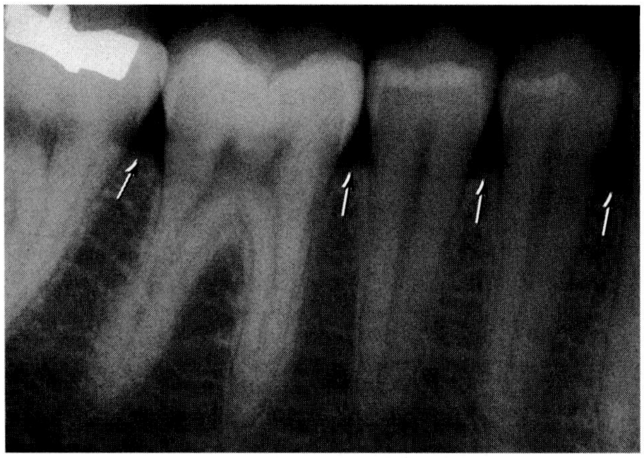

FIGURE 22-20 **Radiograph showing normal periodontium or Case Type I: Gingivitis.** Note the normal radiopaque flat appearance of the lamina dura and thin radiolucent line of the periodontal ligament space.

the posterior region of the oral cavity, the alveolar crest is more flat, smooth, and parallel to an imaginary line drawn between adjacent CEJ (Figure 22–20). The **peridontal ligament space** appears as a thin radiolucent line between the lamina dura and the root of the tooth.

Case Type II: Slight Chronic Periodontitis

Early bone loss up to 30 percent is evident (Figure 22–21). Loss of crestal bone density that often appears as a fuzzy cupping-out of the alveolar crest is the first radiographic indication of periodontal disease (Figure 22–22). The alveolar

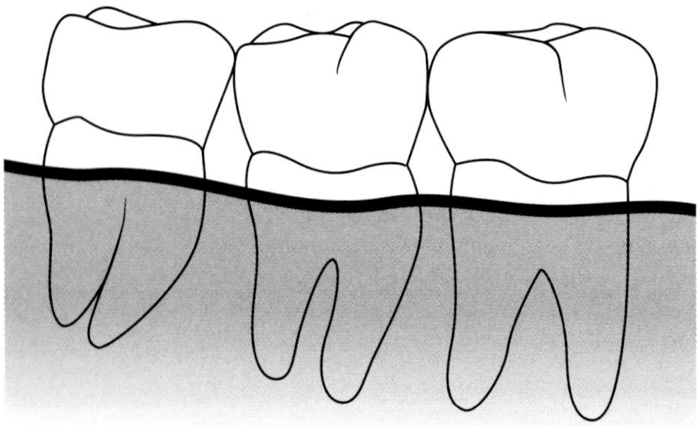

FIGURE 22-21 **Drawing showing Case Type II: Slight Chronic Periodontitis.**

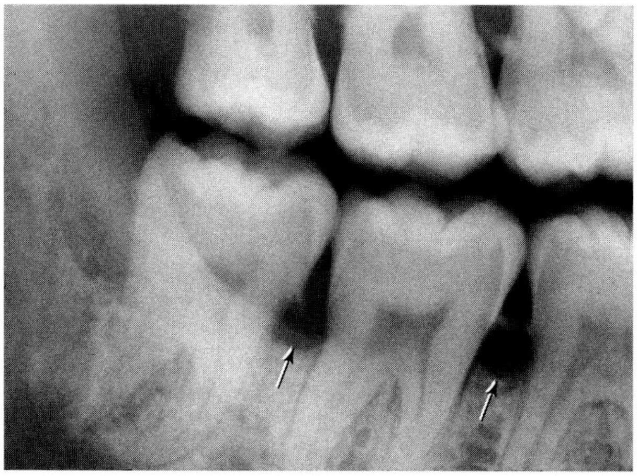

FIGURE 22-22 **Radiograph showing Case Type II: Slight Chronic Periodontitis.** Note the slight radiolucent cupping out of the lamina dura especially visible between the mandibular first and second molars. Radiopaque calculus is visible on the proximal surfaces of the teeth.

crest appears blunted in the anterior region of the oral cavity (Figure 22–23). In the posterior region of the oral cavity - triangulation, a widening of the periodontal ligament space becomes evident at the mesial or distal surface of the tooth.

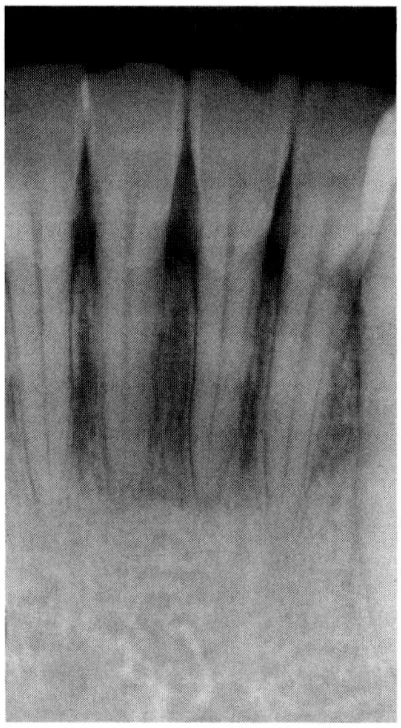

FIGURE 22-23 **Radiograph showing Case Type II: Slight Chronic Periodontitis.** Note the blunting of the lamina dura and slight radiolucent widening of the periodontal ligament space. Slightly radiopaque calculus is visible.

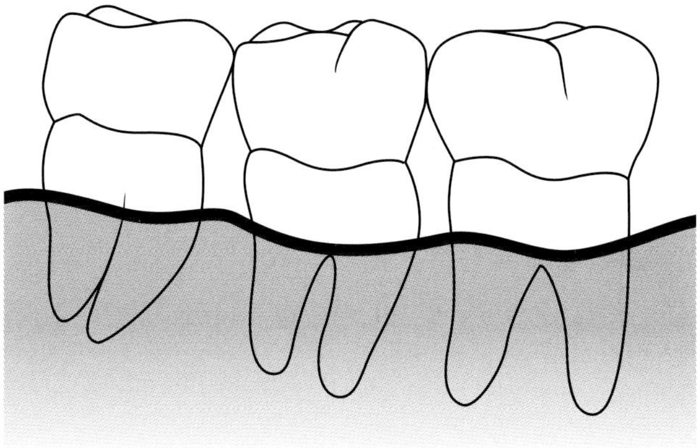

FIGURE 22-24 **Drawing showing Case Type III: Moderate Chronic or Aggressive Periodontitis.**

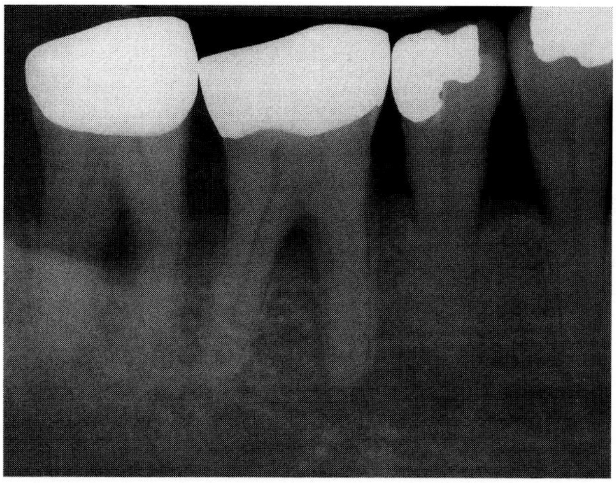

FIGURE 22-26 **Radiograph showing Case Type III: Moderate Chronic or Aggressive Periodontitis.** Note the 30–50 percent bone level resorption and radiolucency in the furca of the mandibular molars indicating furcation involvement.

Case Type III: Moderate Chronic or Aggressive Periodontitis

Moderate bone loss (30 to 50 percent) may appear in both the horizontal and vertical planes (Figures 22–24 and 22–25).

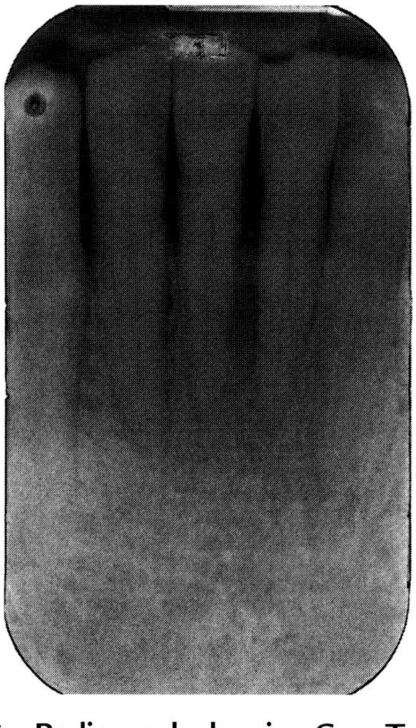

FIGURE 22-25 **Radiograph showing Case Type III: Moderate Chronic or Aggressive Periodontitis.** This radiograph shows the 30–50 percent bone level resorption.

Radiolucencies appear in the furcations of multi-rooted teeth, indicating bone loss in this area (Figure 22–26).

Case Type IV: Advanced Chronic or Aggressive Periodontitis

The advanced stage of periodontal disease (greater than 50 percent bone loss) is characterized radiographically by severe vertical and horizontal bone loss, evidence of furcation involvement, thickened periodontal membranes, and indications of changes in tooth position (Figures 22–27 through 22–29).

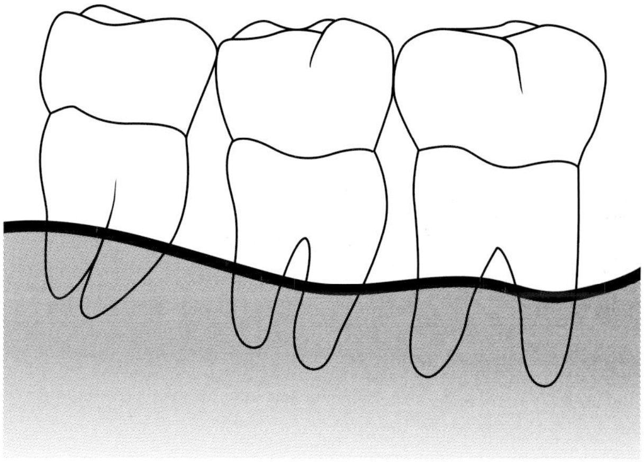

FIGURE 22-27 **Drawing showing Case Type IV: Advanced Chronic or Aggressive Periodontitis.**

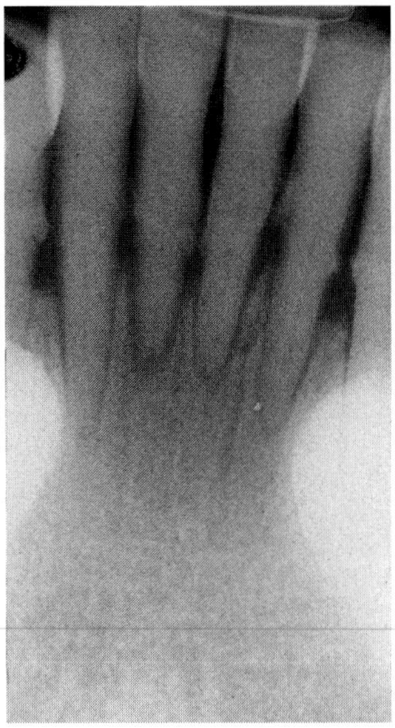

FIGURE 22-28 **Radiograph showing Case Type IV: Advanced Chronic or Aggressive Periodontitis.** Note the 50 percent or greater bone level resorption.

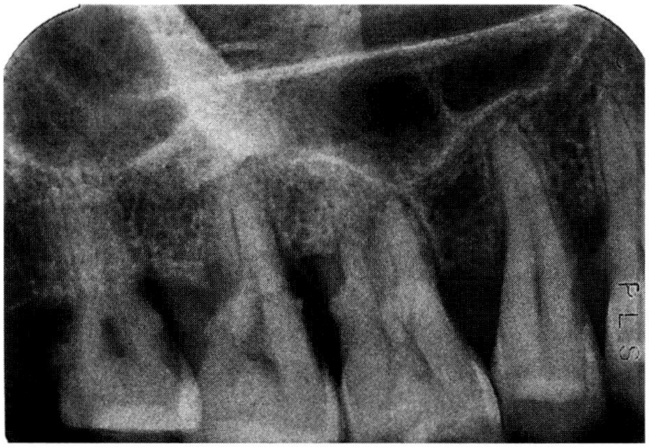

FIGURE 22-29 **Radiograph showing Case Type IV: Advanced Chronic or Aggressive Periodontitis.** Note the 50 percent or greater bone level resorption and obvious furcation involvement.

REVIEW—Chapter Summary

Periodontal diseases are diseases that affect both soft tissues (gingivitis) and bone around the teeth (periodontitis). Properly exposed and meticulously processed radiographs play a key role in the diagnosis and evaluation of periodontal diseases.

The uses of radiographs in the evaluation and treatment of periodontal diseases include imaging the supporting bone; locating predisposing factors; imaging anatomical configurations; evaluating prognosis and treatment intervention needs; and serving as a baseline for identifying and documenting the progression of the disease and the results of treatment. Radiographs are limited in their ability to image periodontal diseases because they are two-dimensional pictures of three-dimensional supporting bone; changes in soft tissue are not imaged; treated disease can not be distinguished from untreated disease; and the actual destruction of bone is more clinically advanced than what is revealed on radiographs.

The ideal radiographs for imaging periodontal diseases are bitewings, particularly vertical bitewings, or periapical radiographs exposed by the paralleling technique. Many practitioners prefer low-contrast images produced with a high kVp setting to better image subtle bone changes.

Radiographs are important aids in identifying changes in the periodontium and can assist in classifying various stages of periodontal disease. The dental hygienist and the dental assistant should possess a working knowledge of normal radiographic appearance of the periodontium to be able to recognize deviations from normal that indicate periodontal disease severity.

RECALL—Study Questions

1. All of the following may be determined from a dental radiograph *except* one. Which one is this *exception?*
   a. Bone loss
   b. Pocket depth
   c. Predisposing factors
   d. Furcation involvement
2. List four uses of radiographs in the assessment of periodontal diseases:
   a. ____________________
   b. ____________________
   c. ____________________
   d. ____________________
3. Which of the following terms describes bone loss that occurs in a plane parallel to the cementoenamel junction of adjacent teeth?
   a. Irregular
   b. Vertical
   c. Horizontal
   d. Periapical
4. Significant bone loss that results in a radiolucency observed in the area between the roots of multi-rooted teeth is called:
   a. Localized bone loss.
   b. Interdental septa.
   c. Predisposing factor.
   d. Furcation involvement.
5. Radiographs may help to locate all of the following predisposing factors *except* one. Which one is this *exception?*
   a. Calculus
   b. Occlusal trauma
   c. Deep pocket
   d. Amalgam overhang

6. Excessive occlusal force may result in a widening of the periodontal ligament space. Widening of the periodontal ligament space is called furcation involvement.
   a. The first statement is true; the second statement is false.
   b. The first statement is false; the second statement is true.
   c. Both statements are true.
   d. Both statements are false.
7. Dental radiographs are important because they document the location and depths of periodontal pockets. Radiographs may serve as a baseline and as a means for evaluating the outcomes of periodontal treatments.
   a. The first statement is true; the second statement is false.
   b. The first statement is false; the second statement is true.
   c. Both statements are true.
   d. Both statements are false.
8. List four limitations of radiographs in the assessment of periodontal diseases:
   a. ____________________
   b. ____________________
   c. ____________________
   d. ____________________
9. Which of the following would be *best* for imaging a generalized periodontal status?
   a. Select periapical radiographs exposed utilizing the bisecting technique.
   b. Select periapical radiographs exposed utilizing the paralleling technique.
   c. Posterior horizontal bitewing radiographs.
   d. Series of vertical bitewing radiographs.
10. A kVp setting of _____ would provide a _____ image that some practitioners prefer for imaging periodontal diseases.
    a. 70; high contrast
    b. 70; low contrast
    c. 90; high contrast
    d. 90; low contrast
11. Alveolar crests pointed in the anterior region and a radiopaque flat, smooth lamina dura 1.5 to 2.0 mm below the CEJ in the posterior region describes:
    a. Case Type I: Gingivitis
    b. Case Type II: Slight Chronic Periodontitis
    c. Case Type III: Moderate Chronic or Aggressive Periodontitis
    d. Case Type IV: Advanced Chronic or Aggressive Periodontitis
12. Radiolucent changes observed on a radiograph such as a fuzzy, cupping-out of the crestal bone and a blunted appearance of the lamina dura in the anterior region describes:
    a. Case Type I: Gingivitis
    b. Case Type II: Slight Chronic Periodontitis
    c. Case Type III: Moderate Chronic or Aggressive Periodontitis
    d. Case Type IV: Advanced Chronic or Aggressive Periodontitis

REFLECT—Case Study

Describe what radiographic changes in the periodontium you would expect to observe on a seven-film series of vertical bitewings on the following patients classified according to the American Academy of Periodontology Disease Classification:

1. Case Type I: Gingivitis
2. Case Type II: Slight Chronic Periodontitis
3. Case Type III: Moderate Chronic or Aggressive Periodontitis
4. Case Type IV: Advanced Chronic or Aggressive Periodontitis

RELATE—Laboratory Application

For a comprehensive laboratory practice exercise on this topic, see E. M. Thomson, *Exercises in Oral Radiography Techniques: A Laboratory Manual,* 2nd ed., Upper Saddle River, NJ: Prentice Hall, 2007. Chapter 12, "Radiographic Interpretation."

BIBLIOGRAPHY

Langlais, R. P. & Kasle, M. J. *Exercises in Oral Radiographic Interpretation,* 3rd ed. Philadelphia: Saunders, 1992.

Langlais, R. P., Langland, O. E., & Nortje, C. J. *Diagnostic Imaging of the Jaws.* Philadelphia: Williams & Wilkins, 1995.

Perry, D. A., Beemsterboer, P., Taggart, E. J. *Periodontology for the Dental Hygienist,* 2nd ed. W. B. Saunders, 2001.

Thomson, E. M. & Tolle, L. A practical guide for using radiographs in the assessment of periodontal disease, Part 2: Interpretation and Future Advances. *Practical Hygiene* 3:2, 1994.

White, S. C. & Pharoah M. J. *Oral Radiology Principles and Interpretation,* 5th ed. St. Louis: Elsevier; 2004.

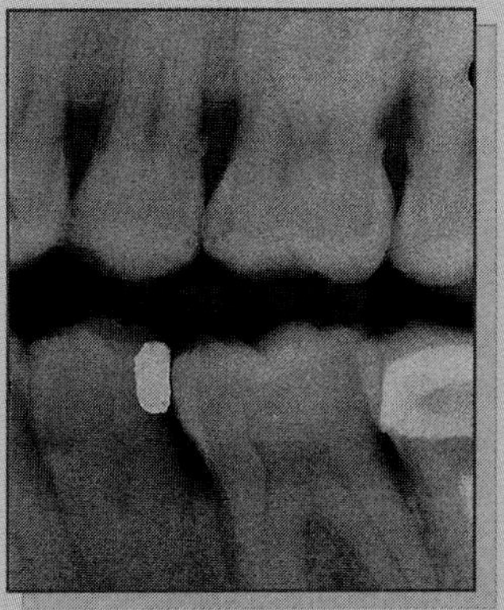

Part VIII • Patient Management and Supplemental Techniques

23

Radiographic Techniques for Children

CHAPTER OUTLINE

■ OBJECTIVES

Following successful completion of this chapter, you should be able to:

1. Define the key words.
2. State the basis for prescribing dental radiographs for children.
3. List the conditions that would indicate radiographs be taken on children.
4. Identify suggested exposure intervals for the child patient.
5. List the factors that determine the number and size of films to be exposed on children.
6. List film size and type suggested for use with primary dentition.
7. List film size and type suggested for use with transitional (mixed primary and permanent) dentition.
8. Identify two types of extraoral radiographs that may be acceptable substitutes for children who cannot tolerate intraoral film placement.
9. Identify adaptations or modifications in standard paralleling and bisecting techniques that aid in radiographic procedures for children.
10. Explain the role occlusal radiographs play in imaging children.
11. Appropriately adjust standard adult exposure settings to apply to children.
12. Explain the roles that the patient management techniques Show-Tell-Do and modeling play in assisting the radiographer with child patient management.

■ KEY WORDS

ALARA (as low as reasonably achievable)
Anodontia
Exfoliation
Lateral jaw projection (mandibular oblique lateral projection)
Modeling
Panoramic radiograph
Pediatric dentistry
Permanent teeth
Primary teeth
Show-Tell-Do
Supernumerary teeth
Transitional mixed dentition

Introduction

Children have the same basic needs for oral health care as do adults. In fact, the best time to prevent dental problems is in childhood. Although the teeth form and begin to calcify in the prenatal stage, much of the rapid growth of teeth and facial bones takes place between birth and six years. Children are at a higher risk for caries that progress more rapidly than in adults. Radiographs play an important role in detecting disease and assessing growth and development for the child patient.

Radiographic techniques and the types of projections used to image the oral cavity of the child patient do not differ significantly from those used for adult patients. However, the child patient presents with unique characteristics such as a smaller oral cavity and behavioral considerations that often require adaptations to standard procedures. The purpose of this chapter is to discuss ways the radiographer can adapt these standard techniques to best image the child's smaller and sometimes more sensitive oral cavity. These adaptations, along with behavior modification strategies can assist the radiographer in gaining the confidence of the child patient to produce the highest quality diagnostic images using the least amount of radiation exposure.

Assessment of Radiographic Need

The indication to expose dental radiographs on a child patient is based on the individual needs of the patient. The evidenced-based selection criteria guidelines, discussed in Chapter 6, have categories for assessing children and adolescents as well as adults (see Table 6–1). Radiographs for the child patient may be indicated for the detection of congenital dental abnormalities, such as **anodontia** (absence of teeth) and **supernumerary** (extra) **teeth;** to assess growth and development and the need for orthodontic intervention; to evaluate third molars; to detect disease such as caries and periodontal diseases; to diagnose pathologic conditions such as an abscess or other infection; and to assess the effect of trauma, such as a fall or accident, not only on the **primary teeth,** but on the developing, unerupted **permanent teeth** as well.

Suggested Exposure Intervals

The American Academy of Pediatric Dentistry (**pediatric dentistry**—*pedia* is Greek for child—is the branch of dentistry that specializes in providing comprehensive preventive and therapeutic oral health care for children), and other oral health and medical organizations, recommend that a child's first professional oral examination be made within 12 months following the eruption of the first primary tooth, usually between six and twelve months of age. Early prevention is key to preventing tooth loss and developing good oral self-care habits. At this early age the teeth can usually be visually inspected clinically without the need for radiographs. Unless an accident, toothache, or other unusual circumstance causes a need for radiographs, the selection criteria guidelines discussed in Chapter 6 (see Table 6–1) suggest that the first radiographic survey may not be necessary until all the primary teeth have erupted, preventing a visual inspection of the proximal (contact) surfaces via a clinical inspection. Patients without evidence of disease and with open interproximal contacts may not require a radiographic exam. Once the teeth have erupted in such a manner that the proximal surfaces can no longer be viewed clinically, and caries are suspected, or the patient presents with high risk factors for caries, such as poor oral self-care or inadequate fluoride exposure, radiographs will need to be exposed.

Film Sizes and Numbers and Types of Projections

Once it has been determined that radiographs are needed, the child's age, size of the oral cavity, and cooperation level must be considered when determining the size and number of films to expose (Table 23–1). While a size #0 or #1 intraoral film is usually used to image a child with primary teeth, the preferred size for **transitional mixed dentition,** where the child presents with a mix of both primary and permanent teeth, is a standard size #2 film. The radiographer should use the largest size film that the child can tolerate. The amount of radiation required does not change with different sizes of intraoral films. Using a size #2 film whenever possible instead of a size #0 or size #1 film will provide more information due to the coverage of a larger area. This is particularly important when imaging permanent teeth that are developing. The choice of film size should be individualized based on anatomical limitations and tissue sensitivity. A smaller size film packet should be selected rather than bending a film to make it fit more comfortably.

The number of films required depends on the needs of the individual (see Table 14–1). When exposing bitewings on a child patient prior to the eruption of the permanent second molar, two horizontal posterior bitewings, one on each side, is recommended. Following eruption of the permanent second molar, four horizontal (or vertical if periodontal disease is suspected) posterior bitewings must be taken to image all proximal contacts of the posterior teeth without overlap.

TABLE 23-1 Considerations for Choosing the Number and Size of Films to Expose on the Child Patient

- Oral health needs
- Willingness to cooperate
- Attention span and emotional state
- Ability to understand and follow directions
- Ability to hold still throughout the exposure
- Size of the opening to the oral cavity
- Size and shape of the teeth and the dental arches
- Sensitivity of the oral mucosa
- Operator's ability to gain patient's trust
- Operator's ability to position the film
- Operator's knowledge of and skill ability to adapt standard techniques

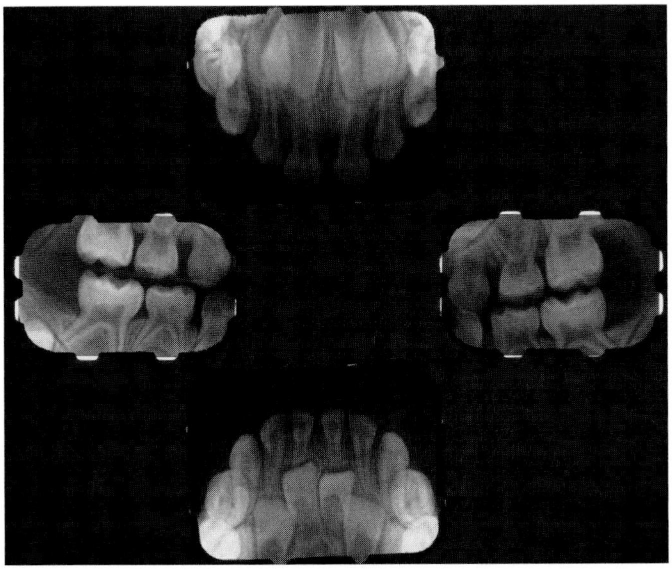

FIGURE 23–1 **Radiographic survey of primary dentition.** One anterior occlusal radiograph in each arch and one posterior bitewing radiograph on each side. (Courtesy D. P. Gutz, DDS, University Nebraska Medical Center, College of Dentistry, Lincoln, NE)

If conditions exist that require additional exposures, the following radiographic full mouth surveys are offered as suggestions.

Primary Dentition

Small oral cavity size, tongue resistance, and gagging can be a problem in small children aged three to six years old. Ideally, it is advisable to expose four films, one anterior occlusal film (see Chapter 15) of each arch (maxilla and mandible) and one posterior bitewing on each side (Figure 23–1).

Transitional (Mixed Primary and Permanent) Dentition

At six years, the first permanent teeth have begun to erupt. Ideally, the survey should include a minimum of twelve radiographs: ten periapical and two bitewing exposures. Periapical films are exposed in each of the four molar and canine regions and in the two incisor regions (Figure 23–2).

Between twelve and fourteen years of age, all the permanent teeth except the third molars have usually erupted. It is during this adolescent period that growth is rapid and metabolic changes occur that heighten the possibility of dental caries and increase the need for preventive oral hygiene care. The full mouth survey recommended for the adolescent is the same as that required for the adult patient, usually fourteen periapical and four bitewing radiographs. (See Chapters 13 and 14.)

Extraoral Radiographs

There may be cases when intraoral radiographs can not be tolerated by the patient. An extraoral technique called a **panoramic radiograph** (see Chapter 28) may be an acceptable substitute. Panoramic radiographs do not image structures with the clarity of intraoral radiographs and therefore, do not reveal details such as early carious lesions. However, these large radiographs are ideal for imaging overall jaw development and the eruption pattern of the teeth (Figure 23–3). Panoramic radiographs are often prescribed to supplement intraoral exposures. The panoramic is usually well tolerated by the child patient. However, the child must be able to hold still for the duration of the exposure (most panoramic machines have a 15–20 second exposure cycle), and the child must

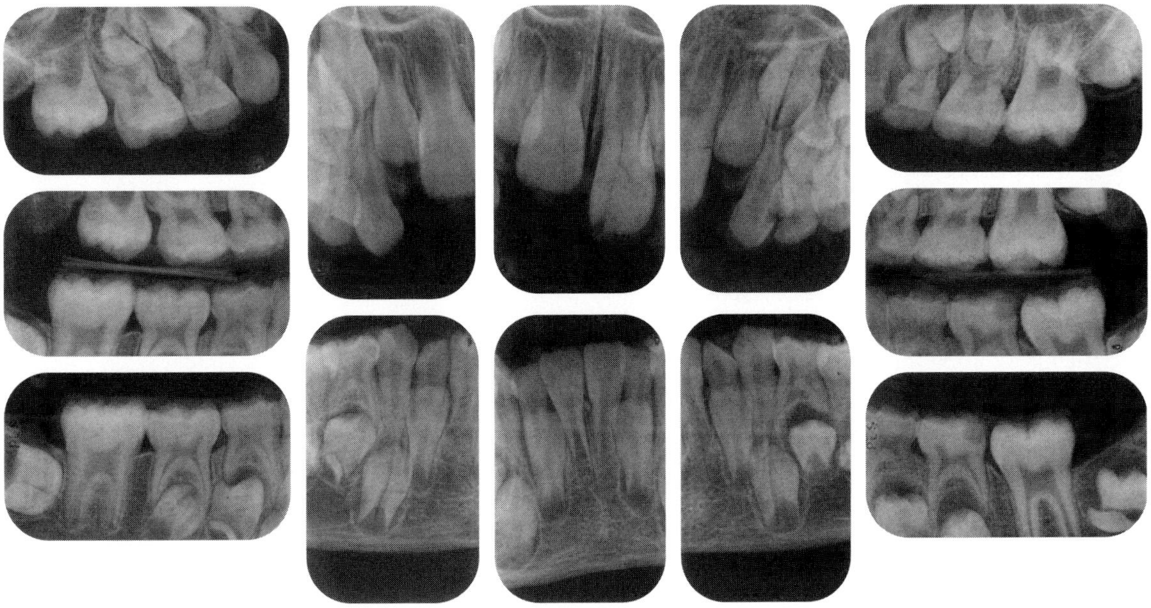

FIGURE 23–2 **Radiographic survey of transitional dentition.** Six anterior periapical radiographs (three on the maxilla and three on the mandible), one posterior periapical radiograph in each quadrant, and one posterior bitewing radiograph on each side.

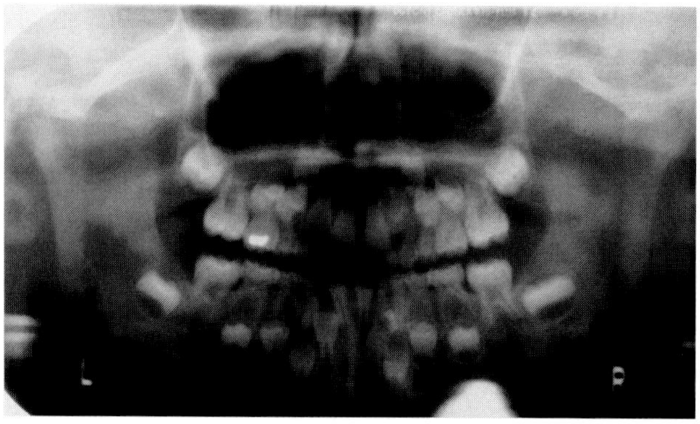

FIGURE 23-3 **Panoramic radiograph of a child with transitional dentition.** Note the overall jaw development and eruption pattern of the teeth.

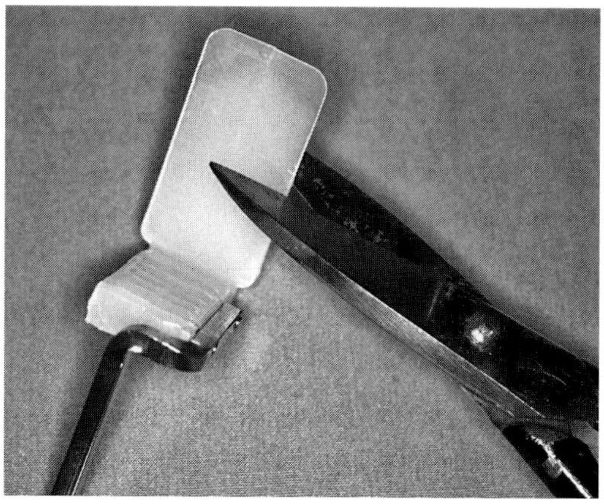

FIGURE 23-4 **Modifying a film holder biteblock for use with the child patient.** (Reprinted from *Dental Hygienist News,* vol. 6, no. 4; E. M. Thomson, "Dental Radiographs for the Child Patient," p. 24, copyright 1993, with permission from The Procter & Gamble Company)

be able to understand and cooperate with the positioning requirements necessary for a diagnostic image (see Chapter 28).

Although largely replaced by the availability of panoramic machines in general practice, the **lateral jaw projection** (also called a mandibular oblique lateral projection) (see Chapter 27) has been especially valuable to use with children (see Figures 27–9 and 27–10). The lateral jaw radiograph is used to examine the posterior region of the mandible with patients who are unable to tolerate intraoral film packet placement. The exposure can be made with any size extraoral film. The lateral jaw technique is described in Chapter 27.

Suggested Radiographic Techniques

Methods for exposing radiographs on children are essentially the same as those for adults. Although either the paralleling or bisecting technique can be employed, the characteristics children present with usually require a slight variation in the vertical angulation. A smaller oral cavity and lowered palatal vault; the tendency toward an exaggerated gag reflex and lack of tongue and muscle control; and sensitive oral mucosa due to growth and the **exfoliation** (shedding) of primary teeth and the eruption of permanent teeth require that the radiographer be creative in improvising on the basic techniques in a manner that will produce diagnostic quality images in the presence of these challenges.

The paralleling method is preferred for use on all patients due to its ability to produce accurate images with little distortion. The greatest challenge of using the paralleling technique with children is placing the film parallel to the long axes of the teeth of interest. Switching to a smaller sized film packet may help with this placement. Often, it is the size and weight of the film holder that the child has difficultly tolerating. Switching to a smaller, lighter film holder, modifying an adult film holder, or designing a custom holder may help the child patient tolerate placement (Figures 23–4 and 23–5).

Once the film packet is positioned, the vertical angulation may still need to be increased slightly (no more than 10 degrees) over the setting used for adult patients. Due to a shallow palatal vault, the film packet will most likely lay flatter in position. Slightly increasing the vertical angulation over perpendicular will help to image the root apices and the unerupted developing permanent teeth (Figure 23–6).

While the bisecting technique produces images with more distortion and magnification than the paralleling technique, its greatest advantage is the ability to produce reasonably acceptable images when parallel film packet positioning is not possible. The bisecting technique with its film packet placement (see Chapter 13) is ideal for use with the child patient.

When the child patient can not tolerate film packet placement in either the parallel or the bisecting relationships, the radiographer can often use the occlusal technique to achieve reasonably acceptable images. While a film size #4 is utilized for

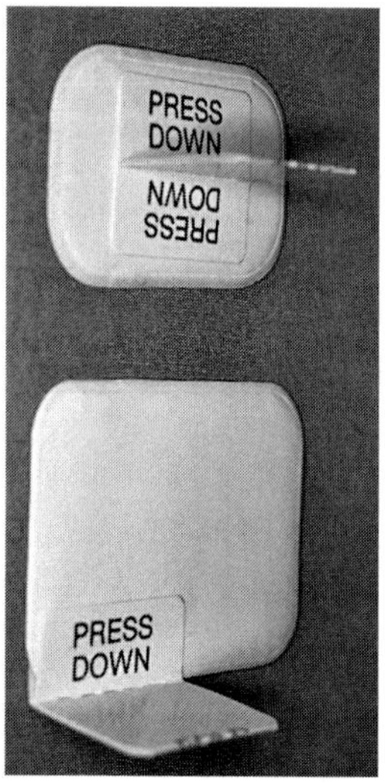

FIGURE 23-5 **Adaptation of film holders for use with the child patient.** Using a bitewing bitetab as a periapical film holder. (Reprinted from *Dental Hygienist News,* vol. 6, no. 4; E. M. Thomson, "Dental Radiographs for the Child Patient," p. 24, copyright 1993, with permission from The Procter & Gamble Company)

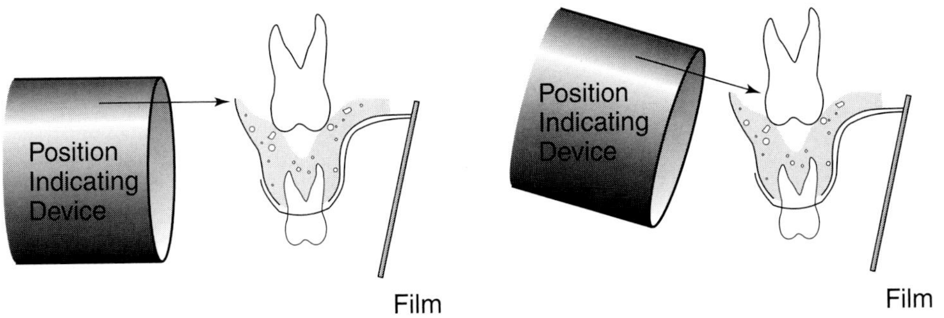

FIGURE 23-6 **Slightly increasing the vertical angulation** will image more of the unerupted developing permanent teeth and compensate for the child's lower palatal vault. (Modified from a drawing reprinted from *Dental Hygienist News,* vol. 6, no. 4; E. M. Thomson, "Dental Radiographs for the Child Patient," p. 24, copyright 1993, with permission from The Procter & Gamble Company)

occlusal radiographs for adults, an intraoral film size #2 can be used with children (Figure 23–7). The flat film packet placement is usually readily accepted by the child patient. The angulation used for the occlusal technique for children differs slightly from the angles used for adults (Table 23–2).

Practice Point

Children can easily understand the directive to bite on the film packet as if it were a graham cracker. Occluding on the flat positioning of a size #2 film packet placed for an occlusal projection is readily accepted by the child patient. It will be up to the radiographer to have the knowledge and skills to align the x-ray beam to produce an acceptable quality radiograph.

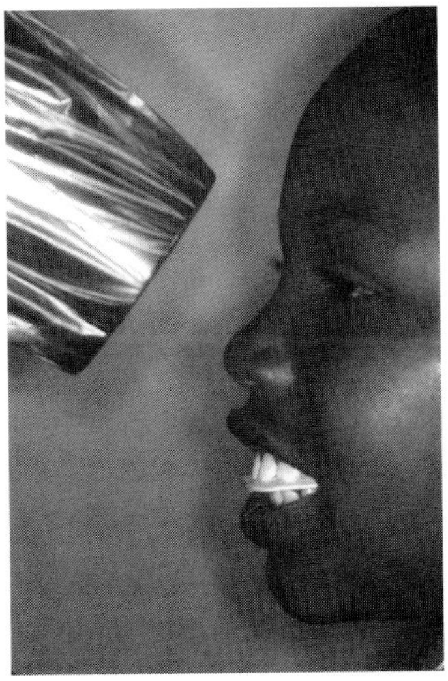

FIGURE 23-7 **Occlusal technique.** Using a size #2 film to expose a maxillary occlusal radiograph.

ALARA Radiation Protection

The child's smaller size places radiation-sensitive tissues closer to the path of the primary beam of radiation. It is imperative that a lead apron and thyroid collar be placed over all patients, including children. Child-sized lead or lead-equivalent protective barriers are available commercially; some are decorated with cartoon figures, making these especially child-friendly. Other **ALARA** (as low as reasonably achievable) (see Chapter 6) protocols that apply to adult patients also apply to children. These include the use of fast film, x-ray beam filtration and collimating devices, and the use of appropriate exposure settings.

As the bone structure of a child is smaller and less dense than that of an adult, less radiation is required to produce an acceptable image. The amount of radiation required for most intraoral exposures can be reduced by about one-third to one-half that required for the same exposure on an adult patient. Reducing the mA setting (amount of radiation) or the exposure time by one-half of that used for adult exposures is appropriate for children under 10 years of age. Exposures on children between the ages of 10 and 15 years can be reduced by approximately one-third. Once the adolescent reaches 15 or 16 years of age, the exposure settings should be the same as for an adult patient.

Patient Management

Obtaining quality radiographs on children can be challenging. The radiographer must be able to communicate and explain the procedure so that the child understands what is expected. The child must be able to follow directions and cooperate with the procedure. The patient management skills of the radiographer should bring out the child's natural curiosity and eagerness to participate.

First impressions are always important and lasting. The child's first experience should be pleasant and informative. Usually it is best to greet and take the child from the reception room to the x-ray room without the parents. The child should be a willing participant in the process. Only in emergencies should a child be forced to undergo dental treatment. If necessary, it is better to

TABLE 23–2 **Recommended Radiographs for the Child Patient**

Dentition Category	Type and Region	Film Size	Number of Films	Film Packet Placement	Vertical Angulation	Horizontal Angulation	Point of Entry	Exposure
Primary dentition (3 to 6 years of age)	Bitewing posterior	#0 or #1	1 on each side	Align the anterior edge of film packet to line up behind the distal half of the primary maxillary or mandibular canine; chose the most mesially located canine.	+5 to +10 degrees	Direct the central rays perpendicularly through the primary first and second molar embrasure.	A spot on the occlusal plane between the primary maxillary and mandibular first molars	Reduce exposure to 1/2 the exposure used for this projection on an adult
Primary dentition (3 to 6 years of age)	Occlusal anterior	#2	1 on each arch	Place long dimension of packet across the mouth (buccal to buccal); white unprinted side toward the arch to be imaged (Figures 23–8 and 23–9).	*Maxilla:* Direct the central rays perpendicular to the imaginary bisector approximately +60 degrees *Mandible:* Direct the central rays perpendicular to the imaginary bisector approximately −30 degrees	Direct the central rays perpendicular to patient's midsagittal plane.	*Maxilla:* Through a point at the tip of the nose toward the center of the film *Mandible:* Through a point in the middle of the chin toward the center of the film	Reduce exposure to 1/2 the exposure used for this projection on an adult
Transitional dentition (7 to 12 years of age)	Bitewing posterior	*Prior to eruption of the permanent second molar:* #1 or #2	*Prior to eruption of the permanent second molar:* 1 on each side	*Prior to eruption of the permanent second molar:* Align the anterior edge of film packet to line up behind the distal half of the primary or permanent maxillary or mandibular canine; chose the most mesially located canine (Figure 23–10).	+10 degrees	*Prior to eruption of the permanent second molar:* Direct the central rays perpendicularly through the primary first and second molar embrasure or, if erupted, the first and second premolar embrasure.	A spot on the occlusal plane between the primary maxillary and mandibular first molars or, if erupted, the first and second premolars to center the film packet within the x-ray beam	Reduce exposure by 1/3 to 1/2 the exposure used for this projection on an adult
		After eruption of the permanent second molar: #2	*After eruption of the permanent second molar:* 2 on each side (1 premolar bitewing and 1 molar bitewing)	*After eruption of the permanent second molar:* Use the same criteria as for the adult patient (see Table 14–3)	+10 degrees	*After eruption of the permanent second molar:* Use the same criteria as for the adult patient (see Table 14–3).	*After eruption of the permanent second molar:* Use the same criteria as the adult patient (see Table 14–3).	Reduce exposure by 1/3 to 1/2 the exposure used for this projection on an adult

Transitional dentition (7 to 12 years of age)	Anterior periapical	#0 or #1	3 on each arch (1 central-lateral, 1 right canine, and 1 left canine)	*Maxillary central-lateral incisors:* Center the film packet to line up behind the primary or, if erupted, permanent central and lateral incisors (Figure 23–11).	*Maxillary central-lateral incisors:* *Paralleling technique*—Direct the central rays toward the film perpendicularly in the vertical dimension. *Bisecting technique*—Direct the central rays toward the imaginary bisector approximately +45 to +50 degrees.	*Maxillary central-lateral incisors:* Direct the central rays perpendicularly through the maxillary left and right primary or, if erupted, permanent central incisor embrasure.	*Maxillary central-lateral incisors:* At the root tips of the central incisors to center the film packet within the x-ray beam	Reduce exposure by 1/3 to 1/2 the exposure used for this projection on an adult
				Mandibular central-lateral incisors: Center the film packet to line up behind the primary or, if erupted, permanent central and lateral incisors (Figure 23–12).	*Mandibular central-lateral incisors:* *Paralleling technique*—Direct the central rays toward the film perpendicularly in the vertical dimension. *Bisecting technique:* Direct the central rays toward the imaginary bisector approximately −20 to −25 degrees.	*Mandibular central-lateral incisors:* Direct the central rays perpendicularly through the mandibular left and right primary or, if erupted, permanent central incisor embrasure.	*Mandibular central-lateral incisors:* At the root tips of the central incisors to center the film packet within the x-ray beam	
				Maxillary canine: Center the film packet to line up behind the primary or, if erupted, permanent canine (Figure 23–13).	*Maxillary canine:* *Paralleling technique*—Direct the central rays toward the film perpendicularly in the vertical dimension. *Bisecting technique*—Direct the central rays toward the imaginary bisector approximately +55 to +60 degrees	*Maxillary canine:* Direct the central rays perpendicularly at the center of the canine.	*Maxillary canine:* At the root tip of the canine to center the film packet within the x-ray beam	

(*continued*)

TABLE 23-2 (*cont.*)

Dentition Category	Type and Region	Film Size	Number of Films	Film Packet Placement	Vertical Angulation	Horizontal Angulation	Point of Entry	Exposure
				Mandibular canine: Center the film packet to line up behind the primary canine, or, if erupted, the permanent canine (Figure 23-14).	*Mandibular canine: Paralleling technique*—Direct the central rays toward the film perpendicularly in the vertical dimension. *Bisecting technique:* Direct the central rays toward the imaginary bisector approximately −25 to −30 degrees	*Mandibular canine:* Direct the central rays perpendicularly at the center of the canine.	*Mandibular canine:* At the root tip of the canine to center the film packet within the x-ray beam	
Transitional dentition (7 to 12 years of age)	Posterior periapical	#1 or #2	*Prior to eruption of the permanent second molar:* 1 in each quadrant (4 molar periapicals)	*Prior to eruption of the permanent second molars:* *Maxillary molar*—Align the anterior edge of film packet to line up behind the distal half of the primary or, if erupted, permanent maxillary canine (Figure 23-15).	*Prior to eruption of the permanent second molars:* *Maxillary molar: Paralleling technique*—Direct the central rays toward the film perpendicularly in the vertical dimension. *Bisecting technique*—Direct the central rays toward the imaginary bisector approximately +30 to +55 degrees	*Prior to eruption of the permanent second molars:* *Maxillary molar:* Direct the central rays perpendicularly through the primary first and second molar embrasure or, if erupted, the first and second premolar embrasure	*Prior to eruption of the permanent second molars:* *Maxillary molar:* At the root tip of the primary first molar, or if erupted, the root tip of first premolar to center the film packet within the x-ray beam	Reduce exposure by 1/3 to 1/2 the exposure used for this projection on an adult

		Mandibular molar—Align the anterior edge of film packet to line up behind the distal half of the primary or, if erupted, permanent mandibular canine (Figure 23–16).	*Mandibular molar: Paralleling technique:* Direct the central rays toward the film perpendicularly in the vertical dimension. *Bisecting technique:* Direct the central rays toward the imaginary bisector approximately −15 to −20 degrees	*Mandibular molar:* Direct the central rays perpendicularly through the primary first and second molar embrasure or, if erupted, the first and second premolar embrasure	*Mandibular molar:* At the root tip of the primary first molar, or if erupted, the root tip of first premolar to center the film packet within the x-ray beam
	After eruption of the second permanent molar: 2 in each quadrant (4 premolar and 4 molar periapicals)	*After eruption of the second permanent molar:* Use the same criteria as the adult patient (see Table 13–5.	*After eruption of the second permanent molar:* Use the same criteria as the adult patient (see Table 13–5).	*After eruption of the second permanent molar:* Use the same criteria as the adult patient (see Table 13–3).	

postpone taking radiographs until the next visit than to cause an unpleasant experience for the child. The child can be told that they will "be bigger" next time and that the procedure will be easier now that they have "practiced" for it. Planting a positive thought is better than risking instilling a fear of dentistry.

Most children react favorably to the authority of a confident, capable operator. Occasionally, a stubborn or frightened child proves difficult to manage. If such a child does not respond to firmness, a parent or older brother or sister may accompany the child into the x-ray room. In fact, if the child is too small to understand instructions or unable to hold the film, a parent or accompanying adult may have to hold the film while it is being exposed. The parent or guardian should be protected with lead, or lead equivalent barriers such as an apron or gloves when they are in the path of the x-ray beam. The radiographer must never hold the film in the mouth of a patient.

Show-Tell-Do

The use of **Show-Tell-Do** (see Chapter 11) is especially useful with children. Children, and adults, can be naturally fearful of the unknown. Orienting the child patient to the radiographic equipment will help to alleviate fear and pique curiosity. The child can be given a film packet to feel and to handle. It may be unwrapped so that the child can see the film. Showing the child different film sizes and then choosing the film size that is "just right" for the child's mouth may assist with cooperation during placement of the film packet intraorally. If a film holder is to be used, the child should be allowed to examine and handle it. The entire procedure should be carefully explained and rehearsed. The terms used to describe the radiographic equipment should be on the level the patient understands. Young children can be told that the x-ray tube head is the "camera" used to take special x-ray pictures of the teeth.

Modeling

Modeling, where the child is given the opportunity to observe the procedure being performed on another patient, is another successful tool the radiographer may apply to alleviate fear of the unknown and gain cooperation. The child may observe an older sibling or parent undergoing the procedure. Of course care should be taken to not subject the child to unnecessary radiation exposure. The child can accompany the radiographer to the protected location of the exposure button and assist in the exposure by watching for, and confirming, that the red exposure indicator lights up.

Communication

Honest communication and good interpersonal skills that are utilized to gain procedure acceptance and cooperation from the adult can also be applied to the child patient (see Chapter 11). Praising the child for his/her cooperation and successful completion of each step of the procedure will encourage more of the same behavior. A young child's attention span can be short, so repeated praise and instructions given again with each exposure is often necessary. Young children can be get fidgety and restless, so when the child is ready, film placement and exposures should be made as rapidly as possible.

Giving the child a job to do, such as listening for the "beep" sound to be sure that the x-ray machine worked, will allow the patient to be a willing participant in the process. Giving the child a sense of control over the procedure will often boost cooperation. However, the radiographer should be careful about which procedures to maintain authority over. Allowing the patient to hold and examine the film holder device is reasonable; giving the child patient permission to place the holder intraorally where he/she wants to may lead to less cooperation.

Many strategies that apply to managing patients with special needs, presented in Chapter 24, will apply to the child patient as well. These include the sequencing of exposures and tips for controlling the gag reflex (see Chapter 24). The easiest and most comfortable exposures, usually radiographs of the maxillary anterior teeth, should be exposed first to gain the child's confidence and to get the child accustomed to having a film in the mouth. Additionally, the anterior films are less likely to excite a gag reflex. Distraction techniques such as telling the child a story during the procedure; asking the child to take a deep breath and hold it while you count down from five to zero, allowing time to make the exposure; and palpating the tissues with an index finger to massage and desensitize sensitive mucosa and familiarize the patient with where the film packet will be are strategies that help make the radiographic experience a comfortable one.

Bitewing, Periapical, and Occlusal Exposures for Children

With few minor exceptions to compensate for the child's smaller mouth, the same technical procedures described in Chapters 13, 14, and 15 are used when exposing radiographs on children. The main difference is in the use of smaller films and shorter exposure times. Additionally, in some areas a slightly steeper vertical angulation than is customary in adults is used to compensate for the flatter palate and shallow floor of the mouth. Other minor changes in technique are listed in Table 23–2 and Figures 23–8 through 23–16.

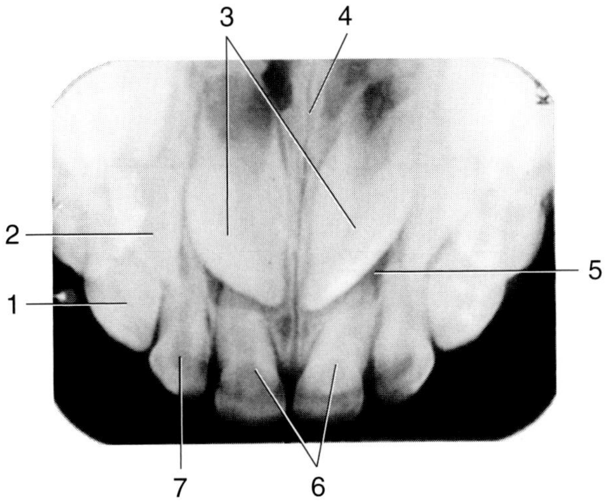

FIGURE 23-8 **Maxillary anterior occlusal radiograph of primary dentition** exposed with size #2 film. Note the: (**1**) primary canine, (**2**) crown of unerupted permanent lateral incisor, (**3**) unerupted permanent central incisors—note that root formation has not started yet, (**4**) thin radiolucent line indicating the location of the median palatine suture, (**5**) partially resorbed root of primary central incisor, (**6**) primary central incisors, and (**7**) primary lateral incisor.

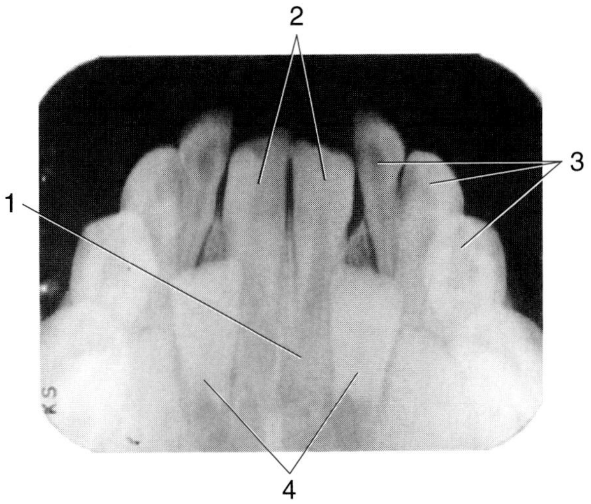

FIGURE 23-9 **Mandibular anterior occlusal radiograph of primary dentition** exposed with size #2 film. Note the: (**1**) alveolar bone, (**2**) partially erupted permanent central incisors, (**3**) primary teeth, soon to be exfoliated, and (**4**) unerupted permanent lateral incisors.

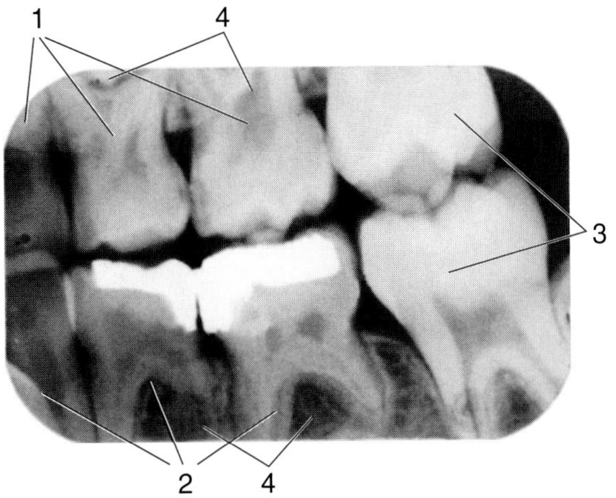

FIGURE 23-10 **Posterior bitewing radiograph of transitional (mixed primary and permanent) dentition** showing the (**1**) primary maxillary canine, first and second molars, (**2**) primary mandibular canine, first and second molars, (**3**) permanent maxillary and mandibular molars. (**4**) Note that this small size film does not adequately image the area of the developing premolars.

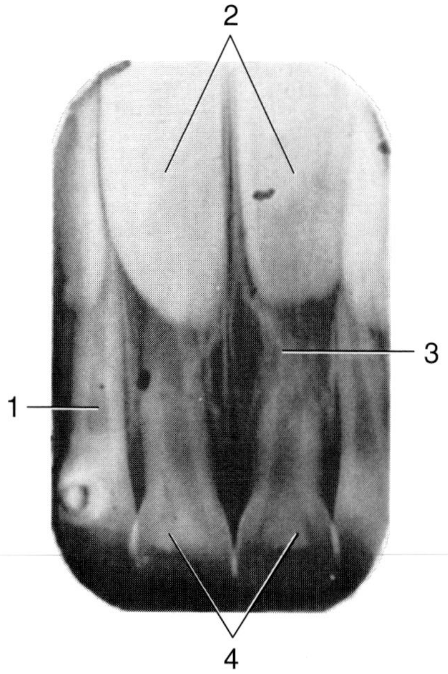

FIGURE 23-11 **Maxillary central-lateral incisors periapical radiograph of transitional (mixed primary and permanent) dentition** showing (**1**) erupted primary lateral incisor, (**2**) crowns of unerupted permanent central incisors, (**3**) roots of primary central incisors showing signs of physiological resorption, and (**4**) primary central incisors.

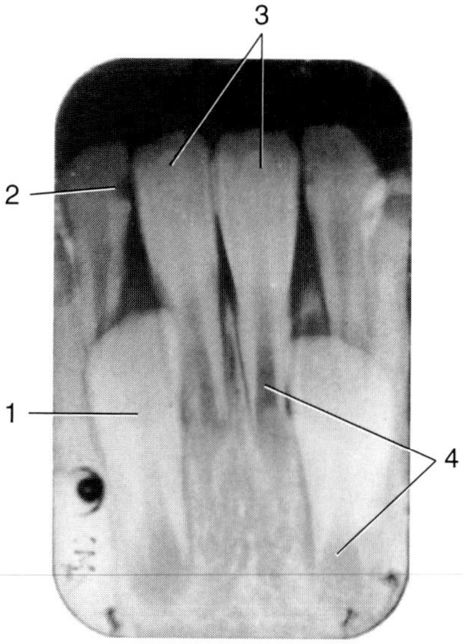

FIGURE 23-12 **Mandibular central-lateral incisors periapical radiograph of transitional (mixed primary and permanent) dentition** showing (**1**) unerupted permanent lateral incisor, (**2**) incipient caries on mesial surface of primary lateral incisor, (**3**) erupted permanent central incisors, and (**4**) large open apex area on all permanent teeth, indicating that root formation is still in progress. Root formation is generally not complete until about two or three years following tooth eruption.

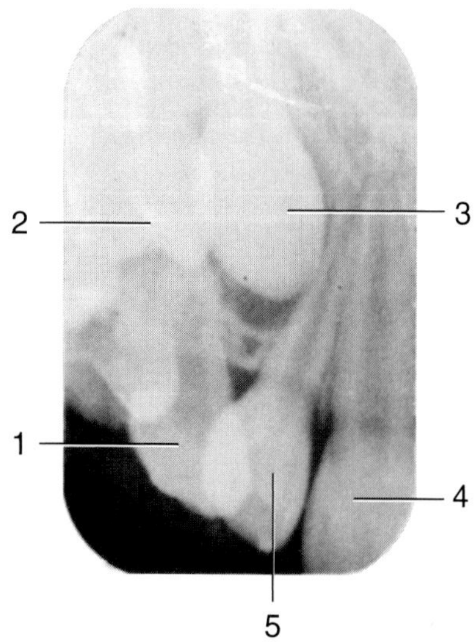

FIGURE 23-13 **Maxillary canine periapical radiograph of transitional (mixed primary and permanent) dentition** showing (**1**) primary canine, (**2**) crown of first premolar, (**3**) unerupted permanent canine with part of crown still in a follicle as indicated by radiolucent area around the tip of the crown, (**4**) erupted permanent central incisor, and (**5**) permanent lateral incisor, which appears to be tipped distally and overlapping with deciduous canine.

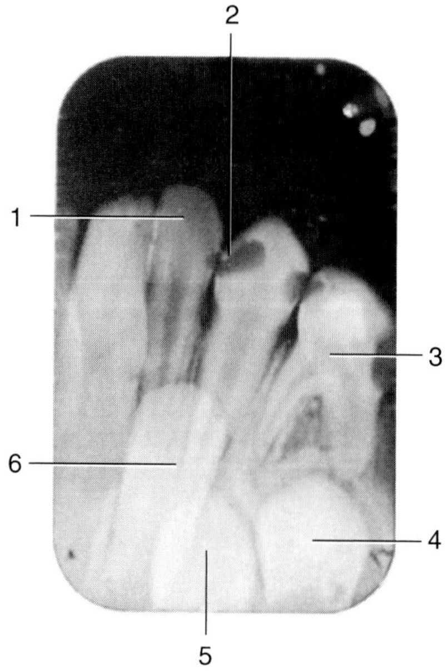

FIGURE 23-14 **Mandibular canine periapical radiograph of transitional (mixed primary and permanent) dentition** showing (**1**) primary lateral incisor, (**2**) radiolucent areas on mesial and distal of primary canine, indicating silicate or acrylic restoration; must be confirmed by visual examination because these filling materials may mimic caries radiographically (see Chapter 21), (**3**) primary first molar, (**4**) unerupted first premolar, (**5**) unerupted permanent canine, and (**6**) unerupted permanent lateral incisor.

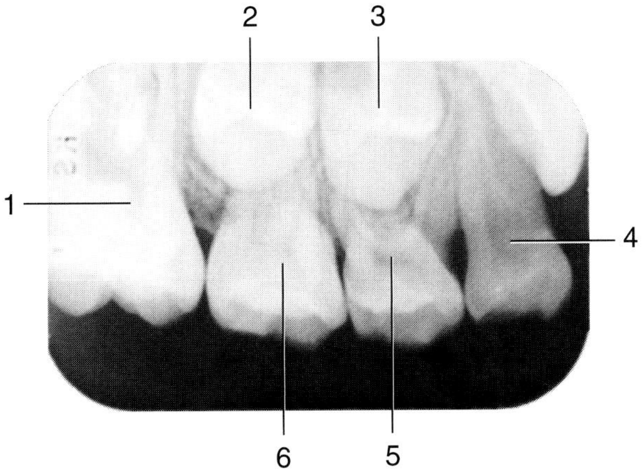

FIGURE 23-15 **Maxillary molar periapical radiograph of transitional (mixed primary and permanent) dentition** showing (**1**) permanent first molar, (**2**) crown of unerupted second premolar, (**3**) crown of unerupted first premolar, (**4**) primary canine, (**5**) primary first molar (note that the roots are almost completely resorbed), and (**6**) primary second molar. Note that the lingual root is superimposed on the crown of the unerupted second premolar.

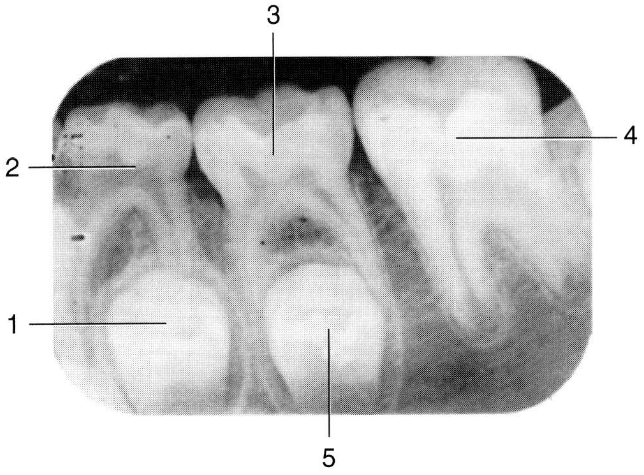

FIGURE 23-16 **Mandibular molar periapical radiograph of transitional (mixed primary and permanent) dentition** showing (**1**) unerupted first premolar, (**2**) primary first molar with partial resorption of distal root, (**3**) primary second molar, (**4**) permanent first molar, and (**5**) unerupted second premolar.

REVIEW—Chapter Summary

Children have the same basic needs for oral health care as do adults. Radiographic techniques and the types of projections used to image the oral cavity of the child patient do not differ significantly from those used for adult patients. However, the child patient presents with unique characteristics, such as a smaller oral cavity and special behavioral considerations that often require adaptation to standard procedures.

Radiographs for the child patient may be indicated for the detection of congenital dental abnormalities, to assess growth and development, and to detect and diagnose diseases and the effect of trauma. Selection criteria guidelines suggest that radiographs on children may not be necessary until all the primary teeth have erupted unless an emergency or suspected pathology exists. Once teeth have erupted in such a manner that the proximal surfaces of the teeth can not be examined clinically for caries, radiographs may need to be exposed.

The number and size of film used for radiographs for the child patient will depend on the child's age, size of the oral cavity, and cooperation level. Film size #0 or #1 is usually used for bitewing radiographs for patients with primary dentition, prior to the eruption of the first permanent molars. Film size #2 is usually used for patients with a transitional (mixed primary and permanent) dentition. Occlusal radiographs may be substituted for periapicals on children with primary dentition if necessary. After the eruption of the permanent second molars, the bitewing and full mouth surveys recommended for the child patient are the same as those recommended for an adult patient.

Panoramic or lateral jaw (mandibular oblique lateral) extraoral radiographs may sometimes be acceptable substitutes for intraoral films on the child patient who can not tolerate intraoral film packet placement.

As with the adult patient, the paralleling method is the technique of choice for use with children; however, film packet placement may be easier with the bisecting method. As the bone structure on a child is smaller and less dense than that of an adult, less radiation is required to produce an acceptable image. Exposure settings for radiographs on children under 10 years of age can be reduced by one-half of that used for adult exposures. Exposure settings for radiographs on children 10 to 15 years of age can be reduced by one-third of that used for adult exposures. Adolescents 15 or 16 years of age and older require the same exposure settings as an adult patient.

Show-Tell-Do and modeling are valuable patient management tools that can aid the radiographer in taking quality radiographic images. Orienting the child patient to the radiographic equipment will help alleviate fear of the unknown. Good communication and demonstration of authority is imperative when interacting with children. Most children react favorably to the authority of a confident, capable operator.

RECALL—Study Questions

1. List five conditions that would indicate the need for dental radiographs on the child patient.
   a. ____________________
   b. ____________________
   c. ____________________
   d. ____________________
   e. ____________________
2. Under which of these conditions would dental radiographs most likely *not* need to be exposed?
   a. When the child presents with poor self-care and suspected caries.
   b. When the child is still under 12 years of age.
   c. When the proximal surfaces of the teeth are visible clinically.
   d. When the child has accidentally fallen and damaged the primary teeth.

3. According to the evidenced-based selection criteria guidelines listed in Table 6–1, which of these intervals is recommended for posterior bitewing radiographs on a 10-year-old child recall patient who presents with good self-care and no evidence of clinical caries?
   a. 6–12 months
   b. 12–24 months
   c. 18–36 months
   d. 24–36 months
4. All of the following need to be considered when deciding what size film to use on a child *except* one. Which one is this *exception?*
   a. Cooperation level
   b. Size of the dental arches
   c. Size of the mouth opening
   d. Amount of plaque present
5. Which film size would be the easiest to position for a bitewing radiograph on a five-year-old patient?
   a. #0
   b. #1
   c. #2
   d. #4
6. Which of the following is the best reason to use the largest size intraoral film that the child will tolerate?
   a. So that a lesser number of films will have to be exposed
   b. To be able to use the paralleling technique
   c. So that the radiation exposure can be reduced
   d. To image an increased amount of the tissues
7. Which of the following is the suggested number and size of projections to use for a three-year-old patient with primary dentition?
   a. Two bitewing and two occlusal radiographs
   b. Two bitewing and two periapical radiographs
   c. Two bitewing and four periapical radiographs
   d. Four bitewing and 10 periapical radiographs
8. Which of the following is the suggested number and size of projections to use for a 10-year-old patient with transitional (mixed primary and permanent) dentition?
   a. Two bitewing and two periapical radiographs
   b. Two bitewing and four periapical radiographs
   c. Four bitewing and 10 periapical radiographs
   d. Four bitewing and 14 periapical radiographs
9. Which of the following is the suggested number and size of projections to use for a 15-year-old patient with permanent dentition?
   a. Two bitewings and six periapical radiographs
   b. Four bitewing and eight periapical radiographs
   c. Four bitewing and 10 periapical radiographs
   d. Four bitewing and 14 periapical radiographs
10. When a child patient can not tolerate film packet placement for exposure of a periapical radiograph, which of the following may sometimes be an acceptable substitute?
    a. Bitewing
    b. Panoramic
    c. Lateral jaw
    d. Both b and c
11. If well tolerated, which of the following techniques will provide the best quality images on the child patient?
    a. Panoramic
    b. Occlusal
    c. Paralleling
    d. Bisecting
12. What slight change in angulation is usually required when using the bisecting technique on a child patient?
    a. Increase the vertical angulation
    b. Decrease the vertical angulation
    c. Direct the horizontal angulation mesiodistally
    d. Direct the horizontal angulation distomesially
13. Which of the following film sizes is recommended for an occlusal radiograph on an 8-year-old patient?
    a. #0
    b. #2
    c. #3
    d. #4
14. The exposure settings for children under the age of 10 years should be:
    a. Reduced by one-half the exposure used for adults.
    b. Reduced by one-third the exposure used for adults.
    c. Three-fourths the exposure used for adults.
    d. The same exposure as used for adults.
15. The exposure settings for children between the ages of 10 and 15 years is:
    a. Reduced by one-half the exposure used for adults.
    b. Reduced by one-third the exposure used for adults.
    c. Three-fourths the exposure used for adults.
    d. The same exposure as used for adults.
16. The exposure settings for children over the age of 16 years is:
    a. Reduced by one-half the exposure used for adults.
    b. Reduced by one-third the exposure used for adults.
    c. Three-fourths the exposure used for adults.
    d. The same exposure as used for adults.
17. Allowing the child patient to observe a sibling or parent undergoing the radiographic procedure may help to alleviate fear of the unknown and promote cooperation. This patient management strategy is called modeling.
    a. The first statement is true. The second statement is false.
    b. The first statement is false. The second statement is true.
    c. Both statements are true.
    d. Both statements are false.
18. When taking a series of periapical radiographs on an 11-year-old patient, which of the following should be placed and exposed first?
    a. Mandibular molar
    b. Mandibular canine
    c. Maxillary molar
    d. Maxillary central-lateral incisors

REFLECT—Case Study

The public health clinic where you have volunteered to work one day a week has just received funding to begin providing oral health care services to children. Currently the exposure times for radiographic projections posted near the x-ray unit control panels list only the following impulse times for adults. Based on what you learned in this chapter, design an exposure setting chart that lists the impulse timer settings that would be appropriate for children. Design your chart to include children of all ages: under age 10, between the ages of 10 and 15, and over age 16. Current settings for adult patients are as follows:

Film speed:	F
PID length:	12-in. (30.5 cm)
mA:	7
kVp:	70

	Impulses		
Bitewings	Adult	Child (under 10 yrs)	Child (10–15 yrs)
Posterior	20	—	—
Anterior	16	—	—
Periapicals			
Maxillary anterior	18	—	—
Maxillary premolar	22	—	—
Maxillary molar	24	—	—
Mandibular anterior	16	—	—
Mandibular premolar	18	—	—
Mandibular molar	20	—	—

RELATE—Laboratory Application

Observe the exposure charts that are used in your clinical facility. Write down the settings that are being recommended for use with adults and with children. How many categories of settings did you find? Are there parameters given for the settings? i.e., are age, size of the patient, or dentition parameters listed to base the settings on? Compare and calculate the difference between the adult and child settings used at your facility. Do the differences match the recommendations presented in this chapter? What is the basis for the recommended settings at your facility? i.e., why were they selected? After analyzing the settings and comparing them to the recommendations in this chapter, write a brief summary that would explain the use of different settings to a concerned parent.

BIBLIOGRAPHY

Eastman Kodak. *Successful Intraoral Radiography.* Rochester, NY: Eastman Kodak, 1998.

Nowak, A. J., Creedon, R. L., & Musselman, R. J. et al. Summary of the conference on radiation exposure in pediatric dentistry. *J. Am. Dent. Assoc.* 103: 426–428, 1981.

Thomson, E. M. Dental radiographs for the child patient. *Dental Hygienist News* 6:19–20, 24, 1993.

White, S. C. & Pharoah, M. J. *Oral Radiology Principles and Interpretation,* 5th ed. St. Louis: Elsevier, 2004.

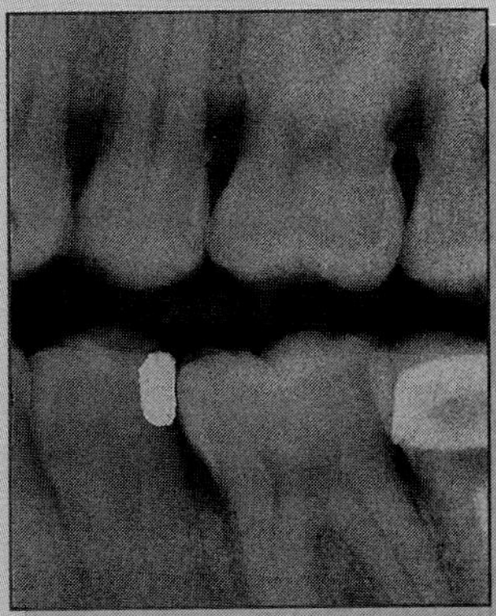

24

Managing Patients with Special Needs

■ OBJECTIVES

Following successful completion of this chapter, you should be able to:

1. Define key words.
2. Discuss five actions for managing the apprehensive patient.
3. Identify the areas of the oral cavity that are most likely to initiate the gag reflex.
4. List the two stimuli that commonly initiate the gag reflex.
5. Describe five methods to reduce psychogenic stimuli to control the gag reflex.
6. Describe four methods to reduce tactile stimuli to control the gag reflex.
7. Discuss ways to manage radiographic procedures for the older adult patient.
8. Discuss ways to manage radiographic procedures for the patient with motor disorders and conditions of involuntary movement.
9. Discuss ways to manage radiographic procedures for the patient with disabilities.
10. Explain necessary radiographs for the cancer patient.
11. Explain necessary radiographs for the pregnant patient.
12. Value the need for cultural sensitivity.

■ KEY WORDS

Angular cheilitis
Apprehensive
Cultural barriers
Disability
Gag reflex
Hypersensitive gag reflex
Speech reading

CHAPTER OUTLINE

Introduction

Each patient presents with unique characteristics. In addition to oral manifestations, the dental radiographer should be familiar with possible medical, physical, psychological, emotional, and cultural conditions that may require additional knowledge and skills to successfully produce diagnostic quality radiographs while practicing ALARA (as low as reasonably achievable) (see Chapter 6).

The purpose of this chapter is to present some of these conditions that the radiographer must manage in order to produce quality radiographs. Additionally, recommendations based on current research for exposure of special conditions will be presented (Table 24–1).

The Apprehensive Patient

Apprehensive means to be anxious or fearful about the future. Apprehensive patients often consider the radiographic procedure to be unpleasant. These patients may have had a negative experience with a past procedure, which causes them to project those negative feelings onto the current radiographer. Therefore, it is important that the apprehensive patient's contact with the dental radiographer be pleasant and reassuring.

It is equally important that the radiographer not project his/her own negative feelings or experiences onto the patient. If the radiographer has personal views regarding the experience as uncomfortable or not necessary, he/she must not assume that the patient shares in those views. Most patients are not apprehensive about radiographic procedures, and the radiographer should not say or do anything that would prompt the patient to become anxious.

To reduce a patient's apprehension, the dental radiographer should:

- **Develop a rapport.** Take the time to explain the procedure and allow the patient to ask questions. A conversation that demonstrates attentive listening and empathy can help relax the patient.
- **Project confidence.** A skilled radiographer who demonstrates confidence will gain the patient's trust and cooperation. A patient's apprehension is increased when the operator appears unsure of him/herself.
- **Maintain authority.** The radiographer should maintain control over the procedure. Be gentle, but firm. The patient who trusts in the radiographer's ability will be less anxious. For example, if film packet placement is uncomfortable, and the radiographer allows the patient to tell the radiographer how to place the film, instead of alleviating patient apprehensiveness, the operator may actually increase it. The patient may now feel responsible for directing the procedure and may become increasingly anxious that the radiographs may not come out right.
- **Be organized.** Progress through the procedure rapidly and accurately. For example, expose the easier maxillary anterior projections first, and then progress to the more difficult posterior areas.
- **Reassure the patient.** Compliment apprehensive patients on their cooperation. Thank them for their cooperation even when the procedure may have been uncomfortable.

A Hypersensitive Gag Reflex

The term gagging means to make an involuntary effort to vomit. Gagging is caused by the **gag reflex,** which is a protective mechanism that serves to clear the airway of obstruction. The receptors for the gag reflex are located in the soft palate and lateral posterior third of the tongue. Two reactions occur prior to the gag reflex. The first is a cessation of respiration and the second is a contraction of the muscles of the abdomen and the throat.

All patients have gag reflexes, but some are more sensitive than others. A **hypersensitive gag reflex** is probably the most troublesome problem the dental radiographer may encounter. Two stimuli that must be diminished or eliminated to reduce gagging are:

1. **Psychogenic stimuli.** Originating in the mind; may result from the suggestion of gagging or as a result of a past experience of gagging.
2. **Tactile stimuli.** Originating from touch; a physical reaction to a feeling of the airway being blocked.

Reducing Psychogenic Stimuli

To help avoid a hypersensitive gag reflex that originates in the patient's mind, the radiographer should apply all of the suggested behaviors just explained for alleviating patient apprehensiveness. If the patient reports a past experience with gagging during the radiographic procedure, or you suspect that a gagging reflex will occur, the following suggestions may help to prevent its occurrence:

- **Do not suggest gagging.** The dental radiographer should not ask the question, "Are you a gagger?" The power of suggestion is a strong psychogenic stimulus and can initiate the gag reflex. Unless the patient brings it up, do not mention it.
- **Empathize.** If the patient brings up the subject of gagging, do not dismiss their concern as "all in the mind." Instead, empathize with their response and explain that there are some tricks and techniques that have been shown to help avoid stimulating the gag reflex and that you will individualize these to help them control their gag reflex.
- **Use the power of suggestion.** When applying these tricks and techniques, explain them to the patient. Letting the patient know that you are altering treatment to help them manage the gag reflex will increase the likelihood of success. The gagging patient will often be embarrassed by their involuntary reaction and most are willing to accept any methods you offer to help them regain control.
- **Apply distraction techniques.** There are many ways to divert the patient's attention away from the oral cavity. This can be done by maintaining an engaging dialogue or telling the patient to think of something pleasant, such as their

TABLE 24-1 **Conditions Prompting Alterations to Radiographic Procedures**

Condition	Anticipated Problem	Management Strategy
Apprehensive	Ability to tolerate film packet placement	Develop a rapport Project confidence Maintain authority Be organized Reassure patient
Hypersensitive gag reflex	Ability to tolerate film packet placement	Do not suggest gagging Empathize Use the power of suggestion Apply distraction techniques Give the patient breathing instructions Reduce tactile stimuli • Radiograph the anterior regions first • Place film firmly and expertly • Confuse the senses • Utilize special products Substitute extraoral radiographs as needed
Elderly	Angular cheilitis (Soft tissue cracking of lips) Decreased muscle function Unsteadiness, tremors Alzheimer's disease (reduced attentiveness to instructions)	Smaller film packet; lighter weight film holder; use of edge cushion products Set exposure to increase radiation and decrease exposure time Utilize caregiver as assistant to stabilize film and/or patient Substitute extraoral radiographs
Motor disorders and conditions of involuntary movement	Ability to remain still throughout the exposure	Set exposure to increase radiation and decrease exposure time Utilize caregiver as assistant to stabilize film and/or patient
Wheelchair-bound	Positioning patient within the range of the x-ray unit extension arm and tube head	Transfer the patient to the dental chair when possible
Visually impaired	Ability to communicate instructions to gain patient cooperation Ability to prevent apprehension of the unknown Patient personal eyewear may be in the path of the central ray	Explain each step of the procedure Use touch to explain equipment and procedures Announce when exiting and entering the room and explain why Allow the patient to wear their familiar eyewear whenever possible; explain the need to remove it; allow the patient to remove glasses
Hearing impaired	Ability to understand and follow directions	Be creative in finding alternate methods of communication
Cancer	Patient hesitant to undergo dental radiographic procedure	Explain the use of evidenced-based selection criteria
Pregnancy	Patient hesitant to undergo dental radiographic procedure	Explain the use of evidenced-based selection criteria Discuss necessary and elective radiographic procedures Explain the need for, and use lead (or lead equivalent) thyroid collar
Culturally diverse	Language, beliefs, traditions and familiar influences can be barriers to care	Exhibit an accepting, non-judgmental attitude Make an effort to understand the culture

favorite vacation. However, if the gag reflex has been identified, it may be better to tell the patient that you are going to give him/her a distraction task to perform. For example, the patient may be instructed to bite hard on the film holder's bite block; raise an arm or clench a fist; or press their head back against the head rest of the treatment chair. Anything that helps to divert the patient's attention from the oral cavity may lessen the likelihood of initiating the gag reflex (Figure 24–1).

- **Give the patient breathing instructions.** A gag reflex is often stimulated by a sense of not being able to breathe. Explain this to the patient and together, plan a breathing exercise that the patient can concentrate on during film packet placement. For example, the patient may be coached to breathe deeply through the nose or the mouth; to hum a familiar song; or to hold the breath while counting to 10 slowly, by which time the radiographer should have completed the exposure.

Reducing Tactile Stimuli

Some patients have an accentuated gag reflex because of hypersensitive pharyngeal tissues. The worst gaggers are patients suffering from chronic sinus problems (postnasal drip). Mucus and saliva accumulate into the nasopharynx area and initiate the gag reflex. The dental radiographer can reduce tactile stimuli by use of the following techniques.

- **Radiograph the anterior regions first.** Anterior films are less likely to initiate the gag reflex. The maxillary molar film is the most likely film placement to initiate the gag reflex. When exposing a series of bitewing radiographs, expose the premolar film before the molar film. It is often easier to prevent a gag reflex than to quell it once excited. Exposing easier films first allows the patient to get used to the procedure, builds acceptance, and will usually permit the radiographer to proceed successfully to the more difficult posterior film packet placements. Additionally, fears from psychic stimuli are most likely to have been forgotten by the time the maxillary molar exposure is made.

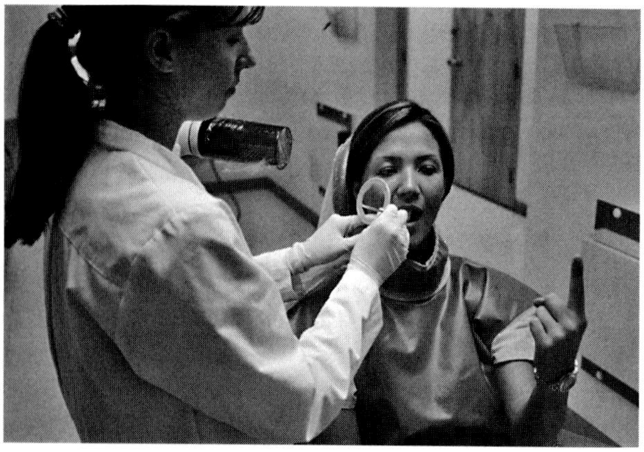

FIGURE 24–1 **Distraction techniques.** To help control a gag reflex, this patient has been given an exercise to bend and straighten her index finger. She has been instructed to keep a steady motion while continuing to watch her finger.

- **Place film firmly and expertly.** For all projections, carry the film into the mouth parallel with the plane of occlusion. When in proper position, rotate the film into place against the appropriate structures. Retain in position without movement. Avoid sliding the film across sensitive oral mucosa (soft tissue lining of the oral cavity).
- **Utilize the bisecting technique.** As you learned in Chapter 12, film packet placement in the oral cavity may be easier with the bisecting technique for patients who present with conditions that prevent parallel film packet placement. Since a gag reflex is sometimes excited by the film packet placement, utilizing the bisecting technique may help prevent gagging.
- **Confuse the senses.** Stimulating the oral mucosa with digital palpation (rubbing with the finger) serves two purposes. When the radiographer places a finger in the area to simulate for the patient where the film packet will be placed, the patient can experience what actual film packet placement will feel like. Second, palpation helps to massage and desensitize the soft tissue to make film packet placement feel less foreign. Another technique that helps confuse the senses and thus lower the risk of gagging is to instruct the patient to rinse with cold water, ice cubes, or antimicrobial oral rinse products just prior to film packet placement. Placing table salt on the middle or tip of the patient's tongue has been shown to be effective at reducing the gag reflex. When introducing any of these agents, care must be taken to first be sure that there are no contraindications for their use. For example, the patient's teeth may be sensitive to cold; and the hypertensive patient (the patient with high blood pressure) may be on a salt-restricted diet.
- **Utilize special products.** A different film holder may be required for use on the patient with a hypersensitive gag reflex. Some film holders are smaller, lighter weight or otherwise more comfortable than others. Additionally, there are products on the market, such as film packet edge protectors that reduce the edge sharpness of the intraoral film packet that some patients report stimulates their gag reflex (Figures 24–2 and 24–3).

Extreme Cases of the Gag Reflex

Occasionally, the radiographer will encounter a patient with a hypersensitive gag reflex that can not be controlled. The radiographer may be able to substitute a smaller sized film, such as a #1 or #0 for the standard #2 size film in some areas. The radiographer should take as many intraoral radiographs as possible and then supplement these with extraoral radiographs.

In rare cases the dentist may prescribe the use a topical anesthetic to numb the areas causing the patient to gag. However, some patients experience an increased anxiety as the result of this numbing sensation, especially in the soft palate and oral

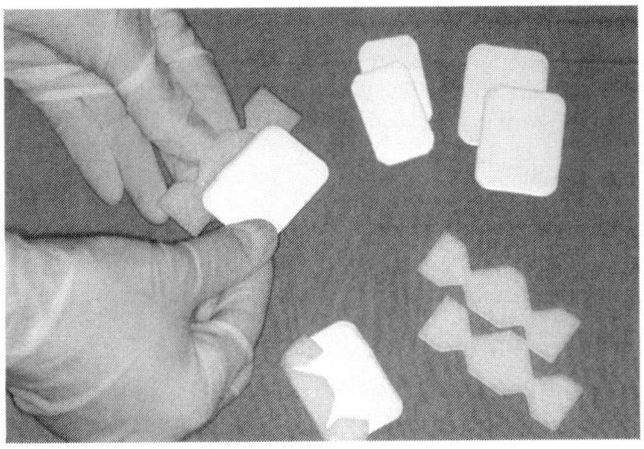

FIGURE 24–2 **Edge protectors.** Applying a commercial product to reduce the edge sharpness of the film.

pharyngeal area. Additionally, the risks and contraindications of the topical anesthetic must be considered.

The Older Adult Patient

Normal changes in the body due to aging do not necessarily mean that all older adult patients will present with unique conditions that require alterations in the radiographic procedure. However, the dental radiographer should be aware that there is an increased incidence of conditions and diseases such as **angular cheilitis** (fissuring and cracking of the soft tissue at the corners of the mouth), missing teeth (see Chapter 25), hearing impairment, arthritis, stroke, and physical impairment that are seen increasingly with aging. Soft tissue changes in the lips may prevent accurate film packet placement. Muscle function that diminishes with aging, resulting in unsteadiness and tremor, may present a barrier to holding still during exposures. Residual effects of stroke, such as paralysis, may involve the ability to move the tongue. Alzheimer's disease—which often results in inattentiveness to instructions, loss of coordination, and other motor abnormalities, including exaggerated reflexes—should be taken into consideration when planning to expose radiographs.

It is important to communicate with the older adult patient to ensure that they can follow instructions for a successful outcome to the radiographic procedure. Some of the alterations suggested above for managing the gag reflex will aid film packet placement for the older adult patient. These include using a smaller, lighter weight film holder, smaller film size, and applying a commercial film packet edge protector.

To assist with possible patient movement that occurs as the result of slight tremors or unsteadiness, the exposure settings may be manipulated to provide the appropriate amount of radiation in the shortest period of time. This is discussed in detail in the next section. If the patient cannot hold still, a caregiver or family member may need to be employed to help steady the patient. The assistant must be offered protective barriers such as lead or lead-equivalent gloves, aprons, or shields. The dental radiographer must never hold the film in the patient's mouth during the x-ray exposure.

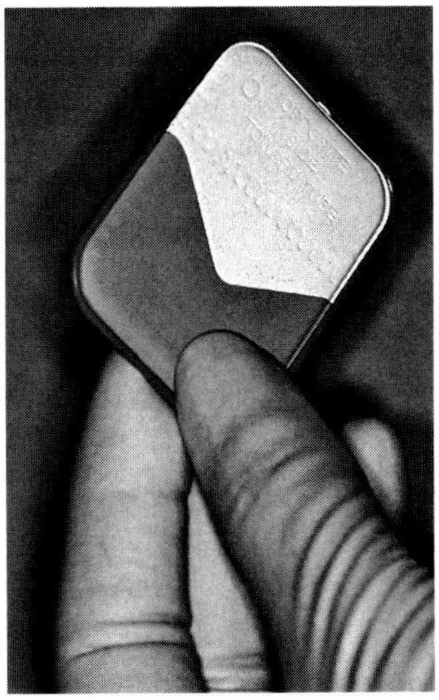

FIGURE 24–3 **Edge protectors.** Film is available with commercially applied edge softeners.

Extraoral radiographs may prove to be an acceptable substitute if the patient's head can be stabilized throughout the duration of the exposure. Head stabilization may be possible with certain panoramic x-ray machines that have secure head positioner guides (see Chapter 28). It is important to note that in later stages of osteoporosis, the loss of stature and spinal deformity that creates a stooping posture will often make the use of the panoramic procedure difficult.

Motor Disorders and Conditions of Involuntary Movement

There are many conditions that present with unsteadiness and tremor that require careful consideration prior to exposing radiographs. In addition to the considerations above, patients who present with Parkinson's disease, Bell's palsy, cerebral palsy, multiple sclerosis, and myasthenia gravis (a neuromuscular disease characterized by weakened muscles, especially of the face and oral cavity) require careful assessment as to their ability to undergo a radiographic examination. If the possibility of movement during the exposure is identified, the exposure settings—the milliamperage (mA) and the exposure time—may be adjusted to decrease the time required for exposure by increasing the amount of radiation generated. As you will recall in Chapter 3, the mA setting controls the amount of radiation generated. By increasing the mA, the x-ray machine will generate more radiation. With this increase in radiation, the exposure time may be decreased (Table 24–2). The guidelines to adjust these settings are explained in Chapter 3.

The Disabled Patient

A **disability** is defined as a physical or mental impairment that substantially limits one or more of an individual's major life activities. The dental radiographer must be prepared to

TABLE 24–2 **Suggested Exposure Times When Changing the mA Setting* for Adult Patients**

	Impulse Setting		
Region to be Radiographed	7 mA	10 mA	15 mA
Maxillary anterior periapical	14	10	7
Maxillary posterior periapical	20	14	9
Mandibular anterior periapical	12	8	6
Mandibular posterior periapical	16	11	8
Anterior bitewing	12	8	6
Posterior bitewing	16	11	8

*F-speed film; 12 in. (20 cm) PID; 70 kVp.

accommodate patients with disabilities. When treating a patient with a disability:

- **Talk directly to the patient.** Do not ask the patient's caregiver questions that should be directed to the patient. For example, do not say to the caregiver, "Can he (or she) stand up?" Instead, speak directly to the patient and say, "Can you stand up?"
- **Offer assistance to disabled patients.** Ask the patient how you can best assist them.
- **Do not ask personal questions about the patient's disability.**

The Wheelchair-bound Patient

The difficulty encountered with the wheelchair-bound patient is getting the patient into position close enough to the x-ray unit (Figure 24–4). Care should be taken to be sure that the extension arm can support the tube head in position without drifting. Unless the patient is in a total-support wheelchair, it may be best to transfer the patient to the dental chair.

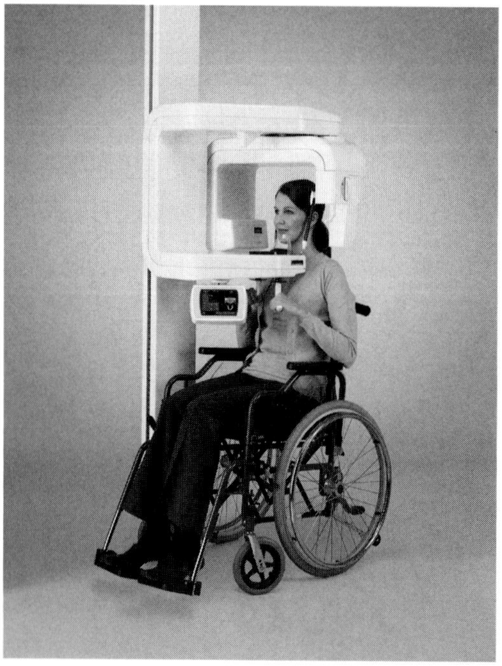

FIGURE 24–4 **Panoramic unit that can accommodate wheelchair-bound patients.** (Courtesy of Planmeca)

Wheelchair patients can be transferred to the dental chair by use of the following techniques:

- **Wheelchair patients who can temporarily support their weight** are transferred to the dental chair by placing the wheelchair alongside the dental chair. Set the brakes of the wheelchair and elevate the dental chair to the height of the wheelchair. Move the dental chair arm from between the chairs. Have the patient move or slide sideways into the dental chair with the caregiver and radiographer assisting.
- **If the patient is unable to support their weight,** the immobile patient may be transferred to the dental chair by radiographer and caregiver. With one taking a position behind the patient and the other facing the patient, the radiographer and caregiver may lift the patient from the wheelchair into the dental chair.

The Visually Impaired Patient

The visually impaired or blind patient requires special consideration during the radiographic procedure. The radiographer must communicate using clear verbal explanations of each step of the procedure before performing it. When taking multiple exposures, it is important to maintain verbal contact to reorient the patient each time you must exit and re-enter the oral cavity. Using touch, the radiographer can demonstrate film packet placement and the feel of the film holder prior to its placement to help eliminate the feeling of anxiety when facing the unknown. Allow the patient to handle the film holder and film packets to get familiar with them if necessary.

The personal eyewear worn by many blind patients may have to be temporarily removed if the glasses will be positioned within the primary beam. Explain the need for this to the patient. Allow the patient to remove his/her own glasses. Immediately following the exposures, allow the patient to resume wearing their personal eyewear.

Maintain communication with the blind patient. Explain why you are leaving the room when you go to the darkroom to process the films. Immediately announce your return to the operatory by speaking directly to the patient.

Practice Point

Never gesture to another person in the presence of a patient who is blind. Blind persons are sensitive to gesture communication and may feel you are "talking behind their back."

The Hearing Impaired Patient

Communication is vitally important to the success of all radiographic procedures. The radiographer must give the patient explicit detailed instructions before, during, and at the end of each film packet placement and exposure. The production of quality radiographs depends on the patient's ability to understand and follow these instructions. Communication with the hearing impaired patient requires that the radiographer be aware of what method of communication works best for the patient. The radiographer should always ask a hearing impaired or deaf patient how he/she prefers to communication. Several options are:

- Use of written instructions.
- Ask a relative or caregiver to act as an interpreter.
- Use of gestures.

If the patient can use **speech reading** (reading lips), face the patient and speak slowly and clearly, allowing the patient to read your facial expressions and gestures. Since a face mask is recommended as PPE (personal protective equipment; see Chapter 9) during radiographic procedures, it is important that the patient and the radiographer agree on the meaning of certain gestures before beginning the procedure (Figure 24–5). In fact, the hearing impaired patient will appreciate the radiographer who takes the time to learn a few of the gestures or sign language he/she uses to communicate.

If the patient uses a hearing aid, it may have to be removed prior to the panoramic radiographic procedure (see Chapter 28). Explain the upcoming radiographic procedures before asking the patient to remove the hearing aid, since communication will be diminished when it is removed.

The Cancer Patient

There is often a concern whenever the necessity arises to expose dental radiographs on any patient who is currently receiving or has recently undergone radiation therapy. The patient is often reluctant to receive additional radiation, no matter how minimal, and the dentist may be hesitant to prescribe dental radiographs. Likewise, the radiographer making the exposure may feel apprehensive about the procedure.

The patient should be told that the concerns for radiation safety are shared. Although the patient may already have received large therapeutic doses of radiation, this is not a contraindication to exposing dental radiographs, provided that they are deemed to be necessary to make an oral diagnosis. The additional radiation that the patient would receive is minimal, and its use is justified if the patient benefits.

Pregnancy

Prior to a research report published by the American Medical Association (AMA) in 2004, the potential effects of dental radiation exposure centered on the possibility of exposure to the developing fetus. Then JAMA (*Journal of the American Medical Association*) published research that investigated the effect on pregnancy outcomes of radiation exposure of the hypothalamus and the pituitary and thyroid glands that suggests that dental radiation exposure is associated with full-term low birth weight infants. More research in this area may lead to altered guidelines on dental radiographs for pregnant females. The American Dental Association (ADA) currently recommends that necessary dental radiographs that help the dentist diagnose and treat oral disease still be exposed on pregnant females; and that elective dental x-rays be postponed for the pregnant female until after delivery. The ADA strongly recommends the use of lead or lead-equivalent thyroid collars in conjuction with lead apron barriers for all patients, and especially for pregnant females and women of child-bearing age.

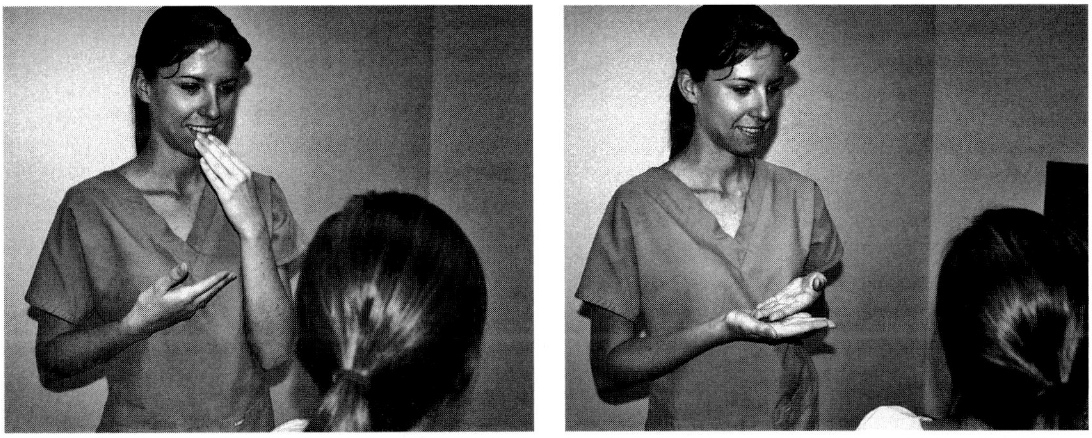

A B

FIGURE 24–5 **Example of signing.** The radiographer is letting this hearing impaired patient know that she is doing a good job cooperating with the radiographic procedure. (**A**) Right hand on chin. (**B**) Drops to left hand open palm. Communicating "Good patient."

Practice Point

Do not confuse the terms "elective" and "unnecessary." The evidenced-based selection guidelines (see Chapter 6) used by dentists to help with the decision to expose radiographs on all types of patients prevent the exposure of unnecessary radiographs. Unnecessary radiographs should never be exposed on any patient. When considering radiographs for the pregnant female, the ADA recommends that elective dental x-rays be postponed until after delivery. While the ADA Council on Scientific Affairs publication "An update on radiographic practices: Information and recommendations" (*J. Am. Dent. Assoc.*, 2001; 132: 234–8) does not define "elective" radiographs, this example is offered to help differentiate elective from unnecessary.

- **Pregnant patient A** presents for dental hygiene services after a one-year time frame. Bitewing radiographs were last taken three years ago. After the assessment it is determined that the patient has periodontal disease. According to the evidence-based selection criteria guidelines (see Table 6–1), this patient should be treatment planned for a set of vertical bitewing radiographs. These radiographs have been determined to be necessary to diagnose and treat this oral condition.
- **Pregnant patient B** presents for a dental consultation to replace a removal partial denture with a fixed bridge. To determine the health of the teeth and the periodontium that will support the bridge, periapical radiographs are necessary. However, the dentist would most likely assess this dental treatment and the need for radiographs as elective at this time, and recommend postponement until after delivery.

The Culturally Sensitive Radiographer

The diversity of culture in today's global society means that the radiographer is more and more likely to find him/herself performing radiographic examinations on patients of a variety of racial, ethnic, and cultural backgrounds. Educating these patients regarding the role radiographs play in the diagnosis and treatment of oral diseases requires that the radiographer be aware of possible **cultural barriers,** such as language, beliefs, traditions, and familiar influences.

Since good communication is the foundation upon which quality radiographs are produced, the radiographer should strive to develop a better understanding of the cultures most likely to be encountered in the community where the oral health care practice is located. To assist in developing cultural sensitivity the radiographer should take into consideration the patient's:

- **Communication style.** Is eye contact considered respectful or a sign of rudeness? Does the patient consider discussing the oral cavity personal and private? Is the patient comfortable having a family member translate personal or sensitive information?
- **Comfortable personal space zone.** Does touch convey acceptance, or is it offensive? Is the patient uncomfortable being treated by a professional of the opposite gender? Does the patient wear certain articles of clothing or spiritual jewelry that they would be uncomfortable removing for the radiographic procedure?
- **Gestures and body language.** Does the hand gesture you use mean the same thing to the patient in his/her culture? Are there hand gestures that you need to use to convey instructions regarding the radiographic procedure considered obscene in another culture?

The dental radiographer who presents an accepting, non-judgmental attitude when presented with diverse cultures is more likely to gain the trust and cooperation of the patient.

REVIEW—Chapter Summary

The dental radiographer must be competent in altering procedures to meet the needs of individual patients. To help manage apprehension, the dental radiographer should develop a rapport with the patient, project confidence, maintain authority, be organized and reassure the patient throughout the procedure.

A hypersensitive gag reflex is probably the most troublesome problem the radiographer encounters. Psychogenic and tactile stimuli must be diminished or eliminated to reduce gagging.

The elderly sometimes present with conditions that require management to produce quality radiographs. Motor disorders and conditions of involuntary movement may be managed by increasing the amount of radiation (mA) and decreasing the exposure time (impulses).

A disability is a physical or mental impairment that substantially limits one or more of an individual's major life activities. The dental radiographer must be prepared to accommodate patients with disabilities.

Patients who have received radiation therapy should be reassured that necessary dental radiographs are justified if the patient benefits. The American Dental Association currently recommends that necessary dental radiographs that help the dentist diagnose and treat oral disease still be exposed on pregnant females; and that elective dental x-rays be postponed for the pregnant female until after delivery.

The dental radiographer who presents an accepting, non-judgmental attitude when presented with diverse cultures is more likely to gain the trust and cooperation of the patient.

RECALL—Study Questions

1. List five actions for managing the apprehensive patient.
   a. ___________________
   b. ___________________
   c. ___________________
   d. ___________________
   e. ___________________
2. A hypersensitive gag reflex that results from a physical reaction to a feeling of the airway being blocked is called a psychogenic stimulus. Eliminating psychogenic and tactile stimuli will prevent a hypersensitive gag reflex.
   a. The first statement is true. The second statement is false.
   b. The first statement is false. The second statement is true.
   c. Both statements are true.
   d. Both statements are false.
3. Dental radiographers who demonstrate confidence, and who tell the patient that gagging is "all in their mind" will experience fewer gagging problems.
   a. The first part of the statement is true, but the second part of the statement is false.
   b. The first part of the statement is false, but the second part of the statement is true.
   c. Both parts of the statement are true.
   d. Both parts of the statement are false.
4. All of the following suggestions help the radiographer avoid exciting a hypersensitive gag reflex *except* one. Which one is this *exception?*
   a. Ask the patient to breathe through the nose.
   b. Ask the patient to rinse with ice water prior to film packet placement.
   c. Ask the patient if they have ever gagged during x-ray exposures.
   d. Ask the patient to press their head against the headrest during the exposures.
5. The film packet placement most likely to initiate the gag reflex is the:
   a. Maxillary premolar
   b. Maxillary molar
   c. Mandibular premolar
   d. Mandibular molar
6. The patient is less likely to gag:
   a. The longer the film stays in the mouth
   b. If they concentrate on the film packet placement
   c. When the film is slid into position over the oral mucosa
   d. While performing a breathing exercise
7. Older adults who present with soft tissue degeneration that makes film packet placement uncomfortable may benefit from all of the following *except* one. Which one is this *exception?*
   a. Increasing the exposure time
   b. Using a smaller sized film packet
   c. Using a lighter weight film holder
   d. Applying an edge protector to the film packet
8. To compensate for slight movement that results from Parkinson's Disease tremors, the radiographer can adjust the exposure settings to:
   a. Decrease the mA and decrease the impulses
   b. Increase the mA and increase the impulses
   c. Decrease the mA and increase the impulses
   d. Increase the mA and decrease the impulses
9. When performing radiographic services for the disabled patient, the radiographer should:
   a. Remove the patient's eyewear for them prior to exposures
   b. Offer to assist the patient in the manner that they want
   c. Communicate with the caregiver instead of talking directly to the patient
   d. Ask personal questions about the patient's disability
10. Unnecessary radiographs may be taken on the cancer patient, but only elective radiographs may be taken on the pregnant female.
    a. The first part of the statement is true, but the second part of the statement is false.
    b. The first part of the statement is false, but the second part of the statement is true.
    c. Both parts of the statement are true.
    d. Both parts of the statement are false.
11. It is ethical practice to take unnecessary radiographs on:
    a. The older adult
    b. The pregnant female
    c. The cancer patient
    d. No one
12. The dental radiographer should consider all of the following to develop sensitivity for the culturally diverse patient *except* one. Which one is this *exception?*
    a. Lowered metal capacities
    b. Personal space zone
    c. Communication style
    d. Culturally different meanings to hand gestures

REFLECT—Case Study

You have just greeted your patient in the reception area, introduced yourself, and asked her to follow you to the operatory, where you will be taking a full mouth series of radiographs. Once seated, you notice that the patient appears apprehensive. As you begin to ready the film packets and film holders needed for the examination, you engage her in a conversation to assess why she appears so nervous. The patient eventually tells you that her last experience taking radiographs could not be completed because she experienced a gagging problem. She states that she was so embarrassed by it that she never went back to that practice.

1. Explain how you would respond to this patient. Include how you would develop a rapport, project confidence, and maintain authority.
2. Prepare a conversation with this patient where your responses reassure her about your ability to perform the procedure; how the procedure today can be different than her past experience; and what techniques you have to help her control the gag reflex.

3. Answer the following questions:
   a. Why should you not tell this patient that gagging is all in her mind?
   b. Which film packet (what area of the oral cavity) should you try placing first, and why?
   c. What is the purpose of thanking and praising the patient for her cooperation with the procedure?
   d. What is the difference between psychogenic and tactile stimuli? Give an example of each.
   e. What is the purpose of asking the patient to do breathing exercises during radiographic exposures?
   f. What is the purpose of rinsing with ice water or placing salt on the tongue?
   g. If you use any of these tricks and techniques, why is it best to tell the patient what trick you are planning to use?

RELATE—Laboratory Application

For a comprehensive laboratory practice exercise on this topic, see E. M. Thomson, *Exercises in Oral Radiography Techniques: A Laboratory Manual,* 2nd ed., Upper Saddle River, NJ: Prentice Hall, 2007. Chapter 7, "Special Patients and Student Partner Practice."

BIBLIOGRAPHY

American Dental Association. Statement on ante partum dental radiography and infant low birth weight. *JAMA,* April 28, 2004. www.da.org/public/media/releases/0404_release03.asp

ADA Council on Scientific Affairs. An update on radiographic practices: Information and recommendations. *J. Am. Dent. Assoc.* 132: 234–238, 2001.

Carl, W. Local and systemic chemotherapy: Preventing and managing oral complications. *J. Am. Dent. Assoc.* 124:119–123, 1993.

Darby, M. L. and Walsh, M. M. *Dental Hygiene Theory and Practice,* 2nd ed. St. Louis: Saunders, 2003.

Hujoel, P. P., Bollen, A., Noonan, C. J., del Aguila, M. A., Ante partum dental radiography and infant low birth weight." *JAMA* 291:16–1993, 2004.

Khan, F. M. *The Physics of Radiation Therapy,* 3rd ed. Philadelphia: Lippincott Williams & Wilkins, 2003.

Langland, O. E. & Langlais, R. P. *Principles of Dental Imaging.* Philadelphia: Lippincott Williams & Wilkins; 1997.

Mettler, F. A. & Upton, A. C. *Medical Effects of Ionizing Radiation,* 2nd ed. Philadelphia: Saunders, 1995.

National Cancer Institute. *Consensus Development Conference on Oral Complications of Cancer Therapies: Diagnosis, Prevention and Treatment.* National Cancer Institute monograph no. 9. Bethesda, MD: National Institutes of Health; 1990.

White, S. C. & Pharoah, M. J. *Oral Radiology Principles and Interpretation,* 5th ed. St. Louis: Elsevier, 2004.

Wilkins, E. M. *Clinical Practice of the Dental Hygienist,* 9th ed. Philadelphia: Lippincott Williams & Wilkins, 2005.

25

Supplemental Radiographic Techniques

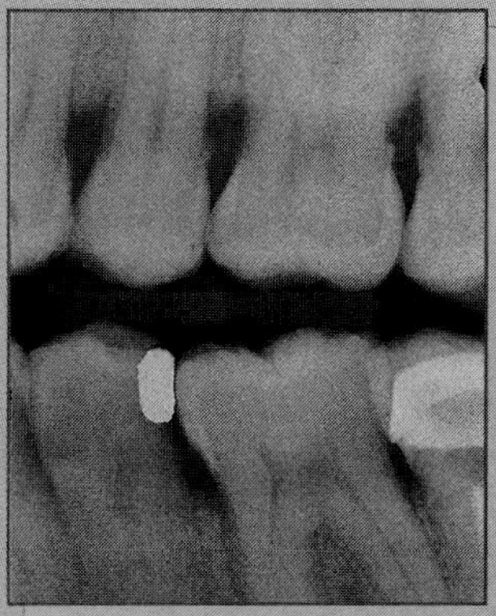

■ OBJECTIVES

Following successful completion of this chapter, you should be able to:

1. Define the key words.
2. Demonstrate the ability to adapt standard techniques appropriately.
3. Demonstrate appropriate adaptations in film packet placement to avoid molar overlap.
4. Explain the need to increase vertical angulation when the patient presents with a shallow palatal vault.
5. Demonstrate knowledge of setting the exposure time based on patient characteristics.
6. Demonstrate the ability to place the intraoral film packet on patients with large maxillary or mandibular tori.
7. Discuss the procedures for film packet placement in patients with edentulous areas.
8. Discuss the procedures for film packet placement during endodontic procedures.
9. List three methods of localization.
10. Utilize the buccal-object rule to identify the location of a foreign object.
11. Describe the difference between a standard molar periapical radiograph and a disto-oblique periapical radiograph.
12. List four reasons to duplicate radiographs.
13. Demonstrate the step-by-step procedures for duplicating radiographs.

■ KEY WORDS

Buccal-object rule
Disto-oblique periapical radiographs
Duplicate radiograph
Duplicating film
Edentulous
Endodontic therapy
Film duplicator
Localization
Root canal treatment
SLOB
Tori
Torus mandibularis
Torus palatinus
Tube shift method
Working radiograph

Introduction

It is important that the dental radiographer possess a working knowledge of radiographic theory and techniques in order to produce diagnostic quality radiographs. However, each patient presents with unique characteristics, some of which may require that the dental radiographer have the knowledge and skills to adapt these ideal procedures to best suit the circumstances. What sets the skilled radiographer apart from the average is the ability to alter techniques and still produce diagnostic images.

The purpose of this chapter is to provide specific information on acceptable alterations of the ideal skills you have learned in this book.

Acceptable Variations in Technique

Anatomical limitations, such as rotation of the teeth, variations in the height of the palate, the presence of unerupted third molars, or excessive root lengths, may require that the radiographer apply acceptable variations in the radiographic technique. Such changes may occur in the horizontal or vertical angulations or in the film packet placement.

Avoiding Overlap

Molars

Because the interproximal surfaces of the molars are in a mesiodistal relationship to the patient's sagittal plane, conventional film packet placement parallel to the buccal surfaces may result in overlapping of the contact areas and closure of the embrasure spaces. To assist with avoiding the occurrence of overlap error, the film packet should be positioned perpendicularly to the embrasures. To achieve this position, the film packet should be placed slightly diagonally, with the front edge of the film a greater distance from the lingual surfaces of the teeth than the back edge of the film (Figure 25–1).

Canine-premolar

The canine periapical and bitewing radiographs will almost always exhibit overlap between the distal of the canine and the mesial of the premolar. This overlap occurs because the curve of the arches in this region superimposes the lingual cusp of the premolar onto the more anterior canine. To help minimize this overlap, the horizontal angulation can be adjusted slightly to direct the central rays of the x-ray beam to intersect the film from the distal. Shifting the PID slightly toward the posterior will help separate these two teeth on the resultant image.

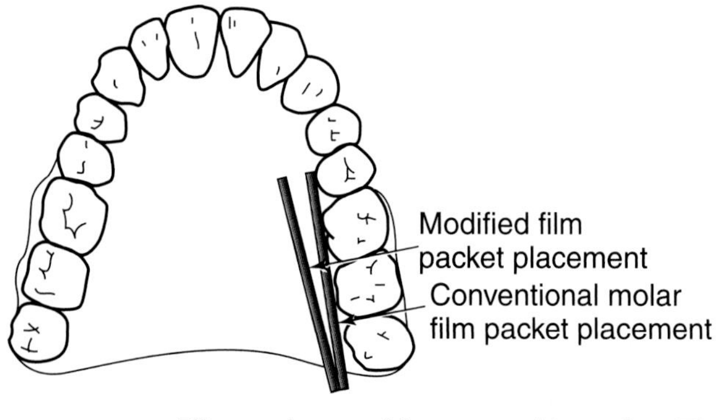

FIGURE 25-1 **Film packet position to avoid overlap.** The anterior portion of the film packet is placed a greater distance away from the lingual surfaces of the teeth.

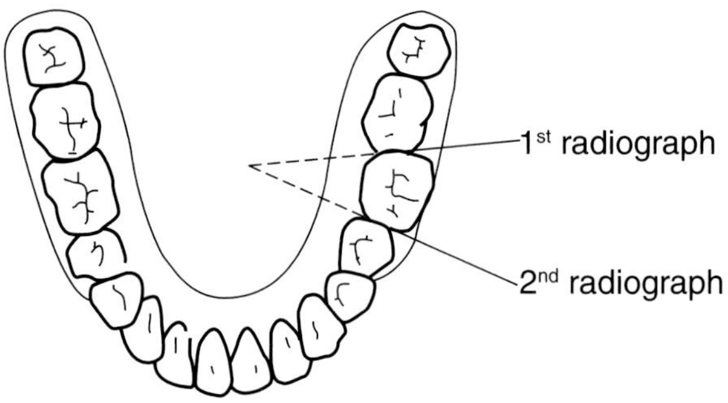

FIGURE 25-2 **Different horizontal angluation is required when teeth are mal-aligned.**

Because the mesial portion of the premolar will often overlap the distal portion of the canine on canine periapical and bitewing radiographs, it is important that the distal portion of the canine be imaged clearly when exposing premolar periapical and bitewing radiographs when taking a series of films.

Mal-aligned or Crowded Teeth

When teeth are mal-aligned or crowded it may be necessary to take additional radiographs at various horizontal angles to image every interproximal area clearly, with no overlap (Figure 25–2). The film packet should be positioned perpendicularly to the embrasures of each tooth as necessary.

Altering Vertical Angulation

Absolute parallelism between the film packet and the long axes of the teeth is sometimes difficult to achieve. If the deviation from parallel does not exceed 15 degrees, the radiograph is generally acceptable (Figure 25–3). This fact can be used to help

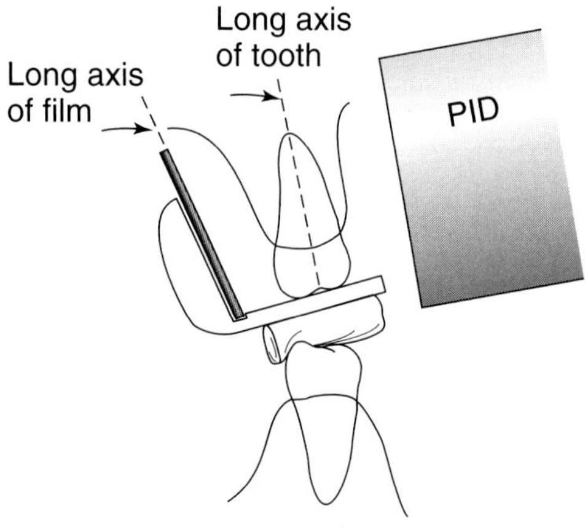

FIGURE 25-3 **Shallow palate.** The tissue edge of the film is shown tipped away from the teeth. When the lack of parallelism is less than 15 degrees, the resultant radiograph will generally be acceptable.

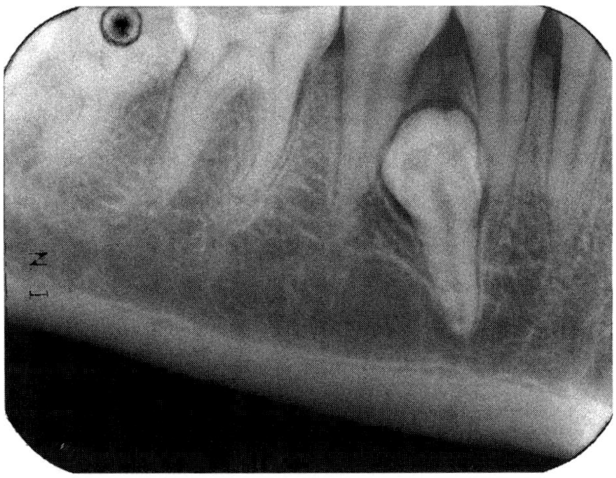

FIGURE 25-4 **Radiograph taken with an increased vertical angulation.** Note the increased coverage of the apical region showing the supernumerary (extra) premolar. The increased vertical angulation used to image more of the apical region cut off a portion of the occlusal region of the teeth.

improve radiographic images when the patient presents with a low palatal vault or when the teeth roots are longer than average. Increasing the vertical angulation by up to 15 degrees over what is indicated will image more of the apical region (see Figure 23–6), desirable when the area of interest is suspected pathology at the root tip, a developing or congenitally missing permanent tooth (Figure 25–4), or simply to compensate for a low palatal vault. When the patient presents with a shallow palate, preventing the film packet from being placed parallel to the teeth, the root tips are often cut off of the image. Increasing the vertical angulation will compensate for the lack of parallelism to a degree (Figure 25–5). It is important to remember that varying the vertical angulation must be slight, no more than 15 degrees, or noticeable distortion will result.

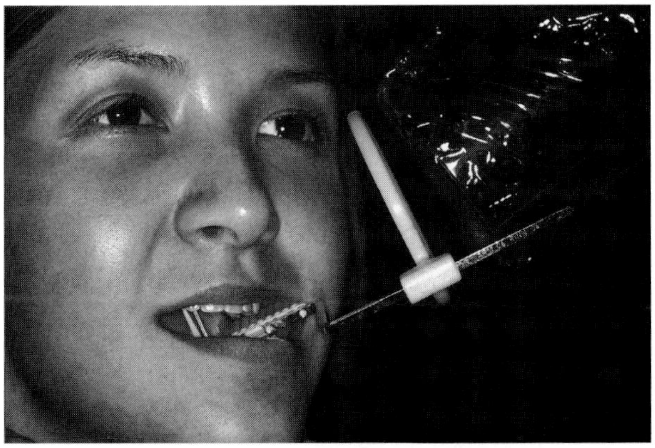

FIGURE 25-5 **Increasing the vertical angulation will increase the periapical coverage on the resultant image.** Note that when applying this alteration, the PID is not aimed directly at the external aiming ring of the film holder in the vertical dimension.

Exposure Factors

Bone and tissue density vary with the age and physical structure of the patient. Moreover, in most patients the bone structures are thinnest in the mandibular incisor region and densest in the maxillary molar region. Thus, for the best radiographs, it may be desirable to make minor changes in exposure time or milliamperage to vary the film density. Making changes in the exposure settings will also allow the radiographer to customize the radiation dose the patient receives. The exposure setting for a child patient, whose bone structures are less dense, should be less than the setting for an adult patient (see Chapter 23). Additionally, patients who present with **edentulous** regions would require less radiation for those areas with missing teeth. Exposure recommendations depend on the characteristics of the patient and the film speed and the type of x-ray equipment in use. Since these exposure recommendations vary widely, recommended settings for all patients and all regions of the oral cavity should be posted next to the x-ray unit control panel for easy reference.

Anatomical Variations

The dental radiographer should be familiar with some of the more common anatomical variations patients may present with. In addition to a shallow palate, patients may present with boney outgrowths on the palate and the lingual surfaces of the mandible, called tori.

Tori

Tori (torus, singular) are commonly seen in the oral cavity. A maxillary torus, called **torus palatinus**, is an outgrowth of bone along the midline of the hard palate. A mandibular torus, called **torus mandibularis** or lingual torus) is an outgrowth of bone along the lingual aspect of the mandible in the canine-premolar area.

A large torus palatinus or torus mandibularis may interfere with film packet placement. Care should be taken when placing the film packet in the presence of tori. In addition to its intrusion into the oral cavity, the oral mucosa covering the tori can be thin and sensitive. The film packet edge should not be placed directly on top of the tori, as this would result in only a partial image of the roots of the teeth. Instead, the film packet should be placed on the far side of the torus (Figure 25–6). When placing the film packet in the presence of mandibular tori, place the film between the torus and the tongue (Figure 25–7). This recommended placement may prove difficult when bitewing tab film holders are used. Positioning the film away from the teeth requires that the patient bite on the very end of the bitewing tab. To aid with proper film placement in such cases, the bite tab would need to be lengthened (see Figure 14–14).

The Edentulous Patient

Preventive radiography is often beneficial to the fully and partially edentulous patient because the normal appearance of the dental ridges may conceal problems underneath. Radiographs benefit the edentulous patient for the following reasons:

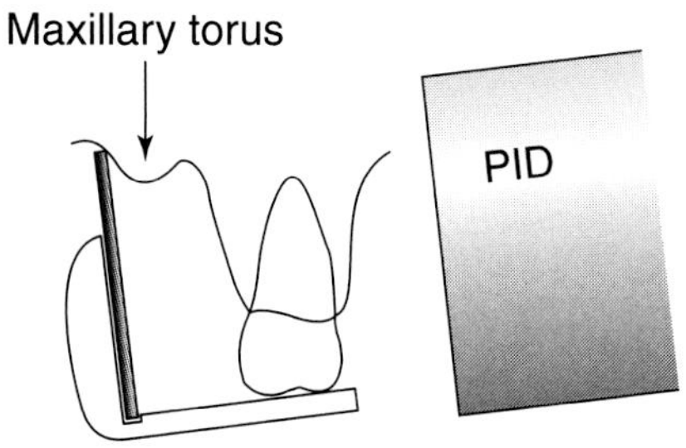

FIGURE 25-6 **Maxillary torus.** Film is shown placed on the far side of the torus away from the teeth.

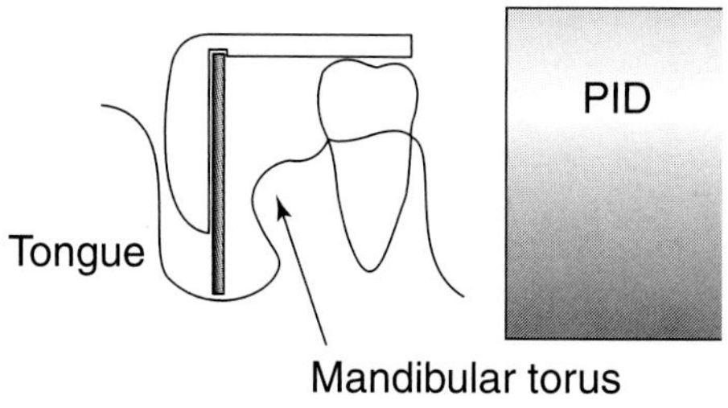

FIGURE 25-7 **Mandibular torus.** Film is shown placed between the torus and the tongue.

- To detect the presence of retained roots, impacted teeth, foreign bodies, cysts, and other pathological lesions.
- To establish the position of the mental foramen before constructing dentures.
- To establish the position of the mandibular canal before implant surgery.
- To determine the condition and quantity of alveolar bone present.

Periapical radiographs may be taken of edentulous areas using either the paralleling or the bisecting technique with minor modifications. Normally, the teeth serve as landmarks to guide film placement. Because these landmarks are not present in the edentulous patient, one must estimate the best film position. Additionally, visualizing and establishing horizontal and vertical planes is more difficult, particularly when the bisecting technique is used. However, in the totally edentulous patient a fair amount of leeway in horizontal angulation is permissible, because the absence of teeth eliminates the problem of overlapping tooth images. The focus of interest is no longer the teeth but the edentulous ridge.

Because it produces the best diagnostic images, the paralleling technique should be the radiographer's first choice. Radiographic detail is improved and dimensional distortion is minimized when film holders can be properly supported with cotton rolls or polystyrene blocks, to position the film packet parallel to the long axis of the edentulous ridge (Figures 25–8 and 25–9). The central rays of the x-ray beam are then directed horizontally and vertically toward the center of the film perpendicular to the mean tangent of the facial side of the ridge and to the plane of the film.

If parallel placement of the film packet remains difficult in an edentulous area, it is better to try utilizing the bisecting technique than to risk taking a poor quality radiograph that would need to be retaken. When utilizing the bisecting technique, the film packet is placed against the lingual surface of the edentulous ridge. The vertical angulation is determined by bisecting the angle formed between the recording plane of the film and an imaginary line through the ridge that substitutes for the long axes of the teeth (Figure 25–10). This position often results in some dimensional distortion; however, acceptable radiographs can still be produced.

Because the edentulous region is less dense, the amount of radiation needed to produce an acceptable radiographic image is less. Exposure settings for edentulous regions should be about 25 percent less than the exposure required for an area where teeth are present.

Overcoming Film Holder Limitations

While film holders with external aiming devices provide an advantage to the operator, their increased size and weight may make these film holders more uncomfortable to place into the correct position. If the film holder can not be placed precisely, the radiographer may be aligning the x-ray beam to the wrong place. The radiographer who possesses the skills necessary to evaluate film packet placement for correctness may still produce a diagnostic quality radiograph by aligning the angles and point of entry to the film packet itself, regardless of the holder's external aiming device. For example, the external aiming ring on the Rinn XCP film holder is an indicator device and does not have to be the absolute "dictator" on where to line up the x-ray beam (see Figure 25–5). The radiographer who can judge the appropriateness of film packet placement can compensate for less than ideal positioning of the film holder.

Endodontic Techniques

Endodontic therapy involves the treatment of the tooth by removing the nerves and tissues of the pulp cavity and replacing them with filling material. Successful endodontic therapy or **root canal treatment** depends on the use of radiographs. A series of films on the same tooth is needed to evaluate various stages of endodontic treatment. The initial film is exposed to determine the preoperative condition and to make a diagnosis. Additional radiographs are made as the work progresses to determine the length of the root; the position of a reamer, broach, or file in the canal; or the position of the sealer and point or points (the tooth may have several canals). And finally, a post-treatment radiograph is needed to make sure that the canal or canals are closed satisfactorily.

Once again, the paralleling technique is the technique of choice. Standard periapical radiographic procedures can be

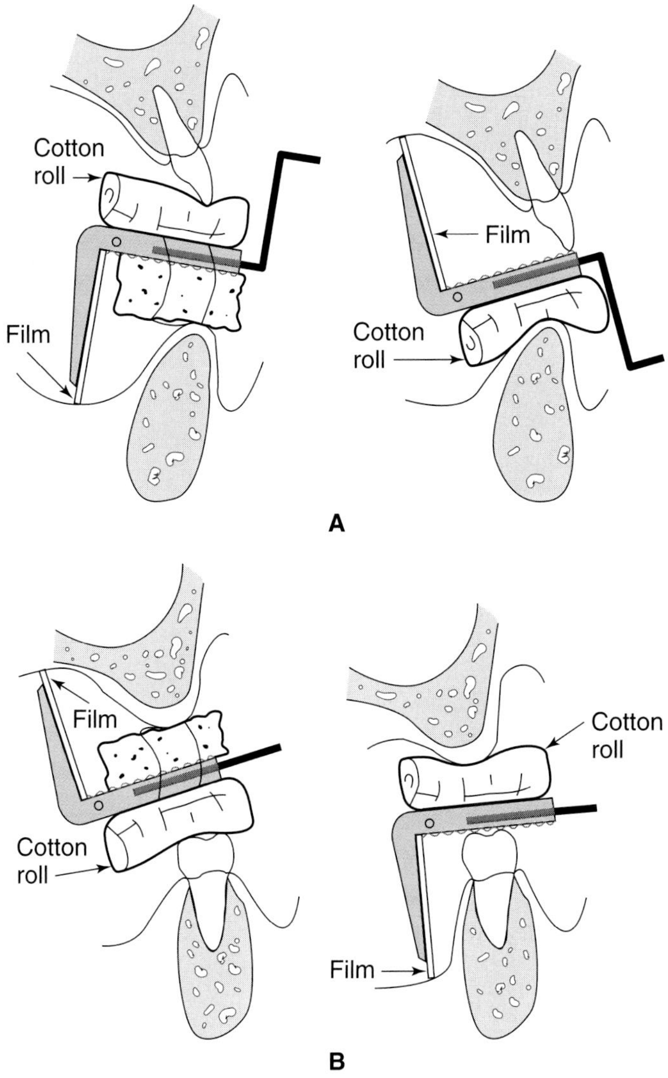

FIGURE 25-8 **Partially edentulous mouth.** Cotton rolls or polystyrene blocks can be used to substitute for missing teeth to help hold the film holder in place. (**A**) Edentulous mandibular anterior region. (**B**) Edentulous maxillary posterior region. (Courtesy of Dentsply Rinn)

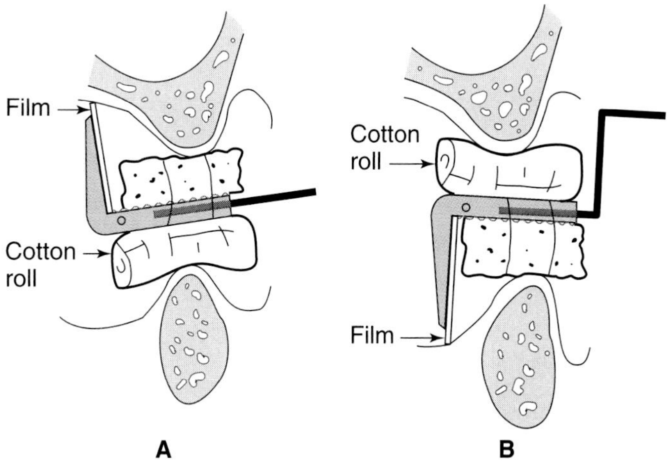

FIGURE 25-9 **Totally edentulous mouth.** When all teeth are missing, cotton rolls, polystyrene blocks, or a combination of both can be used as substitutes for the crowns of the teeth. These will allow the patient to bite and stabilize the film holder. The thickness of the cotton rolls or blocks will determine the amount of film coverage of the edentulous ridges. (**A**) Maxillary anterior region. (**B**) Mandibular posterior region. (Courtesy of Dentsply Rinn)

applied in endodontic radiographic exposures; however, there are some differences. The materials used in endodontic treatment—such as a rubber dam, reamers, broaches, files, or silver or gutta-percha points—often hinder film packet placement. The presence of these materials, that must be left in place during radiographic exposures, makes it impossible for the patient to bite down on the bite block of a film holder in order to hold the film packet in place. The avoidance of distortion or magnification of the image is a major concern in endodontic treatment because the length of each canal must be accurately measured. Therefore the paralleling technique, which consistently produces the least distortion, should be used whenever possible. Although pre-operative and post-operative radiographs are made in the usual manner, some technique modifications are required for the **working radiographs** that are exposed with the rubber dam and instruments in place.

The ideal film holder is one specifically designed to hold the film packet in place for exposure of the working films (Figure 25–11). Other types of film holders may be modified to accommodate film packet retention during endodontic therapy (Figure 25–12). However, it may become necessary to use methods of film packet retention that rely on visual alignment of the PID. Film holders such as the Rinn Snap-A-Ray (Figure 25–13) or the employment of the hemostat (Figure 25–14) or a tongue depressor as a custom-made film holder will allow the patient to help hold the film in place (Figure 25–15).

When imaging multirooted teeth, such as the maxillary premolars and molars, the buccal and lingual root canals will often appear superimposed. The ability to separate the buccal and lingual roots on the image increases the radiograph's value during endodontic procedures. The radiographer can accomplish this through the use of tube head shifting called **localization.**

Methods of Localization

Radiographs are a two-dimensional picture of three dimensional objects. To get that third dimension from a radiographic image, the dental radiographer should be skilled in reading the images. Localization methods help the radiographer to determine whether a structure such as a root canal or a foreign object embedded within the maxilla or mandible is in front of (facial or buccal) or behind (lingual) the teeth. There are three methods of localization.

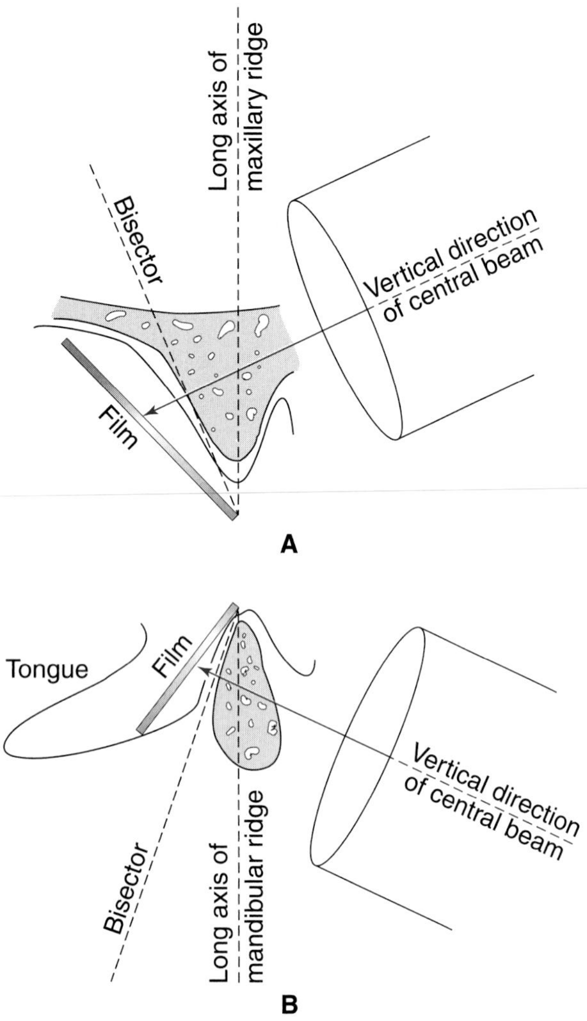

FIGURE 25-10 **Diagrams showing the relationship of the film to the ridge of an edentulous patient.** The film packet lies much flatter in the mouth when teeth are missing. When the rules of bisecting are followed, an imaginary line can be drawn vertically through the ridge to substitute for the long axes of the teeth. The central ray is directed perpendicularly to the bisector to determine the correct vertical angulation. The correct horizontal angulation is difficult to determine when no teeth are present; however, the absence of teeth eliminates the concern over overlapping error. (**A**) Maxillary edentulous ridge, (**B**) Mandibular edentulous ridge.

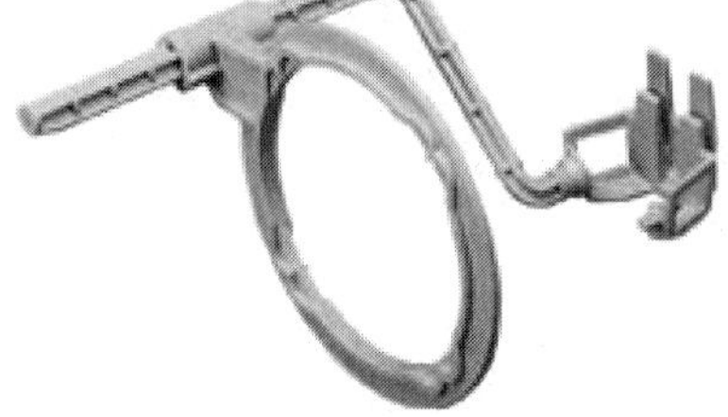

FIGURE 25-11 **Endodontic film holder.** (Courtesy of Dentsply Rinn)

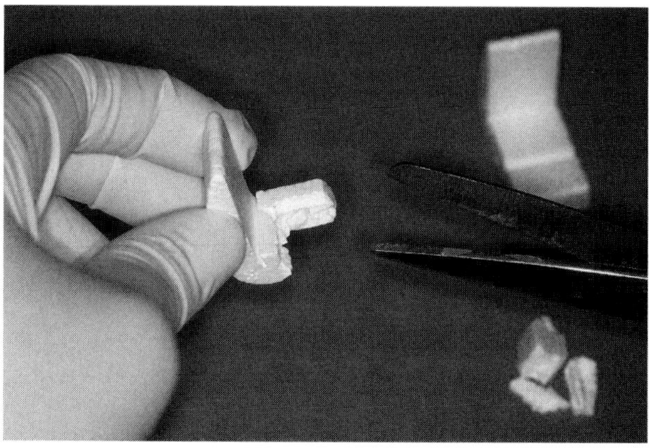

FIGURE 25-12 **Modifying a film holder for use in endodontic therapy.** Removing a portion of this disposable polystyrene film holder will allow the endodontic materials placed in the tooth to remain in place during the exposure.

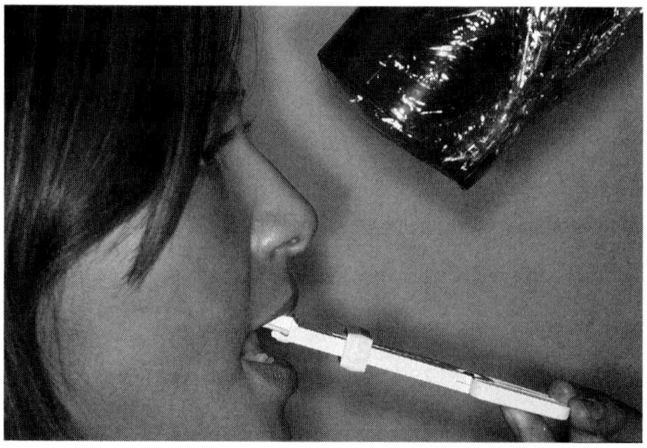

FIGURE 25-13 **Rinn Snap-A-Ray film holder.**

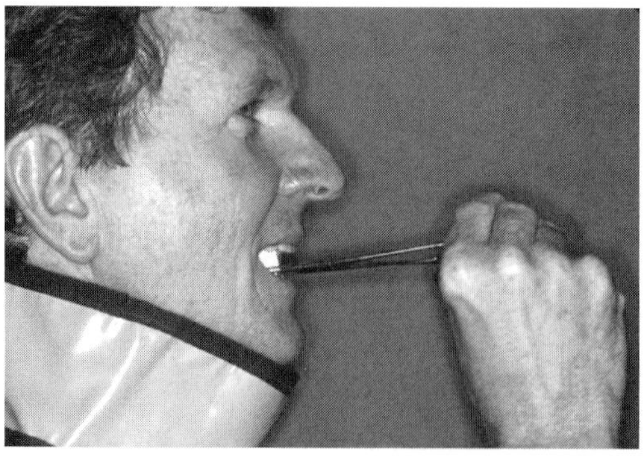

FIGURE 25-14 **Hemostat as a film holder.**

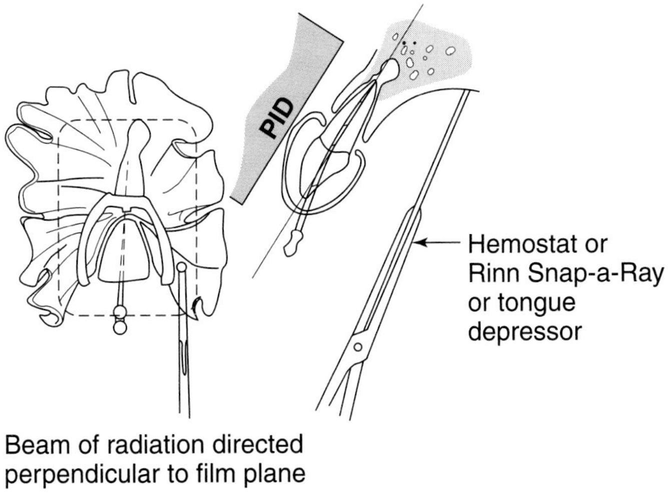

FIGURE 25-15 **Customizing endodontic film holders.** The patient can hold the hemostat or tongue depressor in a parallel position. (Courtesy of J. W. Preece, DDS, University of Texas Health Science Center at San Antonio)

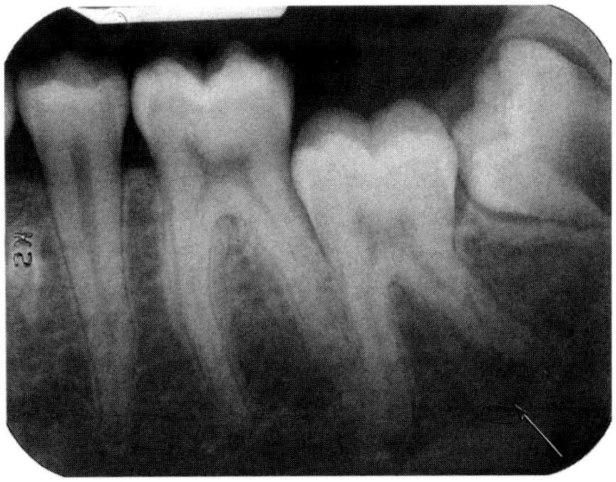

FIGURE 25-16 **Definitive method of localization.** Note the barely visible supernumerary (extra) root on this first molar. Applying the definitive method of localization, it is most likely a buccal root. The buccal position would place this root a greater distance away from the film, resulting in its magnified and less clearly imaged appearance.

Definitive Evaluation Method

The definitive method of localization is based on the shadow casting principles explained in Chapter 4. The principle that an object positioned farther away from the film will be magnified and less clearly imaged is applied with the definitive method. Since intraoral film packet placement positions the film close to the lingual surface of the teeth, those objects on the lingual are more likely to appear clearly on the resultant radiograph. Those objects positioned more toward the buccal or facial surface will be farther away from the film and therefore are more likely to appear magnified and less clearly imaged on the resultant radiograph (Figure 25–16). While true in principle, the definitive method of localization is the least reliable.

Right-angle Method

Once identified on a periapical radiograph, a better way to determine whether or not a foreign object or structure, such as an impacted tooth, is located on the buccal or the lingual is to take an occlusal radiograph. A cross-sectional occlusal radiograph, described in Chapter 15, places the film packet at a right angle to the tooth. In this position the occlusal radiograph will image the object clearly on the buccal or lingual (Figure 25–17).

Tube Shift Method (Buccal-object Rule)

The **tube shift method**, also called the **buccal-object rule**, is the most versatile method of localization (Figure 25–18). To apply the tube shift method, two radiographs are needed. The two

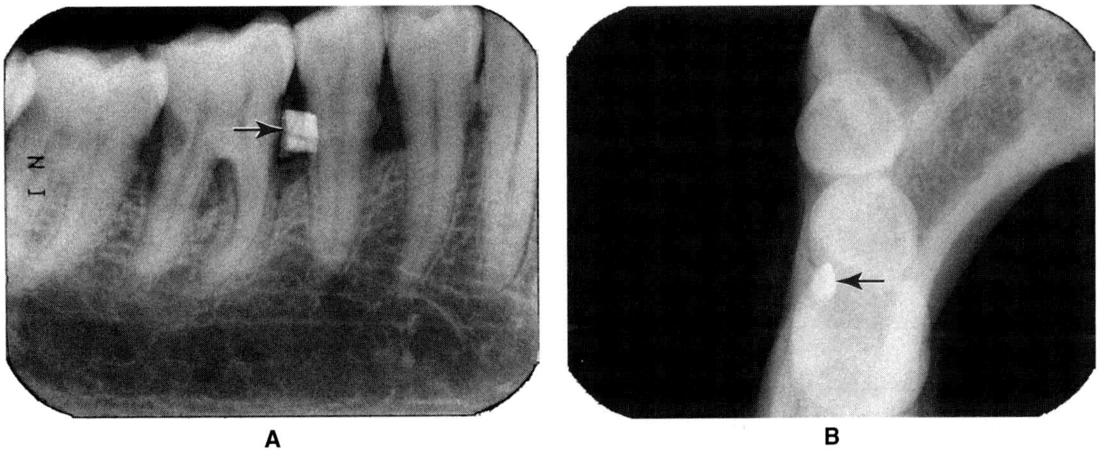

FIGURE 25-17 **Right angle method of localization.** (**A**) A foreign object appears in the periodontal pocket between the second premolar and the first molar. It is impossible to tell from this periapical radiograph whether the object is located toward the buccal or the lingual. (**B**) The occlusal radiograph, placed at a right angle position to the tooth clearly images the object on the buccal side of the pocket.

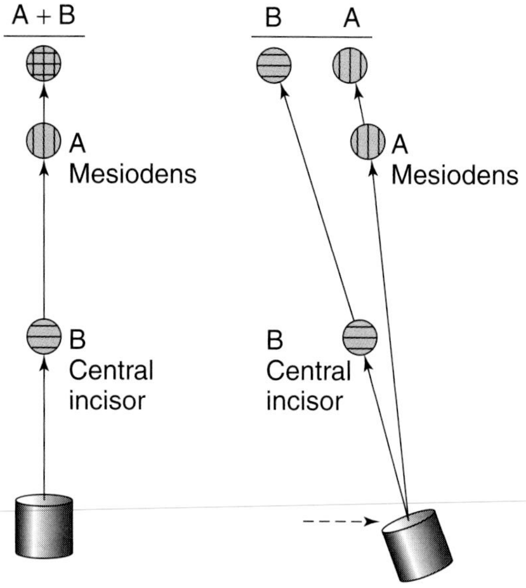

FIGURE 25-18 **Tube shift localization method.** The most lingual object (mesiodens in this case) will move in the same direction as shift of tube. (Courtesy of Eastman Kodak Company and University of Texas Health Science Center at San Antonio. Reproduced with permission from Langland, O. E., Langlais, R. P, & Morris, C. R.: Radiographic localization techniques. *Dent. Radiogr. Photogr.* 52(4): 69-77, 1979).

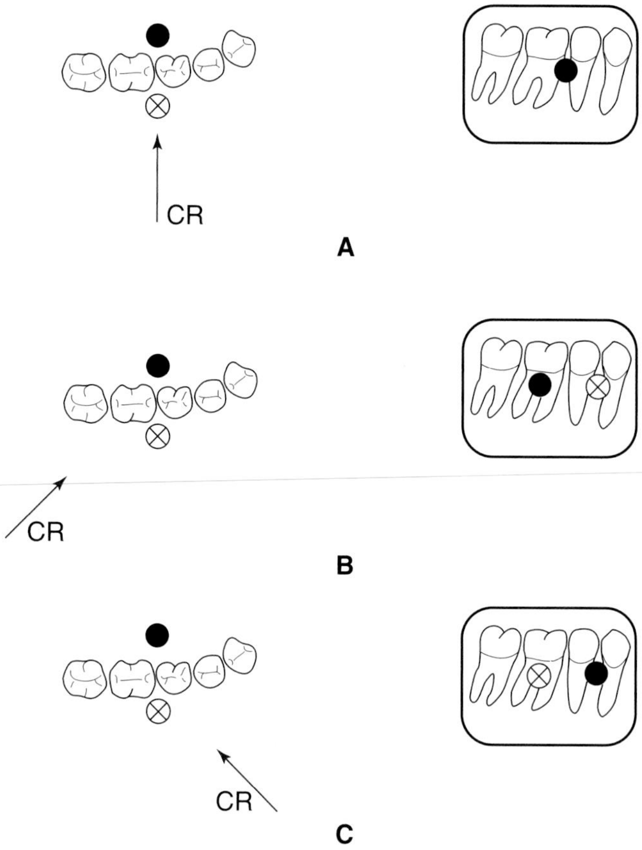

FIGURE 25-19 **Horizontal tube shift.** (**A**) In the original radiograph, buccal and lingual objects are superimposed. (**B**) When the tube head is moved distally, the buccal object appears to move mesially while the lingual object appears to move distally. (**C**) When the tube head is moved mesially, the buccal object appears to move distally, while the lingual object appears to move mesially. (Courtesy of Eastman Kodak Company and University of Texas Health Science Center at San Antonio. Reproduced with permission from Langland, O. E., Langlais, R. P., & Morris, C. R.: Radiographic localization techniques. *Dent. Radiogr. Photogr.* 52(4): 69-77, 1979)

radiographs must have been exposed using either a different horizontal or a different vertical angulation. If a full mouth series of periapicals or a complete set of bitewing radiographs, or a combination of both, are available and the object in question is imaged in more than one film, it is possible to apply the tube shift method to reading the radiographs to determine the buccal or lingual location of the object.

The principle behind the tube shift method is that if the structure or object in question appears to have moved in the same direction as the horizontal (Figure 25–19) or vertical (Figure 25–20) shift of the tube, then the structure or object is located on the lingual. Conversely, if the move is in the opposite direction of the shift of the tube, the structure or object is located on the buccal or facial. The tube shift method is summarized as **SLOB,** which stands for same on lingual–opposite on buccal.

Disto-oblique Periapical Radiographs

Shifting the tube (the PID and tube head) has another useful application. **Disto-oblique periapical radiographs** utilize a tube shift to help image posterior objects such as impacted third molars, especially when the patient can not tolerate posterior film packet placement. Standard vertical and horizontal angulation utilized when exposing periapicals may be altered slightly (no more than 10 degrees) to project posterior objects forward, or anteriorly, onto the film (Procedure Box 25–1).

For example, if an impacted third molar is positioned so far posterior in the oral cavity that the standard film packet placement is not likely to image it, the PID and tube head can be moved to project the impacted tooth forward onto the film (Figure 25–21). By directing the x-ray beam mesially, the posterior object will be projected anteriorly. Since the central rays will intersect the film plane at an oblique angle, there will be slight overlap and distortion of the image (Figure 25–22). However, the focus of disto-oblique periapical radiographs is on identifying an object or structure that may not be imaged in standard periapicals, so this distortion is tolerated.

The maxillary disto-oblique periapical radiograph requires three changes to the standard maxillary molar periapical radiograph. The first and most important step is to shift the horizontal angulation so that the posterior object will be projected forward. Second is to increase the vertical angulation. Most impactions, or foreign objects in the posterior region of the

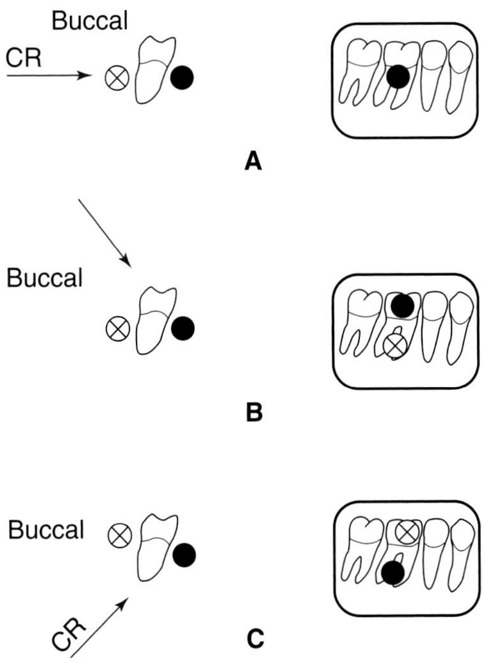

FIGURE 25-20 **Vertical tube shift.** (**A**) In the original radiograph, buccal and lingual objects are superimposed. (**B**) When the tube head is moved superiorly approximately 20 degrees, the buccal object appears to move inferiorally while the lingual object appears to move superiorly. (**C**) When the tube head is moved inferiorly, the buccal object appears to move superiorly while the lingual object appears to have moved inferiorally. (Courtesy of Eastman Kodak Company and University of Texas Health Science Center at San Antonio. Reproduced with permission from Langland, O. E., Langlais, R. P., & Morris, C. R.: Radiographic localization techniques. *Dent. Radiogr. Photogr.* 52(4): 69–77, 1979)

PROCEDURE 25-1

DISTO-OBLIQUE PERIAPICAL RADIOGRAPHS

1. Perform infection control procedures (see Procedure Box 9–2).
2. Prepare unit, patient, and supplies needed according to the procedure for exposing periapicals (see Procedure Box 13–1).
3. Place the film packet into the film-holding device. Place such that the embossed dot will be positioned toward the occlusal/incisal edge (dot in the slot).

Maxillary Disto-oblique Periapical Radiographs

a. Position the film and align the horizontal and vertical angulations for a standard maxillary molar periapical radiograph.
b. From this standard alignment, shift the tube to direct the central rays of the x-ray beam to intersect the film obliquely from the distal by 10 degrees.
c. Increase the vertical angulation by 5 degrees.
d. Check that the film packet is centered in the middle of the x-ray beam.
e. Increase the recommended exposure setting for the standard periapical to the next higher impulse setting.

Mandibular Periapical Radiograph

a. Position the film and align the horizontal and vertical angulations for a standard mandibular molar periapical radiograph.
b. From this standard alignment shift the tube to direct the central rays of the x-ray beam to intersect the film obliquely from the distal by 10 degrees.
c. Check that the film packet is centered in the middle of the x-ray beam
d. No change is made to the standard vertical angulation.
e. No change is made to the standard recommended exposure setting.

4. Make the exposure.

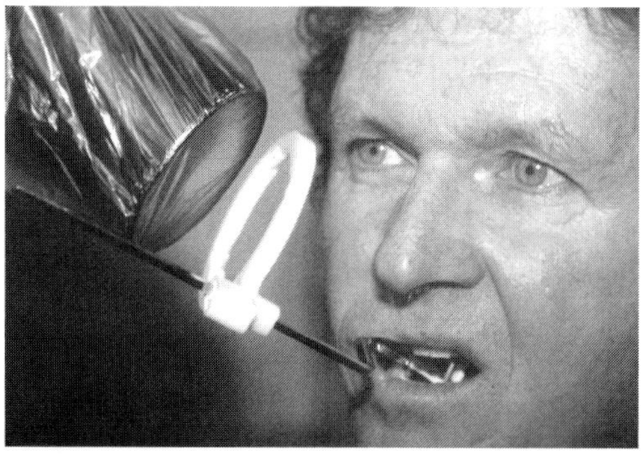

FIGURE 25-21 **Disto-oblique periapaical technique.** The horizontal angulation is shifted 10 degrees from the distal and the vertical angulation is increased 5 degrees.

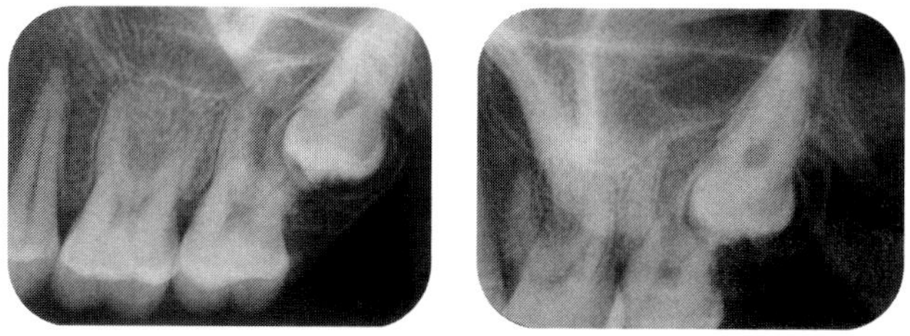

FIGURE 25-22 **Comparision of standard and disto-oblique periapical radiographs.** (**A**) Standard periapical radiograph images a portion of the impacted third molar. (**B**) Disto-oblique periapical radiograph images more of the impacted third molar. Note the overlap and crown portion of the image cut off when shifting the tube horizontally (causing overlap error) and vertically (causing the crowns to be cut off the the image).

maxilla, will be located farther superiorly than the erupted teeth. As discussed at the beginning of this chapter, increasing the vertical angulation will increase the periapical coverage of the image. And finally, the exposure setting for a maxillary disto-oblique radiograph must be increased to the next higher impulse. The oblique angle of the x-ray beam will require a longer passage through the patient's tissues. The increased vertical angulation will most likely direct the x-ray beam through the zygomatic arch. These two changes, in the horizontal and the vertical angulations, necessitate more radiation adequately to expose the film.

The mandibular disto-oblique periapical radiograph requires only the change to the horizontal angulation, to project the impaction or object forward. Most impactions of the posterior mandible will be located at the level of, or higher than, the erupted teeth so no change is required in the vertical angulation. There are no thick bony structures, like the zygoma, to penetrate, so the exposure time does not have to be increased.

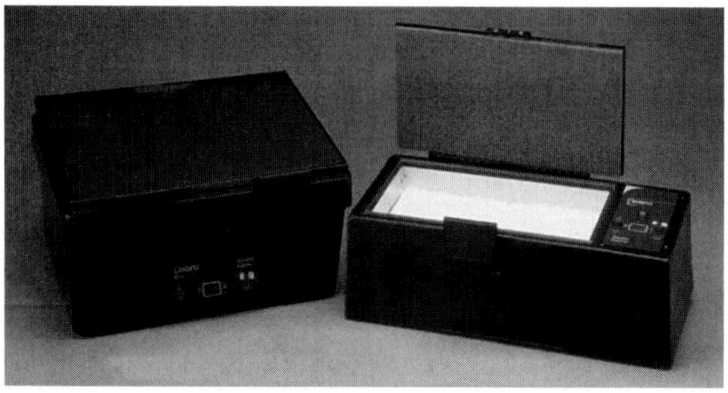

FIGURE 25-23 **X-ray duplicating units.** Contain a built-in ultraviolet fluorescent light source and a timer to permit variations in density. These x-ray film duplicators accommodate duplication of any number of intraoral films up to a full mouth series. Extraoral, panoramic radiographs may also be duplicated. (Courtesy of Densply Rinn)

Film Duplicating Procedure

Original radiographs should remain a part of the patient's permanent record, so there are times when a duplicate radiograph is needed. These include copies for third party payment (insurance companies); when referring the patient to a specialist; when the patient changes dentists or moves; for consultations with other professionals; publications in professional journals or for use in professional study clubs; to accompany biopsies of pathological conditions; and for evidence in legal cases. A **duplicate radiograph** is an identical copy of the original radiograph and may be obtained through the use of two-film intraoral film packets. If a double film packet is not available or the film is an extraoral film, the use of a film duplicator will produce a copy of the original radiograph. Radiographs can be duplicated as often as necessary without additional patient exposure.

Equipment

Duplicating radiographs requires **duplicating film** and a duplicator.

Duplicating Film

Duplicating film is available in sheet form in a variety of sizes. The film is emulsion-coated on one side only. Under a safelight,

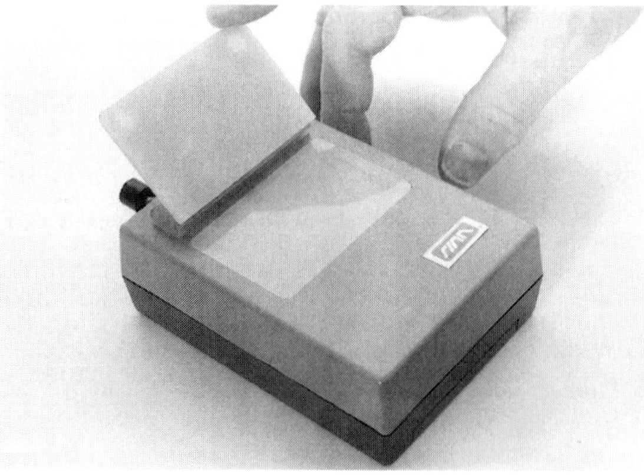

FIGURE 25-24 **Small film duplicator** accommodates film sizes #0, #1, and #2.

the emulsion side looks dull or lighter, while the side without the emulsion coating looks shiny or darker (see Chapter 7). It is possible to duplicate either a single radiograph or a full-mouth series at a single printing.

Film Duplicator

A **film duplicator** is a device that provides a diffused light source (usually ultraviolet) that evenly exposes the duplicating film. The film duplicator may be a commercial model (Figure 25–23) or it may be a photographic printing frame and a light source adapted for this use. Large duplicators accommodate all film sizes, whereas small duplicators may be used only for #2 film and smaller (Figure 25–24).

Procedures for Film Duplication

The process of film duplication is simple and readily learned. All duplication must be done in the darkroom under a safelight (Procedure Box 25–2).

PROCEDURE 25–2

FILM DUPLICATION

1. Select radiographs for duplication (referrals, third party payment, consultations).
2. Prepare duplicator. Raise cover and wipe glass surface with glass cleaner if necessary.
3. Place duplicator mode switch in the VIEW position to turn on the view box as necessary to arrange original radiographs into position for duplicating.
4. Remove the original radiographs from the film mounts prior to duplication. (Leaving the original radiographs in the film mount will prevent close contact between the originals and the duplicating film, resulting in the fuzzy appearance of the duplicate radiograph.)
5. Place original radiographs on the duplicator glass surface with the embossed dots concave (dimple). Placing the "down dot" on the duplicator surface will allow for close contact between the original radiographs and the duplicating films.
6. Place the radiographs near the L or R on the duplicator glass surface to identify the left or right sides respectively on the duplicate images.
7. Turn the duplicator mode switch to the DUPLICATE position to turn off the view box light. Be sure to turn OFF this viewbox light prior to opening the box of duplicating film.
8. Set the timer to the desired exposure time. See the manufacturer's recommendations. If a darker duplicate is desired, decrease the exposure time; if a lighter duplicate is desired, increase the exposure time. (Increasing and decreasing the exposure time from the duplicator light has the opposite effect on the resulting image than increasing and decreasing the x-ray exposure.)
9. Obtain a box of duplicating film.
10. Under safelight conditions, remove a sheet of duplicating film from the box. When duplicating individual films, use scissors to cut duplicating film to the approximate size needed.
11. Place the duplicating film emulsion (light) side down on top of the originals.
12. Close the duplicator cover and secure the latch tightly. (Failure to secure the latch will result in a loss of contact between the originals and the duplicating film, resulting in the fuzzy appearance of the duplicate image.)
13. Depress the exposure button to activate exposure.
14. When the indicator light goes off at the end of exposure cycle, unlatch and raise the cover, remove the duplicating film, and process the duplicating film either automatically or manually.
15. Re-mount the original radiographs and return to the patient's permanent record.
16. Clean the darkroom and replace materials.
17. When the duplicate film exits the processor, label it with the patient's name, date, and any other information necessary. Ensure that the right and left sides of the image are identified appropriately.

REVIEW—Chapter Summary

Anatomical limitations often require alterations in radiographic technique. A skilled radiographer knows how to apply acceptable variations in radiographic technique. The horizontal and vertical angulations may be altered under certain conditions. The exposure times should be adjusted based on the patient's characteristics and the area of the oral cavity to be imaged.

Anatomical conditions that may require an alteration of radiograph techniques include mal-aligned teeth, a shallow palatal vault, the presence of tori, and endentulous regions.

The film holder is an indicating device, not a dictating device. The radiographer who possesses the skills necessary to evaluate film packet placement for correctness may produce a diagnostic quality radiograph by aligning the angles and point of entry to the film packet itself regardless of the holder's external aiming device.

Successful endodontic therapy or root canal treatment depends on the careful attention given to the use of film holders that will permit parallel placement of the film packet.

Modifications or variations in film placement or exposure techniques may be required when certain conditions present. The radiographer who masters the bisecting technique will be prepared for these situations. However, the paralleling technique is the technique of choice because it produces radiographs with the least dimensional distortion.

Localization methods add a third dimension to two-dimensional radiographs. Definitive method is the least reliable method of localization. The right angle method of localization uses a periapical radiograph and a cross-sectional occlusal radiograph. With the tube-shift method of localization, the object in question is located on the lingual if it moves in the same direction as the horizontal or vertical shift of the tube and on the buccal if it moves in the opposite direction as the horizontal or vertical shift of the tube. The tube shift method, or buccal object rule, is summarized as SLOB (same on lingual–opposite on buccal).

Disto-oblique periapical radiographs are useful when the patient can not tolerate posterior film packet placement. Disto-oblique periapical radiographs allow the radiographer to shift the PID and tube head to project posterior objects and structures anteriorly onto the film.

Copies of radiographs are used to send to insurance companies or to another oral health care practice; for use in referrals, consultations with other professionals, or publication in professional journals; or when needed in litigation. Duplicate radiographs are made using a commercially made duplicator and special duplicating film.

RECALL—Study Questions

1. To help avoid molar overlap, the radiographer should place the film packet:
   a. Parallel to the buccal surfaces of the teeth.
   b. Perpendicular to the buccal surfaces of the teeth.
   c. Parallel to the molar embrasures.
   d. Perpendicular to the molar embrasures.
2. To minimize canine-premolar overlap, the radiographer should direct the ray beam slightly from the:
   a. Mesial.
   b. Distal.
   c. Occlusal.
   d. Apical.
3. To compensate for a shallow palatal vault, the vertical angulation may be adjusted to:
   a. Increase by up to15 degrees.
   b. Decrease by up to 15 degrees.
   c. Increase by up to 25 degrees.
   d. Decrease by up to 25 degrees.
4. Which area of the oral cavity would require the highest exposure setting?
   a. Maxillary anterior region
   b. Maxillary posterior region
   c. Mandibular anterior region
   d. Mandibular posterior region
5. The presence of a large mandibular torus may make which of these difficult?
   a. Horizontal angulation
   b. Vertical angulation
   c. Film packet placement
   d. Directing the beam at the center of the film
6. The best film packet placement for a patient with a torus palatinus is:
   a. Between the torus and the tongue.
   b. On the top of the torus.
   c. Near the front of the torus.
   d. Behind the torus.
7. The paralleling technique is the best technique for imaging edentulous areas. The bisecting technique is the best technique when imaging endodontic treatment.
   a. The first statement is true. The second statement is false.
   b. The first statement is false. The second statement is true.
   c. Both statements are true.
   d. Both statements are false.
8. Which of the following radiographs would be the *least* beneficial for the totally edentulous patient?
   a. Occlusal
   b. Periapical
   c. Panoramic
   d. Bitewing
9. The exposure setting for edentulous regions should be:
   a. Decreased by 25 percent.
   b. Decreased by 50 percent.
   c. Increased by 25 percent.
   d. Increased by 50 percent.
10. Which of the following would be the *best* film holder for imaging working radiographs exposed during a root canal procedure?
    a. Rinn XCP
    b. Rinn Snap-A-Ray
    c. Polystyrene block
    d. Endodontic film holder
11. Localization adds which of the following dimensions to two-dimensional radiographs?
    a. Anterior-posterior
    b. Mesial-distal
    c. Buccal-lingual
    d. Inferior-superior

12. Which of the following methods of localization utilizes a cross-sectional occlusal radiograph?
    a. Definitive method
    b. Right-angle method
    c. Tube shift method
    d. Buccal-object rule
13. If the tube shifts to the mesial and the object in question shifts to the distal, the object is located on the lingual. This is an example of the definitive method of localization.
    a. The first statement is true. The second statement is false.
    b. The first statement is false. The second statement is true.
    c. Both statements are true.
    d. Both statements are false.
14. When exposing a disto-oblique periapical radiograph of the maxilla, which of the following changes should be made to the standard periapical radiograph?
    a. 5-degree shift in the vertical angulation
    b. 10-degree shift in the horizontal angulation
    c. 1-impulse increase in the exposure setting
    d. All of the above
15. To project an impacted mandibular third molar anteriorly onto the film, a mandibular disto-oblique periapical radiograph requires a:
    a. 5-degree shift in the horizontal angulation.
    b. 10-degree shift in the horizontal angulation.
    c. 5-degree shift in the vertical angulation.
    d. 10-degree shift in the vertical angulation.
16. List four reasons to duplicate radiographs:
    a. ____________________
    b. ____________________
    c. ____________________
    d. ____________________

REFLECT—Case Study

A patient has presented at your practice today for a consult regarding extensive dental work. This patient has several areas of missing teeth and has expressed an interest in dentures. The dentist has prescribed a full mouth series of radiographs and you are preparing to take the exposures. After performing a cursory exam of the patient's oral cavity you note the following:

Several missing and/or broken down teeth.
Mal-aligned and crowded teeth.
Partially erupted third molars.
Large torus palatinus and torus mandibularis.
A shallow palatal vault.

Consider the following and write out your answers:

1. Describe the alterations in technique you will apply to obtain radiographs in the edentulous areas.
2. Describe the alterations in technique you will apply to avoid overlap error in the areas of mal-aligned and crowded teeth.
3. Identify and describe the technique you will use to best image the partially erupted third molars.
4. Describe the problems you anticipate facing with the presence of large tori and a shallow palatal vault.
5. Identify alterations in techniques that will help you overcome these obstacles.
6. If broken root tips or other foreign objects are identified on the films you take, describe how the interpretation of the films can reveal whether or not the object in question is located on the buccal or the lingual.
7. Describe other methods of localization that can aid in making this determination.
8. Identify reasons why this patient's radiographs may need to be duplicated.

RELATE—Laboratory Application

For a comprehensive laboratory practice exercise on this topic, see E. M. Thomson, *Exercises in Oral Radiography Techniques: A Laboratory Manual,* 2nd ed., Upper Saddle River, NJ: Prentice Hall, 2007. Chapter 7, "Special Patients and Student Partner Practice" and Chapter 13, "Supplemental Radiographic Techniques."

BIBLIOGRAPHY

Del Rio, C. E., Canales, M. L., & Preece, J. W. *Radiographic Technique for Endodontics.* University of Texas Health Science Center at San Antonio, 1982.

Rinn Corporation. *Intraoral Radiography with Rinn XCP/BAS Instruments.* Elgin, IL: Dentsply/Rinn Corporation, 1983.

Thomson, E. M. *Exercises in Oral Radiography Techniques: A Laboratory Manual,* 2nd ed. Upper Saddle River, NJ: Prentice Hall, 2007.

26

Digital Radiography

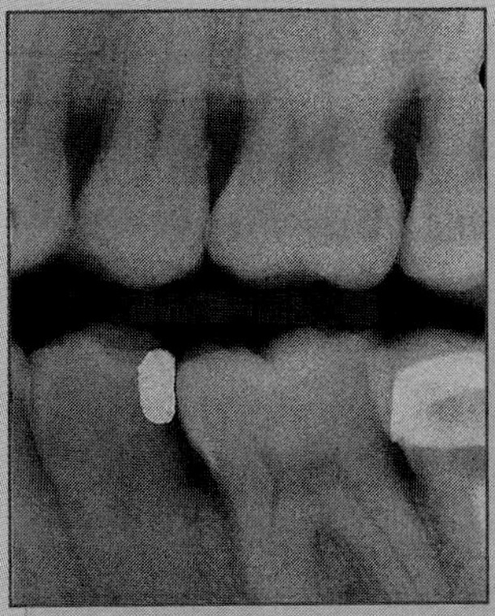

■ OBJECTIVES

Following successful completion of this chapter, you should be able to:

1. Define the key words.
2. Explain the fundamental concept of digital radiography.
3. Differentiate between indirect and direct digital imaging.
4. List the equipment used in digital imaging.
5. List and describe three types of digital sensors.
6. List and describe five software features used to enhance digital image interpretation.
7. Identify and discuss the advantages and disadvantages of digital radiography.

■ KEY WORDS

Analog
Charge-coupled device (CCD)
Complementary metal oxide semiconductor (CMOS)
Digital image
Digital Imaging and Communications in Medicine (DICOM)
Digital radiography
Digital subtraction
Digitize
Direct digital imaging
Gray scale
Indirect digital imaging
Line pair
Photo stimuable phosphor (PSP)
Pixel
Sensor
Spatial resolution

Introduction

Digital technology is revolutionizing the practice of dentistry. Computers and specialized software are being used for business applications such as managing patient records and appointment scheduling, as well as for clinical uses such as intraoral cameras, voice-activated charting systems, and electronic periodontal probes. **Digital radiographs** or filmless imaging is rapidly becoming an integral part of the paperless oral health care practice (Figure 26–1). The introduction of a computer approach to x-rays with instant images has the potential to improve the quality of oral health care while reducing radiation exposure for the patient. While the fundamentals of film-based radiography are necessary, it is important that today's dental assistant and dental hygienist have an understanding of the basic concepts of digital radiography and be prepared to utilize digital technology.

The purpose of this chapter is to present the fundamental concepts of digital radiography, to introduce the types of digital imaging currently available, and to discuss the advantages and disadvantages of digital radiography.

Fundamental Concepts

The term *radiography* is derived from the words radiation and photography, meaning that a radiograph is a photographic image created using radiation. Today, there are many different ways to create images of the patient. Images made within a computer using digital sensors and phosphor plates no longer need the photographic process. The term *imaging* has come to replace the term *radiography* when referring to these images. In radiography, we "take a radiograph," whereas in digital imaging we "acquire an image." Table 26–1 lists several terms pertaining to digital imaging that you should be familiar with.

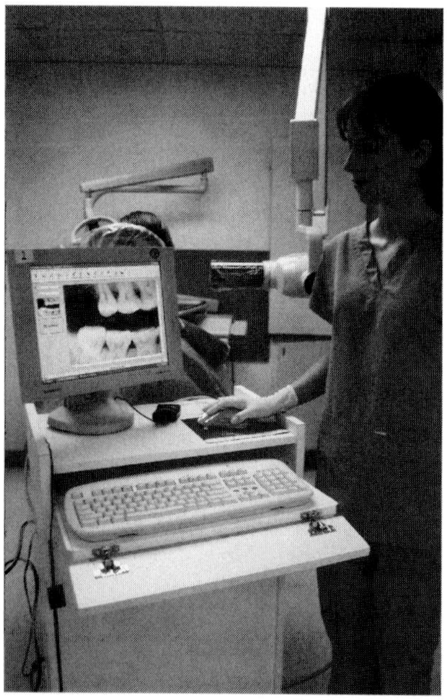

FIGURE 26-1 **Digital intraoral radiographic system.** The radiographic picture is immediately available on the computer monitor.

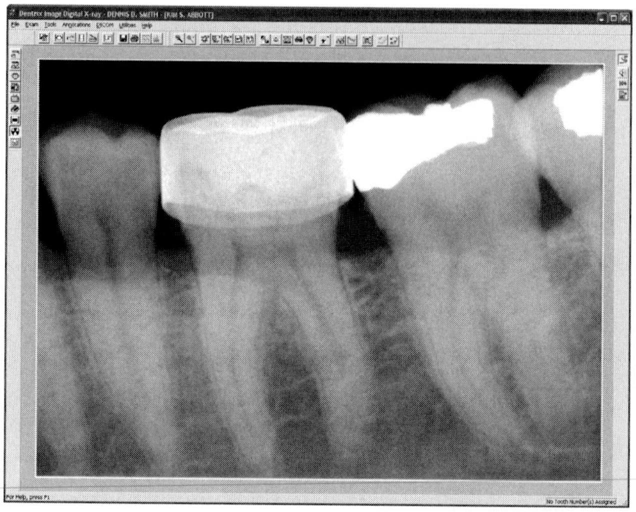

FIGURE 26-2 **An example of a digital radiographic image.** (Courtesy of Dentrix Dental Systems)

The difference between a **digital image** and a radiograph is that a digital image has no physical form. Digital images exist only as bits of information in a computer file which tell the computer how to construct an image on a monitor or other viewing device (Figure 26–2). Digital radiography systems are not limited to intraoral images. Panoramic and cephalometric digital imaging systems are also available.

Methods of Acquiring a Digital Image

There are two methods of acquiring a digital image: **indirect digital imaging** and **direct digital imaging.**

Indirect Digital Imaging

Indirect digital imaging converts radiographs, obtained via conventional film-based radiography, to digital images. An imaging device is used either to scan or photograph the existing radiograph (Figure 26–3). Scanners pass a light beam through the radiograph to an imaging chip that converts the light to a digital image. A device called a transparency adapter can be mounted in the lid of a paper document scanner that will allow the scanner to scan radiographs. Transparency adapters are available as options on many flatbed scanners currently available.

Another method of converting film-based radiographs to digital images is through the use of a digital camera. Existing radiographs can be placed on a viewbox and photographed. The camera scans the image, and then **digitizes** or converts the image so that it can be displayed on the computer monitor.

The quality of an indirect digital image is inferior to a direct digital image because the resultant image is similar to a "copy" of the image versus the "original." However, indirect imaging does offer a way to digitize existing radiographs.

Direct Digital Imaging

In direct digital imaging, no film is used (Procedure Box 26–1). Digital imaging systems used in dentistry replace film with an

TABLE 26-1 **Terminology**

Term	Definition
Analog	Relating to a mechanism in which data is represented by continuously variable physical quantities
CCD	Charge-coupled device. A solid-state detector used in many electronic devices such as video cameras, surgical microscopes, and fax machines. In digital radiography, a CCD is an image receptor found in the intraoral sensor, which converts x-rays to electrons.
Digital radiography	A filmless imaging system that uses a sensor and a computer to acquire, process, store, retrieve, and display the radiographic image
Digital subtraction	A process of digitally merging two images to show changes that occur over time or as the result of treatment intervention. The like images "cancel" each other out, clearly imaging the differences.
Digitize	To convert a film-based image into a digital form that can be processed by a computer
Direct digital imaging	A method of directly obtaining a digital image by exposing an intraoral sensor to x-rays to produce an image that can be viewed on a computer monitor
Gray scale	Refers to the number of shades of gray visible in an image
Indirect digital imaging	A method of obtaining a digital image in which an existing radiograph is scanned or photographed and then converted into a digital image
Pixel	Short for *picture element* (*pix,* plural of *pic*ture and *el,* short for *el*ement); discrete units of information that together constitute an image
Spatial resolution	The discernable separation of closely adjacent image details
Sensor	An electronic or specially coated plate that is sensitive to x-rays. When placed intraorally, the sensor captures the radiographic image when exposed to x-rays.

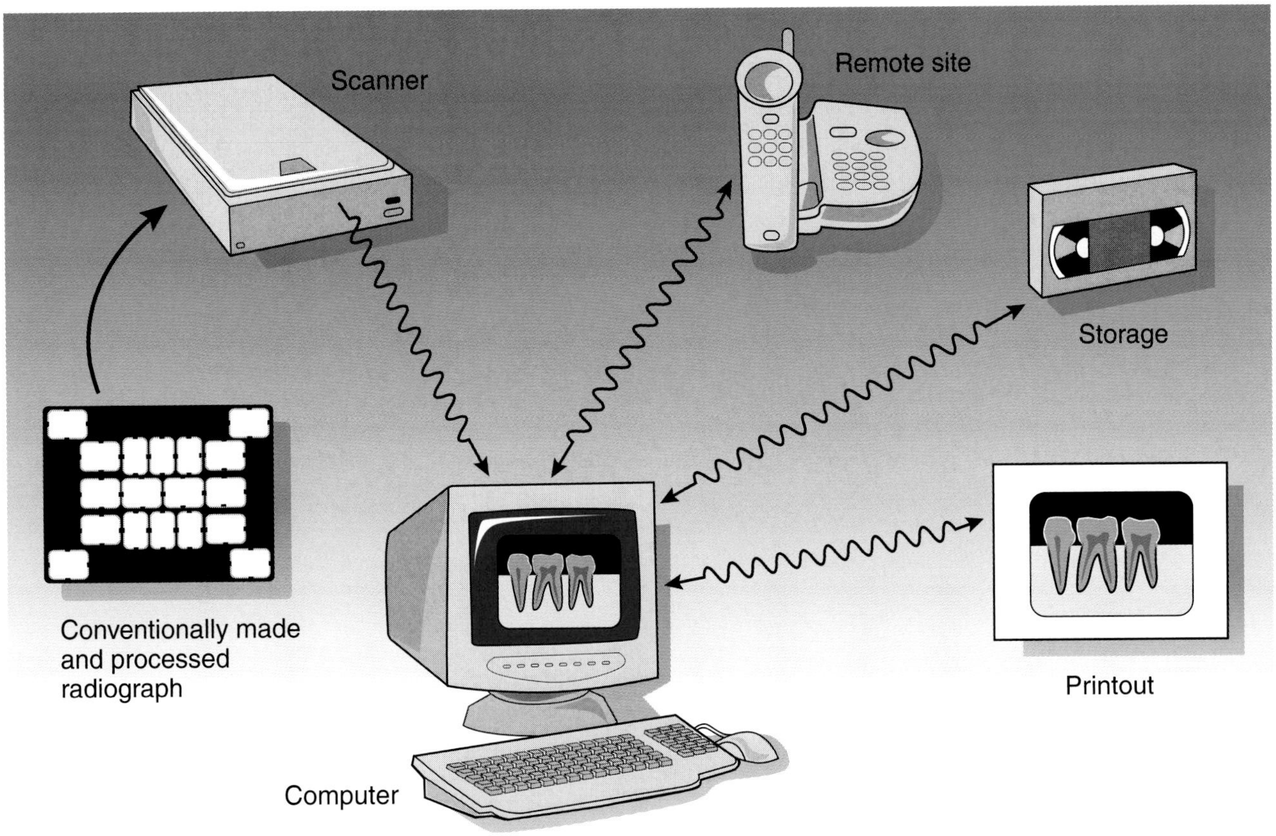

FIGURE 26-3 **Indirect digital imaging.** A film-based radiograph is converted into a digital image by scanning it into the computer. Once converted, the digital image may be electronically stored or transmitted to a remote site (such as a consultant, an insurance company, or a referring dentist).

PROCEDURE 26-1

PROCEDURE FOR OBTAINING DIGITAL IMAGES

Equipment Preparation*

1. Turn on the computer. Using the keyboard or mouse activate the computer exam window and select the type of exam from the task bar. (i.e., bitewings, periapicals, full mouth series)
2. Using the keyboard, type the patient identification information (i.e., name) and date of exam.
3. Wipe the sensor with an intermediate-level disinfectant approved by the sensor manufacturer. Place an FDA-cleared plastic sheath over the sensor (Figures 26–4 and 26–5).

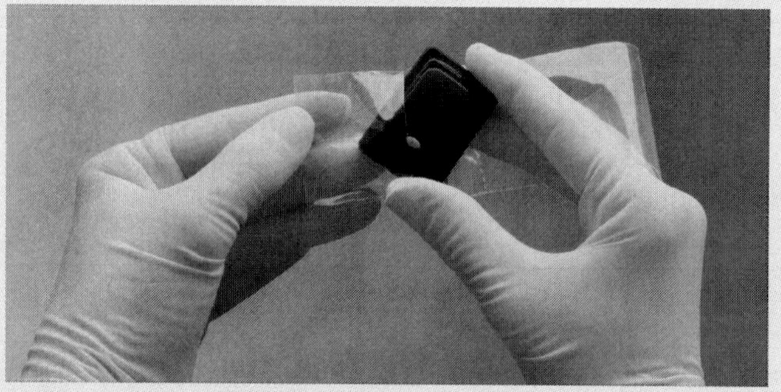

FIGURE 26-4 **Wireless digital sensor.** Wireless sensor being covered with a disposable plastic barrier for placement intraorally. (Courtesy of Schick Technologies, Inc.)

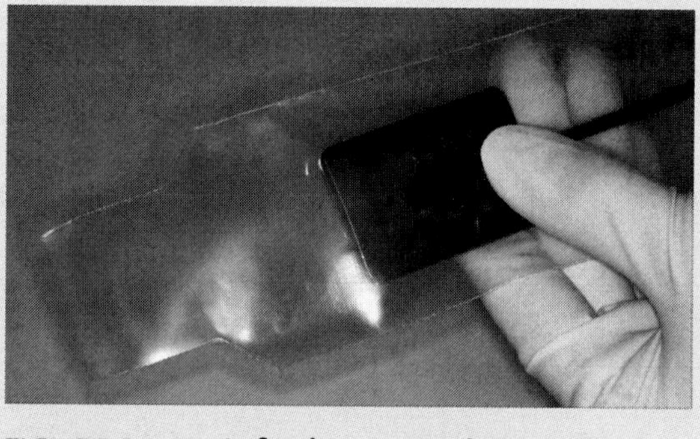

FIGURE 26-5 **Infection control.** A wired digital sensor being covered with a disposable plastic barrier for placement intraorally.

4. Place the sensor into the appropriate bite block and attach to the holding device (Figure 26–6).

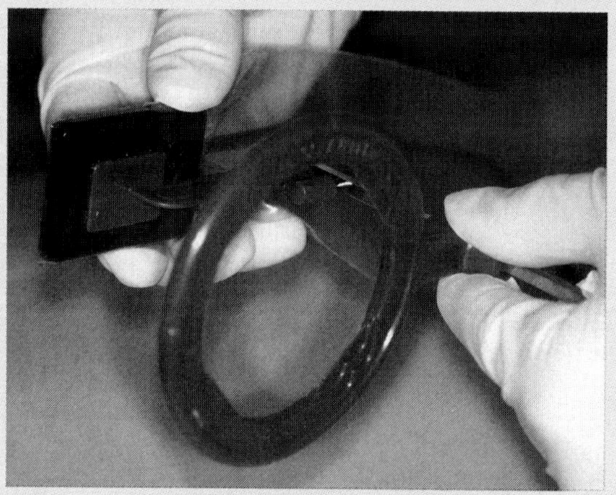

FIGURE 26-6 **Digital sensor.** A wired digital sensor being placed into a special film holder attachment.

5. Turn on the x-ray unit and adjust exposure settings. Reduce exposure settings by one-half those used for F-speed film-based exposures.

*Follow the manufacturer's instructions for your digital system. Only general guidelines concerning patient preparation and sensor placement are included here.

PROCEDURE 26–1 *(cont.)*

Patient Preparation

1. Request that the patient remove objects from the mouth that can interfere with the procedure, and remove eyeglasses.
2. Adjust chair to a comfortable working level.
3. Adjust headrest to position patient's head so that the occlusal plane is parallel to the floor and the midsagittal plane (midline) is perpendicular to the floor.
4. Place the lead apron and thyroid collar on the patient.
5. Perform a cursory inspection of the oral cavity and note possible obstructions (tori, shallow palatal vault, mal-aligned teeth) that may require an alteration of technique or placement of the sensor. Note the patient's occlusion to assist with aligning the sensor with the maxillary or mandibular teeth.

Exposure

1. Place the sensor intraorally into position (Figure 26–7).

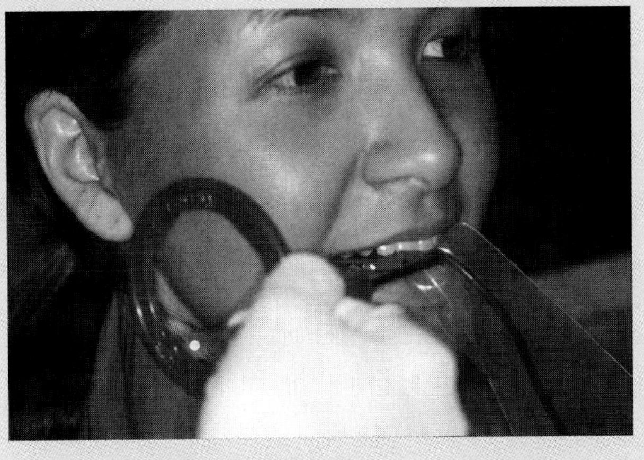

FIGURE 26-7 **Sensor being placed intraorally.**

2. Utilize the paralleling technique to position the sensor parallel to the long axes of the teeth of interest. Align the tube head and PID to direct the central rays of the x-ray beam perpendicular to the sensor. Direct the central rays to the middle (center) of the sensor to avoid cone cut error (Figure 26–8).

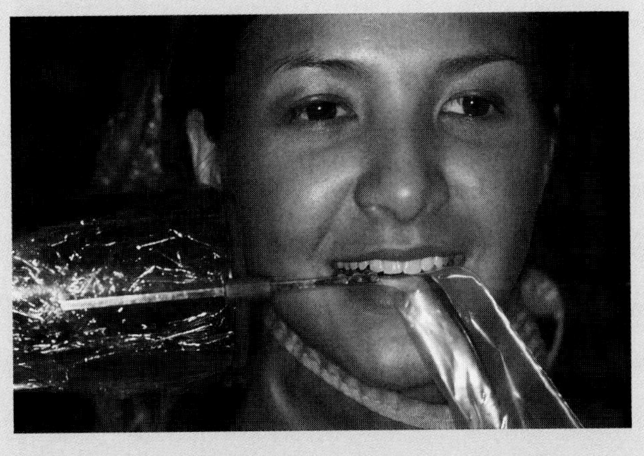

FIGURE 26-8 **PID aligned with sensor held in place by holding device.**

(continued)

PROCEDURE 26–1 *(cont.)*

3. Using the keyboard or mouse, activate the sensor for exposure.
4. Depress the exposure button to expose the sensor.

CCD (Charge-Coupled Device) or CMOS (Complementary Metal Oxide Semiconductor)

5. Wait for the image to appear on the computer monitor and evaluate technique. If a technique error has occurred that compromises diagnostic quality and requires a retake, do the following:
   a. Do not remove the sensor from the patient's oral cavity.
   b. Request that the patient remain still, in position.
   c. Observe the error and decide the corrective action. For example, if a cone cut error has resulted in the posterior section of the image being blank, the appropriate corrective action would be to move the PID toward the posterior to align the central rays of the x-ray beam to the center of the sensor.
   d. Realign the PID to correct. To correct sensor placement errors, request that the patient open slightly, allowing you to perform the corrective action and then occlude on the bite block holding the sensor in this new position.

PSP (Photo Stimuable Phosphor Plate)

5. Remove the sensor (plate) from the patient's oral cavity.
6. Remove the sensor from the holding device.
7. Remove the plastic barrier and clean and disinfect sensor according to manufacturer's instructions.
8. Place the sensor in the special scanner and activate (Figure 26–9).
9. Observe the image on the monitor and evaluate technique. If a technique error has occurred that compromises diagnostic quality, retake the exposure. You may choose to use another prepared sensor or perform the following steps:
   a. Erase the used sensor plate according to manufacturer's instructions.
   b. Repeat the Equipment Preparation, Patient Preparation, and Exposure steps.
10. If the image is satisfactory, remove the sensor from the scanner and erase the used sensor plate according to the manufacturer's instructions. If additional

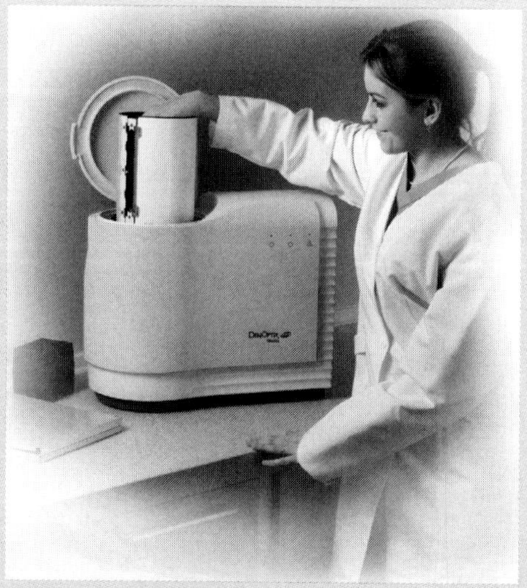

FIGURE 26-9 **PSP sensor system.** Operator placing the exposed PSP sensor plates in to the scanning device. (Courtesy of Gendex Dental Corporation)

PROCEDURE 26–1 *(cont.)*

e. Using the keyboard or mouse, activate the retake window and make the exposure. Repeat step 5 to produce a diagnostic quality image.

6. If the image is satisfactory, remove the sensor from the patient's oral cavity. If additional images are required, reposition the sensor for the next exposure. (It may not be necessary to completely remove the sensor from the patient's oral cavity. Depending on the cooperation of the patient, the sensor may be positioned for the next image without completely removing the sensor from the oral cavity.)
7. Repeat steps 3 through 6 until all exposures are acquired.

images are required, repeat the Equipment Preparation, Patient Preparation, and Exposure steps or use additional sensors.

11. Repeat steps 3 through 10 until all exposures are acquired.

Following Exposure

1. Remove the sensor from the holding device.
2. Remove the plastic barrier and clean and disinfect according to manufacturer's instructions.
3. Save the patient's exam in the archived files. Back up the file on the computer or supplemental storage system.

image detector called a sensor. The **sensor** is a small detector that is placed intraorally in the same manner as a film packet, with the aid of a special film holder attachment (see Figure 26–6). As in conventional radiography, the x-ray beam is aligned to strike the sensor. When the x-rays strike the sensor, an electronic charge is produced on the surface of the sensor. The electronic signal is digitized, or converted into digital form (Figure 26–10). The sensor in turn transmits this information to a computer. Software is used to store the image electronically. The image is displayed within seconds and may be readily manipulated to enhance the appearance for interpretation and diagnosis (Figure 26–11).

Characteristics of a Digital Image

The term digital image is used to distinguish it from an **analog** image. An analog image has been described as being like a painting, with a continuous smooth blend from one color to another. A digital image is like a mosaic, made up of many small pieces put together to make a whole. The digital image is composed of structurally ordered areas called **pixels**. Pixels, short for "picture elements," are tiny dots that make up a digital image. Each pixel is a single dot in a digital image. The more pixels in an image, the higher the resolution and the sharper the image.

Spatial Resolution

The number and size of pixels determines the **spatial resolution** of an image. When the number of pixels is low, the image appears to have jagged edges and is difficult to see. Spatial resolution is measured in terms of line pairs. A **line pair** refers to the greatest number of paired lines visible in 1 mm of an image. For example, a resolution of 10 line pairs/mm would mean that when 10 ruled lines are squeezed into 1 mm of an image, the individual lines can still be seen. The greater the spatial resolution in an image, the sharper it looks.

Gray Scale

Gray scale refers to the number of shades of gray visible in an image. The gray scale of a radiographic image is important for diagnosis of oral conditions. The practitioner most often relies on the radiograph's contrast, its radiolucency and radiopacity, to determine the presence or absence of disease. The ability to record subtle changes in the gray areas of images improves diagnosis. Digital radiographic systems claim the ability to produce up to 65,500 gray levels. However, computer monitors can display only 256 gray levels. A number stored for each pixel determines the number of shades of gray visible. Each pixel has a number from 0 to 255, representing pure black at 0 to pure

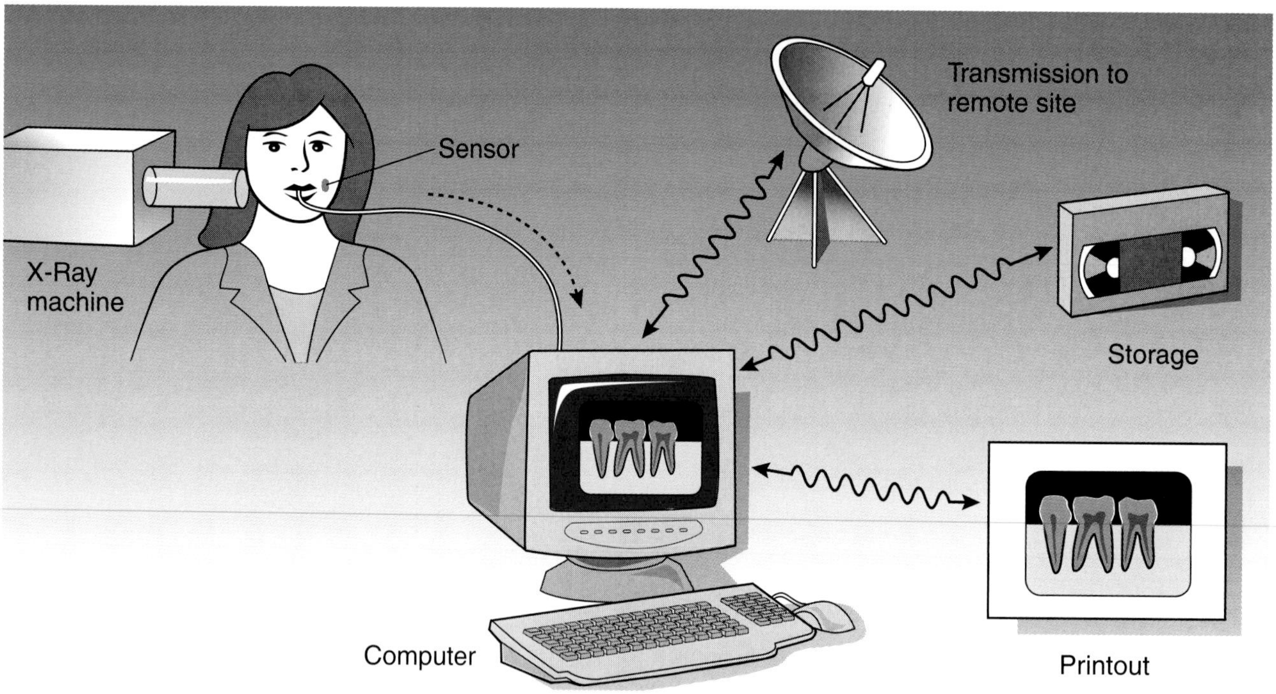

FIGURE 26-10 **Digital imaging system.** The image is captured directly on the sensor that was positioned in the patient's mouth and sent to the computer. The image can then be displayed on the monitor, transmitted electronically over the Internet, stored for future use, or printed as a paper copy if required.

white at 255. Hence there are usually 256 gray levels in an image.

The human eye can distinguish only about 32 shades of gray unaided. However, this does not necessarily mean that the large range of gray scale captured by digital imaging systems is wasted. When aided by the computer software features, which can be utilized to enhance the gray levels, it may be possible detect changes that might be overlooked in film-based images.

The goal of digital imaging systems is to produce high quality diagnostic images. It is the combination of pixels, spatial resolution, and gray scale that determines the quality of the final image. Manufacturers are continuing to improve the capability of digital equipment and software to aid in the early detection of oral diseases.

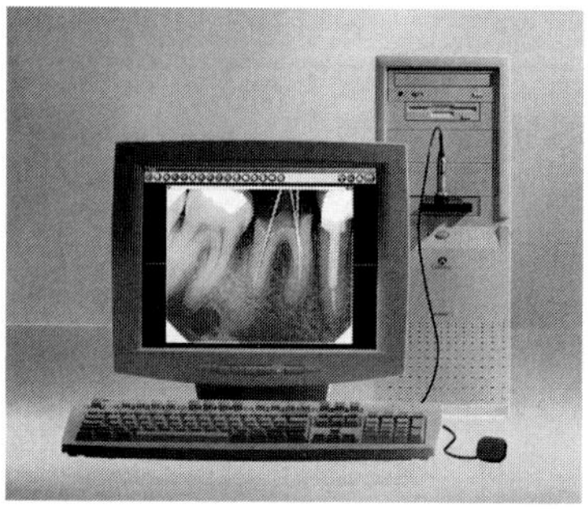

FIGURE 26-11 **Image displayed on computer screen.** The image may be readily manipulated to enhance the appearance for interpretation and diagnosis. (DEXIS x-ray images courtesy of Pro Vision Dental Systems, Inc.)

Uses

The purpose of digital radiography is to produce images that can be used in the diagnosis and treatment of oral conditions. Digital radiography is utilized for the same reasons one would use film-based radiography, including to:

- Detect, confirm, and classify oral diseases and lesions.
- Detect and evaluate trauma.
- Evaluate growth and development.
- Provide information during dental procedures such as root canal therapy and surgery.

Equipment

Digital radiography utilizes a dental x-ray machine, an image detector or sensor, a computer, and specialized software (Figure 26–12).

X-ray Machine

Most digital x-ray systems can be used with existing dental x-ray machines that have electronic timers capable of producing very short exposure times. Older x-ray machines using impulse timers may need to be updated with electronic timers for use with digital systems. An x-ray machine adapted for digital radiography

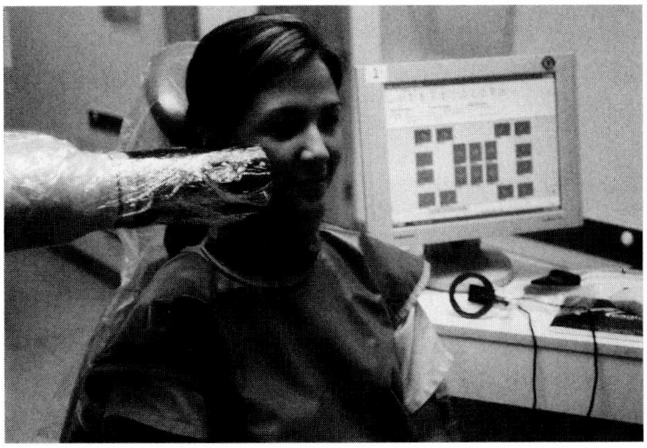

FIGURE 26-12 **Digital radiography system.** An existing dental x-ray unit being utilized with a digital imaging system.

can still be used for conventional film-based radiography. Dental x-ray machines capable of producing low kilovoltage (70 kV or less), low millamperage (5 mA or less) and that have a direct current (DC) curcuit are ideally suited to digital radiography.

Sensor (Image Detector)

In direct digital imaging, an image detector or sensor is used instead of intraoral dental film (Figure 26–13). The sensor is an electronic or specially coated plate that is positioned in the oral cavity in the same manner as an intraoral film packet. When exposed to x-rays, the sensor converts the x-rays into an electronic form that can be read and used in a computer.

Intraoral sensors may be wired or wireless. Wired refers to the fact that the sensor is connected to the computer by a fiber optic cable that records the generated signal. The cable may vary in length from 8 to 35 ft (1.5 to 10.7 m). The shorter the cable, the more limited the range of motion. Wireless sensors use a radio frequency to communicate with the computer and are not connected by a cable (see Figure 26–4).

Sensors are available in different sizes that approximate the different sizes of an intraoral film packet. The sensor design is unique to the manufacturer. Sensors are available with contoured edges (Figure 26–13). and others have been reduced to just over 3 mm in width (thickness), both characteristics designed to enhance patient comfort during sensor placement intraorally.

The three most common types of image detectors available for dental digital imaging are:

1. Charge-coupled device (CCD).
2. Complementary metal oxide semiconductor (CMOS).
3. Photo stimuable phosphor (PSP).

Charge-coupled Device (CCD)

The **charge-coupled device (CCD)** is the most widely used image receptor in dental digital imaging. The CCD, first developed in the 1960s, is not new technology. CCDs are used in video cameras, fax machines, microscopes, and telescopes. The CCD is a solid-state detector made up of a grid of small transistor elements that convert x-rays to electrons. When an x-ray strikes the transistor elements, electrons are trapped in proportion to the number of x-rays striking the element. The individual elements are arranged in a grid formation. Each element represents one pixel in the final image. A pixel serves as a small box or "well" into which the electrons produced by the x-ray exposure are deposited. A pixel is the digital equivalent of a silver halide crystal used in film-based radiography. As opposed to film emulsion that contains a random arrangement of silver halide crystals, pixels are structured in an ordered arrangement. The CCD is 640 by 480 individual pixels in size.

After exposure to x-rays, the elements are read and the electron charges are converted to brightness values and locations to form a digital image. This information is then passed through a wire or communicated wirelessly via radio frequency to a circuit board inside the computer for processing and display on the monitor.

Complementary Metal Oxide Semiconductor (CMOS)

CMOS (complementary metal oxide semiconductor) is a solid-state integrated circuit similar to the CCD. In CMOS technology, individual pixels can be made smaller, and the chip is more durable and less expensive to produce. Additionally, CMOS require less computer power, so the sensor can be connected to the computer using a low power external connection such as

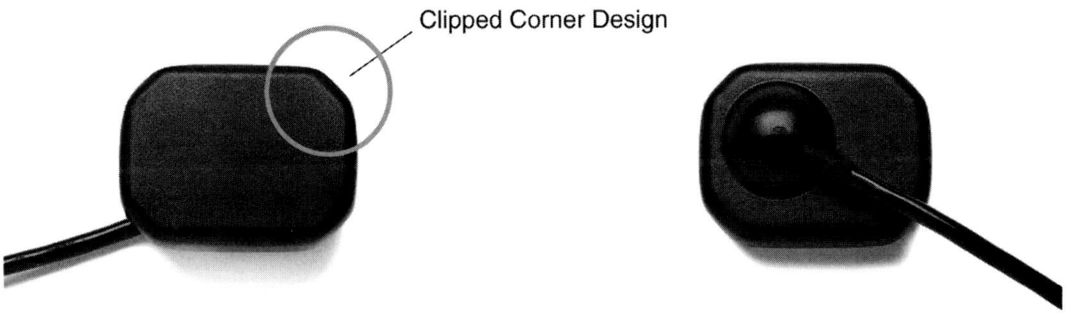

FIGURE 26-13 **Digital wired sensor showing front and back.** (DEXIS x-ray images courtesy of Pro Vision Dental Systems, Inc.)

Universal Serial Bus (USB). These sensors do not require an internal computer circuit card that the CCD sensor needs, making it possible to use a laptop computer system. The use of CCD or CMOS technology depends on the manufacturer. Currently two companies utilize CMOS technology in their sensors (Table 26–2).

Photo Stimuable Phosphor (PSP)

The **photo stimuable phosphor (PSP) sensor** system utilizes completely different technology than CCD and CMOS systems. PSP sensors use rare earth phosphor (barium europium fluorohalide) coated plates. When exposed to x-rays the PSP sensor or plate "stores" the x-ray energy until stimulated by a laser beam. This is done in a separate scanning device where the resulting fluorescent "signal" is read and converted into a digital image (Figure 26–9). This system is similar to film-based radiography in that multiple images are taken and the sensor plates "developed" later. The plates are reusable after they are erased by exposing them to bright light.

A recent study (2005) comparing 17 different digital sensors found that most all produced acceptable images in terms of spatial resolution and gray scale when compared to intraoral film.

Practice Point

The ability to view a digital image immediately allows for quick assessment of diagnostic quality and accurate correction of technique errors. For example, if a technique error results in overlapping or cone cut images, the operator can make the necessary adjustments to the sensor placement or tube head alignment without removing the sensor from the patient's mouth, greatly increasing the likelihood that the corrective action will produce a quality image.

Computer

All digital images require a computer and a monitor to capture and view an image (Figure 26–14). The type and size of computer required depends on the digital imaging software to be used. The computer must have a large enough memory to store the images and be equipped to support visual image displays on a monitor. The computer digitizes, processes, and stores informa-

TABLE 26-2 **Sensor Technology Used by Company**

Company Name and Web Address	Digital System Name	Sensor Technology
Air Techniques, Inc. www.airtechniques.com	ScanX	PSP
Progeny Dental www.progenydental.com	MPSe	CCD
Eastman Kodak Company www.kodak.com	Trophy RVG-ui RVG 6000	CCD CMOS
GE/Instrumentation Imaging www.gehealthcare.com	Sigma	CCD
Gendex www.gendex.com	VisualiX eHD DenOptix	CCD PSP
Integra Medical ww.vipersoft.com	ViperRay	CCD
Owandy/Julie Radio Vision www.owandy.com	DSX 730 USB Upix	CCD CCD
Planmeca Oy www.planmeca.com	Dixi®3	CCD
Provision Dental Supplies www.dexray.com	Dexis	CCD
Schick Technologies www.schicktech.com	CDR CDR (wireless sensor)	CMOS CMOS
Sirona www.sirona.com	Sidexis	CCD
Visiodent www.visiodent.com	RSV VRW (wireless sensor)	CCD CCD

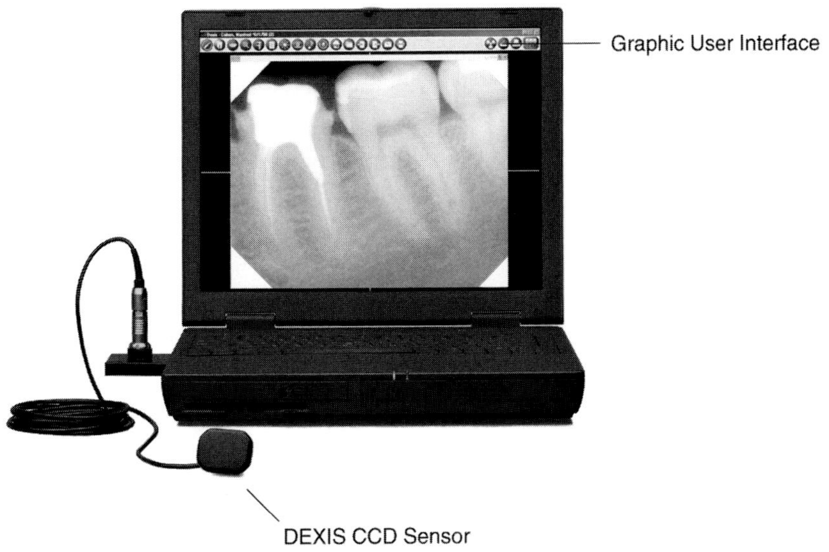

FIGURE 26-14 **Digital imaging system showing a laptop computer and wired sensor.** (DEXIS x-ray images courtesy of ProVision Dental Systems, Inc.)

tion received from the sensor. The monitor allows for immediate viewing. Digital images are usually displayed on a computer monitor within 0.5 to 120 seconds after the sensor is exposed, markedly less time than is required for conventional film processing. The computer may be connected to the Internet to allow for electronic transfer of the images to insurance companies or when referring to other health care specialists. Connecting a printer to the computer will allow the operator to print out a paper copy for the patient record if desired.

Software

Manufacturers of digital radiographic systems provide software programs that when loaded onto the computer will allow the operator to manipulate the images. Digital systems offer a variety of features to aid in viewing and interpreting the images. Some of the features offered by manufacturers of digital software include:

- **Side-by-side displays of images.** Allows the operator to view and compare multiple images on the monitor at one time. This feature is helpful when comparing current images with images taken previously.
- **Magnification.** Allows specific images to be magnified up to four times their original size. This feature is helpful when evaluating subtle changes not easily detected by the unaided human eye.
- **Density and contrast.** Changes can be made to image density and contrast without retaking the radiograph. For example, when an image appears too light, this software tool allows the operator to increase the image darkness.

> **Practice Point**
>
> The ability to increase or decrease digital image density will not compensate for a severely under- or overexposed image. For example, if the exposure setting is too low, the resultant image will be too light. Often a light image will not reveal such subtle changes as an early or incipient carious lesion. If the original image does not detect the radiolucency of the caries because it was underexposed (too light), then merely darkening the image with the digital software density control tool will not "put" the caries into the picture. If it was not detected to begin with, the software will not reveal it.

- **Measurement tools.** Linear and angular measurements can be obtained with a software "ruler" or measuring feature. Measurement tools are useful in measuring the length of root canals in endodontic therapy and for estimating bone loss.
- **Charting.** Many software programs allow the operator to place interpretive notes directly on the radiographic images (Figures 26–15 and 26–16). An arrow or circle may be drawn directly on an area of interest, in much the same manner as an entry would be made on the patient's paper record or chart.
- **Digital subtraction.** This feature allows for comparison of digitally stored images to detect changes over time or prior to and after treatment interventions. **Digital**

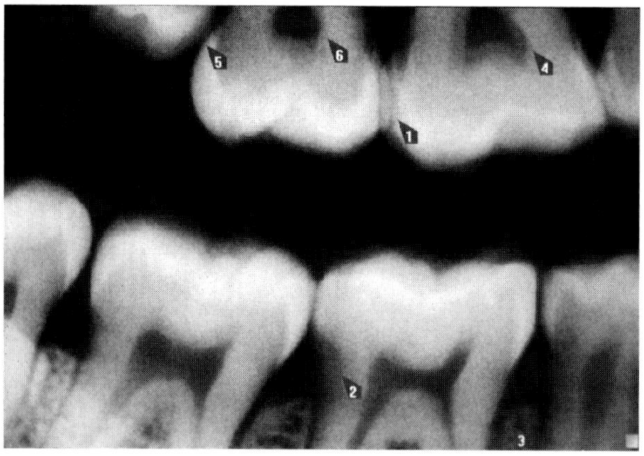

FIGURE 26-15 **Software charting feature.** Digital software that allows the operator to place notes directly on the image.

subtraction merges two radiographic images of the same area, taken at different times. Merged together electronically, those portions of the images that are alike—i.e., did not change over time—will cancel each other out as they are subtracted from each other. The portions of the images where change occurred will stand out conspicuously. Digital subtraction eliminates distracting background information that is similar in both images and highlights the changes (differences). Digital subtraction is an effective method of measuring periodontal changes such as bone loss or regeneration.

For digital subtraction to be effective, the technique used to acquire the two images must be standardized. The positions of the sensor, the patient, and the tube head all must be the same for both images. Altering where the patient bites down on the sensor, the patient's head position, or the horizontal or vertical angulation of the tube head and PID will produce geometric image changes that do not represent actual physical changes. Digital subtraction requires the use of external standardization methods such as custom-made sensor-holder biteblocks specifically designed for the patient or internal standardization such as software that calibrates density and contrast changes that result in exposure fluctuations.

Other features of specialized software promoted by manufacturers include reversing the gray scale, which changes the radiopaque images to radiolucent, and vice versa (Figure 26–17) and colorization, where different densities can be assigned a different color on the monitor. Both of these features have the potential to allow the computer to alert the practitioner to important interpretative findings. However, currently software can not match the ability of a skilled practitioner at interpreting dental disease and deviations from the normal.

Practice Point

The future possibilities of digital imaging software are limitless. Since the computer can record more data than the human eye can detect, in the future software features might be constructed that alert the practitioner to subtle dental disease that may go undetected. For example, the computer could be directed to color all healthy enamel, with a certain level of density, to yellow. Any enamel density that falls below a certain established healthy level could be colored purple. Therefore, when interpreting the image on the computer monitor, the practitioner could easily spot the caries indicated by the purple areas.

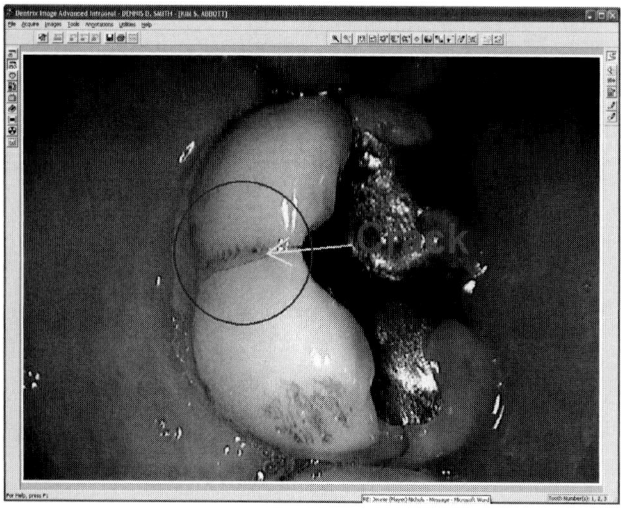

FIGURE 26-16 **Software charting feature.** Digital software that allows the operator to place notes directly on the image. (Courtesy of Dentrix Dental Systems)

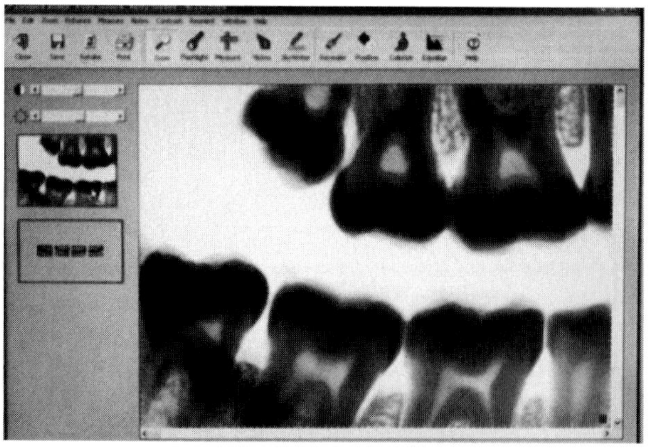

FIGURE 26-17 **Reversing the gray scale.** Digital software can change the image's radiopacities to radiolucencies and vice versa.

Many digital imaging software manufacturers promote colorization tools and other features called sharpen, equalize, enhance, emboss (Figure 26–18), highlight, and spot remover. Some practitioners find these features helpful aids to interpreting images, while others view them as visual gimmicks, since these features currently do not have the power to take the place of the dental practitioner. Interpreting digital images with or without these features requires practice. A practitioner must spend time developing the skills required for interpreting digital images.

Radiation Exposure

The radiation exposure from digital imaging systems can be 50 to 80 percent less than exposures required for film-based dental radiography, depending on the film speed currently in use. Digital imaging sensors are more sensitive to x-rays than conventional dental x-ray film. For example, if a 12-impulse (0.2 second) exposure time is required for a radiograph taken with F-speed intraoral film, the exposure time for this same image acquired utilizing a digital radiography sensor would be approximately 6 impulses (0.1 second). The lower the exposure time, the lower the radiation dose to the patient.

Legal Implications

Because the original digital image can be manipulated, there has been much concern about the legal implications of digital radiographs. It is possible to modify an image to create dental disease where none exists and/or to mask or correct faulty dental restorative work. To address this concern, manufacturers are producing software that will not permit an altered image to be saved except as a copy, clearly labeled as such. One such software feature, called digital watermarking, embeds an invisible ID mark into the image to make fraudulent modification of images too difficult to be practical. Currently many insurance companies opt to accept digital images because the cost savings of doing so greatly exceed the potential for fraud.

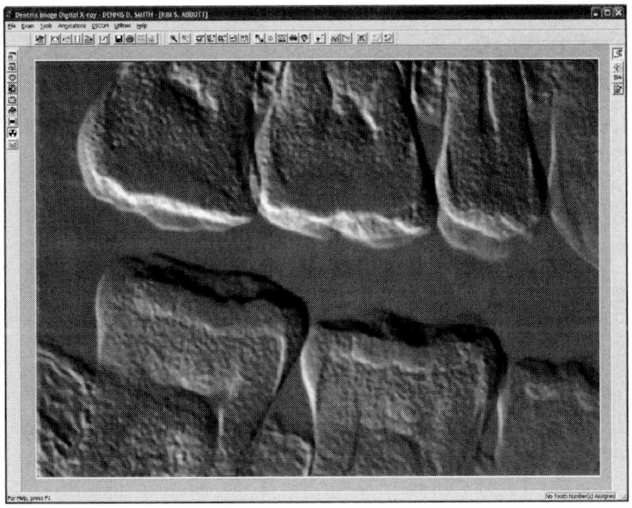

FIGURE 26–18 **Embossing.** An example of a digital software feature that can be used to manipulate the image to aid in interpretation. (Courtesy of Dentrix Dental Systems)

Advantages and Disadvantages

There are both advantages and disadvantages to using digital radiography.

Advantages

Advantages of digital radiography include: less radiation exposure to the patient; a reduction in the time required to obtain the image; the elimination of the photographic process and darkroom; the potential for improved interpretation; the ability to electronically transmit the images, and the opportunity to effectively educate patients on oral health and treatment.

- **Less radiation exposure to the patient.** Digital imaging sensors are more sensitive to x-rays than conventional dental x-ray film, requiring 50 percent less radiation than that required to expose F speed film; 60 percent less radiation than that required to expose E speed film; and 80 percent less radiation than that required to expose D speed film.
- **Instant viewing of the image.** Images are created almost instantaneously, allowing immediate evaluation of the patient's condition. Speed of image viewing allows for diagnosis and treatment of the patient's oral condition in a timely manner. This is especially beneficial during procedures such as endodontic therapy and oral surgery that require working radiographs throughout the treatment. Additionally, when radiograph technique errors result in undiagnostic images, viewing the image on the monitor while the sensor is still in place intraorally will allow the operator to make the correct adjustments with confidence prior to exposing the necessary retakes.
- **Elimination of the photographic process and darkroom.** Digital radiography eliminates the need for dental x-ray film, processing solutions, and the darkroom. The costs of film and processing chemicals are eliminated. Eliminating the darkroom prevents the generation and cost of disposal of hazardous wastes such as used fixer and lead foil from the film packets. Additionally, darkroom processing errors are eliminated.
- **Improvement of the diagnostic image.** The diagnostic image can be manipulated to enhance interpretation. Features such as magnification, density and contrast modification, and others allow the operator to improve the image for better interpretation.
- **Improved gray scale resolution.** An important advantage of digital radiography is the improved gray scale resolution of the image generated. Digital radiography produces up to 256 shades of gray displayed on a computer monitor, compared to the 25 or fewer shades of gray seen on a film-based radiograph. The gray scale resolution is important because

diagnosis is often based on contrast discrimination. The density and contrast of the radiographic image can be manipulated to produce the ideal image from which to diagnose oral conditions.

- **Remote electronic consultation and sending of images.** Digital radiographs can be electronically transmitted via the Internet to other oral health care specialists and insurance companies, reducing the time needed for consulting and payment of treatment. Sending images electronically also eliminates the chance of lost radiographs.
- **Patient education.** Viewing digital images is an effective method of patient education (Figure 26–19). The size of the digitized image on a computer screen (compared with a 2-in. film) makes viewing easier for the patient. Software features, such as a measuring tool to show bone loss, can be used to help the patient see conditions that may be difficult to visualize on a radiograph placed on a viewbox.

Disadvantages

Disadvantages of digital radiography include initial investment costs, technological reliability, learning curve required to read digital images, sensor size, infection control, and legal issues.

- **Initial investment costs.** The cost of purchasing a digital imaging system has dropped significantly over the last several years; however, acquiring a quality system remains a significant investment. The price depends on the manufacturer, the level of computer equipment currently in the office, and auxiliary features, such as multiple sensors in various sizes. The cost of service and maintenance and for training to learn how to use the system must also be considered. Typical start-up costs for a basic dental digital imaging system is estimated at $6,000 to $16,000. This does not include the cost of the x-ray machine.

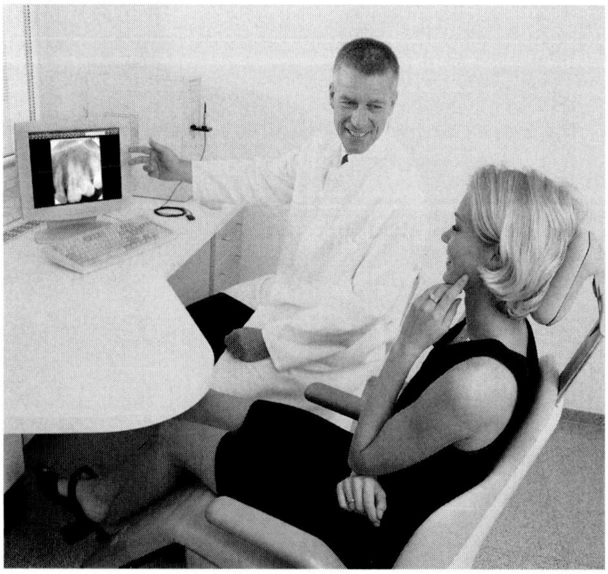

FIGURE 26-19 **Viewing digital images is an effective method of patient education.** (DEXIS x-ray images courtesy of Pro Vision Dental Systems, Inc.)

- **Technology concerns.** A decision an oral health care practice often faces is when to make the change from film-based radiography to digital imaging. Technological advances continue to make available better and more reliable digital imaging systems. When to buy and what type of system to buy can be a difficult decision. Another technological concern is the reliability of the system. Computer crashes, system malfunction, and computer viruses are real risks. While film-based radiographs also have a risk of being misplaced or lost, the risk of loss of computer memory has the potential to wipe out a greater number of records. Additionally, temporary inability to access the images in the computer's memory due to a computer glitch or power failure can delay patient treatment.

  Storage of patient images is also a technological concern. Archival storage (to keep patient records for the time required or recommended by law) and back-up storage (to protect files from computer malfunction) need to be considered. Many manufacturers of digital imaging systems recommend that old images be deleted periodically as newer images are acquired to make room in computer memory for storage of these files. Since radiographic images are a legal part of the patient record, deleting older radiographic images is not recommended (see Chapter 10). Hence, the decision arises of how to store the image files. Floppy disks have been replaced by CDs (compact disks), which are rapidly being replaced by portable storage devices (often referred to as USB drives, flash drives, jump drives, and keychain drives). The media used to store the images will have to be updated continually to the latest storage method to be accessible over time.

  System compatibility may be an issue when the images will be transferred electronically. Currently there is no standard agreed upon between manufacturers of dental digital imaging systems to produce systems that are compatible with each other. Exporting and importing digital images can require complex steps and considerable computer knowledge. The medical community, where digital imaging is more widely utilized, has adopted the **Digital Imaging and Communications in Medicine (DICOM)** standard to allow different systems to interface with each other. As a result, the American Dental Association Informatics Task Group has recommended that this standard be used for dental imaging systems as well. As manufacturers adopt the DICOM standard, the ease with which information can be shared will improve.
- **Learning curve.** Transferring the ability to read radiographs to the ability to read digital images on a computer monitor requires practice. Instead of utilizing a viewbox, digital images are read directly off the computer monitor. The "look and feel" of digital images will take getting used to. New considerations not encountered when reading film-based radiographs include the possibility of not being able to view an entire full mouth series of images on one screen

without switching between views and coping with overhead room lighting reflecting off the monitor screen. Multiple mouse clicks may be needed to view images side by side, especially when viewing radiographs taken on different days and stored in different files on the computer. Viewing digital images will be restricted to the area where the computer and monitor are located.

- **Sensor size.** Sensors are generally thicker (wider) than intraoral film packets. The bulky feel may elicit patient complaints of discomfort or excite a gag reflex. Plastic barrier sheaths placed over the sensor to maintain infection control add additional bulk. Wired sensors require increased operator skill to position accurately and increased patient cooperation to hold in place for exposure (Figure 26–7). The smaller overall dimensions (height and length) of a digital sensor does not allow it to record as large an area as a standard size #2 intraoral film, meaning that more individual images may be needed to image an area entirely. Sensors with contoured edges further limit the amount of image that will be recorded.
- **Infection control.** Digital sensors cannot withstand heat sterilization, and plastic sheaths used as barriers are subject to tearing and are not always totally protective. Additionally, to activate the exposure sequence after placing the sensor intraorally, the computer keyboard and/or mouse must usually be operated. Maintaining infection control when utilizing digital imaging can be difficult. Most manufacturers of digital systems recommend covering the sensor, keyboard, and mouse with disposable plastic barriers that are changed between patients (Figures 26–4, 26–5, and 26–20). The use of an FDA-cleared disposable plastic barrier will help decrease the risk of a breach in asepsis. Additionally, the radiographer is encouraged to ask the manufacturer what intermediate-level disinfectant can be used to clean and disinfect the sensor, keyboard, and mouse when necessary.

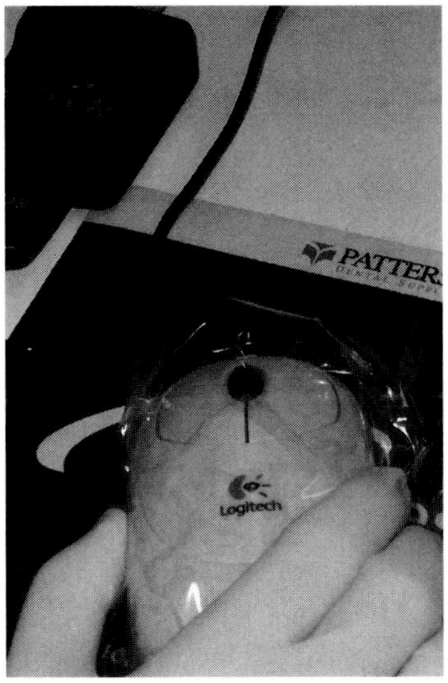

FIGURE 26-20 **Infection control.** A disposable plastic barrier protects the computer mouse.

- **Legal issues.** While software continues to be developed to address the legality of digital images, there remains the question of whether digital radiographs can be used as evidence in court. Digital images carry the possibility that they could have been altered by manipulation. Manufacturers continue to develop software that will guard against fraudulent use of image manipulation, but computer hackers will always be tempted to find ways around software safeguards.

Despite the disadvantages, digital imaging represents a new age of imaging in dentistry. Oral healthcare will continue to adopt this technology; and as improvements and standardizations continue, the oral health care practice of the near future will most likely see a decreased use of film-based radiography.

REVIEW—Chapter Summary

Digital radiography is a method of capturing a radiographic image and displaying it on a computer screen; no film is used and no film processing is required. Digital images have no physical form, but exist as bits of information in a computer file. The computer displays the image on a monitor for viewing.

Indirect digital imaging uses a scanner or digital camera to digitize (convert) a film-based radiograph obtained by conventional methods into a digital image. Direct digital imaging replaces film with a sensor, a small detector that when struck by x-rays produces an electronic signal that is transmitted to a computer for viewing on a monitor.

The digital image is composed of pixels, short for picture elements. Each pixel is a single dot in the digital image. The number and size of pixels determines the spatial resolution and the sharpness of the image. Spatial resolution is measured as line pairs. A line pair refers to the number of paired lines visible in 1 mm of an image. The greater the spatial resolution, the sharper the image appears. Pixels also determine the gray scale of the image. Each pixel has a number from 0 to 255, representing pure black at 0 to pure white at 255. The higher the gray scale, the more likely the image is to record subtle changes in the patient's condition.

Digital imaging is used to detect oral conditions, evaluate growth and development, and provide information during endodontic treatment, oral surgery, and other dental procedures.

Digital imaging utilizes a conventional dental x-ray unit as the radiation source. A sensor or small detector is placed inside the mouth of the patient and the x-ray beam is aimed to strike the sensor. Three types of digital sensors are currently used for digital imaging. The charge-coupled device (CCD) is the most common type of sensor. The pixels on the CCD capture the electrons produced by the x-rays and send this information to the computer via a wire, or wirelessly via radio frequency. The complementary metal oxide semiconductor (CMOS) pixel sensor produces images similar to the CCD. CMOS technology can be attached to the computer via a low power connection such as a Universal Serial Bus (USB). The photo stimuable phosphor (PSP) sensor uses rare earth phosphor (barium europium fluorohalide) coated plates. When exposed to x-rays the PSP sensor "stores" the energy until read later by a special scanner. PSP sensors are not wired to the computer, but are placed into the scanner, which in turn converts the stored energy into a visible image on a monitor. PSP plates must be erased by exposing to bright light before they can be used again.

All digital imaging systems require the use of a computer with enough memory to run the special software and to store the images generated. The images are displayed on the computer monitor. A printer attached to the computer will allow the operator to print hard copies of the radiographic images if desired.

Special software is required to run the digital radiographic systems. Digital software packages often provide programs that allow the operator to manipulate the image. Common features include the ability to view multiple radiographic images on one screen, magnification, and measuring and charting tools. Digital subtraction is a process where two images are merged electronically, canceling out like portions of the image and revealing changes.

Advantages of digital radiography include: less radiation exposure to the patient; a reduction in the time required to obtain the image; the elimination of the photographic process and darkroom; the potential for improved interpretation; the ability to transmit the images electronically, and the opportunity effectively to educate patients on oral health.

Disadvantages of digital radiography include initial investment costs, technological reliability, learning curve required to read digital images, sensor size, infection control, and legal issues

RECALL—Study Questions

For questions 1 to 5, match each term with its definition.

a. analog
b. gray scale
c. line pair
d. pixel
e. spatial resolution

_____ 1. Discrete units of information that together constitute an image.

_____ 2. The discernable separation of closely adjacent image details.

_____ 3. Refers to the number of paired lines visible in 1 mm of an image.

_____ 4. Relating to a mechanism in which data is represented by continuously variable physical quantities.

_____ 5. Refers to the total number of shades of gray visible in an image.

6. A digital radiographic image exists as bits of information in a computer file. The computer transfers this information into an image that appears on the computer monitor.
   a. The first statement is true. The second statement is false.
   b. The first statement is false. The second statement is true.
   c. Both statements are true.
   d. Both statements are false.
7. Digital radiography systems can be used for which of the following?
   a. Bitewing images
   b. Periapical images
   c. Panoramic images
   d. Cephalometric images
   e. All of the above
8. When an existing film-based radiograph is digitized via the use of a special scanner or digital camera, the process is called:
   a. Digital radiography.
   b. Digital subtraction.
   c. Direct digital imaging.
   d. Indirect digital imaging.
9. The smaller the number of pixels in the image the sharper the spatial resolution. Each pixel stores a number representing a different shade of gray.
   a. The first statement is true. The second statement is false.
   b. The first statement is false. The second statement is true.
   c. Both statements are true.
   d. Both statements are false.
10. Digital radiography can be used for which of the following?
    a. To detect caries
    b. To evaluate growth and development
    c. To detect dental disease
    d. To monitor an endodontic procedure
    e. All of the above
11. All of the following are necessary equipment for digital radiography *except* one. Which one is this *exception?*
    a. X-ray machine
    b. Sensor or phosphor coated plate
    c. Computer and monitor
    d. Special software
    e. Darkroom
12. All of the following are digital image receptors *except* one. Which one is this *exception?*
    a. CCD
    b. CMOS
    c. XCP
    d. PSP
13. Which of the following stores the x-ray energy until later stimulation by a laser beam reads the electron signal and converts it into a digital image?
    a. CCD
    b. CMOS
    c. XCP
    d. PSP
14. List five features offered by digital software that can be used to enhance the radiographic image.
    a. ____________________
    b. ____________________
    c. ____________________
    d. ____________________
    e. ____________________
15. Digital radiography requires less radiation exposure to produce an image than film-based radiography because the:
    a. Chemical processing steps are eliminated.
    b. Radiation used for digital imaging is different than radiation used for film-based imaging.
    c. Image detector (the sensor) is more sensitive to x-rays than film.
    d. Computer can control the amount of radiation output better than the operator.

16. All of the following are true regarding digital radiography in comparison to film-based radiography *except* one. Which one is this *exception?*
    a. Provides a more legal document.
    b. Less time is required to obtain a diagnostic image.
    c. Eliminates film and chemical wastes.
    d. Patient radiation is reduced 50 to 80 percent.
    e. Software features enhance interpretation.
17. All of the following are disadvantages of digital radiography when compared to film-based radiography *except* one. Which one is this *exception?*
    a. Initial cost of setting up the system
    b. Being able to magnify the image for diagnosis
    c. Risk of computer crashes and lost files
    d. Learning curve required to transfer interpretation skills
    e. Management of infection control
18. To maintain infection control, most manufacturers recommend that the sensor used in digital radiography be
    a. Packaged for steam sterilization and autoclaved.
    b. Disposed of after use, with biohazard wastes.
    c. Decontaminated with soap and water and disinfected with a high-level disinfectant.
    d. Wiped with an intermediate-level disinfectant and covered with a plastic barrier.
    e. Sanitized and immersed in a chemical sterilant.

REFLECT—Case Study

The oral health care practice where you are employed is considering purchasing a digital radiography system. Using the Internet, search for companies that manufacture and sell dental digital imaging products. From your research, choose two companies and compare their two products. Prepare an analysis to help your practice decide what digital radiography system will be the best choice. Contact the company for brochures or additional information as needed to answer the following questions about each of the products.

a. What are the names of the companies that manufacture the products you chose to compare?
b. What are the names of the digital radiography systems they manufacture/sell?
c. Do these digital systems have special computer requirements, or can they be used with the computer currently in use at your practice?
d. What type of sensor does each offer? How are they alike? How are they different?
e. Are the sensors available in different sizes?
f. Are special sensor holding devices required for positioning the sensor intraorally? Where can these be purchased?
g. What are the infection control guidelines for the sensor? Does the company make custom-sized plastic barriers that fit the sensor?
h. Does software come with the purchase of the digital radiography system? What features are included that will allow the operator to enhance the image for interpretation?
i. Are there built-in safeguards to prevent fraudulent use of altered images?
j. Does the company offer training for your oral health care team to learn to operate the system? Is there training in digital radiographic interpretation? Is there a fee for service and/or maintenance to the system after purchase?
k. Does the company offer articles or reviews of their products by outside agencies that support their marketing claims?
l. Based on what you learned in this chapter, prepare a list of advantages and disadvantages of each of these products.
m. Based on your research, which product would you recommend your practice purchase, and why?

RELATE—Laboratory Application

For a comprehensive laboratory practice exercise on this topic, see E. M. Thomson, *Exercises in Oral Radiography Techniques: A Laboratory Manual,* 2nd ed., Upper Saddle River, NJ: Prentice Hall, 2007. Chapter 15, "Digital Radiography."

BIBLIOGRAPHY

Farman, A. G. & Farman, T. T. A comparison of 18 different x-ray detectors currently used in dentistry. *Oral Surg, Oral Med, Oral Path* 99:485–489, 2005.

Jones, G. A., Behrents, R. C. & Baily, G. P. Legal considerations for digital images. *General Dentistry* 44:242–244, 1996.

Langland, O. E. & Langlais, R. P. Special radiographic techniques. In *Principles of Dental Imaging,* pp. 265–287. Baltimore: Williams & Wilkins, 1997.

Lusk, L. T. Comparison of film-based and digital radiography. *J Practical Hygiene* 7:45–50, 1998.

Mauriello, S. M. & Platin, E. Dental digital radiographic imaging. *J.Dental Hygiene* 75:323–331, 2001.

Palenik, C. J. Infection control for dental radiography. *Dentistry Today,* 23:52–55, 2004.

Tsang, A., Sweet, D., & Wood, R. Potential for fraudulent use of digital radiography. *J. Am. Dent. Assoc.* 130:1325–1329, 1999.

White, S. C. & Pharoah, M. J. *Oral Radiology Principles and Interpretation,* 5th ed. St. Louis: Elsevier, 2004.

PART IX • EXTRAORAL TECHNIQUES

27

Extraoral Radiography

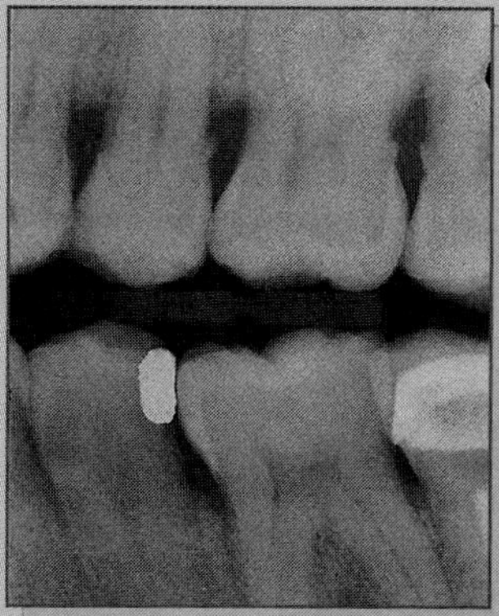

■ OBJECTIVES

Following successful completion of this chapter you should be able to:

1. Define the key words.
2. Describe the purpose and use of extraoral radiographs.
3. Explain the need for proper extraoral film handling.
4. Explain the role intensifying screens play in producing a radiographic image.
5. Match blue- and green-light sensitive film with the appropriate intensifying screen.
6. Explain the role of the extraoral film cassette.
7. Identify the types of projections that can be performed extraorally.
8. State the purpose and describe the technique used to produce a lateral jaw radiograph.
9. State the purpose and describe the technique used to produce a lateral cephalometric radiograph.
10. State the purpose and describe the technique used to produce a posteroanterior cephalometric radiograph.
11. State the purpose and describe the technique used to produce a Waters radiograph.
12. State the purpose and describe the technique used to produce a Reverse-Towne radiograph.
13. State the purpose and describe the technique used to produce a submentovertex radiograph.
14. State the purpose and describe the technique used to produce a transcranial radiograph.

■ KEY WORDS

Acoustic meatus
Ankylosis
Artifacts
Calcium tungstate phosphors
Cassette
Cephalometer
Cephalometric radiographs
Cephalostats
Condyle
Flexible cassette
Frankfort plane
Glenoid fossa
Grid
Intensifying screens
Lateral cephalometric radiograph (lateral skull projection)
Lateral jaw projection (mandibular oblique lateral projection)

- Occipital protuberance
- Panoramic radiographs
- Phosphors
- Posteroanterior cephalometric radiograph (PA projection)
- Rare-earth phosphors
- Reverse-Towne radiograph (open mouth projection)
- Rigid cassette
- Screen film
- Submentovertex radiograph (base projection)
- Temporomandibular disorder (TMD)
- Temporomandibular joint (TMJ)
- Tomography
- Transcranial radiograph (TMJ projection)
- Waters radiograph (sinus projection)

Introduction

Extraoral radiographs are examinations made of the head and facial region using films positioned outside the mouth. These films image large areas of the jaws and skull on a single radiograph. Many types of extraoral radiographs require special equipment not readily available in the general practice dental office. Therefore, the general practice dental assistant and dental hygienist are less likely to be called upon to obtain these valuable radiographs. Even though dental assistants and hygienists may not routinely perform these services, a base knowledge in types of extraoral radiographs; an understanding of what conditions will most likely benefit from which type of examination; and the ability to recognize the different images are valuable skills. Patients may need to be referred to an oral surgeon or to a medical imaging center for examination of a condition affecting the head and facial region. The dental assistant and dental hygienist may be called upon to educate the patient regarding the procedure or may need to assist with scheduling the patient's appointment for the referral. Oral radiographers should be able to communicate professionally with other health care professionals.

Additionally, the patient may present with extraoral images obtained by an oral surgeon, an orthodontist, or a medical imaging facility. The dental assistant and dental hygienist should be able to identify the type of image and be knowledgeable regarding what conditions the image was taken to observe.

The purpose of this chapter is to explain the film types and equipment used for extraoral radiography; to present the purpose and use of seven extraoral radiographs; and to briefly describe the techniques for patient and film positioning.

Purpose and Use of Extraoral Radiographs

The purpose of extraoral radiographs is to examine structures of the skull, the maxilla and mandible, and the temporomandibular joint. Extraoral radiographs are used to:

- Examine large areas of the jaws and skull.
- Study growth and development of bone and teeth.
- Detect fractures and evaluate trauma.
- Detect pathological lesions and diseases of the jaws.
- Detect and evaluate impacted teeth.
- Evaluate **temporomandibular disorder (TMD)**.

Extraoral radiographs may also be substituted for intraoral radiographs when patients cannot or will not open the mouth. Handicapped patients or patients with trismus or TMD may not be able to tolerate the placement of intraoral film. Extraoral radiographs can be used alone or in conjunction with intraoral radiographs. For example, it is common to expose both a panoramic radiograph (see Chapter 28) and intraoral radiographs on the same patient.

The general practitioner is most likely to limit the use of extraoral radiographs to panoramic imaging; the panoramic technique is discussed in detail in Chapter 28. Othodontists, prosthodontists, and oral surgeons are frequent users of extraoral radiographs for diagnosing and treating conditions of the oral cavity and head and facial regions.

- **Orthodontists** use facial profile radiographs, cephalometric headplates ("cephalometric" meaning measuring the head) periodically to record, measure, and compare changes in growth and development of the bones and the teeth.
- **Prosthodontists** use facial profile radiographs to record the contour of the lips and face, and the relationship of the teeth before removal to help in constructing prosthetic appliances that look natural (Figure 27–1).
- **Oral surgeons** use extraoral radiographs extensively to evaluate trauma, to determine the location and extent of fractures, to locate impacted teeth, abnormalities, and malignancies, and to evaluate injuries to the temporomandibular joint.

Extraoral Film

To produce a diagnostic quality radiograph while maintaining a low radiation dose for the patient, extraoral **screen film** (see Chapter 7) must be used in conjunction with a pair of **intensifying screens** housed within a light-tight **cassette**. Because they are extremely light sensitive and not packaged in a protective sealed wrapper like intraoral films, extraoral films must be carefully loaded into a cassette under darkroom safelight illumination (Figure 27–2 and Procedure Box 27–1).

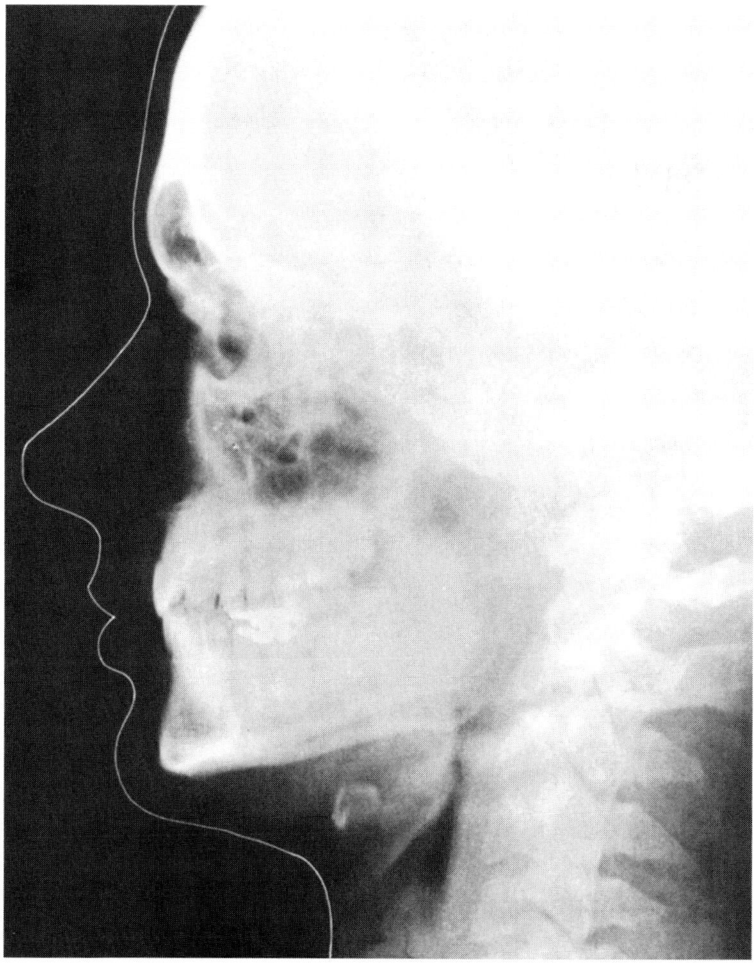

FIGURE 27–1 **Radiograph profile.** Radiograph with outlines of the soft tissues that reveal the patient's profile.

Extraoral films are generally packaged 25, 50, or 100 to a box, so care should be taken to ensure that overhead white lighting is turned off when removing the box cover. Darkroom safelight filter color and bulb wattage must be appropriate for use with extraoral film (see Chapter 8). Because extraoral film is more sensitive than intraoral films, filters that are safe for intraoral film handling may not be safe for extraoral film handling. The type of safelight required for extraoral film can usually be found written on the film package, or by checking with the manufacturer.

Extraoral films should be removed from the box with clean, dry hands. Latex or vinyl treatment gloves should be avoided. Treatment gloves and plastic overgloves increase the risk of generating static electricity. A static charge results in a white light spark that will expose the film, leaving radiolucent **artifacts** (black lines or smudges) on the resultant image (Figure 27–5). Glove powder residue on films will also cause radiolucent artifacts.

Handle films by the edges only. Remove each sheet of film from the box slowly to avoid generating static electricity that will create artifacts on the films inside the box as well as the one being removed. Try to place the film into the cassette without sliding it across the intensifying screens, again to prevent a static discharge. Film should be loaded into the cassette just prior to use. Storing film inside cassettes may increase the likelihood of generating artifacts. Only one film should be loaded into the cassette at a time unless special film made for exposing two films at once is used. Be sure that the film box cover is replaced prior turning on the overhead white light.

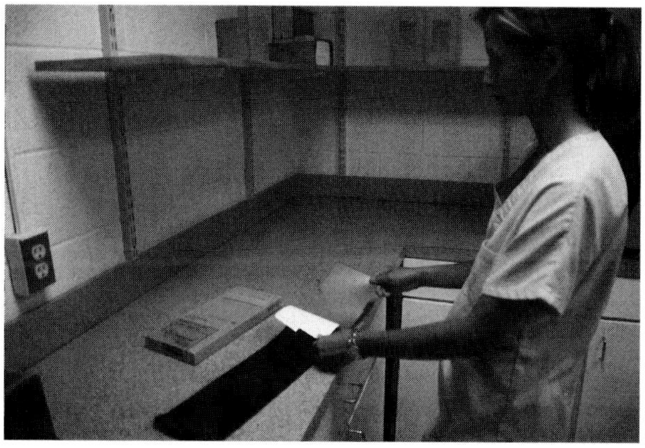

FIGURE 27–2 **Loading film into a flexible cassette.** Extraoral film must be loaded into the cassette under safelight conditions.

PROCEDURE 27-1

LOADING AN EXTRAORAL CASSETTE

1. Obtain the cassette and box of film. Ensure that the film sensitivity matches the intensifying screens used.
2. Open the cassette and inspect to ensure that the hinge and snaps are working. Examine the intensifying screens for debris or scratches. Clean with solution recommended by the manufacturer if necessary.
3. Turn off overhead white light and turn on safelight.
4. Open the package containing the film and slowly pull out one film.
5. Handling the film by the edges only with clean, dry hands, place the film inside the (rigid) cassette (Figure 27–3). When loading the film into a flexible plastic sleeve cassette, pull the screens part way out of the cassette to separate the pair. Slowly slide the film between the folded screens (Figure 27–4). Make sure that the film is seated all the way down to the fold in the screen.

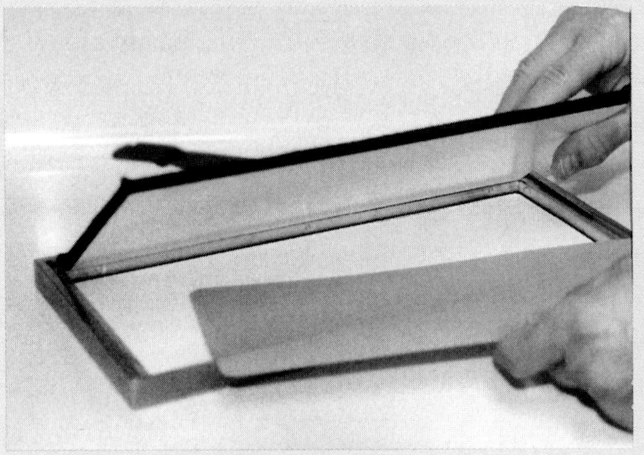

FIGURE 27-3 **Loading a rigid cassette.**

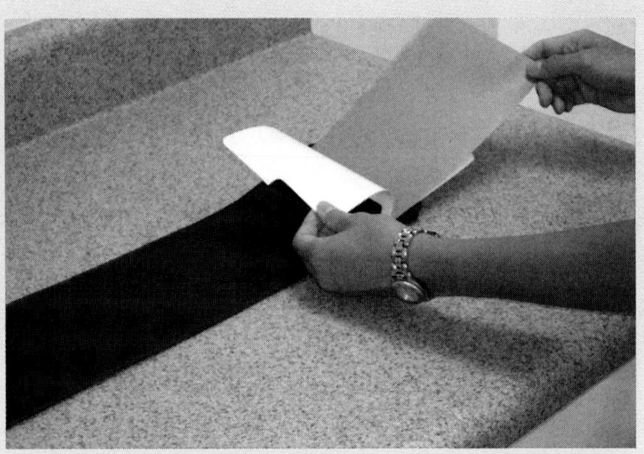

FIGURE 27-4 **Loading a flexible cassette.** Operator is placing an extraoral film between the intensifying screens.

6. Close the cassette and ensure that the hinge is secured (rigid). Close the snaps or Velcro® closures on the flexible cassette. When the cassette is not tightly closed, the film and screen contact is not tight and it causes the radiograph to be blurry.
7. Replace the cover on the film package to protect from white light exposure.
8. Turn on the overhead white light and exit the darkroom.

Intensifying Screens

Intensifying screens transfer x-ray energy into visible light. This visible light, in turn, exposes the screen film. The image produced on an extraoral film results from exposure to this fluorescent light instead of directly from the x-rays. As the name implies, intensifying screens "intensify" the effect of x-rays on film. The use of intensifying screens allows the amount of radiation required to expose the film to be reduced, and thus reduces the amount of radiation the patient is exposed to.

Intensifying screens work in pairs. An intensifying screen is a smooth cardboard or plastic sheet coated with minute fluorescent crystals mixed into a suitable binding medium. Intensifying screens are based on the principle that crystals of certain salts—**calcium tungstate**, barium strontium sulfate, or **rare-earth phosphors** [lanthanum (La) and gadolinium (Gd)]—will fluoresce and emit energy in the form of blue or green light when they absorb x-rays. Each of these fluorescent crystals, also called **phosphors,** gives off blue or green light that varies in intensity according to the x-rays in that part of the image. Screen film is

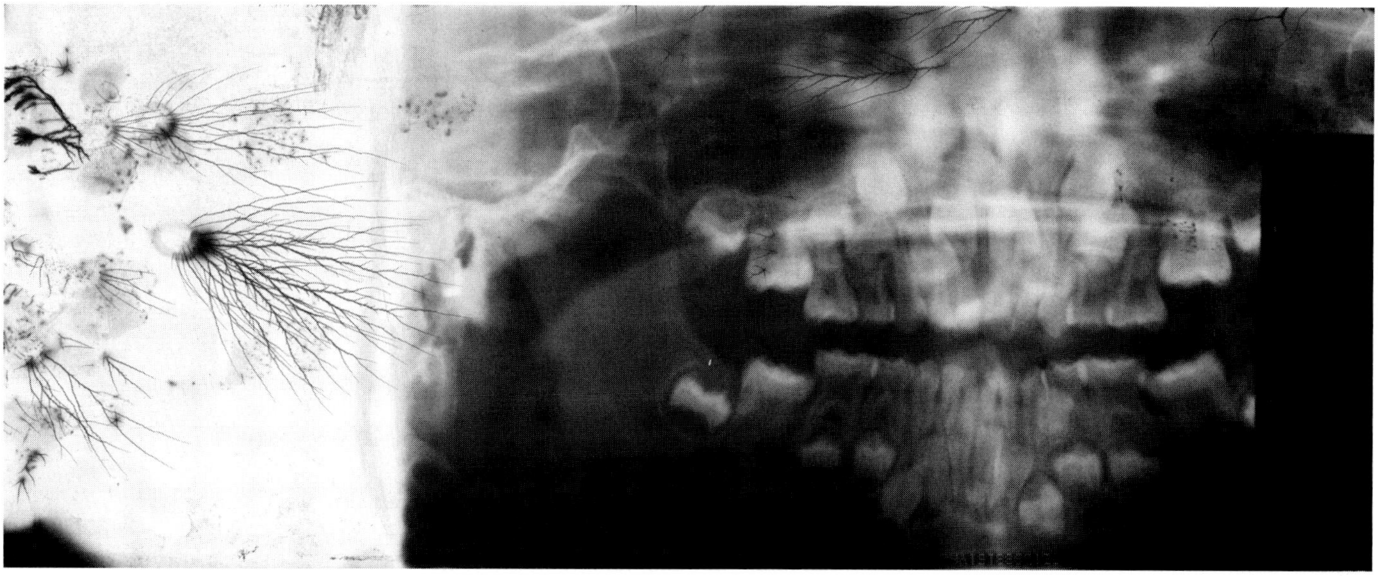

FIGURE 27–5 **Static electricity artifacts.** Blank area on a panoramic film showing static electricity artifacts.

more sensitive to this type of fluorescent light than to radiation. When the film is sandwiched tightly between a pair of two intensifying screens, the x-rays cause the crystals on the screens to fluoresce and return the emitted light to the film emulsion to produce the radiographic image (Figure 27–6).

Rare earth screens emit green light when energized by x-rays and must be paired with green-light–sensitive film. Calcium tungstate screens give off a blue to violet fluorescent light and must be paired with blue-light–sensitive film. Inappropriately interchanging green- or blue-light–sensitive films between calcium tungstate and rare earth screens produces undiagnostic radiographic images.

The use of intensifying screens decreases the amount of radiation required to produce an image. However, the sharpness of the radiographic image also is reduced over the images produced on intraoral films. The sensitivity and image sharpness of different types of intensifying screens varies and depends on the:

- **Size of the crystals.** The larger the crystal size, the less radiation required to produce an image. Larger crystals produce a less sharp image.
- **Thickness of the emulsion.** The thicker the emulsion, the faster the speed of the screen, requiring less radiation to produce an image. Thicker emulsion results in a less sharp image.
- **Type of phosphor used.** Rare earth screens produce a latent image on the film with less radiation exposure than calcium tungstate screens.

Although varying speeds of screens are available, the American Dental Association and the American Association of Oral and Maxillofacial Radiology recommend that the fastest speed

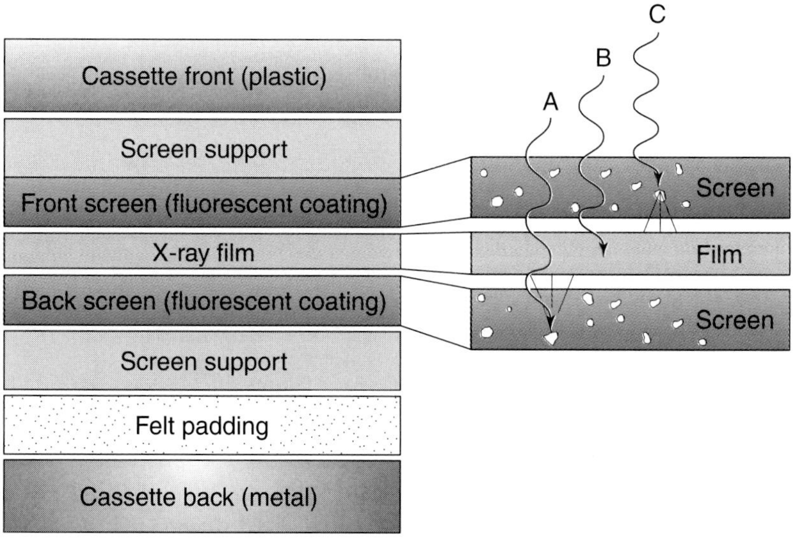

FIGURE 27–6 **Cross section of cassette and diagram showing the effect of x-ray and fluorescent light on the film. X-ray A** strikes a crystal in the screen behind the film, producing light that then forms latent images in the silver halide crystal of the film. **X-ray B** strikes a silver halide crystal in the film, forming a latent image. **X-ray C** strikes a crystal in the screen in front of the film, producing light, which then forms latent images in the silver halide crystals of the film.

screen–film combination be used to reduce the amount of excess radiation exposure to the patient. While reducing the radiation required to produce an image, a large crystal size and a thick emulsion will produce a less sharp radiographic image. The slight reduction in image clarity produced by fast speed screen–film combinations is considered acceptable to reduce the radiation dose to the patient.

Cassettes

The purpose of the cassette is to hold the intensifying screens in close contact with the film and to protect the film from white light exposure. Cassettes are available in a variety of shapes and sizes, depending on the intended use and as recommended by the manufacturer of the dental x-ray unit the cassette will be used with. Cassettes are available as a rigid box or case that may be flat or curved. Rigid cassettes are usually 5 × 7 in. (13 × 18 cm) or 8 10 in. (20 × 25 cm). A typical rigid cassette has a front and back cover joined together with a hinge (Figure 27–7). The front cover is constructed of plastic to permit the passage of the x-ray beam and must be positioned so that it faces the patient. The back cover is constructed of heavy metal to absorb remnant x-rays. A pair of intensifying screens lines the inside of the front and back covers of the cassette.

Flexible plastic sleeve cassettes are most often used for exposing panoramic radiographs (see Figure 28–10). **Flexible cassettes** measure 5 or 6 × 12 in. (13 or 15 × 30 cm) and are composed of a plastic sleeve with intensifying screens inside. The paired intensifying screens are usually joined together at one end, folding the screens so that a film may be inserted in between. Snaps or Velcro® closures seal the cassette to prevent white light from leaking in. When the film is placed inside and the cassette is closed, the film will be held tightly between the two intensifying screens (Figure 27–4).

Care of Cassettes and Intensifying Screens

Extraoral cassettes and intensifying screens should be inspected periodically. Rigid and flexible cassette hinges and snaps should be checked to ensure light tightness to prevent film fog. Cassettes should be checked for warping to ensure close screen–film contact. Poor screen–film contact results in an image of reduced sharpness (blurry image). Defective cassettes should be repaired or replaced.

Intensifying screens should be examined for cleanliness and scratches. Debris present on the screens will block the light given off by the crystals and result in radiopaque artifacts on the resultant radiographic image. Screens may be carefully cleaned as needed with solutions recommended by the manufacturer. However, overuse of chemical cleaning may cause scratches and should be avoided. A scratched or damaged screen will not produce the light needed to expose the film and will result in radiopaque artifacts.

Grids

Grids are sometimes used in extraoral radiography to absorb scattered x-rays that contribute to film fog that reduces image constrast (Figure 27–8). Radiation that strikes the patient's tissues has the potential to be deflected back toward the film, reexposing it. A **grid** is a mechanical device composed of thin strips of lead alternating with a radiolucent material (usually plastic). The grid is placed between the patient and the film in order to absorb scattered x-rays and reduce film fog to improve image contrast. However, the use of a grid requires an increased dose of radiation, usually double the dose of radiation required when not using a grid. The use of a grid with its increased radiation dose to the patient must be carefully weighed against the diagnostic benefits. For example, when exposing radiographs to assess growth and development, a grid may be contraindicated. However, when evaluating the extent of a tumor, the increased image contrast obtained by using a grid may be justified.

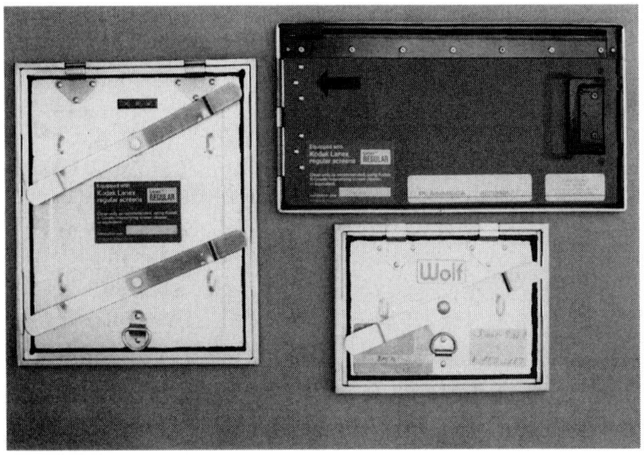

FIGURE 27-7 **The back side of three rigid cassettes of various sizes.**

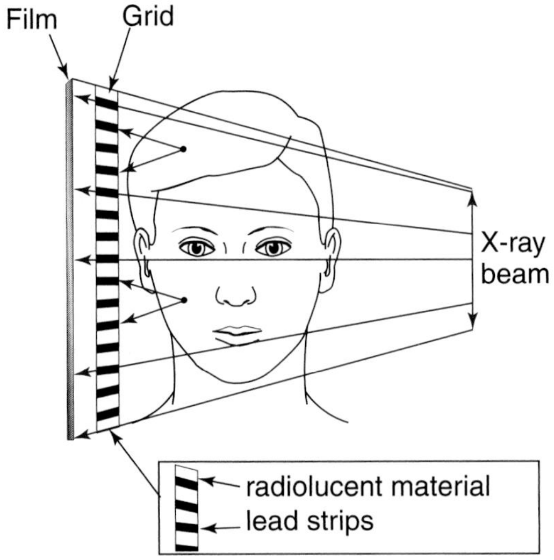

FIGURE 27-8 **Grid used to absorb back scattered radiation.** A device placed between the patient and the film that absorbs scattered x-rays to reduce film fog.

Film Identification

Extraoral films do not have the embossed identification dot that intraoral films have to aid in identifying the left and right sides of the image. Extraoral films are best identified by fastening an identification letter or plate to one of the corners of the front of the cassette. Special lettering sets, made of lead, are available for this purpose. The letters R (for right) and L (for left) can be placed on the front of the cassette prior to exposure. These identifications become visible on the processed radiograph. Identification plates can be used to image the patient's name and date of exposure directly on the film. Commercial film identification imprinters are available that permanently image pertinent data on the processed film (Figure 27–9).

Exposure Factors

The exposure factors for extraoral techniques vary considerably. The settings depend largely on the intensifying screen–film combination, which plays a similar role to intraoral film speed in determining appropriate exposure settings. The patient's size and tissue density and the target–film distance also must be considered. Refer to the x-ray equipment and film and screen manufacturers' recommendations to determine appropriate mA, kVp and impulse settings.

Extraoral Radiographic Techniques

There are many techniques for exposing radiographs of the head and face. It is not within the scope of this book to describe every available technique. The seven projections discussed in this chapter are the most common extraoral radiographs in which the x-ray source and the film receptor remain still and in position during exposure. The panoramic radiograph, which requires movement of the x-ray source and the film during exposure, is discussed in Chapter 28. The following extraoral projections will be presented here: (1) lateral jaw (mandibular oblique lateral); (2) lateral cephalometric (lateral skull); (3) posteroanterior cephalometric (PA); (4) Waters (sinus); (5) reverse-Towne (open mouth); (6) submentovertex (base); and (7) transcranial (TMJ).

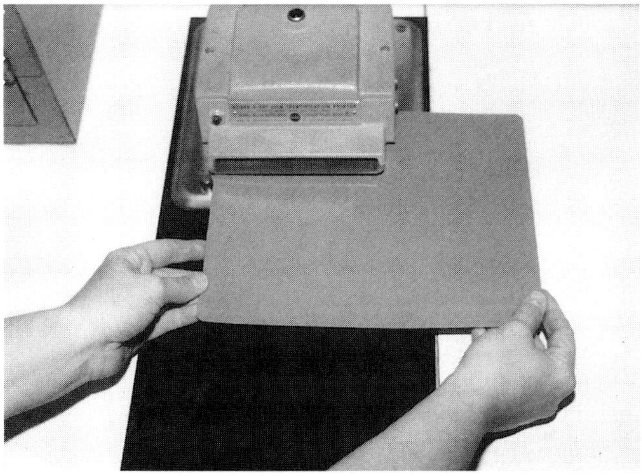

FIGURE 27-9 **Film identification printer** for imprinting permanent identification information on the radiographic image.

Lateral Jaw Radiograph (Mandibular Oblique Lateral Projection)

The **lateral jaw projection** (Figure 27–10), also known as the **mandibular oblique lateral projection,** is the most common extraoral radiograph made with a conventional x-ray unit used for exposing intraoral films. Lateral jaw projections have been largely replaced by **panoramic radiographs,** but are still taken when greater image detail is needed or when panoramic equipment is not available.

Purpose

The lateral jaw radiograph is used to examine the posterior region of the mandible. It is especially valuable to use with children (Figures 27–10 and 27–11), with patients who have fractures or swelling, and with patients who are unable to tolerate placement or hold intraoral films in place. The lateral jaw radiograph is often made to evaluate the condition of the bone and to locate impacted teeth or large lesions.

Film Placement

The cassette is positioned flat against the cheek and centered over the mandibular first molar area (Figure 27–12.) The front edge of the cassette should protrude slightly beyond the tip of the nose and the chin. The patient presses the tube side of the cassette firmly against the cheek with the palm of one hand and the thumb is placed under the lower edge of the cassette.

Head Position

The head is tilted (about 10 to 20 degrees) toward the side to be examined and the chin is protruded. This helps to move the side that is not being imaged up and out of the way to avoid superimposition of the left and right sides.

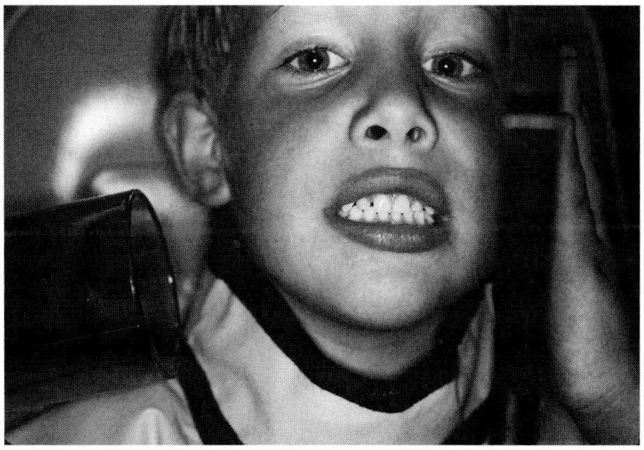

FIGURE 27-10 **Lateral jaw radiograph being exposed on a child.**

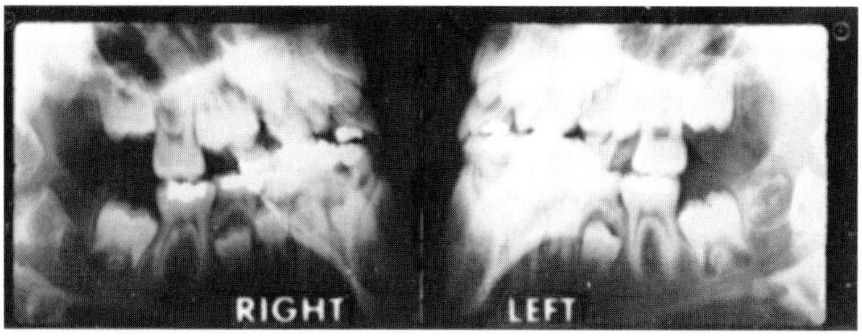

FIGURE 27-11 **Lateral jaw radiograph of a child with a mixed dentition.**

Central Ray Alignment

The central ray is directed toward the first molar region of the mandible from a point slightly underneath the opposite side of the mandible (Figure 27–12). The central ray should be directed as close to perpendicular to the horizontal plane of the film as possible. Figure 27–13 shows four possible centers of interest on the radiograph; the ramus area, the molars, the premolars, and the incisors. To change the center of interest, one varies the angle at which the film is held against the face and the direction of the central ray. The beam of radiation is directed perpendicularly to the desired area, usually at the level of the occlusal plane. Before making the exposure, ask the patient to thrust the mandible forward so that the vertebrae will not be superimposed on the mandibular structures.

Lateral Cephalometric Radiograph (Lateral Skull)

Cephalometric radiographs may be either lateral skull projections (Figure 27–14) or frontal (posteroanterior) (Figure 27–15). The word "cephalometric" means measurement of the head. Cephalometric radiographs are made by placing the patient's head in a **cephalometer.** The cephalometer is a device used to standardize the placement of the head during exposure for a series of identical exposures. Most orthodontists require cephalometric radiographs before treatment, at various stages of treatment, upon completion of treatment, and often as a follow-up procedure. Either conventional x-ray machines modified for cephalometric exposures or special units may be used (Figure 27–16). Devices called **cephalostats** stabilize the patient's head parallel to the film and at right angles to the direction of the beam of radiation. The cassette with intensifying screen is aligned in a definite relationship to the cephalostat so that the patient's head is between it and the source of radiation.

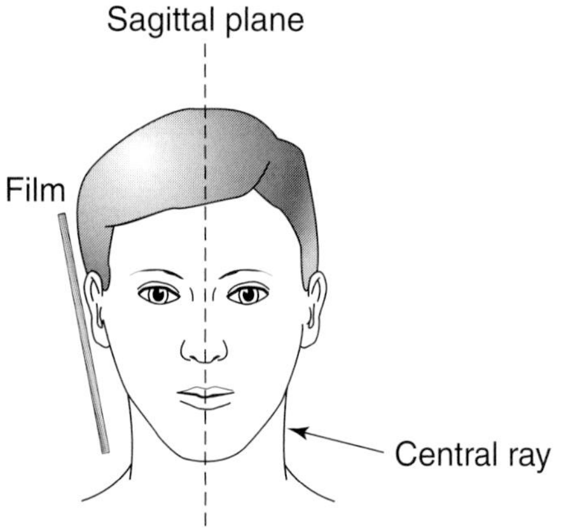

FIGURE 27-12 **Lateral jaw technique.** Note that the central ray is directed at the cassette slightly underneath the opposite side of the mandible.

The lateral cephalometric radiograph, also called a lateral skull projection, shows the entire skull from the side. It is so named because the x-ray beam passes through the skull from side (lateral) to side (Figure 27–17).

Purpose

The purpose of the lateral skull cephalometric projection is to evaluate growth and development, trauma, pathology, and developmental abnormalities. It also reveals the facial soft tissue profile when a filter is placed between the tube and the patient to remove some of the x-rays to enhance the image of the soft tissue profile of the face. It is the projection most often used by orthodontists. Prosthodontists and oral surgeons use lateral cephalometric radiographs to establish pre-treatment and post-treatment records.

Film Placement

An 8 × 10 in. (21 × 26 cm) cassette is positioned vertically in a holding device.

Head Position

The head is positioned with the left side of the face next to the cassette. The midsagittal plane is parallel to the cassette. Ear rods attached to the cephalostat are used to stabilize the patient's head (Figure 27–14).

Facial Soft-tissue Profile

If a facial soft tissue profile is desired, a wedge filter is placed over the anterior side of the beam at the tube head. The filter absorbs some of the x-rays in the anterior region and results in the soft tissue outline of the patient's face on the radiograph (Figure 27–1).

Central Ray Alignment

The central ray is directed toward the **acoustic meatus** (opening of the ear) and perpendicularly toward the center of the film (Figure 27–18).

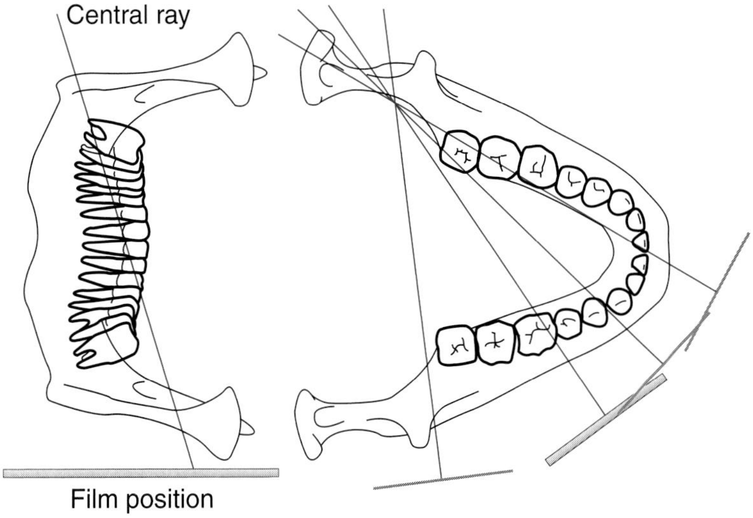

FIGURE 27-13 **X-ray beam direction for the lateral jaw projection.** X-rays strike the film obliquely in the vertical plane but should be perpendicular in the horizontal plane. A true lateral projection of an entire side of the jaw is not possible because the image of the opposite side would be superimposed on it. The lateral jaw projection must be made with some oblique angulation. The beam of radiation can be directed toward the area of interest from two basic directions-underneath the mandible opposite the side being radiographed or behind the mandible opposite the side being radiographed. (Reproduced with permission from Wuehrmann, A. H. & Manson-Hing, L. R. *Dental Radiology,* 5th ed. St. Louis: Mosby, 1981)

Posteroanterior Cephalometric Radiograph (PA Projection)

The posteroanterior radiograph or (PA projection) shows the entire skull in the posteroanterior plane. The PA cephalometric radiograph is so named because the x-ray beam passes through the skull in a posterior-to-anterior direction.

Purpose

The purpose of the PA cephalometric projection is to examine facial growth and development, disease, trauma, and developmental abnormalities. Because the right and left sides of the bony and facial structures are not superimposed on each other, this survey is often used to supplement the lateral survey.

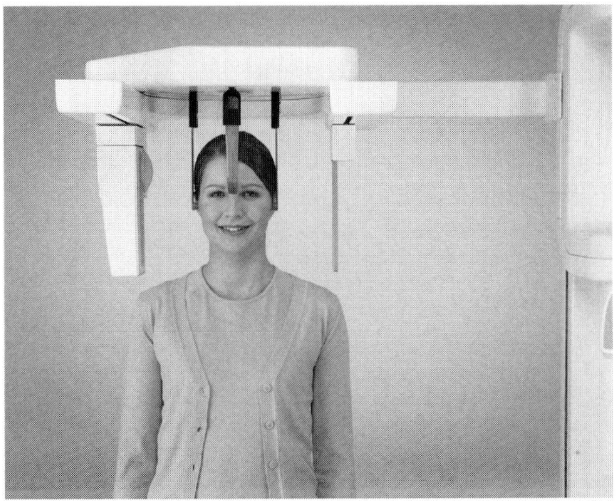

FIGURE 27-14 **Patient positioned for a lateral cephalometric radiograph.** A cephalostat is used to position the head to achieve standardization and to establish a fixed relationship among the x-ray tube, the patient's head, and the film cassette. Ear rods are used to stabilize and maintain the head position. The central ray passes through both ear rods from the target–film distance of 60 in. (1.52 m) or more. (Courtesy of Planmeca)

Film Placement

An 8 × 10-inch (21 × 26-cm) cassette with intensifying screen is held in position vertically by a holding device.

Head Position

The patient faces the cassette. The patient's head is centered in front of the cassette so that the forehead and nose touch the face of the cassette (Figure 27–19).

Central Ray Alignment

The central ray is directed perpendicular to the film toward the **occipital protuberance** (the large bump that can be felt by palpating the occipital bone near the base of the skull) (Figure 27–19).

Waters Radiograph (Sinus Projection)

The **Waters radiograph** is also known as the **sinus projection.** It is similar to the posteroanterior cephalometric radiograph except

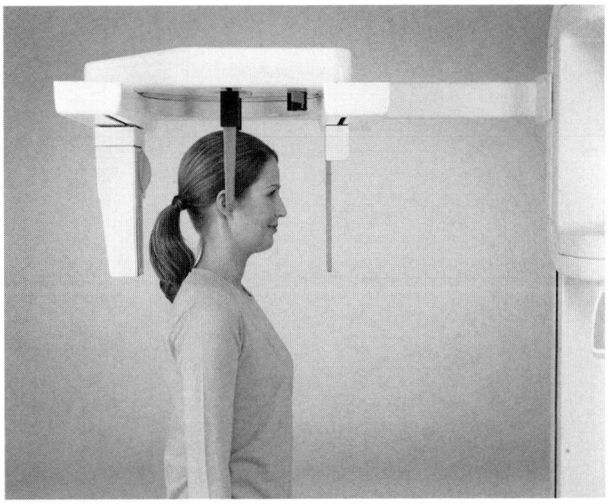

FIGURE 27-15 **Patient positioned for posterior-anterior (frontal) radiograph.** (Courtesy of Planmeca)

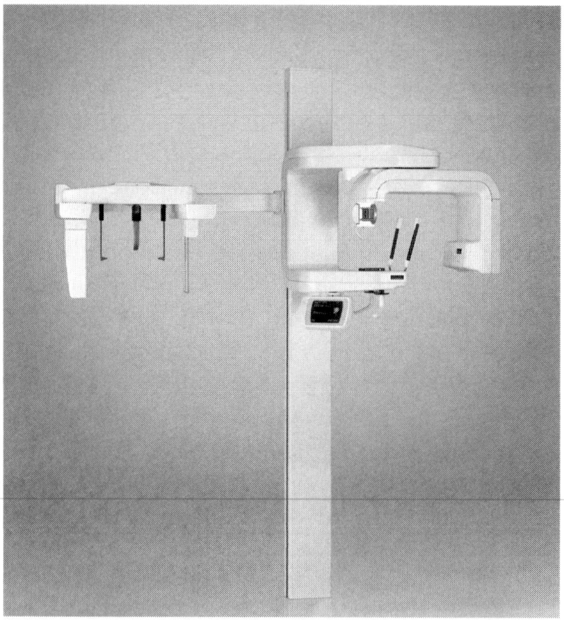

FIGURE 27-16 **A combination panoramic and cephalometric dental x-ray unit.** (Courtesy of Planmeca)

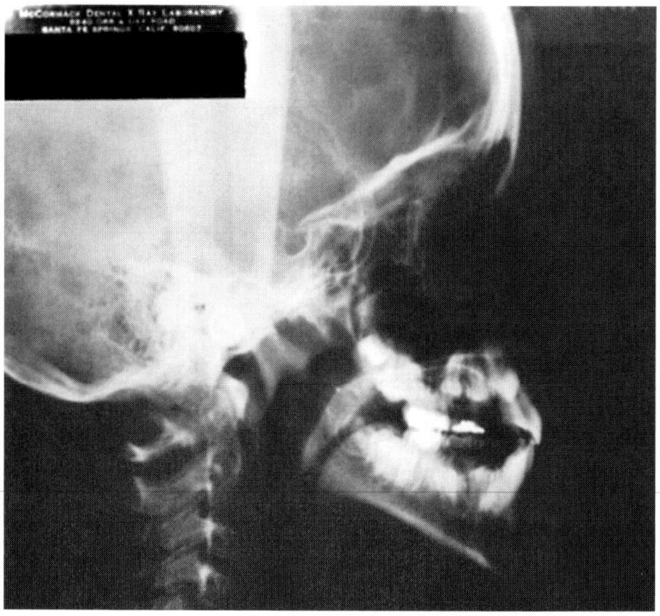

FIGURE 27-17 **Lateral cephalometric radiograph.** (Courtesy of McCormack Dental X-ray Laboratory)

that the center of interest is focused on the middle third of the face (Figure 27–20).

Purpose

The Waters radiograph is particularly useful to evaluate the maxillary, frontal, and ethmoid sinuses.

Film Placement

An 8 × 10 inch (21 × 26 cm) cassette with intensifying screen is held in position vertically by a holding device.

Head Position

The patient faces the cassette. The patient's head is centered on the cassette with the mid-sagittal plane perpendicular to the floor. The chin touches the cassette and the nose is positioned about 0.75 in. (18 mm) from the cassette.

Central Ray Alignment

As in the posteroanterior cephalometric radiograph, the central ray is directed perpendicular to the center of the film through the occipital protuberance. The target–film distance is usually a minimum of 36 in. (0.9 m) (Figure 27–19).

Reverse-Towne Radiograph (Open Mouth Projection)

Purpose

The **Reverse-Towne radiograph**, also referred to as an **open mouth projection**, is used to examine fractures of the condylar neck of the mandible (Figure 27–21).

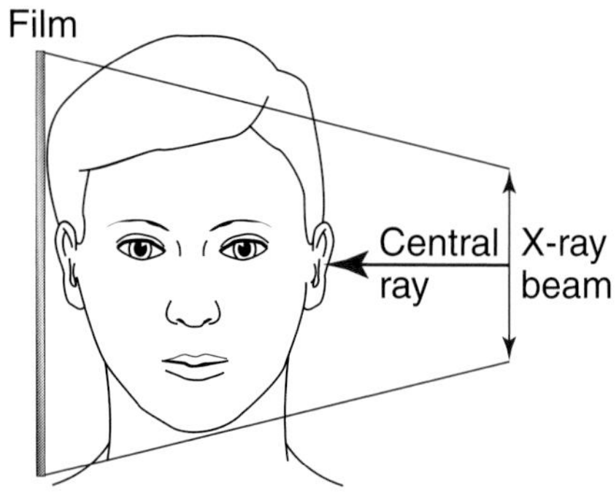

FIGURE 27-18 **Lateral cephalometric technique.** The central ray is directed at 0 degree vertical angulation through the acoustic meatus of the ear and perpendicular to the cassette.

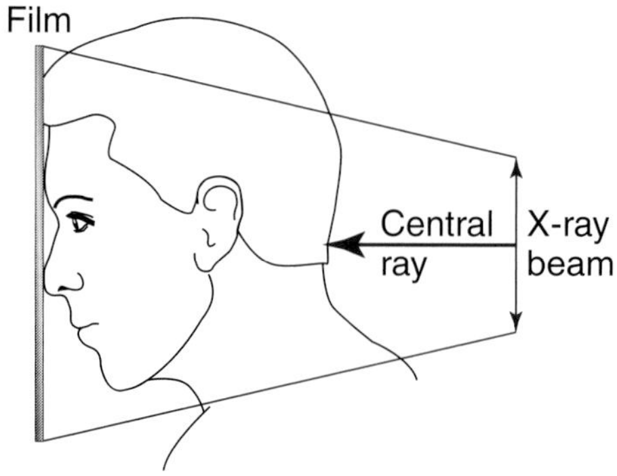

FIGURE 27-19 **Posteroanterior cephalometric technique.** The nose and forehead touch the cassette. The central ray is directed at the occipital protuberance at a vertical angulation of 0 degrees and perpendicular to the cassette.

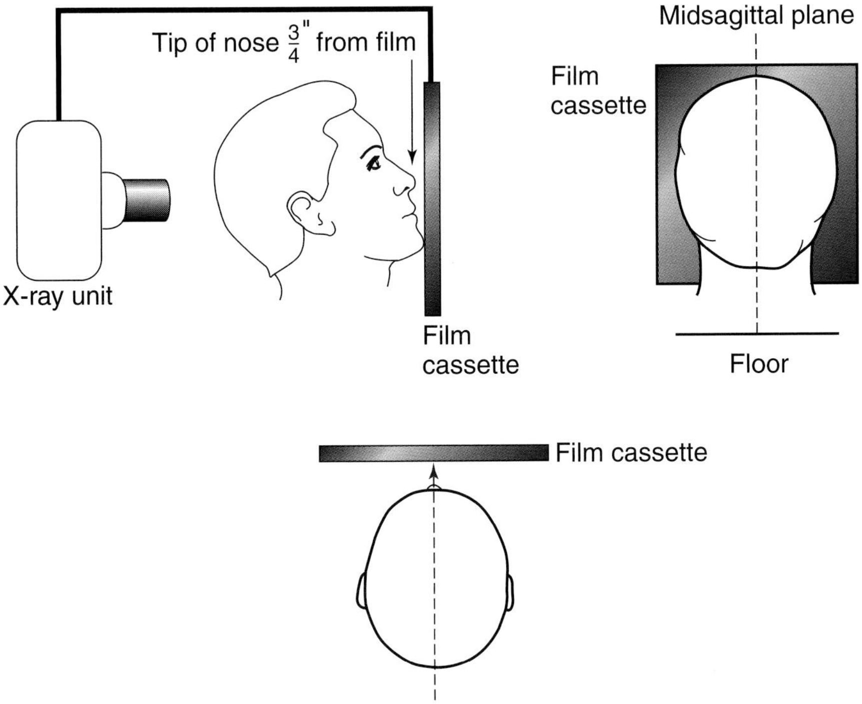

FIGURE 27-20 **Waters technique.** The chin touches the cassette and the nose is positioned about 0.75 in. (18 mm) from the cassette. The central ray is directed perpendicular to the center of the cassette through the occipital protuberance.

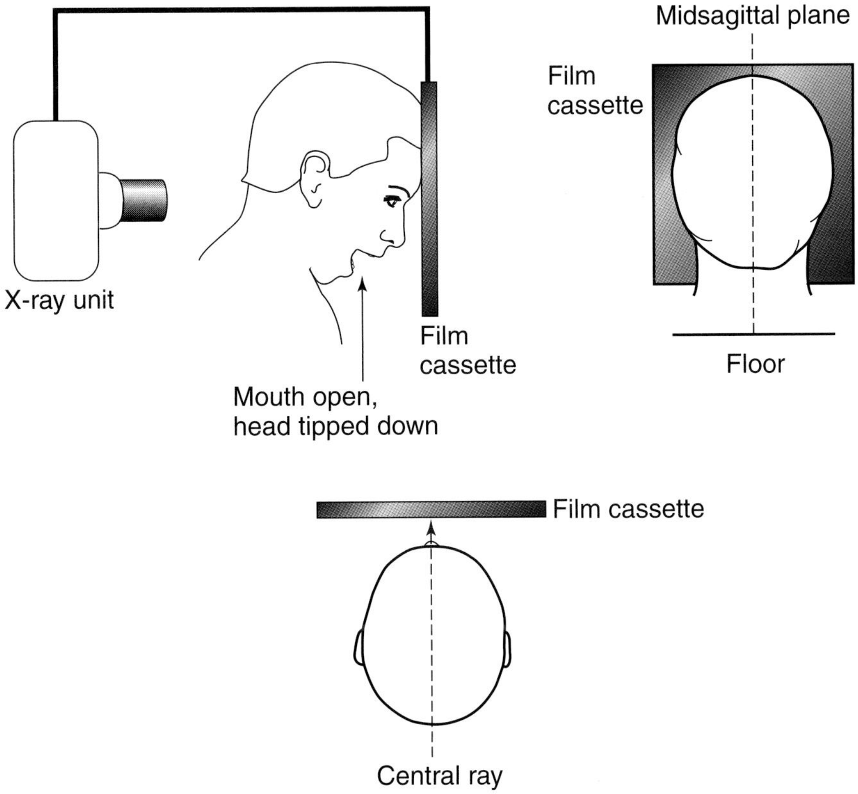

FIGURE 27-21 **Reverse-Towne projection.** The patient faces the cassette with the midsagittal plane perpendicular to the floor. With the mouth wide open, the patient's head is tipped down until the chin touches the chest. The top of the forehead rests against the cassette.

Film Placement

An 8 × 10 inch (21 × 26 cm) cassette with intensifying screen is held in position vertically by a holding device.

Head Position

The patient faces the cassette with the midsagittal plane perpendicular to the floor. With the mouth wide open, the patient's head is tipped down until the chin touches the chest. The top of the forehead rests against the cassette.

Central Ray Alignment

The central ray is directed perpendicular to the center of the film through the occipital protuberance. The target–film distance is usually a minimum of 36 in. (0.9 m) (Figure 27–21).

Submentovertex Radiograph (Base Projection)

Purpose

The **submentovertex radiograph** is used to show the base of the skull (**base projection**), the position and orientation of the condyles, the sphenoid sinus, and fractures of the zygomatic arch (Figure 27–22).

Film Placement

An 8 × 10 in. (21 × 26 cm) cassette with intensifying screen is held in position vertically by a holding device.

Head Position

The patient's head and neck are extended backward so the vertex (top) of the head touches the center of the cassette. The midsagittal plane is perpendicular to the floor. The **Frankfort plane** (see Figure 28–14) is vertical and parallel with the film.

Central Ray Alignment

The central ray is directed perpendicular to the film from below the mandible through the center of the head (Figure 27–22).

Transcranial Radiograph (TMJ projection)

Purpose

The transcranial radiograph (TMJ projection) aids in diagnosing **ankylosis** (a stiffening of the temporomandibular joint caused by fibrous or bony union), malignancies, fractures, and tissue changes caused by arthritis. A radiograph, or series of radiographs, showing the TMJ in both open and closed positions is essential for diagnosis.

The **temporomandibular joint (TMJ)** is very difficult to examine radiographically because the head of the mandibular **condyle** articulates with the **glenoid fossa** in an area where the structure of the temporal bone is extremely dense. There are several ways to take a transcranial radiograph. As the area to be examined is relatively small, a common practice is to take several exposures on one large film. Sections of the film are covered with lead so that only one part of the film is exposed each time. Thus three or four exposures, with the head of the condyle in a different position each time, can be made consecutively on the same film (Figure 27–23).

Film Placement

An 8 × 10 inch (21 × 26 cm) cassette with intensifying screen is held in position against the ear and centered over the acoustic meatus (opening of the ear) (Figure 27–24).

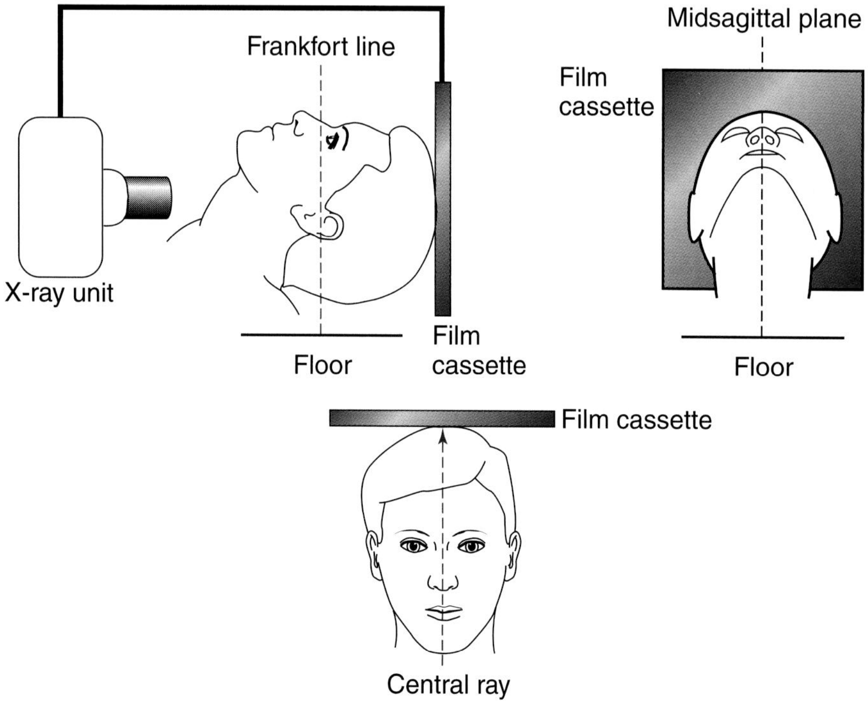

FIGURE 27–22 **Submentovertex projection.** The patient's head and neck are extended backward so the vertex (top) of the head touches the center of the cassette. The midsagittal plane is perpendicular to the floor. The Frankfort line is vertical and parallel with the film.

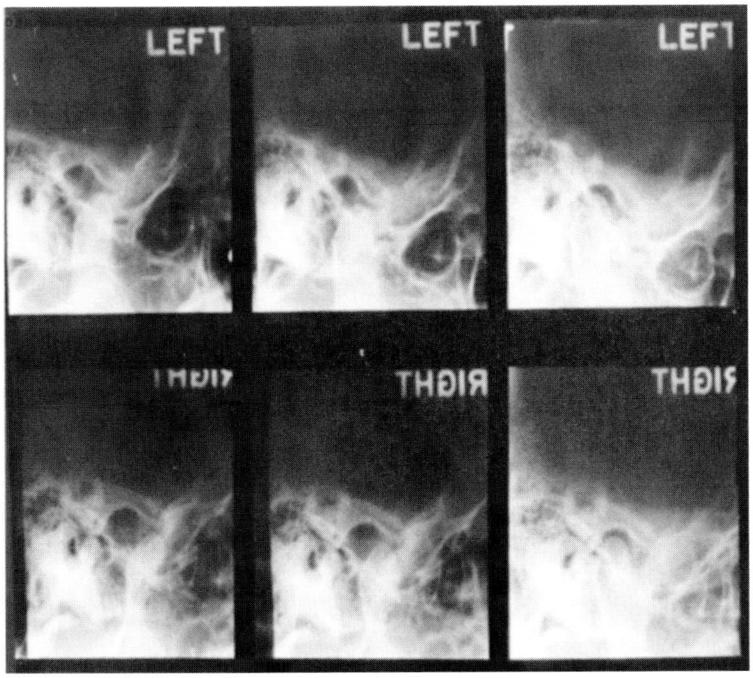

FIGURE 27-23 **Serial radiographs of the temporomandibular joint** showing the head of the condyle in the glenoid fossa with the mouth closed, in the at-rest position, and with the mouth open. (Courtesy of McCormack Dental X-ray Laboratory)

Head Position

The midsagittal plane of the patient's head is positioned perpendicular to the floor and parallel to the cassette.

Central Ray Alignment

Exposures are often made with the mouth closed and the teeth in occlusion, at rest with the teeth slightly separated, and with the mouth fully open (Figure 27–23). Because the transcranial projection is made from the opposite side, the central ray has to pass first through a series of bones and soft structures. Therefore, the exposure requires extreme care and accuracy in adjusting the cassette to the head position and directing the PID so that the x-rays will strike the film at the best angle.

The central ray should be directed toward the center of that part of the film not covered with lead at +25 degrees vertical angulation. The point of entry for the central ray is located about 2 1/2 in. (6.4 cm) higher and slightly in front of the acoustic meatus (opening of the ear).

The disadvantage of this technique is that it is difficult to stabilize the patient's head and prevent movement. Moreover, without special equipment, it is difficult to repeat the exposure and get identical results. Better results are often obtained through the use of **tomography**, a technology in which the x-ray source and film–screen combination move in relationship to each other (Figure 27–25). Panoramic radiography is based on the principles of tomography discussed in Chapter 28.

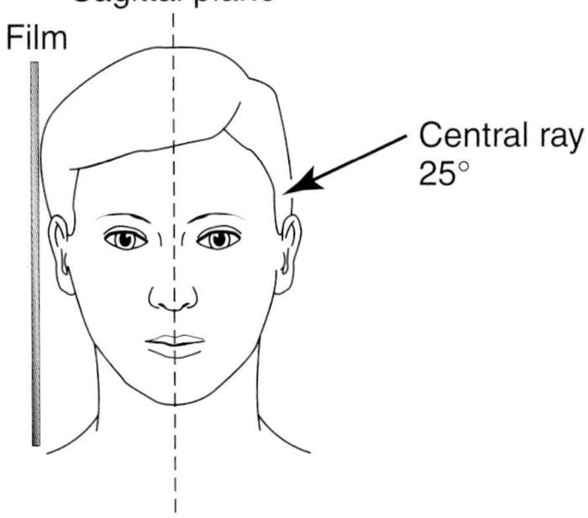

FIGURE 27-24 **Transcranial technique.** The central ray is directed at a vertical angulation of about +25 degrees to the center of the film not covered by lead. The point of entry is located about 2.5 in. (6.4 cm) higher and slightly in front of the acoustic meatus of the ear.

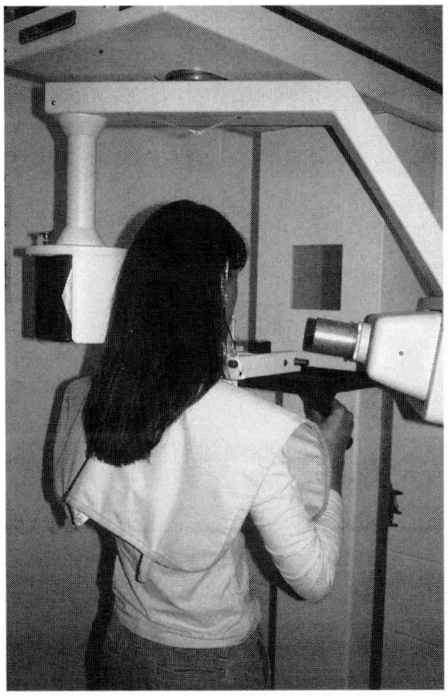

FIGURE 27-25 **A combination panoramic and TMJ imaging dental x-ray unit.**

REVIEW—Chapter Summary

Extraoral radiographs image large areas of the head and facial regions. Extraoral films are useful in examination of large areas of the jaws and skull; to study growth and development of bone and teeth; in the detection of fractures, pathological lesions, and diseases of the jaws; in assessment of impacted teeth; and in evaluation of temporomandibular disorders (TMD). Orthodontists, prosthodontists, and oral surgeons are major users of extraoral films.

Extraoral screen film is used in conjunction with a pair of intensifying screens housed in a light-tight cassette. Extraoral film is more sensitive than intraoral film. Careful handling of the film is needed to avoid static electricity and glove powder artifacts.

Intensifying screens transfer x-ray energy into visible light that in turn exposes screen film to produce an image. Intensifying screens intensify the effect of x-rays on the film resulting in a reduced dose of radiation required to produce an image.

Faster speed intensifying screens have larger sized fluorescent crystals (phosphors) and thicker emulsion, but a slightly less sharp image. Rare earth phosphor screens are faster than calcium tungstate screens. Rare earth screens emit green light and must be paired with green-light–sensitive film. Calcium tungstate screens emit blue light and must be paired with blue-light–sensitive film. The use of fast speed screen–film combinations is recommended to produce acceptable images at a reduced radiation dose to the patient.

Cassettes hold the intensifying screens in close contact with the film in a light-tight rigid case or a flexible plastic sleeve. Cassettes and intensifying screens should be examined periodically to ensure optimum performance. Dirty or scratched screens will result in radiopaque artifacts that compromise the radiographic image.

Grids are devices used to absorb scatter radiation that will fog the film and compromise image contrast. The use of grids requires increased radiation exposure and so they are not usually recommended with extraoral images used to assess growth and development.

Special lettering sets or commercial film imprinters are used to label and identify extraoral film. Exposure settings for extraoral techniques depend on the intensifying screen–film combination used, the patient's size and tissue density, and the target–film distance.

The purpose and technique for exposing the following extraoral radiographs are presented: lateral jaw (mandibular oblique), lateral cephalometric (lateral skull), posteroanterior cephalometric (PA), Waters (sinus), Reverse-Towne (open mouth) submentovertex (base) and transcranial (TMJ).

RECALL—Study Questions

1. For which of these purposes are extraoral radiographs least suitable?
   a. For detection of interproximal caries
   b. For locating impacted teeth
   c. For viewing the sinuses
   d. For determining the extent of a fracture
2. Which of these surveys is most frequently ordered by the orthodontist?
   a. Transcranial
   b. Lateral cephalometric
   c. Waters
   d. Reverse-Towne
3. The general practitioner is most likely to use which of these extraoral radiographs?
   a. Posteroanterior cephalometric
   b. Reverse-Towne
   c. Panoramic
   d. Submentovertex
4. What size film is generally used in cephalometric radiography?
   a. 5×7 in. (13×18 cm)
   b. 8×10 in. (20×25 cm)
   c. 5×12 in. (13×30 cm)
   d. 6×12 in. (15×30 mm)
5. Black artifacts on extraoral films may result from each of the following *except* one. Which one is this *exception?*
   a. Static electricity
   b. Glove powder residue
   c. Rapidly removing films from the packaging
   d. Scratched intensifying screens
6. Intensifying screens will:
   a. Increase x-ray intensity.
   b. Increase image detail.
   c. Reduce exposure time.
   d. Decrease processing time.
7. What term describes the crystals used in the emulsion of intensifying screens?
   a. Phosphors
   b. Halides
   c. Sulfates
   d. Bromides
8. Fast intensifying screens have ____________ sized crystals and ____________ thickness of emulsion.
   a. large, decreased
   b. large, increased
   c. small, decreased
   d. small, increased
9. Rare-earth intensifying screens require less radiation to produce a quality image. Rare-earth intensifying screens emit blue light when energized by x-radiation.
   a. The first statement is correct. The second statement is incorrect.
   b. The first statement is incorrect. The second statement is correct.
   c. Both statements are correct.
   d. Both statements are incorrect.
10. Unsharp (blurry) images result from which of the following?
    a. Film and screens not in close contact.
    b. Faulty (not tight) hinge on rigid cassette.
    c. Not closing the cassette tightly.
    d. All of the above.
11. Which of these radiographs would best image an impacted mandibular third molar?
    a. Lateral cephalometric
    b. Bitewing
    c. Lateral jaw
    d. Reverse-Towne

12. Which of these radiographs would best image the maxillary sinus?
    a. Transcranial
    b. Waters
    c. Periapical
    d. Posteroanterior cephalometric
13. "The patient presses the tube side of the cassette firmly against the cheek, centered over the mandibular first molar area. The front edge of the cassette protrudes slightly beyond the tip of the nose and the chin." This describes the film placement for which of these radiographs?
    a. Submentovertex
    b. Lateral jaw
    c. Posteroanterior cephalometric
    d. Waters

REFLECT—Case Study

Consider the following patients and conditions. Which of the seven extraoral radiographs described in this chapter might be the *best* recommendation for these cases? (*Note:* Radiographs of the skull are difficult to interpret due to the numerous structures that exist in a very small area. These structures often appear superimposed over each other, requiring multiple views to obtain a good diagnosis. Therefore, in some of these cases, while there is usually a *best* answer, there may be more than one correct answer.)

1. A 20-year-old patient presents with pain and swelling from an impacted third molar. The patient can open only 10 mm. No panoramic unit is available. What is an alternate extraoral projection type that can be used to assess with diagnosis for this patient?
2. A 13-year-old patient presents for an orthodontic consultation. Occlusal (teeth) and facial disharmonies (soft tissue relationships) need to be assessed prior to treatment intervention.
3. A difficult extraction case presents with a severely decayed maxillary molar. During the extraction procedure, the root tip fractures and is possibly lost in the ethmoid sinus.
4. A medically compromised patient suffered a seizure and fell. A fractured mandibular condyle is suspected.
5. A 69-year-old patient presents with a history of degenerative joint disease that may be affecting the temporal mandibular joint. An examination for the purpose of diagnosing ankylosis (a stiffening of the TMJ) is planned.
6. A patient presents for extraction of several badly decayed teeth, following which the prosthodontist will construct a maxillary full denture and a mandibular partial denture for the patient.

RELATE—Laboratory Application

Because intensifying screens fluoresce visible light when energized by x-radiation, you can perform this experiment to confirm what types of intensifying screens are available for use at your facility:

Open the cassette to expose the intensifying screens and place on the counter or operatory chair, face up. No film is needed. Place the x-ray tube head directly over the opened cassette and aim the PID so that x-rays will strike the exposed intensifying screens. Set the exposure factors on the x-ray machine to the recommended settings for posterior molar periapicals. Then increase the exposure time significantly, to a full second, for example. Stand at least six feet away from the tube head at a 90- to 135-degree angle (see Figure 3–7) or remain behind a barrier that allows visual contact with the screens during the exposure (see Figure 3–6). Depress the exposure button and observe the intensifying screens. Make note of the color, either blue or green, of the light emitted during exposure. Match the color observed with what you learned about calcium tungstate screens and rare-earth screens.

Next, perform an inventory on the extraoral films available for use at your facility. Does the film, either blue-light–sensitive or green-light–sensitive, match the screens? Use the information learned in this chapter to explain why this is important.

BIBLIOGRAPHY

Farman, A. G., Nortje, C. J., & Wood, R. E. *Oral and Maxillofacial Diagnostic Imaging.* St. Louis: Mosby, 1993.

White, S. C. & Pharoah, M. J. *Oral Radiology Principles and Interpretation,* 5th ed. St. Louis: Elsevier, 2004.

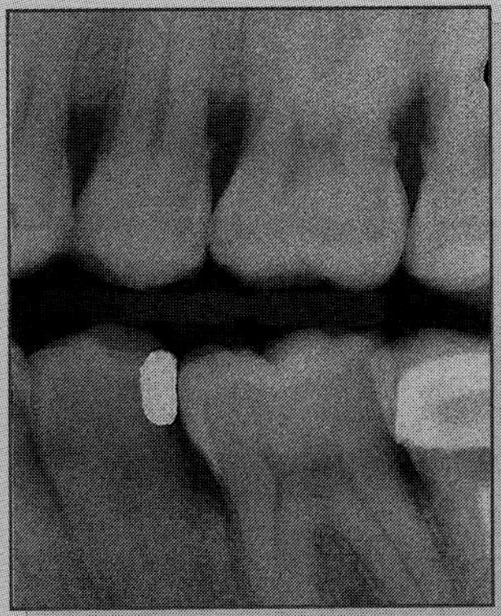

28

Panoramic Radiography

■ OBJECTIVES

Following successful completion of this chapter, you should be able to:

1. Define the key words.
2. State the purpose and use of panoramic radiography.
3. Compare the advantages and disadvantages of panoramic versus intraoral radiographic surveys.
4. Explain the principle of tomography.
5. Differentiate between a conventional intraoral x-ray unit and a panoramic x-ray machine.
6. Explain the concept of the focal trough.
7. Identify the three dimensions of the focal trough.
8. List the four basic components common to most panoramic x-ray machines.
9. Identify the planes used to position the arches correctly within the focal trough.
10. Match the head-positioning errors with the characteristic appearances that image on the panoramic radiograph.
11. List patient preparation errors and describe the appearance that results on the panoramic radiograph.
12. List exposure and film handling errors and describe the appearance that results on the panoramic radiograph.
13. List and identify the anatomic landmarks of the maxilla and surrounding tissues as viewed on a panoramic radiograph.
14. List and identify the anatomic landmarks of the mandible and surrounding tissues as viewed on a panoramic radiograph.
15. List and identify soft tissue images as viewed on a panoramic radiograph.
16. List and identify three air space images as viewed on a panoramic radiograph.
17. List and identify machine part artifacts as viewed on a panoramic radiograph.
18. List and identify ghost image artifacts as viewed on a panoramic radiograph.
19. Identify in sequence the basic steps in operating a panoramic x-ray unit.

■ KEY WORDS

Ala-tragus line
Cassette holder (drum)
Focal trough
Frankfort plane
Ghost image
Glossopharyngeal air space
Head positioner guides
Midsagittal plane
Nasopharyngeal air space
Negative shadows
Palatoglossal air space
Panoramic
Panoramic radiography
Rotational center
Rotational panoramic radiography
Split image
Tomographs
Tomography

Introduction

The panoramic radiograph is probably the most common extraoral projection used in general oral health care practice. **Panoramic radiography** refers to a technique for producing a broad view image of both the maxilla and mandible on a single radiograph. Placing an elongated screen film varying in width from 5 to 6 in. wide and 12 in. long (13 to 15 cm wide and 30 cm long) in a rigid or flexible cassette that is positioned extraorally will produce an image of the entire dentition, the surrounding alveolar bone, the sinuses, and the temporomandibular joints on a single film (Figure 28–1).

The purpose of this chapter is to explain the fundamental concepts of panoramic radiography and to describe the operational procedures of panoramic x-ray machines. Normal anatomy of the maxilla and mandible, soft tissue images, and air space images are also presented.

Purpose and Use

The term **panoramic** means "wide view." Panoramic radiography is descriptive of the wide view of the maxilla and mandible produced on a single film. Panoramic radiographs play a valuable role in:

- Examining large areas of the face and jaws.
- Locating impacted teeth or retained root tips.
- Evaluating trauma, lesions, and diseases of the jaws.
- Assessing growth and development.

Panoramic image quality has improved over the last 15 years suggesting that panoramic radiographs may aid in the evaluation of large caries and moderate periodontal diseases. However, panoramic imagery is not as sharp and detailed as the images produced by intraoral radiographs. When specific conditions or diseases are suspected, intraoral radiographs are often prescribed in conjunction with panoramic radiographs (see Table 6–1).

Advantages and Disadvantages of Panoramic Radiography

The greatest advantage of panoramic radiographs is that they image a greater area and provide an increased amount of diagnostic information when compared to a full mouth series of individual films with a reduced amount of radiation dose to the patient (Table 28–1). Additionally, the broad image produced by a panoramic radiograph is easy for patients to understand, aiding in the explanation of the diagnosis and the proposed

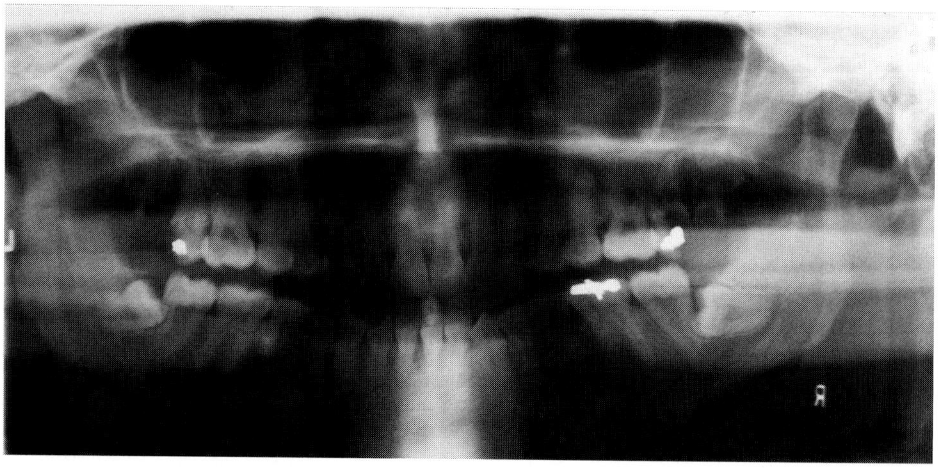

FIGURE 28–1 **Panoramic radiograph.** Provides a broad view of the dental arches. Note, however, the inherent image distortion as the panoramic view broadens the arches.

Table 28–1 Advantages and Disadvantages of Panoramic Radiographs

Advantages

- Increased coverage of supporting structures of the oral cavity.
- Reduced patient radiation dose over an intraoral full mouth series of radiographs.
- Can be performed in less time than the exposure of a full mouth series of radiographs.
- Simple procedure to perform.
- Minimal patient discomfort.
- May be performed on patients who can not tolerate placement of an intraoral film packet.
- Requires minimal patient instruction and cooperation.
- Infection control protocol minimized.
- Mounting time is eliminated.
- Aids in explaining treatment plan to patients.

Disadvantages

- Increased image distortion.
- Reduced image sharpness.
- The amount of vertical and horizontal distortion is not constant—it varies from one part of the radiograph to another.
- Increased occurrence of overlapping of the proximal contact areas, especially in the premolar region.
- Focal trough size and shape limits imagery to only those structures which "fit" into the image layer. Teeth with labial or lingual tilting may not image well.
- The size and shape of the focal trough is pre-determined by the manufacturer, therefore not all patients will image equally as well.
- Superimposition of structures (e.g., the spinal column) may make interpretation difficult.
- Soft tissue shadows present on the resulting image may mimic pathology.
- Ghost images present on the resulting image may hide pathology.
- Not useful in detecting incipient carious lesions.
- Not useful in detecting early periodontal changes.
- Simple procedure may be overused inappropriately.
- Length of exposure time may limit its use on young children and other patients who cannot remain still throughout the exposure cycle
- Cost of panoramic unit is significant.

treatment plan in a manner that is clear and understandable. Panoramic procedures are relatively easy to perform, requiring less time than a full mouth series. The simple procedure demands less patient cooperation and because the film is not placed intraorally, there is less discomfort, making the panoramic procedure an acceptable substitute, under certain conditions, for patients who can not tolerate intraoral procedures. Because of the relative ease with which panoramic radiograph may be obtained, there may be a tendency to overuse this diagnostic tool. It is important to note that research on the use of panoramic radiographs cautions against using panoramic images as a screening film for occult disease (diseases that may exist without signs or symptoms).

The greatest limitation of panoramic radiographs is image quality. Magnification, distortion, and poor definition are inherent with panoramic techniques. **Ghost images, negative shadows,** and other artifacts can make interpreting panoramic images difficult. Further compromising the ability to obtain quality images is the difficulty associated with positioning the patient within the **focal trough** (area of image sharpness). Manufacturers design panoramic x-ray machines to be able to image the average patient. However, patients whose dental arches do not fall into this average range may be more difficult to image.

Fundamentals of Panoramic Radiography

Panoramic radiography is based on the principle of **tomography**. Tomography is a special radiographic technique used to show images of structures located within a selected plane of tissue, while blurring structures outside the selected plane. Tomography produces images by utilizing a narrow beam of x-rays to image a curved layer or slice of tissue. Radiographs made using the tomography technique are called **tomographs.** A familiar medical tomograph is a CT scan (computed tomograph). Tomographic x-ray equipment is often utilized for imaging temporomandibular disorder (TMD).

During intraoral and conventional extraoral radiography (see Chapter 27), the x-ray source and the film remain stationary. During tomography and **rotational panoramic radiography,** the x-ray source and film move in relationship to each other to focus the x-ray beam on a select layer of interest while blurring out structures not located in this precise image layer. Panoramic x-ray machines operate with the patient positioned between the tube head and the cassette that holds the film. The exposure is made as the tube head and cassette rotate slowly around the patient's head during the operational cycle (usually about 15 to 20 seconds), recording a selected image within the focal layer.

The film within the cassette and the tube head move in directions opposite of each other while the patient stands or is seated in a stationary position (Figure 28–2). Through the use of a series of rotational points or centers (differing according to the unit manufacturer), the x-ray beam is directed toward the moving cassette to image a select plane of dental anatomy (Figure 28–3). The **rotational center,** which is defined as the axis on which the tube head and the cassette rotate, is the functional focus of the projection. Unlike the concentric or rectangular beam of x-radiation of intraoral radiography, the x-rays emerge from a narrow vertical slit opening in the tube head and are constricted to form a narrow band. The radiation beam then passes vertically through the patient toward the cassette and through another vertical slit in the cassette holder to expose the film that is moving or rotating past (Figure 28–4). By making use of this narrow opening in the tube head, the x-ray beam is collimated and much less tissue is irradiated as the x-rays pass through the patient to the slit in the cassette holder. This results in a panoramic radiograph showing a well-defined image of a curved layer of tissue including the teeth and supporting structures.

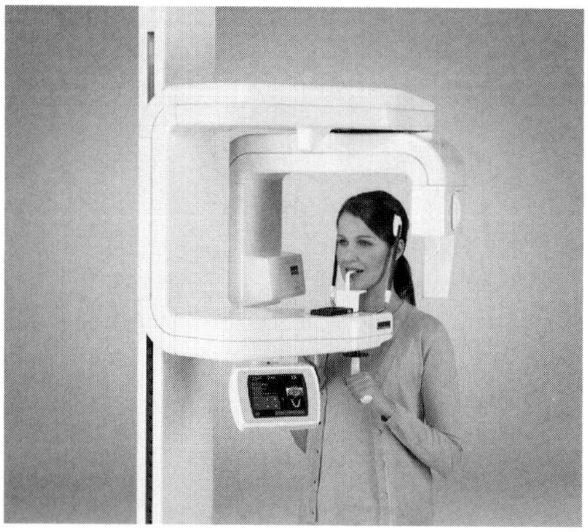

FIGURE 28-2 **Panoramic x-ray unit.** (Courtesy of Planmeca.)

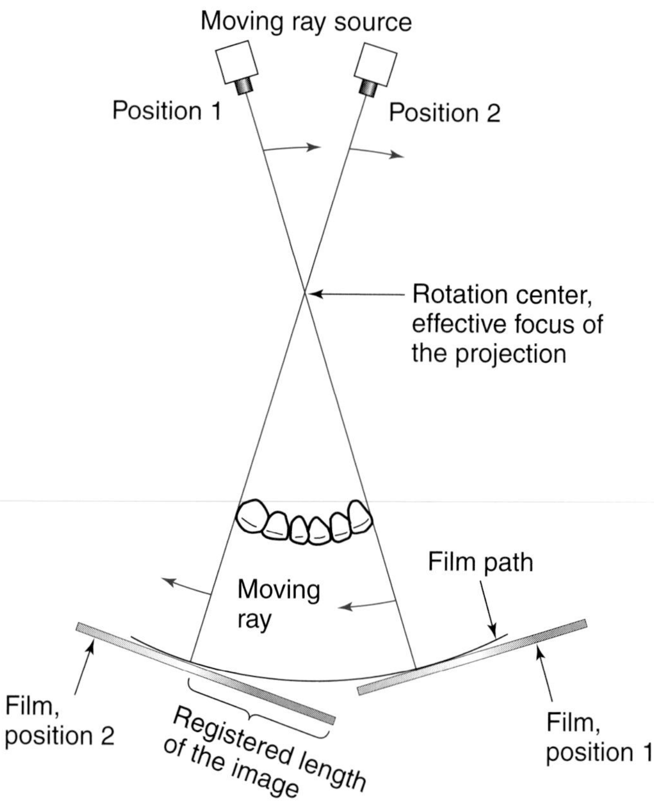

FIGURE 28-3 **Panoramic radiography.** Diagram showing the relationship of the moving x-ray beam as it passes through the center of rotation in a horizontal plane toward the path of the moving x-ray film. As the beam scans the object (the dental arches), a continuous image is registered on the moving film. (From presentation Panoramic radiography by American Dental Association in cooperation with the University of Texas Health Science Center at San Antonio, 1983. Panelists C. R. Morris, W. D. McDavid, J. W. Preece, R. P. Langlais, B. J. Glass, and O. E. Langland)

Panoramic machines are available with differing rotational centers (Figure 28–5).

1. **Double-center rotation.** The exposure begins as the tube head pivots around one side of the dental arches. When the exposure reaches the midline, the radiation is temporarily stopped and the rotation center is shifted. From the new pivot point, the exposure begins again to expose the opposite side to complete the image (Figure 28–5A). Because the radiation output shuts off during the switch to the second rotation center, a **split image** results, where a blank, or clear area is in the middle of the film (Figure 28–6).
2. **Triple-center rotation.** Three centers of rotation are used (Figure 28–5B). Although the examination contains three separate segments, the x-ray beam can be shifted from one center to the other with minor interruption, and a continuous image results on the film.

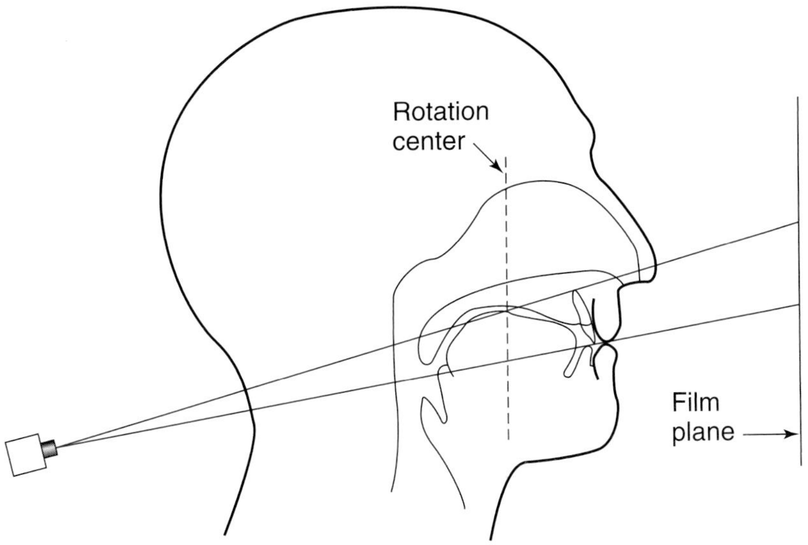

FIGURE 28–4 **Rotational center.** Diagram showing the relationship in a vertical plane of the tube head to the center of rotation and the film as the moving x-ray beam passes through the patient's head toward the moving film. (From presentation Panoramic radiography by American Dental Association in cooperation with the University of Texas Health Science Center at San Antonio, 1983. Panelists C. R. Morris, W. D. McDavid, J. W. Preece, R. P. Langlais, B. J. Glass, and O. E. Langland)

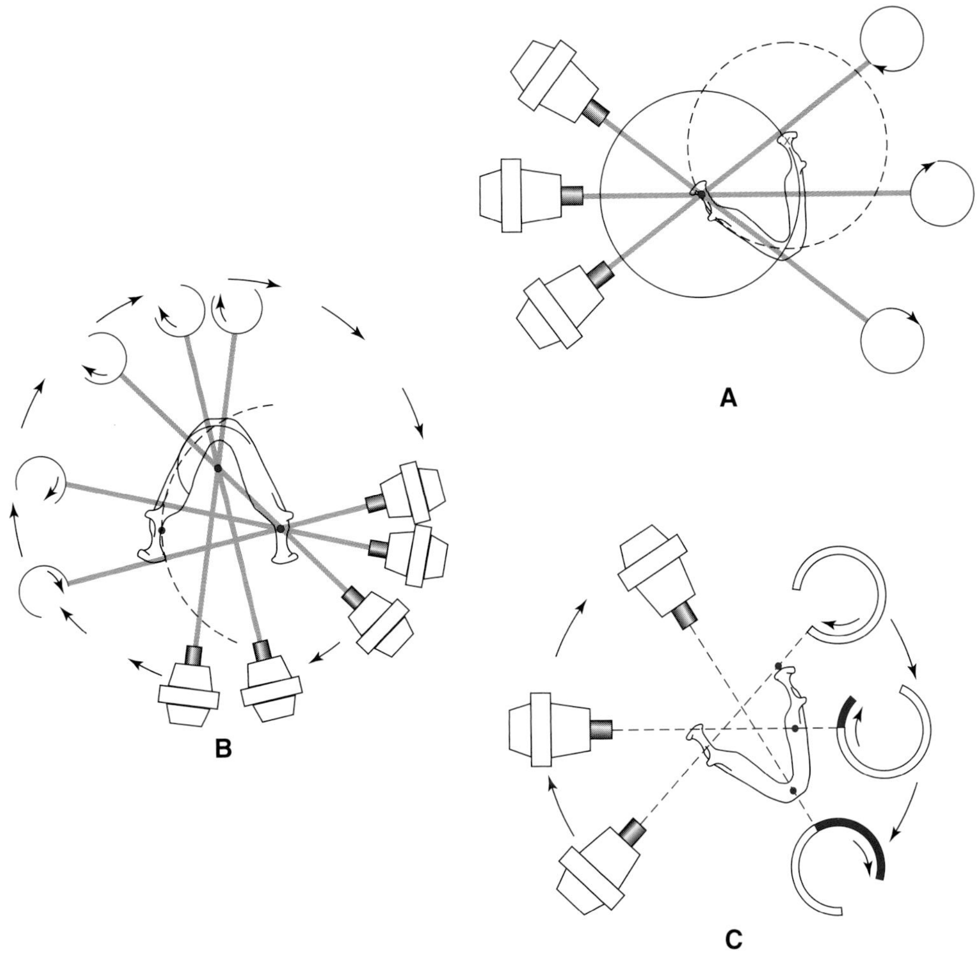

FIGURE 28–5 **Rotational centers.** (**A**) Double-center rotation system. (**B**) Triple-center rotation system. (**C**) Moving-center rotating system. (Reproduced with permission from L. R. Manson-Hing, *Principles of Panoramic Radiography.* Springfield, IL: Thomas, 1976)

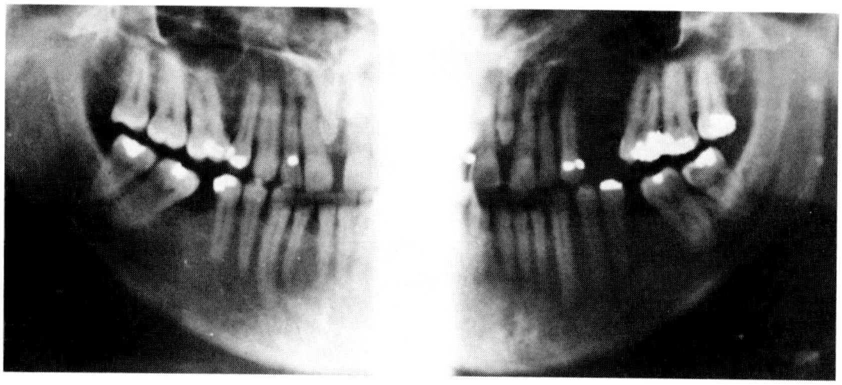

FIGURE 28-6 **Split image panoramic radiograph.** The blank/clear area in the center of the film and the duplication of tooth structures in the incisor regions result when the radiation is momentarily stopped and the rotation center shifts position.

3. **Moving-center rotation.** Most panoramic machines available today utilize a continuous moving-center rotation. The elliptical pattern made by the machine shown in Figure 28–5C very closely matches the arc of the teeth and jaws. A continuous image is produced on the film. Both horizontal and vertical magnification of the image are relatively constant, and this system allows adjustment of the size of the elliptical path to match the varying size of the patient's dental arches.

It is important to be aware that the projections in the horizontal (Figure 28–3) and the vertical (Figure 28–4) directions do not have the same focus of projection. In the horizontal plane, it is at the center of rotation, whereas in the vertical plane it is located at the target in the tube head. This difference in the location of the foci of projection accounts for the fact that a degree of image distortion is characteristic of rotational panoramic radiographs (Figure 28–1).

Concept of the Focal Trough

The focal trough is a theoretical concept used in rotational panoramic radiography to determine where the dental arches, the sinuses, or other areas that are to be examined should be positioned in order to achieve the clearest image. The focal trough (Figure 28–7) is that area between the x-ray source and the film that will be imaged distinctly on the panoramic radiograph. Theoretically, a plane extends through this trough, and objects in that plane are recorded with diagnostic sharpness (Figure 28–8). Objects located at various distances from the plane become less sharp as they get farther from the plane.

Size and Shape of the Focal Trough

The focal trough is three-dimensional, and its actual shape varies depending on the equipment used. The main factor that determines the width of the focal tough is the distance from the functional center of rotation to the object (the structures to be radiographed). As a general rule, the width of the focal trough increases whenever the distance from the rotational center to the object is increased. The width of the focal trough and distance from the rotation center is controlled by the speed of the moving cassette. This means that the manufacturer can program the width and the shape of the focal trough to conform to the shape of an average dental arch by varying the speed of the moving cassette.

The drawings in Figure 28–9 show variations in the shape of the focal trough produced by panoramic x-ray machines having a double-center rotation, a triple-center rotation, and a moving-center rotation.

The double-center rotation system (Figure 28–9A) trough is wide both anteriorly and posteriorly, with the distal ends of the trough curving medially. The inward curving is unfavorable to obtaining the best sharpness in the temporomandibular joint areas. Triple-center and moving-center rotation systems have focal troughs that are wide in the posterior and narrow anterior regions. The clinical implication of this is that the anterior teeth must be positioned accurately to be imaged correctly. The moving-center rotation system has the widest trough in the posterior region, facilitating temporomandibular joint imaging.

Panoramic X-ray Machines

Although considerable differences exist in the size and configuration of modern panoramic x-ray units, the operational procedures are similar and relatively simple (Procedure Box 28–1). Many units require that the patient stand during the exposure;

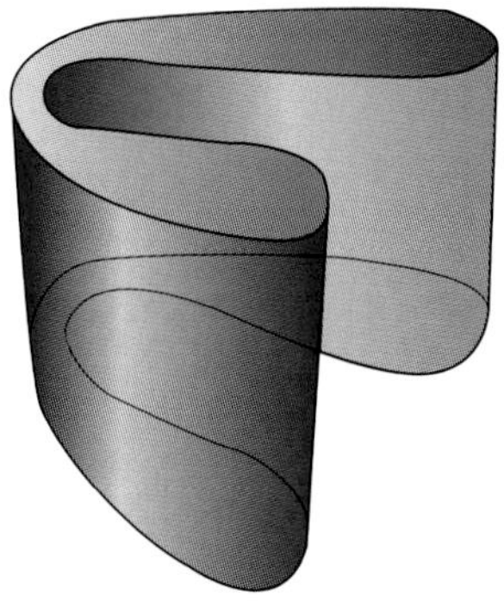

FIGURE 28-7 **Diagram of the focal trough.** (Reproduced with permission from L. R. Manson-Hing, *Principles of Panoramic Radiography.* Springfield, IL: Thomas, 1976)

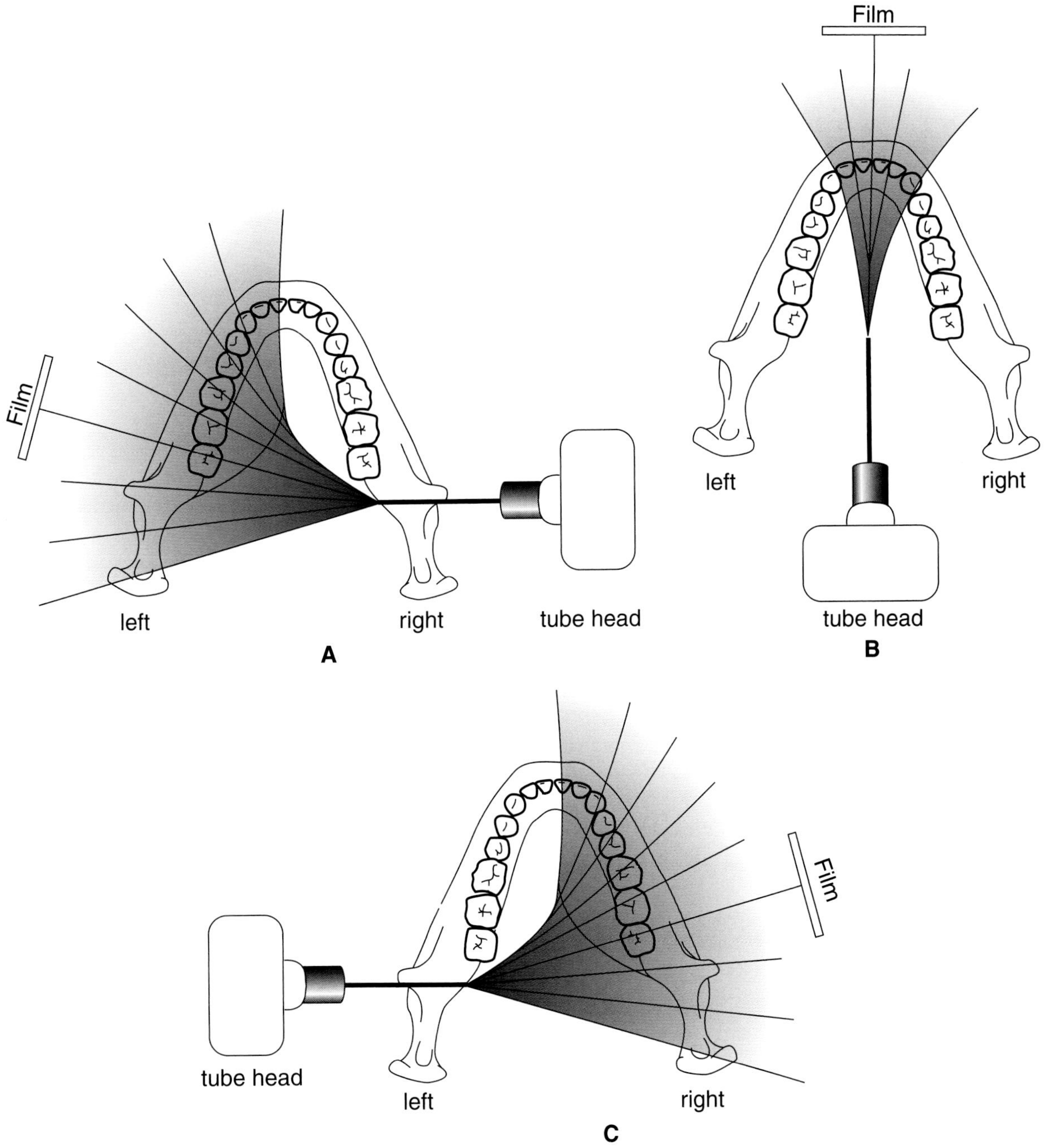

FIGURE 28-8 **Plane of focus within the focal trough.** The x-ray beam is focused on imaging the structures that are positioned closest to the film. As the tube head and film rotate, the x-ray beam is re-focused to image the next section of anatomy. (**A**) Illustrated here is one moment in the continuous exposure. At this precise moment, the tube head is positioned on the right side, allowing the x-ray beam to penetrate the right side, then continue on to penetrate the left side and carry the images of the structures penetrated to the film. At this moment the right side is farther from the film than the left side. At this moment in the exposure sequence, the left side will be imaged on the film, while the right side will be blurred out as a ghost image. (**B**) As the tube head and film rotate, the x-ray beam now penetrates the back of head (and the cervical vertebrae), then continues on to penetrate the anterior teeth. Since the anterior teeth at this moment are closer to the film, the cervical vertebrae will most likely appear magnified and blurred out as a ghost image, while the anterior teeth will be more distinctly recorded onto the film. (**C**) As the tube head and film continue to rotate to the opposite side, the x-ray beam now penetrates the left side first, blurring it out of the image. The right side is now closer to the film, so it will be imaged more clearly.

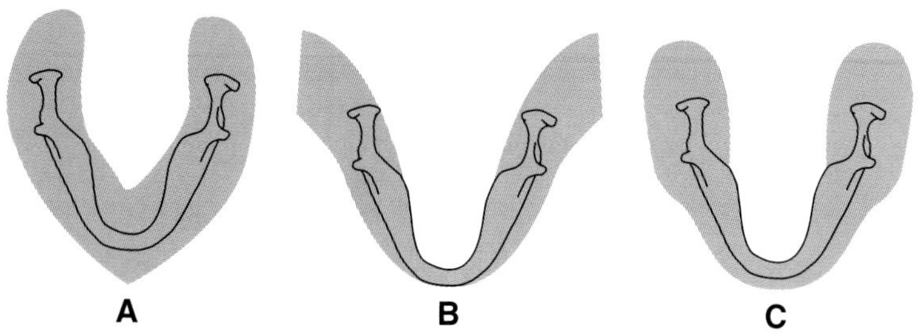

FIGURE 28–9 **Variations in the shape of the focal trough** produced by panoramic x-ray machines having (**A**) double-center rotation, (**B**) triple-center rotation, and (**C**) moving-center rotation. (Reproduced with permission from L. R. Manson-Hing, *Principles of Panoramic Radiography.* Springfield, IL: Thomas, 1976)

others call for the patient to be seated. When seated, the patient is usually positioned to face the radiographer. The patient faces away from the radiographer when positioned into a unit requiring the patient to stand. Panoramic radiographs require the use of either a rigid or flexible cassette with intensifying screens. The extraoral film selected for use must match the type of screen used (see Chapter 27).

All panoramic x-ray units have four basic components:

1. Rotational x-ray tube head
2. Cassette holder (drum)
3. Head positioner guides
4. Exposure control panel

The x-ray tube used in panoramic x-ray machines generates electrons to produce x-ray energy similar to x-ray units used for intraoral exposures. The panoramic tube head is in a fixed vertical position with the short PID pointing up slightly, about negative 8 degrees. The opening of the PID is collimated with a lead diaphragm in the shape of a narrow vertical slit opening. The tube head and PID will rotate around the back of the patient's head while the cassette with film rotates around the front. The x-ray beam strikes the patient's tissues from the back of the head.

The cassette with film must be attached to the unit so that it will rotate in relation with the tube head. Each unit manufacturer provides specific instructions for attaching the cassette to the unit (Figure 28–10).

Since the focal trough is determined and set by the unit manufacturer, every panoramic machine will have **head positioner guides** to aid the radiographer in positioning the patient. Most units are equipped with: a bite block or forehead rest that allows the radiographer to correctly determine how far forward the patient should be positioned; side positioner guides or a mirror for determining the correct alignment of the **mid-saggital plane**; and a chin rest to correctly locate how far up or down the arches should be positioned. Some units have beams of light that when turned on to shine on the patient's face will guide the operator to finding each of the three dimensions (Figure 28–11).

The exposure control panel will usually allow the radiographer to select the mA and kVp as recommended by the manufacturer. The size of the patient and density of the tissues to be imaged will determine what settings are used. The kVp controls the penetrating ability of the beam, so it is often adjusted up when exposing larger patients or denser tissues, and adjusted down when exposing children and edentulous patients. The exposure time is pre-set by the manufacturer and varies from 15 to 20 seconds to complete the cycle. To activate the exposure, the radiographer must depress the exposure button and hold for the duration of the cycle.

Patients should be protected with a lead barrier when undergoing the panoramic exam. The thyroid collar must be removed from the lead apron for use during a panoramic exposure. Due to the position of the tube head and PID, the thyroid collar would get in the way of the primary beam and block the radiation from reaching the tissues. Lead aprons are available without a thyroid collar and there are cape-style aprons made especially for panoramic use (see Figures 6–12 and 28–12).

Importance of Correct Head Positioning

Positioning of the patient's head and dental arches in the focal trough is necessary for diagnostic images. Correct head positioning will vary, depending on whether the area of interest is in the region of the temporomandibular joints, the sinuses, or the teeth and their supporting structures. Because the focal trough is pre-determined by the panoramic unit manufacturer, the radiographer must refer to the manufacturer's instructions when positioning the patient. Each manufacturer provides an instruction manual that must be carefully read and followed. It is the radiographer's responsibility to position the patient's dental arches in relation to the focal trough to avoid images that are magnified, diminished, or blurred.

Most panoramic x-ray machines have guides such as a head positioner, chin rest, or beams of light that shine on the patient's face to aid the radiographer in positioning the patient within the focal trough (Figures 28–11 and 28–12). Since the focal trough or area of image sharpness is three dimensional (Figure 28–7), the patient's dental arches must be positioned in the correct: forward or back position; left or right position; and up or down position.

The radiographer must be able to determine the location of three facial landmarks to position the patient correctly. (1) The midsaggital plane (see Figure 12–8) that divides the patient's head into a right and left side must be positioned perpendicularly to the floor. (2) The **ala-tragus line**—an imaginary plane or line from the ala (a wing-like projection at the side of the nose) to the tragus (the cartilaginous portion in front of the acoustic meatus of the ear)—must be positioned approximately 5 degrees down (toward the floor). (3) When the ala-tragus line is positioned

PROCEDURE 28–1

PANORAMIC RADIOGRAPHIC PROCEDURE*

Cassette and Film Preparation

1. Examine cassette for proper function. Check hinge for wear. Check for light-tight seal.
2. Examine intensifying screens for quality. Check for scratches and need of cleaning.
3. Obtain a box of extraoral film. Ensure that the film sensitivity matches the screen type used (see Chapter 27).
4. Turn off white overhead light and turn on safelight. (Ensure that safelight color filter recommended by the film manufacturer is in use.)
5. Remove the cover from the box of film and carefully, with clean, dry hands, remove one sheet of film from the box. Remove sheet of film slowly to avoid generating static electricity.
6. Handling the film by the edges only, load the film into the cassette. (When using a flexible cassette, ensure that the film is inserted between the screens and is seated all the way down to the fold in the screens). Close tightly, securing the hinge (rigid cassette) or snaps (flexible cassette). Replace the cover on the box of film prior to turning on overhead white light or leaving the darkroom.

Unit Preparation

1. Clean and disinfect with appropriate disinfectant all surfaces that will come in contact either directly or indirectly with the patient, such as the:
   a. Forehead rest
   b. Chin rest
   c. Side head positioner guides
   d. Patient support handles
   e. Chair (sit-down units)
2. Select sterile or disposable bite block or cotton roll.
3. Attach the cassette onto the cassette holder (drum) of the unit according to the manufacturer's instructions. Ensure that the cassette is placed so that the exposure will begin at the appropriate edge of the film.
4. Turn the machine on to check that it is operational. Raise or lower the overhead assembly, and swing the head positioner out of the way (if necessary) so that the patient can be positioned.

Patient Preparation

1. Inform patient of the need for the panoramic radiograph. Explain the procedure, answer patient concerns/questions regarding the procedure, and obtain patient's consent.
2. Request that the patient remove eyeglasses, necklaces, hair barrettes, facial jewelry (tongue, lip piercing adornments), removable dental appliances and any other material which may interfere with the radiographic procedure such as chewing gum or a jacket with thickly padded shoulders.
3. Place the lead (or lead-equivalent) apron without a thyroid collar over the patient. Ensure that the lead apron will not impede the rotation of the unit.

Patient Positioning

1. To position the arches into the focal trough's anterior/posterior dimension, instruct the patient to bite on the bite guide with the anterior teeth occluding edge to edge, or to place the chin completely forward into the chin rest or against the forehead rest.

(continued)

PROCEDURE 28–1 (*cont.*)

2. To position the arches into the focal trough's lateral (right-left) dimension, close the head positioner guides or instruct the patient to view reflection in the mirror (on some units) and align the mid-saggital plane perpendicular to the floor. Utilize unit light beams if available.
3. To position the arches into the focal trough's superior-inferior dimension adjust the patient's chin up or down until the Frankfort plane is parallel to the floor or until the ala-tragus line is approximately positive 5 degrees to the floor. (Some panoramic x-ray units have indicator lines scribed on the head positioner guides or projected as a beam of light from the unit to align either the Frankfort plane or the ala-tragus line to obtain correct superior-inferior patient positioning in the focal trough.)

Exposure

1. Select the appropriate kVp and mA for the patient. Refer to posted exposure settings or use the manufacturer's recommendations.
2. Instruct the patient to place the tongue up against the hard palate and to close the lips around the bite guide or cotton roll. (Asking the patient to swallow will assist with correct placement of the tongue and lips.)
3. Instruct the patient to remain still throughout the exposure cycle.
4. Take a position behind a protective barrier or an adequate distance away from the x-ray source and depress the exposure button for the duration of the cycle. You should be able to watch the procedure during the exposure from a protected location (see Figure 3-6) to ensure that the patient does not move and that the rotation of the unit continues unhindered. If patient movement occurs or the unit contacts the patient or lead apron, release the exposure button to stop the process. The cassette should be removed from the unit and the procedure should start over, beginning with a new film.
5. When the exposure cycle is complete, swing the head positioner out of the way (if necessary) so that the patient can be released. Remove the lead apron. Return glasses, earrings, or appliances to the patient.
6. Return the head positioner and overhead assembly to the closed position and turn off unit. Discard the disposable bite guide or prepare autoclavable bite guide for sterilization. Clean and disinfect with appropriate disinfectant all surfaces which came in contact either directly or indirectly with the patient such as the:
   a. Forehead rest
   b. Chin rest
   c. Side head positioner guides
   d. Patient support handles
   e. Chair (sit-down units)

Processing

1. Remove the cassette from the cassette holder or drum.
2. Proceed to the darkroom. Turn off the overhead white light and turn on the safelight. Open the cassette and remove the film from between the intensifying screens. Handle the film with clean, dry hands by the edges only. Use care to avoid sliding the film across the screens in such a manner that would generate static electricity or scratch the screens or the film.
3. Manually or automatically process the film according to the manufacturer's instructions.**

*The procedures for taking panoramic radiographs are similar on most panoramic machines. As the complexity of the controls and head holder adjustments varies from unit to unit, the radiographer should read the manufacturer's instructions carefully before attempting to operate an unfamiliar machine.

**Prior to processing, a film identification printer may be utilized to permanently label the film with the patient's name, the date of exposure and other information (see Figure 27–8).

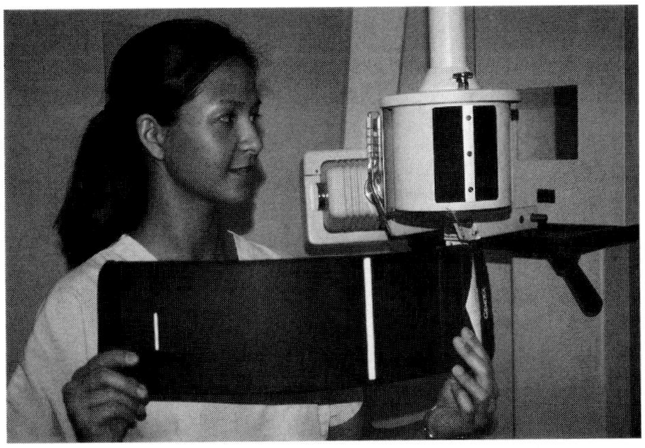

FIGURE 28-10 **Radiographer preparing to attach flexible cassette to the cassette holder (drum).** Note the markings on the outside of the cassette that indicate the correct direction for attaching the cassette to the unit.

correctly, the **Frankfort plane**—an imaginary plane or line from the orbital ridge (under the eye) to the acoustic meatus of the ear—will be parallel to the floor. Some panoramic machines utilize guides that aid the radiographer in locating the ala-tragus line while others focus on the Frankfort plane. The radiographer should be able to utilize either landmark (Figure 28–13).

When the arches are correctly positioned within the focal trough, all teeth and supporting structures are imaged and there is less unequal magnification and unsharpness over all parts of the radiographic image (Figure 28–14). If the patient has been positioned incorrectly, the resultant radiographic image will exhibit unique errors that are characteristic of the positioning mistake made. It is important that the radiographer be able to identify what causes common panoramic image errors to be able to apply the appropriate corrective action.

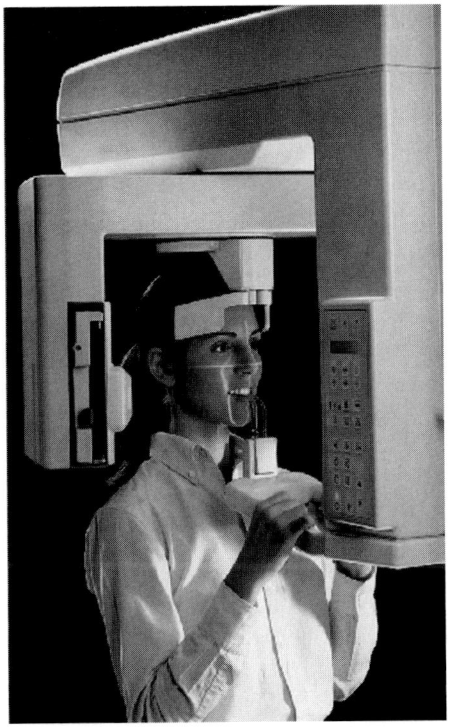

FIGURE 28-11 **Head positioner guides.** Beams of light shine on the patient's face to aid the radiographer in positioning the arches in the focal trough. (Courtesy of Gendex Dental Corporation)

Panoramic Imaging Errors

In addition to patient positioning mistakes, panoramic errors may result from film and unit preparation mistakes; patient preparation and cooperation problems; and incorrectly exposing and processing the film. Since positioning the patient within the focal trough is paramount to producing diagnostic quality radiographic images, the radiographer should possess a working knowledge of the characteristic appearance of errors made in this important step.

Positioning Errors

Positioning the patient too far forward in the focal trough results in all of the anterior teeth appearing blurred and diminished, particularly in width (Figure 28–15). Consequently, when the patient is too far back toward the tube head, the anterior teeth will appear blurred and magnified (Figure 28–16). Most panoramic machines have relatively narrow focal troughs in the anterior region, requiring precision in locating the forward and backward dimension of image sharpness. Panoramic machines will have a forehead rest or may require the patient to bite on a biteblock to position the arches correctly in this dimension. The radiographer should request that the patient bring the incisors into an edge-to-edge position on the biteblock or on a cotton roll for better visualization.

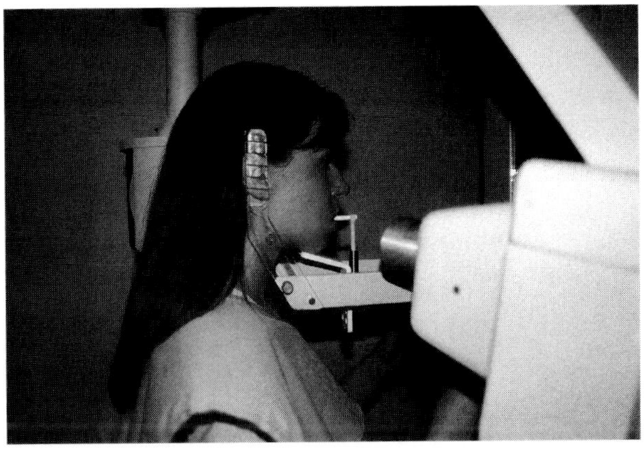

FIGURE 28-12 **Head positioner guides.** The panoramic machine uses a biteblock to aid the radiographer in locating the correct forward and back dimension of the focal trough; side positioner guides to aid with locating the correct left and right dimension; and a chin rest to aid with locating the correct up and down dimension. Note the cape-style lead apron without a thyroid collar for use with panoramic exposures.

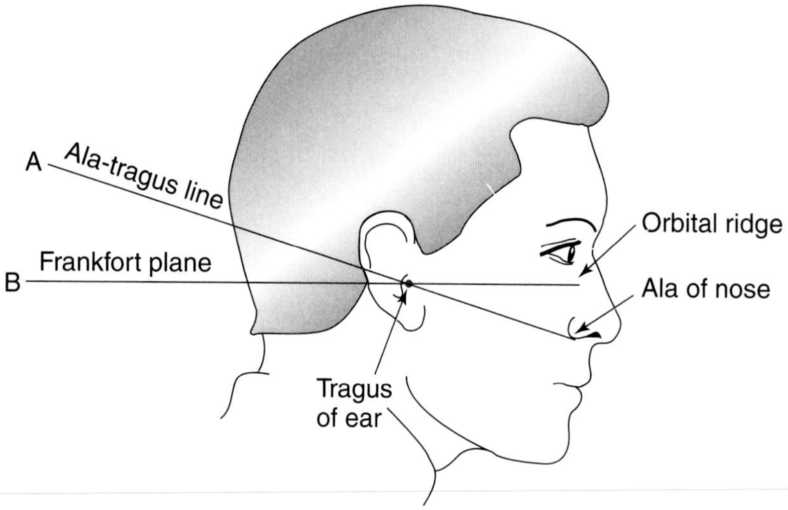

FIGURE 28–13 **Landmarks used to position the patient.** (**A**) Ala-tragus line. (**B**) Frankfort plane.

If the patient's head is rotated, turned, or tipped to the left or to the right, the teeth on the side closer to the film will appear diminished, whereas those on the side closer to the center of rotation appear enlarged (Figure 28–17). When the patient is positioned too far to the left, the teeth on the right appear magnified, whereas when the patient is positioned too far to the right, the teeth on the left appear magnified.

If the patient's chin is tipped too low (Frankfort plane angled downward and ala-tragus line angled downward greater than 5 degrees), the resultant image will appear as an exaggerated smile (Figure 28–18). The mandibular condyles slant inward and the nasopharyngeal air space appears larger and darker, reducing the quality of the image. The appearance of a reversed smile (frown) results when the patient's chin is raised too high (Figure 28–19). Tipping the chin up causes the bottom of the nasal cavity and the hard palate to widen into a radiopaque band that obscures the apices of the maxillary teeth. Tipping the chin up or down will also cause the anterior teeth to be positioned outside the focal trough, often resulting in the appearance of root resorption.

Another patient positioning error results when the patient is not standing or sitting up straight (Figure 28–20). When the patient is slumped over in position, the radiation (which enters the patient from behind) is attenuated by the compressed vertabrae, resulting in a wide radiopacity superimposed over the anterior teeth.

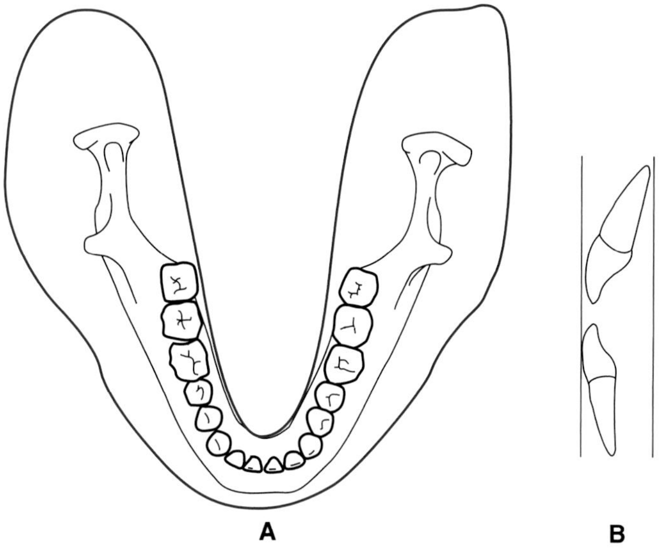

FIGURE 28–14 **Correct positioning.** The arches are positioned correctly within the focal trough in all three dimensions: (**A**) Anterior-posterior and left-right; and (**B**) superior-inferior (up-down).

Patient Preparation Errors

It is important to remember that the x-ray beam rotates around the patient from behind. Any objects made of metal or other dense material located here, such as a necklace, earrings, or hair adornments will be in the path of the primary beam and result in radiopaque artifacts on the film. These items, along with the patient's glasses, dental appliances, patient napkin chain, oral piercings and other facial jewelry, must be removed prior to exposure. Additionally, the thyroid collar must be removed from the lead apron for panoramic exposures. There are occasions when the clothing the patient is wearing may interfere with the rotation of the tube head. Thickly padded shoulders of jackets or dresses need to be assessed to ensure that they won't impede the progression of the film cassette drum during the rotational cycle.

Patient understanding of the procedure and their cooperation are necessary to produce quality images. The patient must hold still, in position, throughout the exposure. The patient should be requested to rest the tongue against the palate and close the lips around the bite guide. The open air space between the tongue and the roof of the mouth (palatoglossal air space) will create a large radiolucency on the image that will obscure the root apices of the maxillary teeth. Raising the tongue to the palate utilizes the soft tissue image of the tongue to "fill in" this airspace and create a more even density to the image. Additionally, open lips

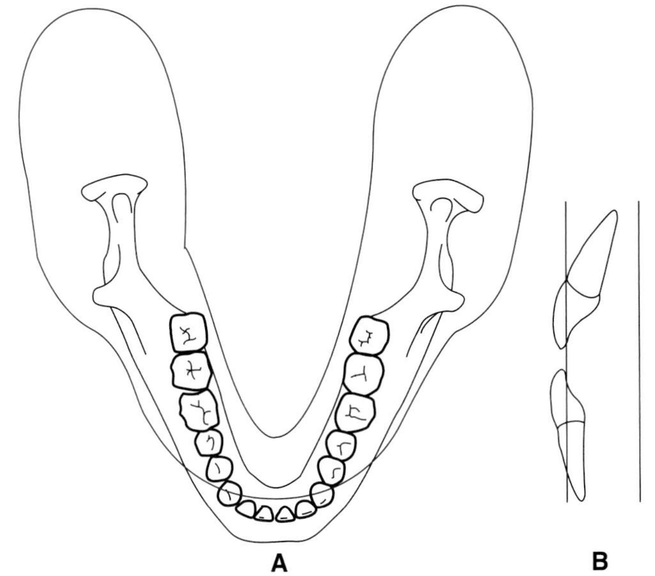

FIGURE 28–15 **Incorrect positioning: too far forward (arches positioned away from the x-ray tube head and toward the film).** (**A**) The arches are positioned too far forward (placing the anterior teeth farther away from the x-ray tube head and closer to the film). (**B**) The anterior teeth are outside the focal trough and will appear blurred and diminished.

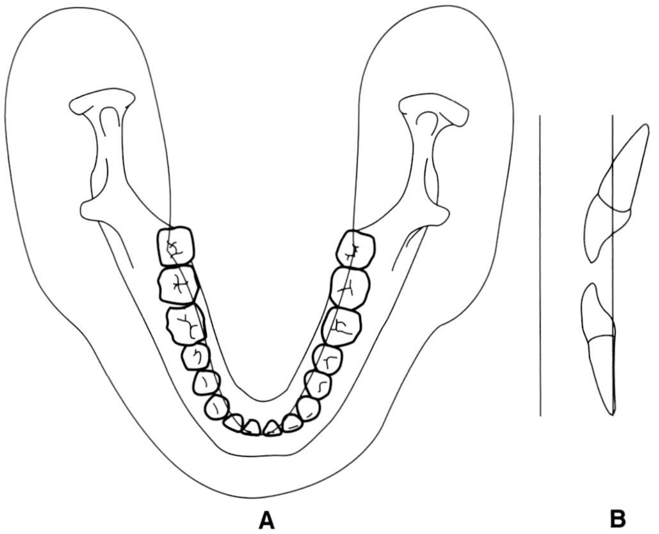

FIGURE 28–16 **Incorrect positioning: too far backward (arches positioned toward the x-ray tube head and away from the film).** (**A**) The arches are positioned too far backward (placing the anterior teeth closer to the x-ray tube head and farther away from the film). (**B**) The anterior teeth are outside the focal trough and will appear blurred and magnified.

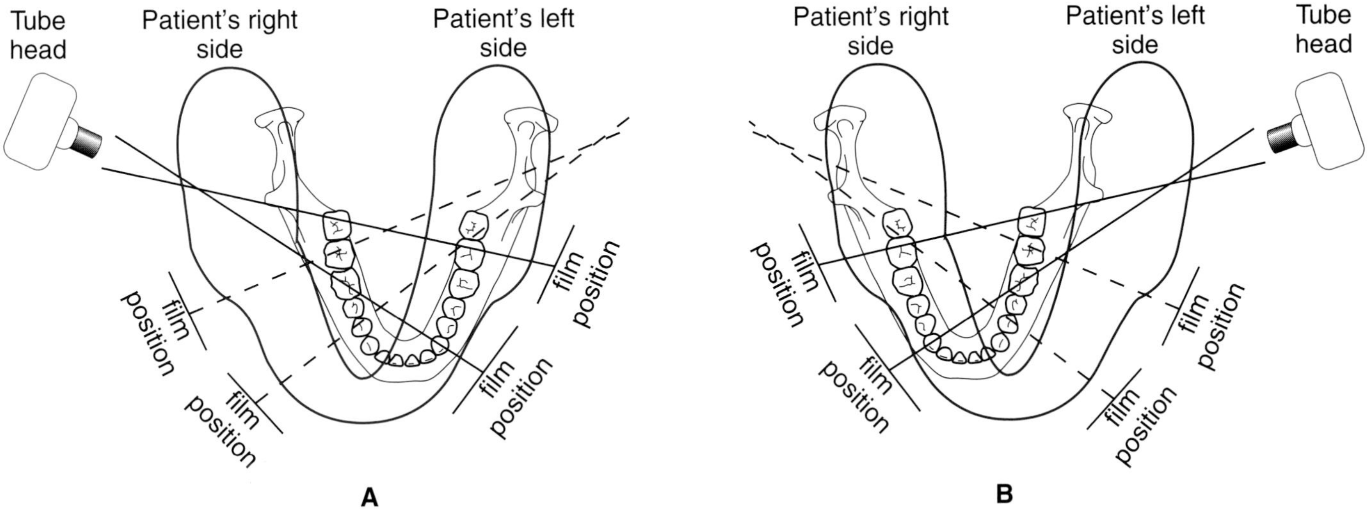

FIGURE 28–17 **Incorrect positioning: patient's head is rotated.** Diminution will be apparent on the side mal-positioned closer to the film, and magnification will be apparent on the side mal-positioned farther away from the x-ray tube head. (**A**) The patient is positioned rotated to the left (making the left side closer to the film and the right side farther away from the x-ray tube head). The teeth on the left will appear blurred and diminished, and the teeth on the right side will appear blurred and magnified. (**B**) The patient is positioned rotated to the right (making the right side closer to the film and the left side farther away from the x-ray tube head). The teeth on the right will appear blurred and diminished and the teeth on the left side will appear blurred and magnified.

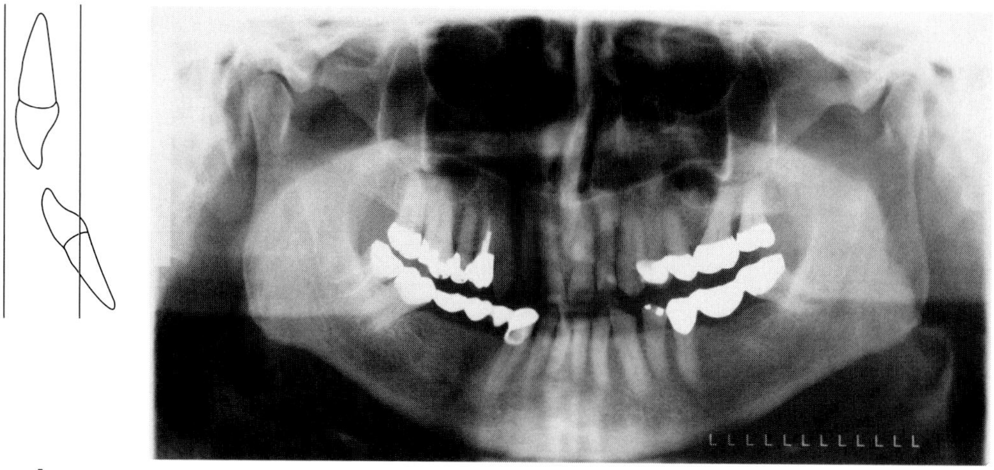

A B

FIGURE 28–18 **Incorrect positioning: patient's chin too low.** (**A**) The root apices of the mandibular anterior teeth slant out of the focal trough. (**B**) Note the characteristic exaggerated "smile" appearance and the pronounced radiolucent air space.

will create an image that mimics fracture lines across the anterior teeth. Closing the lips together on the biteblock avoids this appearance (Figure 28–21).

Exposure and Film Handling Errors

Careful attention to exposure settings and film handling will avoid errors that result in undiagnostic radiographs. Consideration should be given to the following. Exposure settings for the panoramic unit should be posted near the control panel to avoid over- or underexposing the film. Extraoral film requires careful handling to avoid static electricity artifacts (see Figure 27–3). Darkroom safelighting must be appropriate for light-sensitive extraoral film. Cassettes should be inspected to ensure a tight contact between film and intensifying screens. Blurry images result when the film and screens are not in tight contact. Intensifying screens must be free of scratches that would result in a loss of image and radiopaque artifacts.

Careful loading of flexible plastic sleeve cassettes must ensure that the film is seated all the way down at the fold in the pair of intensifying screens. Failure to correctly load the film into the cassette will result in a loss of part of the image.

All panoramic units have special instructions on how to load the film cassette onto the film drum of the unit. The manufacturer's instructions must be followed to avoid positioning the film so that only a portion gets exposed (Figure 28–10).

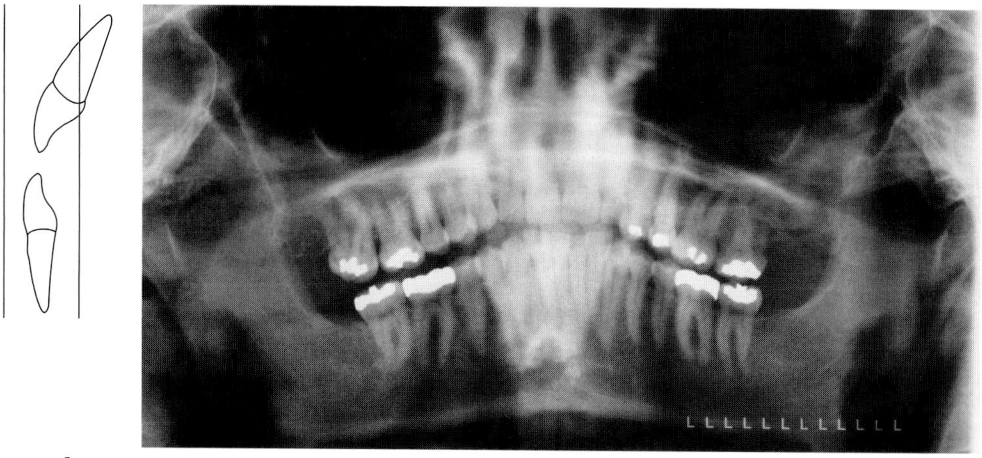

A B

FIGURE 28–19 **Incorrect positioning: patient's chin too high.** (**A**) The root apices of the maxillary anterior teeth slant out of the focal trough. (**B**) Note the characteristic "frown" appearance and the widened appearance of the hard palate.

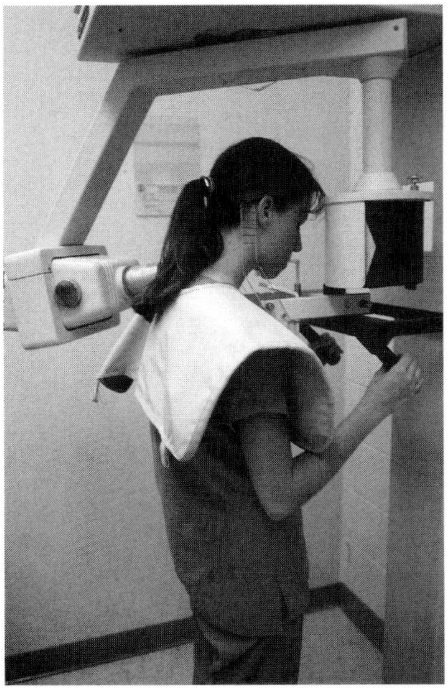

FIGURE 28-20 **Incorrect patient positioning.** Patient not standing up straight. Compare with the correct straight posture illustrated in Figure 28-11.

Normal Panoramic Anatomical Landmarks

The principles of panoramic radiography result in the formation of a unique image. The superimposition of anatomical structures and the broadening of the arches produces unusual anatomical relationships in the panoramic image not seen in intraoral radiographs. In the panoramic radiograph, the mandible and maxilla as well as the spine are imaged as if they were split vertically in half down the midsagittal plane, with each half folded outward. The split cervical spine appears twice, beyond the mandibular rami at the extreme right and left edges of the radiograph. Many structures will appear broadened and wider in the same way that a map of the world flattens and broadens the images of a globe.

To develop the skills needed to recognize normal anatomic structures viewed on the panoramic radiograph, the radiographer should build on his/her knowledge of how normal anatomy appears on intraoral films and transfer this knowledge to the panoramic image. For example, when viewing the maxillary posterior area on a panoramic image, the radiographer can visualize a periapical taken in this same area. Since the radiographer would be able to identify anatomical landmarks most likely to be imaged here (e.g., the zygomatic arch and maxillary sinus) on an intraoral film, he/she can expect to see these landmarks here on the panoramic image as well. Of course the panoramic radiograph will image more structures of the head and facial regions than intraoral films. The structures listed here are those anatomical landmarks that commonly appear on the panoramic image.

Anatomic Landmarks of the Maxilla and Surrounding Tissues (Figures 28-22 and 28-23)

Mastoid Process

The mastoid process of the temporal bone is located posterior and inferior to the temporomandibular joint (TMJ). On a panoramic radiograph, this structure appears as a rounded radiopacity.

Styloid Process

The styloid process appears as a long, narrow radiopaque spine that extends downward, from the inferior surface of the temporal bone, just anterior to the mastoid process.

External Auditory Meatus

The external auditory meatus (external acoustic meatus), a round opening in the temporal bone located anterior and superior to the mastoid process, appears as a round radiolucency.

Glenoid Fossa

The glenoid fossa (mandibular fossa) is a concave, depressed area of the temporal bone located anterior to the external auditory

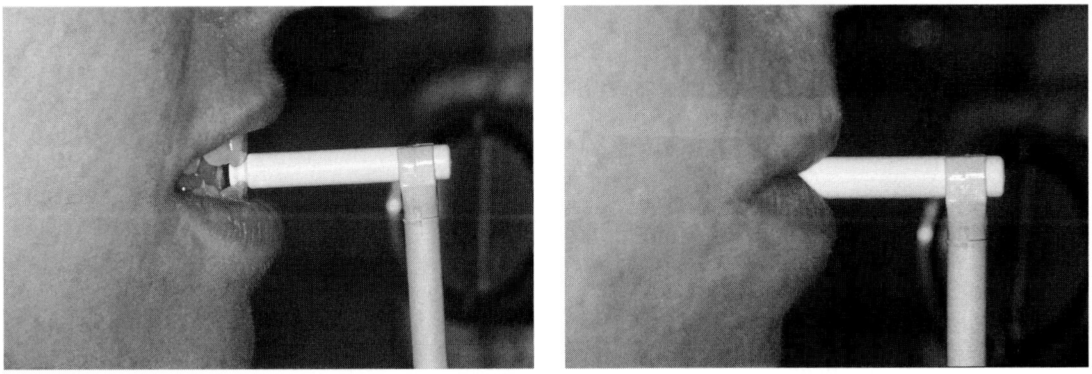

A B

FIGURE 28-21 **Positioning of lips on the biteblock.** (**A**) The lips incorrectly open on the biteblock. (**B**) The lips correctly positioned closed around the biteblock. Note the narrow, slit opening in PID in the background.

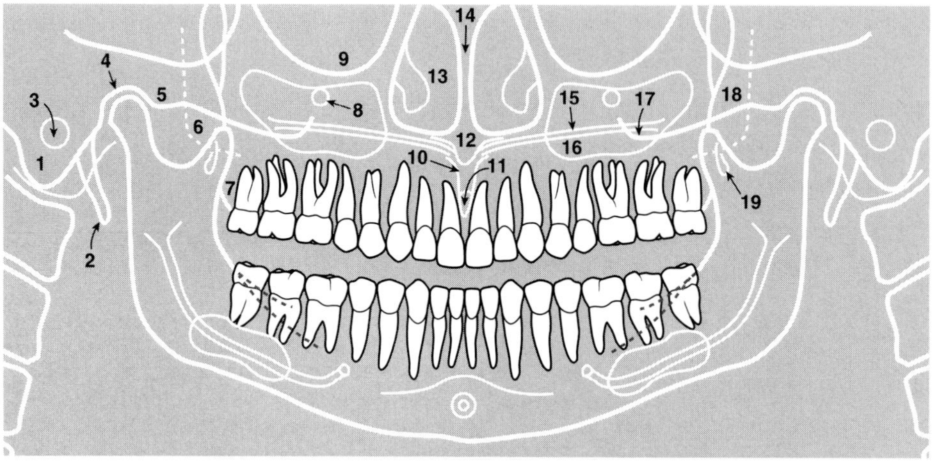

FIGURE 28-22 **Drawing of panoramic radiograph showing the maxilla and surrounding normal anatomic landmarks.** (**1**) Mastoid process, (**2**) styloid process, (**3**) external auditory meatus, (**4**) glenoid fossa, (**5**) articular eminence, (**6**) lateral pterygoid plate, (**7**) maxillary tuberosity, (**8**) infraorbital foramen, (**9**) orbit of the eye, (**10**) incisive canal, (**11**) incisive foramen, (**12**) anterior nasal spine, (**13**) nasal cavity, (**14**) nasal septum, (**15**) hard palate, (**16**) maxillary sinus, (**17**) zygomatic process of the zygoma, (**18**) zygoma, and (**19**) hamulus.

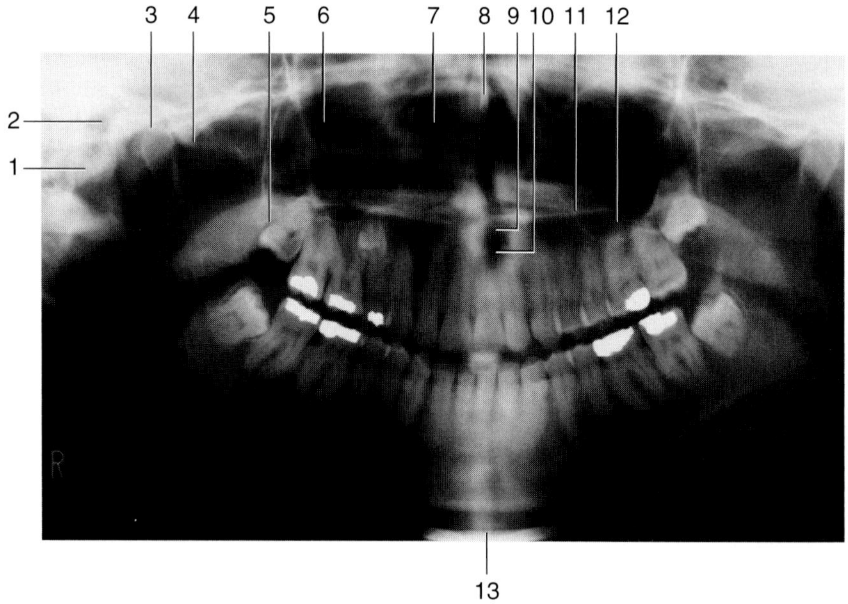

FIGURE 28-23 **Panoramic radiograph showing the maxilla and surrounding normal anatomic landmarks.** (**1**) Mastoid process, (**2**) external auditory meatus, (**3**) glenoid fossa, (**4**) articular eminence, (**5**) maxillary tuberosity, (**6**) orbit of the eye, (**7**) nasal cavity, (**8**) nasal septum, (**9**) incisive canal, (**10**) incisive foramen, (**11**) hard palate, (**12**) maxillary sinus, and (**13**) chin rest (machine part artifact).

meatus. The head of the mandibular condyle rests in the glenoid fossa. On a panoramic radiograph, this landmark appears as a concavity superior to the mandibular condyle.

Articular Eminence

Just anterior to the glenoid fossa is the articular eminence (articular tubercle), a rounded projection of the temporal bone. On a panoramic radiograph, this landmark appears as a rounded radiopaque bony projection.

Lateral Pterygoid Plate

The lateral pterygoid plate appears as a radiopaque wing-like bony projection of the sphenoid bone located posterior to the maxillary tuberosity.

Maxillary Tuberosity

The maxillary tuberosity appears as a radiopaque rounded prominence distal to the third molar region.

Infraorbital Foramen

The infraorbital foramen, a small round opening in the maxilla, appears as a round radiolucency inferior to the border of the orbit.

Orbit of the Eye

The orbit, the bony cavity of the eye socket, appears as a large round radiolucency with radiopaque borders superior to the maxillary sinuses. Often, only the inferior border of the orbit is visible as a radiopaque line.

Incisive Canal

The incisive canal (nasopalatine canal) is a Y-shaped passageway that extends from the floor of the nose to the hard palate lingual to the central incisors. On a panoramic radiograph, this landmark appears as a tunnel-like radiolucency with radiopaque borders located between the maxillary central incisors.

Incisive Foramen

The incisive foramen (nasopalatine foramen), an opening in bone located in the anterior midline of the hard palate directly posterior to the maxillary central incisors, appears as a round pea-shaped radiolucency between the roots of the maxillary central incisors.

Anterior Nasal Spine

The anterior nasal spine, a pointed bony projection of the maxilla located at the most anterior point of the floor of the nasal cavity, appears as a V-shaped radiopacity located at the intersection of the floor of the nasal cavity and the nasal septum.

Nasal Cavity

The nasal cavity (nasal fossa), a pear-shaped compartment of bone located superior to the maxilla, appears as a large radiolucency above the maxillary incisors.

Nasal Septum

The nasal septum, a vertical bony wall that separates the right and left nasal fossae, appears as a vertical radiopacity that divides the nasal cavity into two parts.

Hard Palate

The hard palate a bony wall that separates the oral cavity from the nasal cavity, appears as a horizontal thick radiopaque band superior to the maxillary teeth.

Maxillary Sinus

The maxillary sinuses consist of two paired cavities located within the maxilla apical to the maxillary posterior teeth. On a panoramic radiograph, these appear as paired radiolucent cavities apical to the maxillary posterior teeth.

Zygomatic Process of the Maxilla

The zygomatic process of the maxilla, a bony process of the maxilla that extends laterally to articulate with the zygoma, appears as a J- or U-shaped radiopacity located apically to the maxillary first molar.

Zygoma

The zygoma (malar bone) is the cheekbone that articulates with the zygomatic process of the maxilla. On a panoramic radiograph, this structure appears as a thick radiopaque band that extends posteriorly from the zygomatic process of the maxilla.

Hamulus

The hamulus (hamular process) appears as a very small radiopaque hook-like process of bone that extends downward and slightly backward from the medial pterygoid plate of the sphenoid bone.

Anatomic Landmarks of the Mandible and Surrounding Tissues (Figures 28–24 and 28–25)

Mandibular Condyle

The mandibular condyle appears as a radiopaque rounded bony process extending from the posterior superior border of the ramus of the mandible that articulates with the glenoid fossa of the temporal bone.

Mandibular Notch

The mandibular notch (coronoid notch or sigmoid notch) appears as a concavity of bone located posterior to the coronoid process on the superior border of the ramus of the mandible.

Coronoid Process

The coronoid process appears as a large radiopaque triangular prominence of bone located on the anterior superior ramus of the mandible.

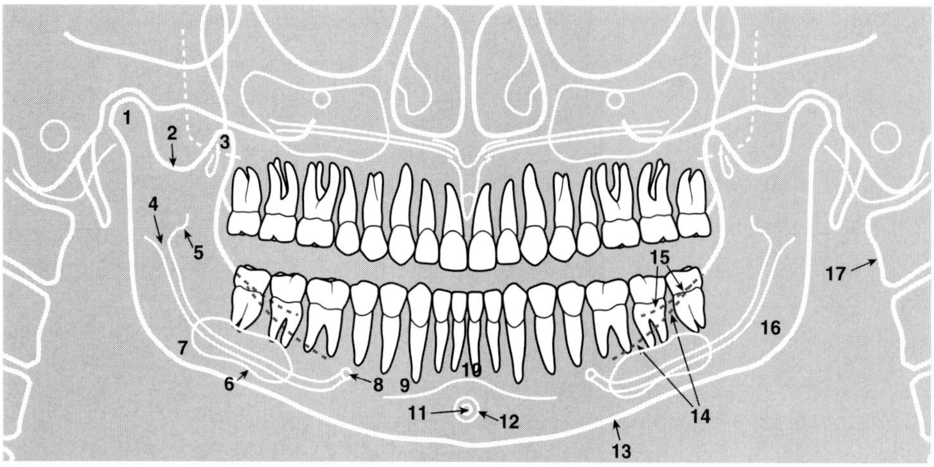

FIGURE 28–24 **Drawing of panoramic radiograph showing the mandible and surrounding normal anatomic landmarks.** (**1**) Mandibular condyle, (**2**) mandibular notch, (**3**) coronoid process, (**4**) mandibular foramen, (**5**) lingula, (**6**) submandibular fossa, (**7**) mandibular canal, (**8**) mental foramen, (**9**) mental ridge, (**10**) mental fossa, (**11**) lingual foramen, (**12**) genial tubercles, (**13**) inferior border of the mandible, (**14**) mylohyoid ridge, (**15**) oblique ridge, (**16**) angle of the mandible, (**17**) cervial spine.

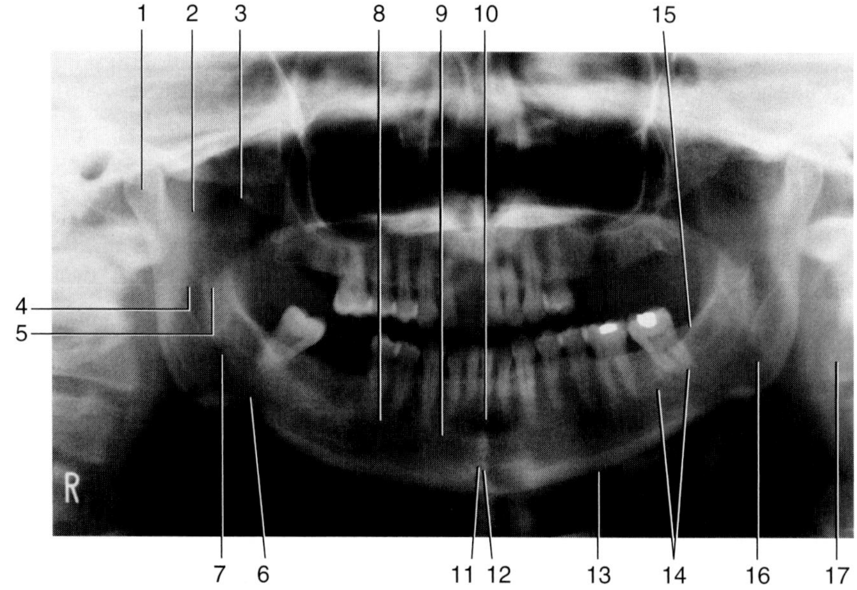

FIGURE 28–25 **Panoramic radiograph showing the mandible and surrounding normal anatomic landmarks.** (**1**) Mandibular condyle, (**2**) mandibular notch, (**3**) coronoid process, (**4**) mandibular foramen, (**5**) lingula, (**6**) submandibular fossa, (**7**) mandibular canal, (**8**) mental foramen, (**9**) mental ridge, (**10**) mental fossa, (**11**) lingual foramen, (**12**) genial tubercles, (**13**) inferior border of the mandible, (**14**) mylohyoid ridge, (**15**) oblique ridge, (**16**) angle of the mandible, (**17**) cervial spine.

Mandibular Foramen

The mandibular foramen, an ovoid opening in the bone on the lingual aspect of the ramus of the mandible, appears as a round radiolucency located in the center of the ramus of the mandible.

Lingula

The lingula (meaning "little tongue") is a small tongue-shaped projection of bone located anterior and adjacent to the mandibular foramen. On a panoramic radiograph, this landmark appears as a small radiopacity anterior to the mandibular foramen.

Mandibular Canal

The mandibular canal, a long tunnel-like passageway extending from the mandibular foramen on the medial aspect of the ramus of the mandible to the mental foramen on the lateral aspect of the body of the mandible, appears as a radiolucent tube outlined by two thin radiopaque lines representing the walls of the canal.

Mental Foramen

The mental foramen, an opening through which the mental nerve and related blood vessels emerge on the lateral aspect of the body of the mandible, appears as a small round radiolucent area near the roots of the mandibular premolars.

Mental Ridge

The mental ridge, appears as a thick radiopaque band representing the prominence of bone located on the external surface of the mandible and extends anteriorly from the premolar area to the midline.

Mental Fossa

The mental fossa appears as a radiolucent depressed area of bone in the region of the roots of the mandibular incisor teeth.

Lingual Foramen

The lingual foramen, a very small round opening located in the center of the genial tubercles on the lingual side of midline of the mandible, appears as a small round radiolucency located inferior to the apices of the mandibular incisor teeth.

Genial Tubercles

The genial tubercles, four small projections of bone located on the lingual surface of the midline of the mandible, appear as a radiopaque donut-shaped circle surrounding the lingual foramen.

Inferior Border of the Mandible

The inferior border of the mandible, composed of the thick cortical bone that outlines the lower border of the mandible, appears as a dense radiopaque band.

Mylohyoid Ridge

The mylohyoid ridge, a ridge of bone running diagonally downward and forward on the lingual aspect of the ramus of the mandible to near the apices of the molar roots, appears as a dense radiopaque band.

Submandibular Fossa

The submandibular fossa, a concavity in the mandible where the salivary glands are located, appears as a diffuse radiolucenct area below the mylohyoid ridge and the roots of the mandibular molars.

Oblique Ridge

The oblique ridge, a diagonal ridge of bone on the lateral aspect of the mandible that runs downward and forward from the anterior border of the ramus to the level of the cervical portion of the molar and premolar roots, appears as a dense radiopaque band.

Angle of the Mandible

The angle of the mandible, the area at the posterior and inferior corners of the mandible, where the body of the mandible meets and joins the ascending ramus of the mandible.

Cervical Spine

On a panoramic radiograph, the cervical spine appears as a radiopaque area beyond the rami of the mandible at the extreme right and left edges of the radiograph.

Soft Tissue Images Viewed on the Panoramic Radiograph (Figures 28–26 and 28–27)

The panoramic radiograph is unique in that some soft tissue structures (e.g., tongue, soft palate, lipline, and ear) attenuate the beam of radiation enough to become visible on the radiograph.

Tongue

When positioned correctly, resting on the palate, the soft tissue image of the tongue should be minimally visible. When visible the radiopaque dorsal side of the tongue appears superimposed over the ramus. The tongue appears broadened and much wider than it appears clinically.

Soft Palate

The soft palate, located posterior to the hard palate, separating the oral cavity from the nasal cavity, appears as a diagonal radiopaque structure above and posterior to the maxillary tuberosity.

Lipline

The appearance of the lipline on a panoramic radiograph can be avoided if the patient is instructed to close the lips together around the bite guide or cotton roll used to position the patient into the focal trough and to separate the arches (Figure 28–21).

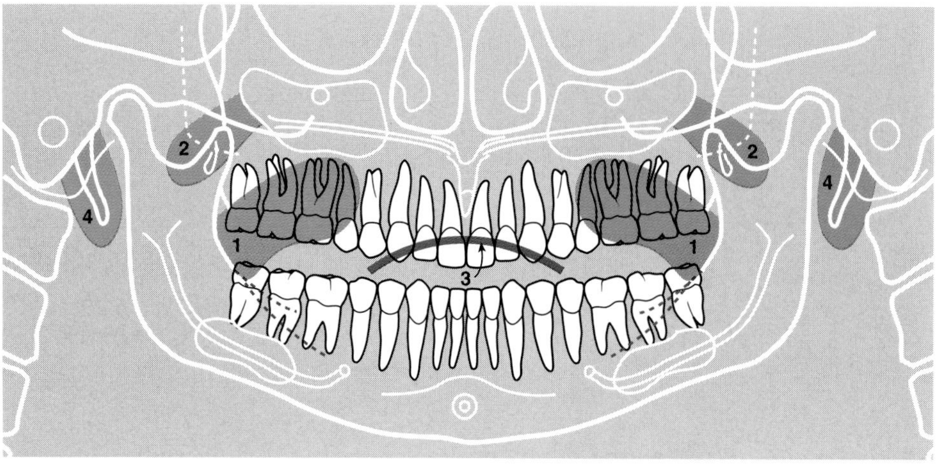

FIGURE 28-26 **Drawing of panoramic radiograph showing soft tissue images.** (**1**) Tongue, (**2**) soft palate, (**3**) lipline, and (**4**) ear.

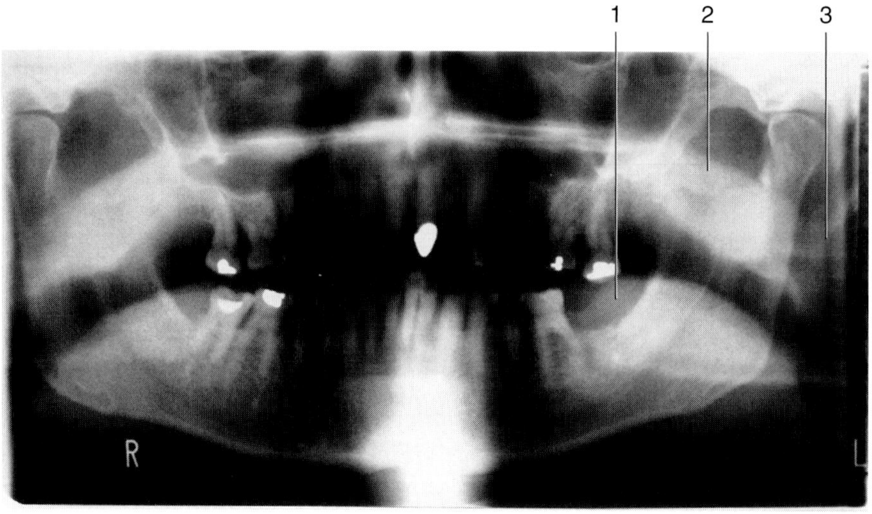

FIGURE 28-27 **Panoramic radiograph showing soft tissue images.** (**1**) Tongue, (**2**) soft palate, and (**3**) ear.

When imaged, the outline of the patient's lips appears as a radiopacity superimposed over the anterior teeth.

Ear

On a panoramic radiograph, the ear appears as a radiopaque area that is superimposed over the styloid process, anterior and inferior to the mastoid process.

Air Space Images Viewed on the Panoramic Radiograph (Figures 28-28 and 28-29)

Air does not attenuate the beam of radiation as much as hard or soft tissue. For this reason, air spaces appear radiolucent (black) on a panoramic radiograph. Air spaces that may be imaged include the palatoglossal, nasopharyngeal, and glossopharyngeal air spaces. The radiolucencies produced by these landmarks often are so dark that they may obscure other structures, compromising the diagnostic ability of the panoramic radiograph. Careful positioning of the patient into the focal trough will help minimize the appearance of these negative shadows. The term negative shadow implies to these radiolucencies because they are shadows of "nothing."

Palatoglossal Air Space

The **palatoglossal air space** (glossopalatine air space) appears as a radiolucency between the palate and the tongue. When the patient is instructed to rest the tongue against the hard palate, the

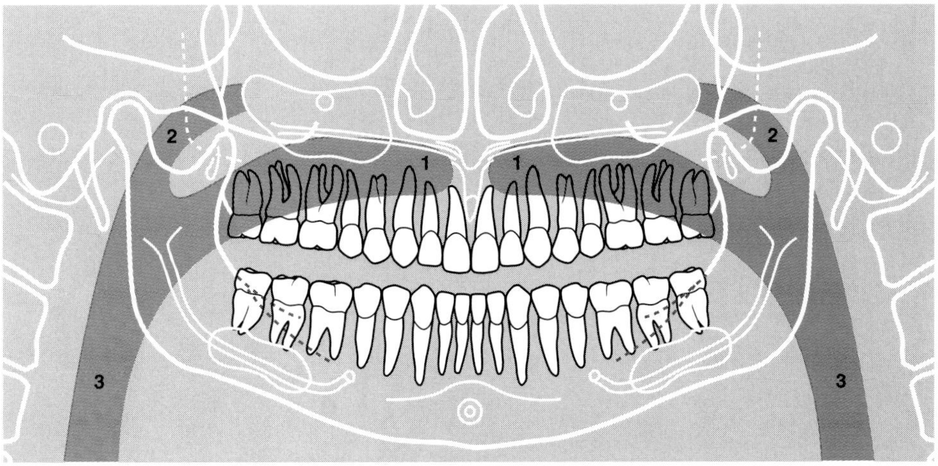

FIGURE 28–28 **Drawing of panoramic radiograph showing air space images.** (**1**) Palatoglossal air space, (**2**) nasopharyngeal air space, and (**3**) glossopharyngeal air space.

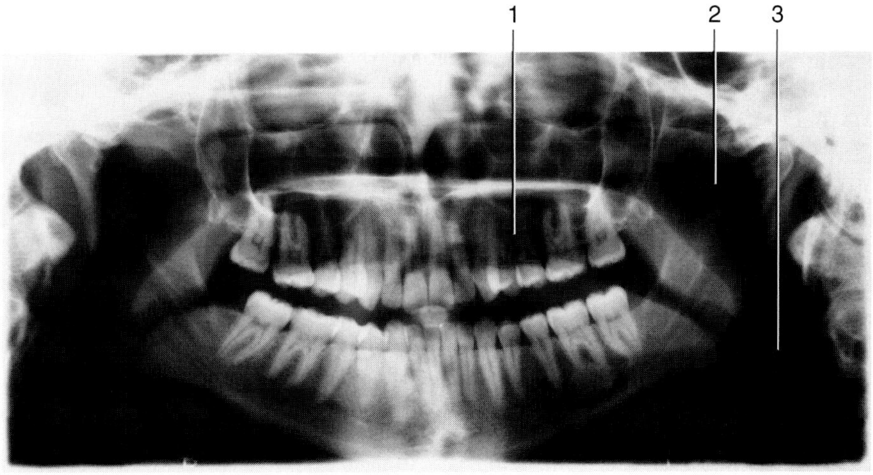

FIGURE 28–29 **Panoramic radiograph showing air space images.** (**1**) Palatoglossal air space, (**2**) nasopharyngeal air space, and (**3**) glossopharyngeal air space.

palatoglossal air space negative shadow is minimized. If the tongue is not correctly positioned against the palate during exposure, the radiolucency appears superimposed on or above the apices of the maxillary teeth.

Nasopharyngeal Air Space

The **nasopharyngeal air space** is the radiolulcency located posterior to the nasal cavity. The negative shadow it creates on the image often appears as a diagonal radiolucent area located superior to the radiopaque soft palate. This negative shadow is emphasized when the patient's chin is incorrectly tipped down.

Glossopharyngeal Air Space

The **glossopharyngeal air space** (oropharyngeal air space) is the portion of the pharynx located posterior to the tongue and oral cavity. The negative shadow it creates on the image appears as a vertical radiolucent band superimposed over the ramus of the mandible.

Images of Machine Parts Viewed on the Panoramic Radiograph (Figures 28–23, 28–30, and 28–31)

Unique to the panoramic image is the appearance of machine parts. The chin rest, side head positioner guides and the bite block are often imaged on the resultant radiograph. Care should

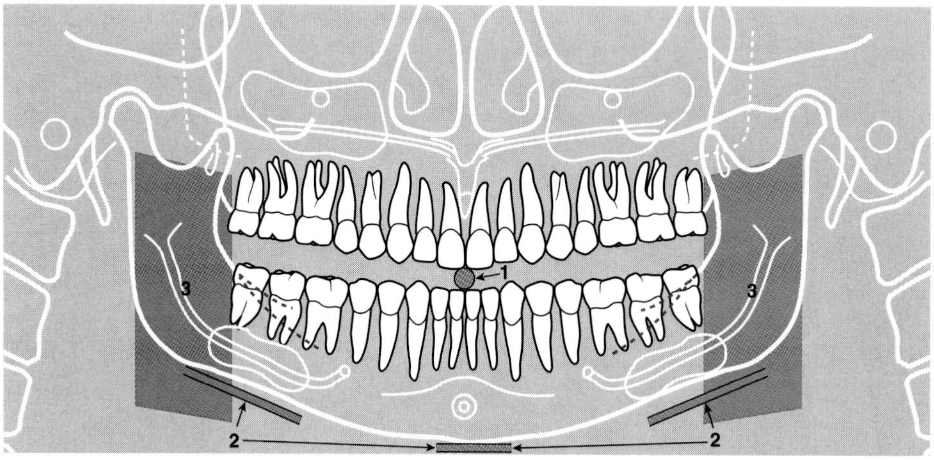

FIGURE 28-30 **Drawing of panoramic radiograph showing images of machine parts.** (**1**) Biteblock, (**2**) chin rest, (**3**) side positioner guides.

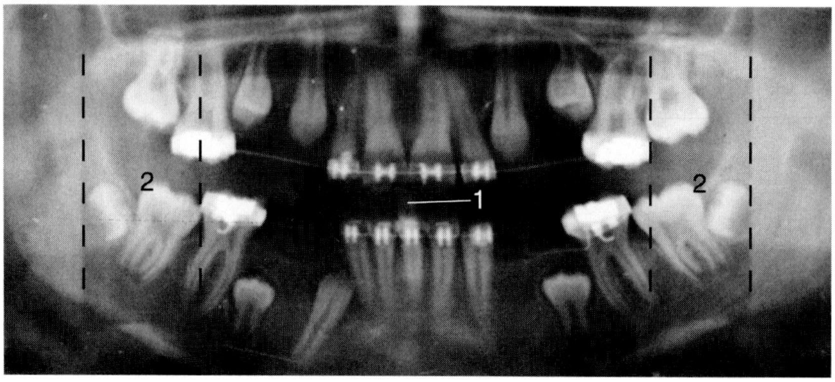

FIGURE 28-31 **Panoramic radiograph showing images of machine parts.** (**1**) Biteblock, (**2**) side positioner guides.

be taken to identify these artifacts so that they are not confused with normal anatomical landmarks or the presence of disease.

Ghost Images Viewed on the Panoramic Radiograph (Figures 28–32 and 28–33)

The rotation of the panoramic tubehead and the use of a focal trough to isolate slices or layers of the image creates ghost images on the resultant panoramic radiograph. Ghost images are mirror or second images of structures that are penetrated by the x-ray beam twice. Consider that when the x-ray tube head is on the patient's right side, the x-ray beam penetrates the right side first. Since this right side is closest to the x-ray source and farthest from the film, the structures here are blurred and diminished out of the image. Instead, the beam continues through the patient to the left side, which is at that moment closer to the film and inside the focal trough (Figure 28–8). As the tube head rotates around the back of the patient, the x-ray beam enters the back of the head and "re-focuses" on imaging the anterior teeth. Because the anterior teeth at that moment are closest to the film, and in the focal layer, they are being imaged onto the film and the back of the skull is being blurred out. As the beam continues around the patient to the left side, the blurring out and re-focusing continues along the predetermined focal layer. In principle those structures outside the focal trough should not be imaged on the film. However, a magnified, unsharp image called a ghost image often appears. For example, when viewing a panoramic image of the patient's right mandible, a ghost image of the left mandible can be observed superimposed over the actual right mandible, as a mirror image (Figures 28–32 and 28–33). Ghost images appear on the opposite side of the image than the actual structure and will often appear larger (more magnified) and higher (due to the slight negative vertical angulation of the PID). Being aware of ghost images will assist the radiographer in interpreting panoramic radiographs.

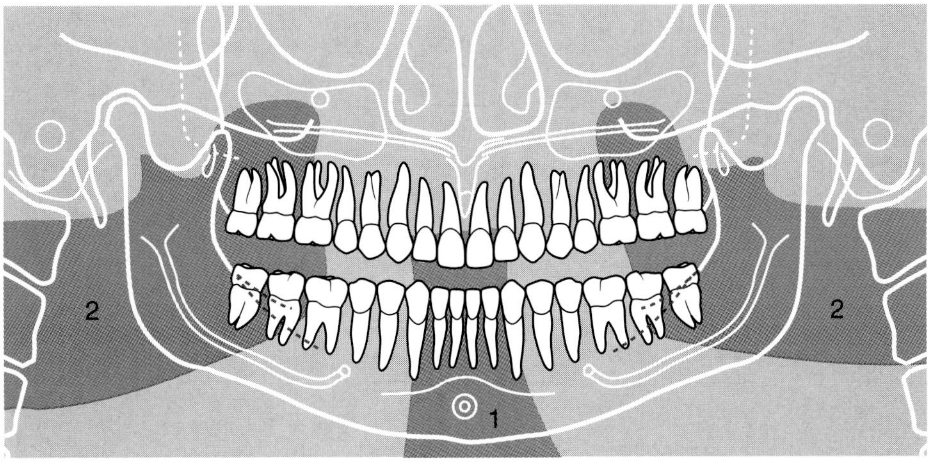

FIGURE 28-32 **Drawing of panoramic radiograph showing ghost images.** (**1**) Ghost image of the spinal column (cervical vertebrae), (**2**) ghost image of the opposite side mandible.

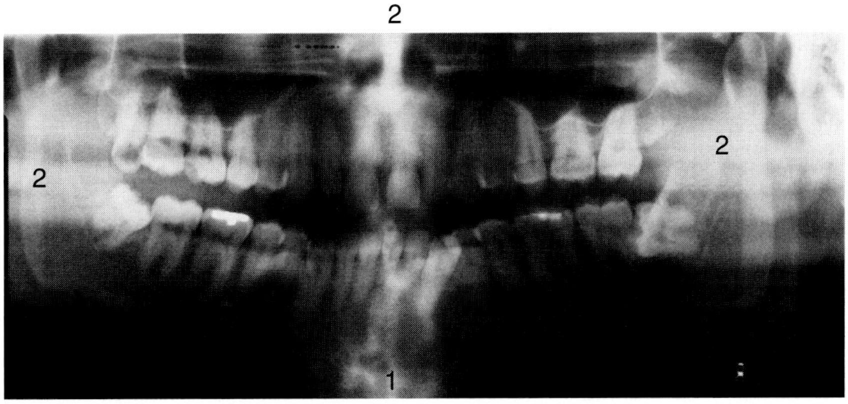

FIGURE 28-33 **Panoramic radiograph showing ghost images.** (**1**) Ghost image of the spinal column (cervical vertebrae), (**2**) ghost image of the opposite side mandible.

REVIEW—Chapter Summary

Panoramic radiography produces a broad view image of both the maxilla and the mandible on a single film. Panoramic radiographs are valuable in examining large areas of the face and jaws; locating impacted teeth or retained root tips; evaluating trauma, lesions, and diseases of the jaws; and assessing growth and development.

The greatest advantage of the panoramic radiograph is that it can image a greater area and provide an increased amount of diagnostic information when compared to a full mouth series of intraoral films. The greatest disadvantage of the panoramic radiograph is the image magnification and distortion that make interpreting the image difficult.

Panoramic imagery is based on tomography where a slice or layer of tissue can be imaged with relative clarity, while blurring out other structures not of interest. During the panoramic exposure, the film and the x-ray tube head move slowly (about 15–20 seconds cycle) in opposite directions around the patient's head. The patient remains still during the exposure, either in a standing or sitting position (depending on the unit type). Through the use of a series of rotational points or centers, the x-ray beam is directed toward the moving cassette to image a select plane of dental anatomy. The rotational center is defined as the axis on which the tube head and the cassette rotate. Manufacturers of panoramic machines use a double-center rotation, a triple-center rotation, or a moving-center rotation. Double-center rotation units produce a split image radiograph where the center of the film is blank/clear where the radiation momentarily shut off while the system shifted between the two rotation centers. Most modern panoramic units utilize a moving-center rotation and a continuous image.

The focal trough is the area between the x-ray source and the film where structures will be imaged clearly on the radiograph. Structures positioned outside the focal trough will be blurred out of the image. The focal trough is three-dimensional and the size and shape is determined by the unit manufacturer. Each unit manufacturer provides instructions and head positioner guides to aid the radiographer in positioning the patient within the focal trough.

All panoramic units have: (1) a rotational x-ray tube head; (2) a cassette holder (drum); (3) a head positioner guides; and (4) an exposure control panel. The PID is collimated to a narrow slit opening, allowing the x-ray beam to fan out to expose a slice of tissue as the tube head rotates around the patient's head. The x-ray beam penetrates the patient from the back of the head.

Positioning the patient's head within the focal trough is key to producing a diagnostic image. Most panoramic units have a forehead rest, chin rest or bite block to aid the radiographer in positioning the arches in the correct anterior–posterior dimension; side head positioner guides, a mirror, or beams of light that shine on the patient's face to determine the correct left–right dimension; and a chin rest or light beams to aid in locating the ala-tragus line or Frankfort plane to determine the correct superior–inferior dimension of the focal trough.

Panoramic errors result in characteristic image appearances. Positioning the arches too far forward in the focal trough produces blurred and diminished anterior teeth; positioning the arches too far back in the focal trough produces blurred and magnified anterior teeth. Positioning the arches too far to the lateral (tipping or turning the head to the right or left) results in diminished teeth on the side closer to the film and magnified teeth on the side closer to the center of rotation. Positioning the patient's chin too far down results in an image with an exaggerated "smile." Positioning the patient's chin too far up results in an image with an exaggerated "frown."

Panoramic errors also result from patient preparation mistakes. All metal or dense material objects, such as a necklace, earrings, oral piercings and other facial jewelry, must be removed prior to exposure. The patient must be instructed to rest the tongue against the palate and to close the lips around the biteblock during the exposure to minimize the appearance of these structures on the radiograph. Accurate exposure settings and careful film handling will avoid errors that result in undiagnostic radiographs.

The skilled radiographer should be able to identify normal radiographic anatomy of the maxilla and the mandible, including soft tissue images and air spaces that appear on a panoramic radiograph. The radiographer should be able to identify artifacts such as machine parts and ghost images as they appear on a panoramic radiograph.

RECALL—Review Questions

1. A panoramic radiograph is valuable when diagnosing each of the following *except* one. Which one is this exception?
   a. A cyst
   b. An impacted molar
   c. Recurrent caries
   d. A supernumerary tooth
2. Which of these is an advantage of a panoramic radiograph when compared to an intraoral radiograph?
   a. More structures are imaged
   b. The image is magnified
   c. Distortion is eliminated
   d. Definition is improved
3. Which of these is a disadvantage of a panoramic radiograph when compared to an intraoral radiograph?
   a. More teeth are shown on a panoramic film
   b. Ghost images appear on a panoramic film
   c. The sinuses may be shown on a panoramic film
   d. The temporomandibular joints may be shown on a panoramic film
4. What is the term given to the technique where a slice of tissue is exposed distinctly, while structures outside the designated area are blurred out of the image?
   a. Ghost image
   b. Artifact
   c. Focal trough
   d. Tomography
5. Which of the following panoramic machines must stop the radiation exposure to shift to the next pivotal point?
   a. Double-center rotation
   b. Triple-center rotation
   c. Moving-center rotation
6. Which of the following rotational centers results in a split-image panoramic radiograph?
   a. Double-center rotation
   b. Triple-center rotation
   c. Moving-center rotation
7. What is the term given to the area where structures will be imaged with relative clarity, while structures outside this area are blurred out of the image?
   a. Ghost image
   b. Artifact
   c. Focal trough
   d. Tomography
8. All of the following are components of most panoramic x-ray machines *except* one. Which one is this *exception?*
   a. Rotational x-ray tube head
   b. Cassette holder (drum)
   c. Head positioner guides
   d. Round collimated PID
9. Which of the following must be pre-set by the manufacturer of the panoramic x-ray machine?
   a. mA
   b. kVp
   c. Exposure time
   d. Head position guides
10. Which of the following planes is utilized to position the patient correctly within the superior-inferior (up-down) dimension?
    a. Ala-tragus line
    b. Frankfort plane
    c. Midsaggital plane
    d. Both (a) and (b)
11. Which of the following positioning errors results in anterior teeth that are blurry and diminished in size?
    a. Too far forward in the focal trough
    b. Too far backward in the focal trough
    c. Too far to the left in the focal trough
    d. Too far to the right in the focal trough
12. When the arches are rotated to the left, the teeth on the right side will be positioned closer to the film. The teeth closest to the film will appear blurry and magnified.
    a. The first statement is true. The second statement is false.
    b. The first statement is false. The second statement is true.
    c. Both statements are true.
    d. Both statements are false.

13. Which of the following positioning errors results in an exaggerated "smile" appearance of the arches?
    a. Midsaggital plane tipped to the left
    b. Midsaggital plane tipped to the right
    c. Chin tipped too far up
    d. Chin tipped too far down
14. The appearance of a large radiolucency that obscures the maxillary teeth apices results when:
    a. The lips are not closed around the bite block during exposure.
    b. The tongue is not resting on the palate during exposure.
    c. The lead thyroid collar gets in the way of the primary beam.
    d. Facial jewelry (e.g., oral piercing) is not removed prior to exposure.
15. Which of the following appears radiolucent on a panoramic radiograph?
    a. Nasal cavity
    b. Nasal septum
    c. Nasal spine
    d. Hard palate
16. Which of the following appears radiopaque on the panoramic radiograph?
    a. External auditory meatus
    b. Zygomatic process of the maxilla
    c. Mental fossa
    d. Mandibular foramen
17. Which of the following could be called a negative shadow?
    a. Tongue
    b. Ghost image
    c. Glossopharyngeal air space
    d. Bite block
18. List three air spaces that may be imaged on panoramic radiographs:
    a. ____________________
    b. ____________________
    c. ____________________
19. List three machine parts that may be imaged on panoramic radiographs:
    a. ____________________
    b. ____________________
    c. ____________________
20. What is the term given to a structure that is imaged a second time, with less sharpness and on the opposite side?
    a. Ghost image
    b. Focal trough
    c. Split image
    d. Tomograph

REFLECT—Case Study

You have to expose a panoramic radiograph on the following patients today. Each of these patients presents with a characteristic that will make positioning the patient for the procedure a challenge. Carefully review each of the patient descriptions and answer the following questions:

1. What patient positioning step do you anticipate having a problem with?
2. What error is most likely to occur?
3. What will the image look like?
4. How can you prevent this error from occurring or minimize the result on the image?
5. Write out the specific steps you plan to take to produce a diagnostic quality image.

Case A
A hyperactive 10-year-old child who seems to be having difficulty paying attention to your directions.

Case B
A young adult with multiple facial piercings, including a tongue ring and several earrings.

Case C
A young woman with fashionable hair extensions gathered into a large ponytail.

Case D
A middle-aged man who wears partial dentures that when removed reveal missing anterior teeth.

Case E
An older woman with osteoporosis who exhibits a pronounced stooped posture as a result of collapsed vertebrae.

RELATE—Laboratory Application

For a comprehensive laboratory practice exercise on this topic, see E. M. Thomson, *Exercises in Oral Radiography Techniques: A Laboratory Manual,* 2nd ed., Upper Saddle River, NJ: Prentice Hall, 2007. Chapter 14, "Panoramic Radiographic Technique."

BIBLIOGRAPHY

Eastman Kodak. *Successful Panoramic Radiography.* Rochester, NY: Eastman Kodak, 2000.

Farman, A. G., Nortje, C. J. & Wood, R. E. *Oral and Maxillofacial Diagnostic Imaging.* St. Louis: Mosby, 1993.

Langland, O. E., Langlais, R. P., & McDavid W. D. et al. *Panoramic Radiology,* 2nd ed. Philadelphia: Lea & Febiger, 1989.

White, S. C. & Pharoah, M. J. *Oral Radiology Principles and Interpretation,* 5th ed. St. Louis, Elsevier, 2004.

Answers to Study Questions

Chapter 1: 1. c, 2. a, 3. d, 4. e, 5. b, 6. d, 7. c, 8. b, 9. c, 10. c, 11. a, 12. d, 13. Use Table 1–2 to list uses, 14. a.

Chapter 2: 1. a, 2. Use chapter information and Figure 2–1 to draw diagram, 3. d, 4. c, 5. b, 6. c, 7. a, 8. a, 9. d, 10. b, 11. d, 12. Use chapter information to list properties, 13. a, 14. b, 15. d, 16. b, 17. Use chapter information to list sources, 18. c.

Chapter 3: 1. c, 2. b, 3. 0.5, 0.75, 20, 6, 4. a, 5. d, 6. a, 7. b, 8. Use chapter information to list conditions, 9. Use chapter information and Figure 3–11 to draw and label diagram, 10. c, 11. c, 12. b, 13. d, 14. a, 15. b, 16. a, 17. c, 18. d, 19. c.

Chapter 4: 1. Use chapter information to list criteria, 2. a, 3. c, 4. b, 5. c, 6. a, 7. b, 8. d, 9. a, 10. d, 11. b, 12. c, 13. d, 14. a, 15. a.

Chapter 5: 1. a, 2. c, 3. a, 4. d, 5. c, 6. b, 7. b, 8. d, 9. As low as reasonably achievable, 10. Use chapter information to list responses, 11. c, 12. a, 13. a, 14. b, 15. d, 16. c, 17. d, 18. d, 19. c, 20. d.

Chapter 6: 1. d, 2. d, 3. b, 4. c, 5. a, 6. c, 7. b, 8. d, 9. d, 10. c, 11. a, 12. b, 13. b, 14. c, 15. c, 16. b.

Chapter 7: 1. a, 2. d, 3. c, 4. b, 5. b, 6. c, 7. c, 8. b, 9. a, 10. d, 11. a, 12. a.

Chapter 8: 1. b, 2. c, 3. a, 4. a, 5. c, 6. d, 7. b, 8. d, 9. a, 10. c, 11. b, 12. b, 13. d, 14. Used fixer, lead foil, discarded radiographs, 15. a, 16. c, 17. b, 18. a, 19. b, 20. c, 21. d.

Chapter 9: 1. d, 2. a, 3. b, 4. Use chapter information to list items, 5. c, 6. b, 7. c, 8. b, 9. d, 10. a.

Chapter 10: 1. d, 2. a, 3. d, 4. b, 5. Use chapter information to list aspects, 6. c, 7. Use chapter information to list items, 8. c, 9. a, 10. d, 11. b, 12. d, 13. c, 14. a.

Chapter 11: 1. d, 2. Use chapter information to list aspects, 3. a, 4. a, 5. c, 6. d, 7. b, 8. a, 9. d, 10. c, 11. b, 12. Use chapter information to list responses.

Chapter 12: 1. c, 2. a, 3. d, 4. b, 5. a, 6. b, 7. c, 8. a, 9. d, 10. d. 11. Use chapter information to list contraindications, 12. c, 13. a, 14. b, 15. c, 16. c, 17. d.

Chapter 13: 1. c, 2. b, 3. a, 4. b. 5. c, 6. d, 7. d, 8. a, 9. c, 10. b, 11. c, 12. a, 13. c, 14. b, 15. d, 16. d, 17. b, 18. a, 19. b.

Chapter 14: 1. c, 2. b, 3. b, 4. c. 5. d, 6. a, 7. c, 8. a, 9. d, 10. c, 11. d, 12. c, 13. d, 14. d.

Chapter 15: 1. d, 2. d, 3. a, 4. b, 5. b, 6. a, 7. c, 8. c, 9. d.

Chapter 16: 1. d, 2. c, 3. a, 4. d, 5. c, 6. b, 7. c, 8. a, 9. d, 10. b, 11. c, 12. d, 13. a, 14. c.

Chapter 17: 1. c, 2. Use chapter information to list objectives, 3. d, 4. b, 5. a, 6. d, 7. b, 8. d, 9. c.

Chapter 18: 1. Use chapter information to list advantages, 2. d, 3. d, 4. b, 5. d, 6. c, 7. a, 8. d, 9. b, 10. c, 11. a, 12. b, 13. d.

Chapter 19: 1. c, 2. d, 3. b, 4. b, 5. a, 6. d, 7. a, 8. c, 9. d, 10. b, 11. a, 12. c, 13. b, 14. d, 15. c, 16. b, 17. a.

Chapter 20: 1. b, 2. a, 3. d, 4. d, 5. c, 6. c, 7. b, 8. a, 9. b, 10. c, 11. d, 12. c, 13. a.

Chapter 21: 1. b, 2. d, 3. a, 4. b, 5. c, 6. a, 7. a, 8. c, 9. b, 10. d, 11. c, 12. a, 13. b, 14. b.

Chapter 22: 1. b, 2. Use chapter information to list uses, 3. c, 4. d, 5. c, 6. a, 7. b, 8. Use chapter information to list limitations, 9. d, 10. d, 11. a, 12. b.

Chapter 23: 1. Use chapter information to list conditions, 2. c, 3. b, 4. d, 5. a, 6. d, 7. a, 8. b, 9. d, 10. c, 11. c, 12. a, 13. b, 14. a, 15. b, 16. d, 17. c, 18. d.

Chapter 24: 1. Use chapter information to list actions, 2. b, 3. a, 4. c, 5. b, 6. d, 7. a, 8. d, 9. b, 10. d, 11. d, 12. c.

Chapter 25: 1. d, 2. b, 3. a, 4. b, 5. c, 6. d, 7. a, 8. d, 9. a, 10. d, 11. c, 12. b, 13. d, 14. d, 15. b, 16. Use chapter information to list reasons.

Chapter 26: 1. d, 2. e, 3. c, 4. a, 5. b, 6. c, 7. e, 8. d, 9. b, 10. e, 11. e, 12. c, 13. d, 14. Use chapter information to list features, 15. a, 16. b, 17. d.

Chapter 27: 1. a, 2. b, 3. c, 4. b, 5. d, 6. c, 7. a, 8. d, 9. a, 10. d, 11. c, 12. b, 13. b.

Chapter 28: 1. c, 2. a, 3. b, 4. d, 5. a, 6. a, 7. c, 8. d, 9. c, 10. d, 11. a, 12. d, 13. d, 14. b, 15. a, 16. b, 17. c, 18. palatoglossal, nasopharyngeal, glossopharyngeal, 19. chin rest, side head positioner guides, 20. a.

Glossary

Abscess: A localized pus formation often accompanied by swelling and pain. When involving an infected tooth, an abscess is usually located near the apex of the roots. May be chronic or acute. Appears radiolucent when large enough to be visible on a radiograph.

Absorbed dose: The amount of energy deposited in any form of matter, such as teeth, soft tissues, treatment chair, air, and so forth, by any type of radiation (alpha or beta particles, x- or gamma rays, etc.). The units for measuring the absorbed dose are the gray (Gy) and the rad (radiation absorbed dose).

Absorption: The process through which radiation imparts some or all of its energy to any material through which it passes.

Acetic acid: A chemical in the fixer solution that provides the acid medium to stop further development by neutralizing the alkali of the developer.

Acidifier: A chemical (acetic acid) in the fixer solution that neutralizes the alkali in the developer solution and stops further action of the developer.

Acoustic meatus: The opening at the center of the ear. Located directly over the temporal bone. Observed on extraoral radiographs as a small radiolucent circle.

Acquired immune deficiency syndrome: *See* AIDS.

Activator: A chemical (usual sodium carbonate) in the developer solution that causes the emulsion on the radiographic film to swell. Initiates the reducing action of the developing agents. Sodium carbonate makes the developer alkaline.

Acute: Having a rapid onset, short, severe course, and pronounced symptoms. Opposite of chronic.

Acute radiation syndrome: Symptoms of the short-term radiation effects after a massive dose of ionizing radiation.

Added filtration: Added to the inherent filtration built into the x-ray machine. Added filtration is in the form of thin disks of pure aluminum, which can be inserted between the x-ray tube and the lead collimator when the inherent filtration is not sufficient to meet modern radiation safety requirements.

Advanced caries: A classification of proximal surface caries. Category where caries has progressed all the way through the enamel, to or through the dentinoenamel junction (DEJ) but less than halfway through the dentin toward the pulp

AIDS (acquired immune deficiency syndrome): The end stage of an infection with the human immunodeficiency virus (HIV). A complex disease that interferes with the body's immune system.

Ala: The wing of the nose. The depression at which the nostril connects with the cheek. Used as a facial landmark in dental radiography.

ALARA: As low as reasonably achievable. Adopted as a culture and attitude of professionals who work with ionizing radiation to minimize radiation exposure and risks.

Ala-tragus line: An imaginary plane or line from the ala of the nose (a winglike projection at the side of the nose) to the tragus of the ear (the cartilaginous projection in front of the acoustic meatus of the ear). Important in determining the correct position of the patient's head.

Alpha particle: A common form of particulate (corpuscular) radiation. Alpha particles contain two protons and two neutrons, and are positively charged.

Alternating current (AC): A flow of electrons in one direction, followed by a flow in the opposite direction.

Aluminum equivalent: The thickness of aluminum affording the same degree of attenuation, under specified conditions, as the material in question.

Alveolar (crestal) bone: That portion of the maxillary or mandibular bone that immediately surrounds and supports the roots of the dentition.

Alveolar process: The most coronal portion of the alveolar bone. Appears radiopaque when visible on a radiograph.

Alveolus: In dentistry, that part of the alveolar bone that forms the bony socket in which the roots of the tooth are held in position by fibers of the periodontal ligament.

Amalgam: Metallic restorative material.

Amalgam tattoo: The bluish-purple color of the gingival tissue caused by fragments of amalgam under the tissue.

Ameloblastoma: An odontogenic tumor of enamel origin that does not undergo differentiation to the point of enamel formation.

Amelogenesis imperfecta (enamel hypoplasia): A hereditary enamel deficiency of the teeth. Believed to be caused by a generalized disturbance of the ameloblasts (enamel-producing cells). The remaining tooth structures are not affected. On radiographs, such teeth lack the radiopaque image of enamel.

American Dental Assistants Association (ADAA): Professional organization for the purpose of promoting the dental assisting profession in ways that enhance the delivery of quality oral healthcare to the public.

American Dental Association (ADA): Professional organization of dentists committed to the public's oral health through professional advancement, research, education, and the development of standards of care.

American Dental Hygienists' Association (ADHA): Professional organization for the purpose of advancing the art and science of dental hygiene by ensuring access to quality oral healthcare and increasing awareness of the cost-effective benefits of prevention.

Amperage: The strength of an electric current measured in amperes.

Ampere (A): The unit of intensity of an electric current produced by 1 volt acting through a resistance of 1 ohm.

Analog: Relating to the mechanism in which data is represented by continuously variable physical quantities.

Anatomical order: The order in which the teeth are arranged in the dental arches.

Angle of mandible: The area at the posterior and inferior corners of the mandible, where the body of the mandible meets and joins the ascending ramus of the mandible.

Angstrom: A unit of measurement that describes the wavelengths of certain high-frequency radiation. One angstrom unit (AU, or Å) measures 1/100,000,000 of a centimeter. Most wavelengths used in dentistry vary from about 0.1 AU to a maximum of 1.0 AU.

Angular chelitis: Fissuring and ulcerations at the corners of the mouth.

Angulation: The direction in which the central ray and the PID of the x-ray machine are directed toward the teeth and the film. *See* Horizontal angulation, Negative angulation, Positive angulation, and Vertical angulation.

Ankylosis: A stiffening of a joint, such as the TMJ caused by a fibrous or bony union. In dentistry the term can also apply to a union of the tooth to the alveolus caused by mineralization and hardening of the fibers of the periodontal ligament.

Anode: The positive electrode (terminal) in the x-ray tube. Tungsten block, normally set at a 20-degree angle facing the cathode, imbedded in the copper portion of the terminal.

Anodontia: A congenital absence of teeth. Any tooth in the dental arch may fail to develop. The teeth most frequently absent are the third molars, the premolars, and the maxillary lateral incisors.

Anomaly: A deviation from the normal.

Anterior nasal spine: The most anterior point on the floor of the nasal cavity. Located at the mid-sagittal plane.

Antihalation coating: A dye added to the non-emulsion side of duplicating film to prevent backscattered ultraviolet light from coming through the films and creating an unsharp image.

Antiseptic: Refers to agents used on living tissues to destroy or stop the growth of bacteria.

Apical foramen: The opening to the pulp canal at the apex (terminal end) of the root of the tooth. A three-rooted tooth would have three apical foramina.

Apprehensive: To be anxious or fearful about the future.

Area monitoring: The routine monitoring of the level of radiation in an area such as a room, building, space around radiation-emitting equipment, or outdoor space.

Arrested caries: Caries that are no longer active.

Artifacts: Images on the film other than anatomy or pathology that do not contribute to a diagnosis of the patient's condition.

Asepsis: The absence of septic matter, or freedom from infection.

Atom: The smallest particle of an element that has the properties of that element. Atoms are extremely minute and are composed of a number of subatomic particles. *See* Proton, Electron, and Neutron.

Atomic number (also called Z number): The total number of protons in the nucleus of an atom.

Atomic weight (also called A number or mass number): The total number of protons and neutrons in the nucleus of an atom.

Attenuation: In radiography, the process by which a beam of radiation is reduced in energy when passing through matter.

Attitude: The position assumed by the body in connection with a feeling or mood.

Automatic processing unit: A machine that develops, fixes, washes and dries radiographic film.

Autotransformer: A special single-coil transformer that corrects fluctuations in the current flowing through the x-ray machine.

Background radiation: Ionizing radiation that is always present. Consists of cosmic rays from outer space, naturally occurring radiation from the earth, and radiation from radioactive materials.

Backscatter: Radiation that is deflected by scattering processes at angles greater than 90 degrees to the original direction of the beam of radiation.

Barrier: Any material that is used to prevent the transmission of infective micro-organisms to the patient.

Barrier envelope: Plastic envelopes used to seal intraoral film packets to protect from contact with fluids in the oral cavity during exposure.

Base material: A thick layer of cement used as a cavity preparation under a restoration. Base material often appears slightly more radiopaque than dentin.

Beam indicating device (BID): *See* Positioning indicating device (PID).

Benign: Non-cancerous. Not usually an immediate threat to overall health.

Beta particle: A form of particulate radiation. High-speed negative electrons.

Binding energy: The internal energy within the atom that holds its components together.

Bisecting technique (bisecting-angle or short-cone technique): An exposure technique in which the central beam of radiation is directed perpendicular to an imaginary line that bisects the angle formed by the recording plane of the film and the long axes of the teeth.

Bisector: The imaginary line that bisects the angle formed by the film and teeth. *See* Bisecting technique.

Biteblock: A plastic or polystyrene device that functions to hold the x-ray film in position while it is being exposed. The patient occludes and holds the film in place by biting on the biteblock.

Bite extension: That portion of the biteblock that allows the patient to occlude in such a way that film packet will be positioned parallel to the long axes of the teeth.

Bitetab: An extension, usually made out of heavy paper, that is attached at the center of the film packet and on which the patient bites to stabilize the film during a bitewing exposure.

Bitewing radiograph: An intraoral radiograph that shows the crowns of both the upper and lower teeth on the same film.

Bloodborne pathogens: Pathogens present in blood that causes disease in humans.

Bremsstrahlung radiation: *See* general radiation.

Buccal caries: Caries that involves the buccal surface of a tooth.

Buccal-object rule: Principle that structures portrayed in two or more radiographs exposed at different angles will appear to shift positions.

Calcium tungstate phosphors: Barium strontium sulfate salt crystals that are used in intensifying screens. When x-rays are absorbed, the crystals fluoresce and emit energy in the form of blue light.

Calculus: Calcified microbial plaque.

Canal: A tube-like passageway through bone that contains nerves and blood vessels. Appears radiolucent in radiographs.

Cancellous bone: *See* Trabecular bone.

Canthus: The angle at either end of the slit that separates the eyelids. The inner canthus is nearest the nose. The outer canthus is farthest from the nose.

Carcinoma: Malignant growth of epithelial cells. A form of cancer.

Caries: Disease of the calcified tissues of the teeth. The inorganic portion is demineralized and the organic tissues are destroyed.

Cassette: A rigid or flexible extraoral film holder. Cassettes contain a pair of intensifying screens.

Cassette holder (drum): That part of a panoramic x-ray machine where the cassette is positioned for exposure.

Cathode: The negative electrode (terminal) in the x-ray tube. The cathode consists of a tungsten filament wire that is set in a molybdenum focusing cup that directs the cathode stream toward the target on the anode.

Cemental (root) caries: Caries that develops on the roots of teeth between the enamel border and the free margin of the gingiva.

Cementoenamel junction (CEJ): The area where the enamel covering of the tooth crown meets the cementum covering of the tooth root.

Cementoma: A tumor derived from the periodontal ligament of a fully developed and erupted tooth, usually a mandibular incisor. Early cementomas are radiolucent and appear identical to radicular cysts. In the later stages of development, calcification occurs and cementomas appear as radiopaque masses surrounded by a radiolucent line. The teeth associated with cementomas are vital and need no treatment.

Cementum: One of the four basic tooth structures. The thin layer of dense tissue that covers the root of a tooth. Because the cementum layer is thin, it is generally radiographically indistinguishable from dentin. When the condition of hypercementosis presents, the overgrowth of cementum will appear radiopaque and bulbous.

Central ray: The central portion of the primary beam of radiation.

Cephalometer: A headholder or precision instrument used to stabilize the patient's head during exposure. Holds the head parallel to the film and at right angles to the radiation beam.

Cephalometric radiographs: Lateral and posteroanterior extraoral radiographs. Frequently used in orthodontic and prosthodontic treatments.

Cephalostat: A device used to stabilize the patient's head in a plane that is parallel to the film and at right angles to the central rays of the x-ray beam. Ear rods that can be placed into the openings of the acoustic meatus of the ear help to accomplish this.

Cervical burnout: A radiolucency often observed on the mesial and distal root surfaces near the cementoenamel junction. The radiolucent appearance is caused by the concave shape of the root at the cervical line and may be mistaken for caries.

Chairside darkroom: A light-tight box with a filter cover used to rapidly process working radiographs. Usually in the operatory where the patient is being treated.

Chairside manner: Refers to the conduct of the dental radiographer while working at the patient's chairside.

Chairside processing: Refers to the use of a chairside processor to rapidly obtain working radiographs. Often necessary during endodontic procedures.

Characteristic radiation: A form of radiation originating from an atom following removal of an electron or excitation of the atom. The wavelength of the emitted radiation is specific for the element and the particular energy levels involved.

Charge-coupled device (CCD): A CCD is a solid-state detector used in many electronic devices such as video cameras and fax machines. A CCD is used as the image receptor found in digital sensors. Converts x-rays to electrons that are sent to a computer via a wire, or wirelessly via radio frequency.

Clearing time test: Quality control test to determine the efficacy of fixer solution.

Code of ethics: A professional organization's principles to assist members in achieving a high standard of ethical practice.

Coherent scattering: Radiation that is scattered when a low-energy x-ray passes near an atom's outer electron. Approximately 8 percent of interactions of matter with the dental x-ray beam are the result of coherent scattering.

Coin test: Quality control test used to determine the adequacy of safelighting in the darkroom.

Collimation: The restriction of the useful beam to an appropriate size. Intraoral beam diameter is collimated to 2 3/4 in. (7 cm) at the skin surface.

Collimator: A diaphragm, usually lead, designed to restrict the dimensions of the useful beam.

Communication: The process by which information is exchanged between two or more persons.

Complementary metal oxide semiconductor (CMOS): A solid-state integrated circuit similar to the CCD. Used in digital radiography as an image receptor in the intraoral sensor. Converts x-rays to electrons that are sent to a computer via a wire, or wirelessly via radio frequency.

Composite (composite resin): Tooth-colored material used for restorations.

Compton effect (Compton scattering): An attenuation process for x- and gamma radiation in which a photon interacts with an orbital electron or an atom to form a displaced electron and a scattered photon (x-ray) of reduced energy.

Computed tomography (CT): Radiographic imaging technique that images an isolated "slice" of tissue while blurring out other structures.

Concrescence: Condition where the cementum of adjacent teeth is joined together.

Condensing osteitis: Term used to describe the formation of compact sclerotic bone. Such areas of hardened bone are frequently seen on dental radiographs and appear more radiopaque than the surrounding bone areas. Such areas are generally irregular in shape or location.

Condyle: A rounded knob or projection on a bone, usually where that bone articulates (joins) with another bone. The condyle of the mandible articulates with the glenoid fossa (depression) of the temporal bone.

Confidentiality: Private information, such as dental records, that is protected by law from being shared with non-privileged individuals.

Cone: Older term used to describe the positioning indicating device (PID) or beam indicating device (BID).

Cone cut: A term used to describe a technique error in which the central beam is not directed toward the center of the film. This produces a blank area in that part of the radiograph that was not reached by the radiation.

Consumer-Patient Health Act: Action that sought to establish minimum standards for personnel who administer radiation in medical and dental radiographic procedures. Passed and signed into law to protect patients from unnecessary radiation.

Contact points: The area of a tooth surface that touches another tooth. This generally refers to the mesial surface of one tooth making contact with the distal surface of the tooth adjacent to it in the dental arch. The spot where the teeth actually touch is the contact point and the area between the contact point and the gingiva (gum) is called the embrasure.

Contamination: The soiling by contact or mixing.

Contrast: The visual differences between shades ranging from black to white in adjacent areas of the radiographic film. A radiograph that shows few shades has a short-scale or high contrast. A radiograph that shows many variations in shade has a long-scale or low contrast. High kilovoltage produces a radiograph with long-scale contrast. Low kilovoltage produces a radiograph with short-scale contrast.

Control factors: *See* Exposure factors.

Control panel: That portion of the x-ray machine that houses the major controls. Includes the line switch, timer, milliamperage and kilovoltage selectors, and the exposure button.

Coronoid process of the mandible: The pointed, anterior process on the upper border of the mandible.

Cortical bone: The solid, outer portion of the dense, compact bone. Appears very radiopaque on radiographs.

Coulombs per kilogram (C/kg): Système Internationale unit for measuring exposure. A coulomb is a unit of electrical charge (equal to 6.25×10^{18} electrons). The unit C/kg measures electrical charges (ion pairs) in a kilogram of air.

Cross-contamination: To contaminate from one place or person to another place or person.

Cross-sectional technique: An occlusal radiographic technique in which the central ray is directed perpendicular to the film.

Crown: That portion of the tooth covered with enamel. "Clinical crown" refers to the entire portion of a tooth that is visible in the oral cavity. May also refer to a metallic or porcelain or combination of metal and porcelain restoration.

Crystal: Term used to refer to the silver halide combinations that are present in the film emulsion. Larger crystals require less radiation exposure to produce an image. However, larger crystal size may result in slightly less image resolution.

Cultural barriers: When language, beliefs, traditions, and familiar influences become obstacles to the patient achieving optimal oral health.

Cumulative effect: The theory that radiation-exposed tissues accrue damage and may function at a diminished capacity with each repeated exposure.

Cyst: An epithelium-lined sac containing fluid or other fibrous or solid material which appear radiolucent. Common cysts observed on dental radiographs are dentigerous, follicular, radicular (apical or periapical), and residual.

Darkroom: A light-tight room with special safelighting where x-ray film is handled and processed.

Daylight loader: A light-shielded compartment attached to an automatic processor so films can be unwrapped in a room with white light.

"Dead-man" switch: A switch so constructed that a circuit-closing contact can only be maintained by continuous pressure by the operator.

Decay: The radioactive disintegration of the nucleus of an unstable atom by the emission of particles, photons of energy, or both.

Definition: Sharpness and clarity of the outline of the structures in a radiographic image. Poor definition is generally caused by movement of the patient, film, or the tube head during exposure.

Dens in dente: A developmental anomaly in which the enamel invaginates within the body of the tooth.

Density: The overall darkening or blackening of the radiographic image as determined by the amount of light transmitted through a film. The simplest way to increase or decrease the density of a radiograph is to increase or decrease the milliamperage and exposure time (milliampere/second).

Dentigerous cyst: A cyst derived from the enamel organ and always associated with the crown of a tooth.

Dentin: One of the four basic tooth structures. The chief tissue of the tooth that surrounds the pulp. Dentin is covered by enamel on the crown of the tooth and by cementum on the root. Appears slightly less radiopaque than enamel.

Dentinoenamel junction (DEJ): The junction between the dentin and enamel of a tooth.

Dentinogenesis imperfecta: A hereditary condition characterized by imperfectly formed dentin that has an opalescent or amber color.

Dentition: Teeth. The term dentulous refers to areas of the jaws having teeth.

Deterministic (non-stochastic): Observable adverse biological effects caused by radiation exposure. The severity of change in tissues depends on the radiation dose.

Developer: The chemical solution used in film processing that makes the latent image visible.

Developing agent: Elon and hydroquinone, substances that reduce the halides in the film emulsion to metallic silver. Elon brings out the details and hydroquinone brings out the contrast in the film.

Diagnosis: The art of differentiating and determining the nature of a problem or disease.

Diaphragm: *See* Collimator.

Digital image: Radiographic image that exists as bits of information in a computer file. Special computer software constructs an image on a monitor for viewing.

Digital imaging: A method of producing a filmless radiographic image using a sensor (instead of film) and transmitting the electronic information directly into a computer, which serves to acquire, process, store, retrieve, and display the radiographic image.

Digital Imaging and Communications in Medicine (DICOM): A joint committee formed in 1983 by the American College of Radiology and the National Electrical Manufacturers Association to create a standard method for electronic transmissions of digital images, the goal of which is to achieve compatibility and ease exchange of electronic information between digital image systems.

Digital radiography: A filmless imaging system. The terms digital imaging and digital radiography are often used interchangeably.

Digital subtraction: Using a computer to superimpose two standardized radiographic images, causing the like areas of the image to "cancel" each other out, leaving only the changes visible.

Digitize: To convert an image into a digital form that can be processed by a computer.

Dilaceration: A sharp bend in the tooth root.

Direct current (DC): Electric current that flows continuously in one direction. Similar to current produced in batteries. Ideal for use with digital imaging.

Direct digital imaging: A method of directly obtaining a digital image by exposing an intraoral sensor to x-rays to produce an image that can be viewed on a computer monitor.

Direct supervision: Means the dentist is present in the office when the radiographs are taken on patients.

Direct theory: States that cell damage results when ionizing radiation directly hits critical areas within the cell.

Disability: A physical or mental impairment that substantially limits one or more of an individual's major life activities.

Disclosure: The process of informing the patient about the risks and benefits of a treatment procedure.

Disinfect: A term used to describe those efforts made to reduce disease-producing microorganisms to an acceptable level.

Disinfection: The act of disinfecting.

Distomesial projection: When the projection angle of the x-ray beam is directed from distal to mesial, resulting in overlapping error.

Disto-oblique periapical radiographs: Periapical radiographs that utilize a tube shift to help image posterior objects such as impacted third molars. Shifting the tube to the distal, causing the x-rays to be directed from the distal aspect, will project the posterior object forward onto the film.

Distortion: The variation in the true size and shape of the object being radiographed.

Dosage: The radiation absorbed in a specified area of the body measured in grays (Gy) or rads.

Dose: The amount of absorbed radiation in grays or rads at any given point. Dose may refer to absorbed dose, depth of the dose, entrance dose, or surface dose.

Dose equivalent: Compares the biological effects of various types of radiation. Dose equivalent is defined as the product of the absorbed dose times a biological effect qualifying factor. Since the qualifying factor for x-rays is one, the absorbed dose and the dose equivalent are equal. The units for measuring the dose equivalent are the sievert (Sv) and the rem.

Dose rate: The radiation dose received per unit of time.

Dose-response curve: Graph produced when radiation dose and the resultant biological response are plotted.

Dosimeter: A radiation measuring device.

"Dot in the slot": Saying used to prompt the radiographer to position the embossed film identification dot into the slot of the film holder to position the dot away from the area of interest.

Double exposure: Using the same film packet to expose two radiographs. Results in an overexposed, double image error.

Drum: *See* cassette holder.

Duplicate radiograph: A copy made of a radiograph. Useful in referrals, consultations, and for submitting to insurance companies for payment of dental treatment.

Duplicating film: A photographic film similar to x-ray film. Duplicating film is exposed by the action of infrared and ultraviolet light rather than by x-rays. Used to duplicate x-ray films in a contact-printer-type x-ray duplicating unit.

Edentulous: Without teeth. Areas of the jaws with no teeth.

Effective dose equivalent: Aids in making more accurate comparisons between different radiographic exposures. Compensates for the differences in area exposed and the tissues that may be in the path of the x-ray beam. Measured in microsieverts (μSv).

Electric current: The flow of electrons through a conductor.

Electrical circuit: A path of electrical current.

Electrode: Either of two terminals of an electric source. In the x-ray tube, either the anode or the cathode.

Electromagnetic radiation: Forms of energy propelled by wave motion as photons. This is a combination of electric and magnetic energy. Has no charge, mass, or weight and travels at the speed of light. Differ in wavelength, frequency, and properties. For convenience, electromagnetic radiations are arranged in diagrammatic form as the electromagnetic spectrum.

Electromagnetic spectrum: Types of electromagnetic energies arranged in diagrammatic form on a chart. Include radio and television waves, infrared waves, visible light, ultraviolet waves, x-rays, gamma rays, and cosmic radiations. The longer wavelengths are measured in meters and the shorter ones in centimeters or angstroms.

Electron: A small, negatively charged particle of the atom containing much energy and little mass.

Electron cloud: A mass of free electrons that hovers around the filament wire of the cathode when it is heated to incandescence. The number of free electrons increases as the milliamperage is increased.

Element: In chemistry, a simple substance that cannot be decomposed by chemical means.

Elon: Developer reducing agent that converts exposed silver halide crystals to black metallic silver. Builds up gray tones in the image.

Elongation: Refers to a distortion of the radiographic image in which the tooth structures appear longer than the anatomical size. Often caused by insufficient vertical angulation of the central beam.

Embrasure: The space between the sloping proximal surfaces of the teeth. The space may diverge facially, lingually, occlusally, or apically. The interdental papillae normally fill most of the apical embrasures.

Empathy: The ability to share in another's emotions or feelings.

Emulsion: The gelatinous coating on radiographic film containing silver halide crystals.

Enamel: One of the four basic tooth structures. The dense, hard substance that covers the dentin of the crown of the teeth. Appears very radiopaque on the radiograph.

Endodontic therapy: The treatment of the tooth by removing the nerves and tissues of the pulp cavity and replacing them with filling material.

Energy: The ability to do work and overcome resistance.

Energy levels (electron shells or orbits): A term used in chemistry and physics to denote spherical levels containing the electrons of the atom.

Ethics: A sense of moral obligation regarding right and wrong behavior.

Exfoliation: Shedding of primary teeth.

Exostosis: A bony growth projecting outward from the surface of a bone or tooth. Occasionally encountered on the palate or the lingual surface of the mandible as tori.

Exposure: A measure of ionization produced in air by x- or gamma radiation. The units of exposure are coulombs per kilogram (C/kg) and the roentgen (R).

Exposure button: Key pad or switch that activates the x-ray production process.

Exposure chart: A chart listing the exposure factors (milliamperage, exposure time, and kilovoltage) for each radiographic procedure.

Exposure factors: Settings for milliamperage (mA), exposure time, and kilovoltage (kVp).

Exposure incident: An incident that involves contact with blood or other potentially infectious materials that results from procedures performed by oral healthcare personnel.

Exposure time: The time interval, expressed in seconds or impulses, that x-rays are produced.

Extension arm: Flexible arm from which the tube head of the x-ray machine is suspended.

External aiming device (indicator ring): An indicating component of some film holders that is used to aid in aligning the x-ray beam to the film.

External auditory meatus (foramen): An opening in the temporal bone located superior and anterior to the mastoid process.

External oblique ridge: *See* Oblique ridge.

External resorption: Tooth structure lost through a resorptive process. Characterized by tooth roots that appear shorter than normal, but can also occur anywhere along the tooth root. Resorption of the roots of primary teeth in response to the erupting permanent teeth is considered normal. Pathologic external resorption may be associated with an impacted or unerupted tooth, a tumor, or trauma. Often the cause is idiopathic (unknown).

Extraoral: Outside the mouth.

Extraoral film: Designed for use outside the mouth.

Extraoral radiograph: A radiograph exposed outside the mouth. More sensitive to light exposure than intraoral film.

Extraoral radiography: Radiographic examinations made of the head and facial region using films positioned outside the mouth. Requires the use of a cassette and intensifying screens.

FAQs: Stands for frequently asked questions.

Federal Performance Act of 1974: Requires that all x-ray equipment manufactured or sold in the United States meet federal performance standards.

Filament: The spiral tungsten coil in the focusing cup of the cathode of the x-ray tube.

Film badge: A monitoring device containing a special type of film which, when properly developed and interpreted, gives a measurement of the exposure received during the time the badge was worn.

Film contrast: *See* Contrast.

Film duplicator: A device that provides a diffused light source (usually ultraviolet) that evenly exposes the duplicating film.

Film feed slot: Opening in an automatic film processor where the film is inserted for processing.

Film fog: An overall darkening of the radiograph caused by old or contaminated processing solutions, exposure to chemical fumes, faulty safelight, or scatter radiation.

Film hanger: A stainless steel hanger equipped with clips used to hold films during manual processing.

Film holder: Device used to hold and stabilize an intraoral film packet in the mouth.

Film loop (bitewing loop): Cardboard loop used as a film holder in bitewing radiography. The patient bites on the tab portion to hold the film in position during exposure.

Film mount: Plastic or cardboard holder with frames or windows that display films for viewing.

Film mounting: The placement of dental radiographs in a film mount.

Film packet: Intraoral film packaged in a moisture-proof outer plastic or paper wrap. May contain one or two films, wrapped in dark protective paper on either side, and a thin sheet of lead foil on the back side of the film(s).

Film recovery slot: Opening in an automatic film processing unit where the finished radiograph exits at the completion of the processing cycle.

Film speed: The sensitivity of the film to radiation exposure. Fast film speed requires less radiation to produce an image. Slow film speed requires more radiation to produce an image.

Filter: Absorbing material, usually aluminum, placed in the path of the beam of radiation to remove a high percentage of the low energy (longer wavelength) x-rays.

Filtration: The use of absorbers for selectively absorbing or screening out low-energy x-rays from the primary beam. *See* Added filtration, Inherent filtration, and Total filtration.

Fixer: A solution of chemicals that stops the action of the developer and makes the image permanently visible.

Fixing agent: Sodium thiosulfate, also known as "hypo" or hyposulfite of sodium. It is one of several chemical ingredients in the fixer solution and functions to remove all unexposed and any remaining undeveloped silver bromide grains from the emulsion.

Flexible cassette: Plastic sleeve cassette. Flexible cassettes are placed to wrap around the drum of certain types of panoramic x-ray machines.

Floor (border) of the maxillary sinus: Dense bone indicating the walls of the maxillary sinuses. Appears radiographically as a thin radiopaque line.

Focal spot: Small area on the target on the anode toward which the electrons from the focusing cup of the cathode are directed. X-rays originate at the focal spot.

Focal trough: That area between the x-ray source and the film that will be imaged distinctly on the panoramic radiograph. The size and shape of the focal trough vary with each panoramic x-ray machine.

Focusing cup: A curved device around the cathode wire filament that is designed to focus the free electrons toward the tungsten target of the anode.

Follicular (eruptive) cyst: A cyst associated with the enamel follicle.

Foramen: A naturally formed hole or passage through a bone or tooth, often the opening for a canal through which blood vessels and nerves pass. Appears radiolucent radiographically.

Foreign body: Any object or material not normally found in the area.

Foreshortening: Distortion of the radiographic image in which the tooth structures appear shorter than their actual anatomical size. Most often caused by excessive vertical angulation of the central beam.

Fossa: A depression or hollow area on a tooth or bone. If large enough, will appear as a radiolucent area on a radiograph.

Fracture line: A break in a bone or a tooth. Appears radiolucent radiographically.

Frankfort plane: An imaginary plane or line from the orbital ridge (under the eye) to the acoustic meatus of the ear.

Frequency: The number of crests of a wavelength passing a given point per second.

Fresh film test: Quality control test used to monitor the quality of each new box of film.

Frontal bone: Cranial bone that forms the forehead.

Full-mouth survey: The complete radiographic examination of the arches in which all teeth are imaged at least once, usually consists of 14 to 22 periapical and bitewing radiographs.

Furcation involvement: Bone loss between the roots of multi-rooted teeth.

Fusion: A condition where the dentin and one other dental tissue of adjacent teeth are united.

Gag reflex: A protective mechanism that serves to clear the airway of obstruction.

Gamma rays: A form of electromagnetic radiation with properties identical to x-rays. Usually produced spontaneously in the form of emission from radioactive substances.

Gelatin: Component of the film emulsion in which the halide crystals are suspended.

Gemination: A single tooth bud that divides and forms two teeth.

General radiation: Also called bremsstrahlung (which means "braking" in German) radiation. The stopping or slowing of the electrons of the cathode stream as they collide with the nuclei of the target atoms.

Generalized bone loss: Bone loss that occurs throughout the dental arches.

Genetic cells: The cells contained within the testes and ovaries, containing the genes.

Genetic effects: Radiation effects that are passed on to future generations.

Genetic mutations: Changes in the genetic material of cells that passes from one generation to another.

Genial tubercles: Anatomical landmark situated near the midline on the lingual surface of the mandible about halfway between the alveolar crest and the inferior border of the mandible. Appear radiographically as a small doughnut-shaped, radiopaque ring. The lingual foramen is located in the center of this ring.

Geometric factors: Factors that relate to the relationships of angles, lines, points, or surfaces that contribute to the quality of radiographic image definition.

Ghost image: Mirror or second image of a structure that is penetrated twice by the x-ray beam observed on panoramic radiographs.

Gingivitis: Inflammation of the gingiva.

Glenoid fossa: Depression on the temporal bone. The condyle of the mandible fits into this fossa to form the temporomandibular joint. Seen only on extraoral radiographs.

Globulomaxillary cyst: Type of nonodontogenic cyst arising between the maxillary lateral incisor and the canine.

Glossopharyngeal air space: Open space posterior to the tongue that continues into the oral-pharyngeal (throat) region. Appears as a radiolucest negative shadow on a panoramic radiograph.

Granuloma: A tumor or neoplasm made up of granulation tissue. Often follows an abscess. Usually round or oval and surrounded by a fibrous capsule. Appears radiolucent on a radiograph.

Gray (Gy): Système Internationale unit for measuring absorbed dose. One Gy equals 100 rads; 1,000 milligrays equals 1 Gy.

Gray scale: Refers to the total number of shades of gray visible in an image.

Grenz rays: *See* Soft radiation.

Grid: A device used in extraoral radiography to prevent scatter radiation from fogging the film.

Gutta percha: Endodontic filling material.

Half-value layer (HVL): Thickness of a specified material that, when introduced into the path of a given beam of radiation, reduces the exposure rate by half.

Halide: A compound of a halogen (astatine, bromine, chlorine, fluorine, or iodine) with another element or radical. Dental film emulsion is primarily, about 90 to 99 percent, silver bromide and 1 to 10 percent silver iodide.

Hamulus (hamular process): A very small hooklike process of bone that extends downward and slightly backward from the sphenoid bone. Appears radiopaque and can occasionally be seen posterior to the maxillary tuberosity.

Hard radiation: Rays of high energy and extremely short wavelengths. Essential for dental radiography.

Hardening agent (hardener): Potassium alum, one of the chemicals of the fixing solution. Functions to shrink and harden the wet emulsion.

Head positioner guides: Device used on panoramic and cephalometric x-ray machines to stabilize the patient's head in the correct position.

Health Insurance Portability and Accountability Act of 1996 (HIPAA): Federal law designed to provide patients with more control over how their personal health information is used and disclosed. A patient will usually be asked to sign a notice that indicates how their radiographs may be used and their privacy rights under this law.

Hepatitis B (HBV): Form of viral hepatitis. May be transferred between patient and oral healthcare professionals via contact with blood. Hepatitis B vaccine in a series of three doses is recommended to achieve immunity.

Herringbone pattern (also called tire-track pattern): Image produced on a radiograph when the film packet is placed in the mouth backwards. The embossed pattern in the lead foil produces this image when exposed.

Horizontal angulation: Direction of the central beam in a horizontal plane. Incorrect horizontal angulation results in overlapping the proximal structures.

Horizontal bitewing radiograph: Bitewing radiograph placed in the oral cavity with the long dimension of the film packet positioned horizontally. Considered the traditional placement for most patients.

Horizontal bone loss: Bone loss that occurs in a plane parallel to the cementoenamel junctions of adjacent teeth.

Horizontal placement: Act of positioning the film packet in the patient's oral cavity. In horizontal placement, the widest dimension of the film is positioned horizontally.

Human immunodeficiency virus (HIV): A type of retrovirus that causes AIDS (acquired immunodeficiency syndrome).

Hydroquinone: Reduces (converts) exposed silver halide crystals to black metallic silver. Slowly builds up black tones and contrast.

Hypercementosis: An excessive development of cementum that makes the tooth root appear bulbous. Most frequently observed on premolars. Appears radiopaque.

Hypersensitive gag reflex: Exaggerated gag response that is overly sensitive.

Identification dot: Small circular embossed mark on the corner of intraoral x-ray film. Used to determine the patient's right or left side when viewing radiographs.

Idiopathic resorption: Of unknown original. *See* External resorption and Internal resorption.

Immunization: Method, such as vaccines, of inducing resistance to an infectious disease.

Impacted tooth (impaction): A tooth embedded in alveolar bone in such a manner that its eruption is prevented. An impaction may be partial or total.

Impulse: Measure of exposure time. There are 60 impulses per second.

Incandescence: Stage when the tungsten filament in the cathode becomes red hot and glows. Free electrons are liberated and swarm around the glowing wire to form the electron cloud.

Incipient (enamel) caries: Caries beginning to appear or exist.

Incisive canal cyst: A type of non-odontogenic cyst arising in the incisive canal.

Incisive (anterior palatine) foramen: Maxillary landmark situated at the midline of the palate immediately behind the central incisors from which the nasopalatine nerve and vessels emerge. Shape varies but is usually observed as a round pea-shaped radiolucency. Incorrect horizontal angulation superimposes the incisive foramen over the apex of the root of the central incisor where it may then be mistaken for an abscess or a cyst.

Indicator ring: *See* External aiming device.

Indirect digital imaging: Method of obtaining a digital image in which an existing radiograph is scanned or photographed and then converted into a digital image.

Indirect theory: States that cell damage results indirectly when x-rays cause the formation of toxins in the cell such as hydrogen peroxide. Toxins in turn cause the cell damage.

Infection control: The prevention and reduction of disease-causing (pathogenic) microorganisms.

Infectious waste: Waste (such as blood, blood products, and contaminated sharps) that may contain pathogens.

Inferior border of the mandible: Dense layer of cortical bone that forms the lower portion of the body of the mandible. Appears very radiopaque on the radiograph.

Informed consent: Permission given by a patient after being informed of the details of a treatment procedure.

Inherent filtration: Filtration built into the x-ray machine by the manufacturer. This includes the glass x-ray tube envelope, the insulating materials of the tube head, and the materials that seal the port.

Intensifying screen: Plastic sheet coated with calcium tungstate or rare earth fluorescent salt crystals. Positioned in a cassette. When exposed to radiation, the fluorescent salts glow, giving off a blue (calcium tungstate) or green (rare earth) light. Produces a latent image faster than is possible when radiation alone is used.

Intensity: Intensity is the total energy of the x-ray beam. Intensity of the x-ray beam is the product of the number of x-rays (quantity) and energy of each x-ray (quality) per unit of area per time of exposure.

Interdental septa: Alveolar bone between adjacent teeth.

Internal oblique ridge: *See* Oblique ridge.

Internal resorption: Tooth structure lost through a resorptive process. Typically appears as a radiolucent widening of the root canal, representing the resorption process taking place from the inside out. Often the cause is idiopathic (unknown).

Interpersonal skills: Techniques that increase successful communication with others.

Interpret: To explain or to disclose meaning.

Interpretation: The ability to read what is revealed by the radiograph.

Interproximal: Between two adjacent tooth surfaces.

Interproximal caries: *See* proximal caries

Interproximal radiograph: *See* Bitewing radiograph.

Intraoral: Inside the mouth.

Intraoral film: Film that is placed in the oral cavity for exposure.

Intraoral radiograph: A radiograph produced when the film is placed within the mouth and exposed.

Intraosal radiography: Radiographic examinations where films are placed inside the mouth.

Inverse square law: States that the intensity of radiation is inversely proportional to the square of the distance from the source of the radiation to the point of measurement.

Inverted Y: Radiographic landmark made up of the lateral wall of the nasal Fossa and the anterior-medial wall of the maxillary sinus often observed near the canine-premolar region.

Ion: An electrically charged particle, either negative or positive.

Ion pair: A pair of ions, one positive and one negative.

Ionization: The formation of ion pairs.

Ionizing radiation: Radiation that is capable of producing ions.

Irradiation: The exposure of an object or a person to radiation. Term can be applied to radiations of various wavelengths, such as infrared rays, ultraviolet rays, x-rays, and gamma rays.

Irreparable injury: Following exposure to radiation, injury that results in damage that is not repaired during the recovery period. May give rise to later long-term effects of radiation exposure.

Isotope: Alternate form of an element, having the same number of protons but a different number of neutrons inside the nucleus. Many isotopes are radioactive.

Kilovolt (kV): A unit of electromotive force, equal to 1,000 volts. High kilovoltage is essential for the production of dental x-rays.

Kilovolt peak (kVp): The crest value in kilovolts of the potential difference of a pulsating generator.

Kinetic energy: Energy possessed by a mass because of its motion.

Labial mounting method: Radiographs mounted so that the embossed dot is convex. The viewer is reading the radiograph as if standing in front of, and facing, the patient. Recommended by the American Dental Association and the American Academy of Oral and Maxillofacial Radiology over the lingual mounting method.

Lamina dura: A thin, hard layer of cortical bone that lines the dental alveolus. Appears as a thin, radiopaque line around the roots of the teeth on dental radiographs.

Latent image: The invisible image produced when the film is exposed to x-ray photons. Image remains invisible until the film is processed.

Latent period: The time between exposure to radiation and the first clinically observable symptoms. Latent means hidden.

Lateral cephalometric radiograph: Extraoral radiograph of the side of the skull often used by orthodontists at various stages of treatment. Made by placing the patient's head in a cephalometer. Also called a lateral skull projection.

Lateral fossa: Slight decreased thickness (concavity) in bone between the maxillary lateral incisor and the maxillary canine.

Lateral jaw projection: Extraoral radiograph of the posterior mandible. Also called mandibular oblique lateral projection.

Lateral skull projection: *See* Lateral cephalometric radiograph.

Law of B and T (Bergonie and Tribondeau): States that "the radiosensitivity of cells and tissues is directly proportional to their reproductive capacity and inversely proportional to their degree of differentiation."

Lead apron: Protective barrier made of lead or lead-equivalent materials. Shields patients' gonadal areas from radiation during dental x-ray exposures.

Lead equivalent: The thickness of a material that affords the same degree of attenuation to radiation as a specified thickness of lead.

Lethal dose: The amount of radiation that is sufficient to cause the death of an organism.

Liable: To be legally obligated to make good any loss or damage that may occur.

Light-tight: Securing an area against all sources of white light. Characteristic of a darkroom.

Line pair: Refers to the number of paired lines visible in 1 mm of an image. The more line pairs visible, the better the spatial resolution in an image.

Line switch: Toggle switch that is used to turn the x-ray machine on or off.

Lingual caries: Caries that involves the lingual surface of a tooth.

Lingual foramen: A very small opening through which a branch of the incisive artery emerges. Located in the center of the genial tubercles on the lingual side of the mandible. *See* Genial tubercles.

Lingual mounting method: Radiographs are mounted so that the embossed dot is concave. The viewer is reading the radiograph as if standing behind the patient.

Localization: Methods to provide a third dimension to two-dimensional radiographs. Assists the radiographer in determining whether an object is located on the facial (buccal) or lingual.

Localized bone loss: Bone loss that occurs in isolated areas.

Long-scale contrast: Low-contrast image. A radiographic image with many shades of gray. Produced with high kilovoltage.

Mach band effect: An optical illusion that occurs along boundaries of sharp contrast. There appears to be a darker band along the edge of radiolucent areas and, similarly, a lighter band along the edge of radiopaque areas. The mach band effect is an edge enhancement, created in the eye, which does not result from an actual density change in the film emulsion

Magnetic resonance imaging (MRI): Technique for obtaining cross-sectional images of the human body. Does not use x-rays. Machine generates a magnetic field. Certain atoms within the body react to this magnetic field, and an image is produced.

Magnification (enlargement): Enlargement of the structures imaged on a radiograph over the actual size. Enlargement is greatest when the target of an x-ray machine is closer to the structures of interest, and is decreased when distance is greater.

Malignant: Tendency to progress in virulence and spread. Condition that may result in death.

Mal-posed tooth: A tooth not in its normal location.

Malpractice: Improper practice. Malpractice results when one is negligent.

Mandible: Lower arch (jaw).

Mandibular canal: Long canal extending from the mandibular foramen on the medial aspect of the ramus of the mandible to the mental foramen on the lateral aspect. Carries nerves and blood vessels that supply most of the teeth in the mandible. Appears radiolucent, with thin radiopaque lines above and below outlining the cortical bone that lines the canal.

Mandibular foramen: Small opening on the lateral side of the body of the mandible. Usually observed near the apices of the premolars.

Mandibular oblique lateral projection: *See* Lateral jaw projection.

Mastoid process: Large rounded protuberance of the temporal bone located behind the ear.

Maxilla: Upper arch. The maxillae are actually two bones, a right and left maxilla.

Maxillary sinus: Large radiolucent cavity observed within the maxilla apical to the maxillary posterior teeth.

Maxillary tuberosity: A radiopaque prominence of bone on the distal portion of the maxillary alveolar ridge.

Maximum permissible dose (MPD): The maximum accumulated dose that persons who are occupationally exposed may have at any given time of their life. It is the dose of ionizing radiation that, in the light of present knowledge, is not expected to cause detectable body damage. Currently established at 0.05 Sv per year (5 rem/year) whole body.

Mean tangent: Average point where several curved surfaces touch if a ruler is held against them. The labial or buccal surfaces of all teeth have their most prominent point toward the lips or the cheeks and curve toward the mesial or distal. A mean tangent would be established by using a small ruler or any straight edge (such as a tongue depressor) and attempting to align as many of the teeth as possible. Occasionally, four or even five of the posterior teeth will touch the ruler at some point. Used to establish correct horizontal angulation, which requires that the central ray of the x-ray beam be directed at right angles to the mean tangent

Median palatine suture: An irregular line formed by the junction of the palatine processes of the right and left maxillae. Appears as a thin radiolucent line running vertically between the roots of the maxillary incisors.

Mental foramen: An opening through which the mental nerve and related blood vessels emerge on the lateral aspect of the body of the mandible; exact location varies. When imaged on radiographs, appears as a small round radiolucent area near the roots of the mandibular premolars. Should not be mistaken for an abscess, cyst, or other pathological condition.

Mental fossa: A depression on the labial aspect of the mandibular incisor area.

Mental ridge: Raised ridge of bone located in the anterior region on the lateral surface of the mandible.

Mesiodens: A supernumerary tooth located in the maxillary midline.

Mesiodistal projection: When the projection angle of the x-ray beam is directed from mesial to distal resulting in overlapping error.

Microsievert (μSv): One millionth of a seivert. *See* Seivert.

Midsagittal plane (midsagittal line): An imaginary vertical line or plane passing through the center of the body that divides it into a right and left half. Important orientation line in determining the ideal position of the patient's head during radiographic exposures.

Milliampere (mA): One thousandth of an ampere. Milliamperage determines the number of electrons available at the filament. *See* Ampere.

Milliampere second (mAs): The relationship between the milliamperage and the exposure time in seconds. When one is increased, the other must be correspondingly decreased to maintain film density.

Modeling: Technique used to orient children to the radiographic procedure. Child is given the opportunity to observe procedure being performed on another, such as a sibling or parent. May help to alleviate fear of the unknown and gain patient cooperation.

Moderate caries: A classification of proximal surface caries. Category where caries penetrate over halfway through the enamel toward the dentinoenamel junction (DEJ), but does not reach the DEJ.

Molecule: Chemical combination of two or more atoms that forms the smallest particle of a substance that retains the properties of that substance.

Monitoring: Use of any of several devices to determine whether an area is within safe radiation limits or whether a person's exposure is within permissible limits. *See* Area monitoring and Personnel monitoring.

Motion: Movement of the film, patient, or tube head during radiographic exposure that results in a less sharp image.

Mount: To place radiographs in a film mount for viewing and interpretation.

MRI: *See* Magnetic resonance imaging.

Mylohyoid ridge: Raised ridge of bone running diagonally downward and forward on the medial aspect of the ramus of the mandible to near the apices of the molar roots. Parallels the (external) oblique ridge, but on the lingual surface and about 1/4 in (6 mm) lower. Appears radiopaque when observed on a radiograph.

Nasal bones: Bones that make up the upper bridge of the nose.

Nasal conchae: Thin bony extensions of the nasal wall.

Nasal fossa (cavity): Large air space divided into two paired radiolucencies by the radiopaque nasal septum. Visible above the roots of the maxillary incisors.

Nasal septum: Dense cartilage that separates the right nasal fossa from the left. Appears as a vertical radiopaque line separating the paired radiolucencies of the nasal cavity

Nasal spine: V-shaped projection from the floor of the nasal fossa in the midline. Appears as a triangle-shaped radiopacity.

Nasopharyngeal air space: Open space superior to the soft palate. Appears as a radiolucent negative shadow on a panoramic radiograph.

Negative angulation (negative vertical angulation): Achieved by pointing the tip or end of the PID upward from a horizontal plane.

Negative shadows: Term given to the radiolucencies produced on a panoramic radiograph as a result of more radiation reaching the film in the areas of air spaces. Negative shadows are shadows of "nothing."

Negligence: Failure to use a reasonable amount of care that results in injury or damage to another.

Neutron: One form of particulate (corpuscular) radiation or subatomic particle. A neutron has no electric charge and has about the same mass as a proton.

Nonmetallic restoration: Restoration containing no metal. May appear radiolucent, or radiopaque when radiopaque fillers have been added to the restorative material.

Nonodontogenic cyst: Cyst that arises from epithelium other than that associated with tooth formation.

Nonstochastic: *See* Deterministic.

Nonthreshold dose response curve: A graph showing the relationship between the dose of exposure and the response of the tissues, indicating that any amount of radiation, no matter how small, has the potential to cause a biological response.

Nonverbal communication: Communication achieved without words. Includes gestures, facial expressions, body movement, and listening.

Nutrient canal: Small tube-like passageway through bone that contains blood vessels and nerves. Appears radiolucent in radiographs.

Nutrient foramen: Occasionally imaged on a radiograph as a tiny radiolucent dot indicating the small opening in the tube-like passageway of a nutrient canal.

Object-film distance: Distance between the object being radiographed and the film.

Oblique ridge: Diagonal ridge of bone on the lateral aspect of the mandible that runs downward and forward from the anterior border of the ramus to the level of the cervical portion of the molar and premolar roots. Sometimes referred to as the external oblique ridge. The internal oblique ridge appears faintly parallel to the external oblique ridge. The internal oblique ridge is not identified as an anatomical structure, but as a landmark only.

Occipital bone: Forms the posterior part of the skull.

Occipital protuberance: A bulge or prominence at the center of the outer surface of the occipital bone. The location of this protuberance can be determined by palpating the back of the patient's head.

Occlusal caries: Caries found on the occlusal (chewing) surface of posterior teeth.

Occlusal plane: Plane between the maxillary and the mandibular teeth.

Occlusal radiograph: Radiograph produced by placing the film against the incisal or occlusal plane. The patient stabilizes the film packet by biting down on it. In addition to the teeth, occlusal radiographs may show surrounding maxillary or mandibular structures. Depending on the film placement and angle of exposure, cross-sectional or topographic radiographs are produced. *See* Cross-sectional technique and Topographical technique.

Occlusal trauma: Excessive or repetitive force against the teeth that results in a response.

Occupational exposure (infection control definition): A worker (oral healthcare professionals) coming in contact with blood, saliva, or other infectious material that involves the skin, eye, or mucus membrane.

Odontogenic cyst: A cyst that arises from epithelial cells associated with the development of a tooth.

Odontoma: A tumor of odontogenic origin in which enamel and dentin are formed. May contain soft tissues that appear radiolucent and a hard calcified mass, sometimes resembling a tooth, which appears radiopaque. Compound odontoma refers to odontogenic tissues that resemble teeth. Complex odontoma denotes odontogenic tissues arranged in a haphazard manner with no resemblance to tooth formation. Compound-complex odontoma is a mixture of the two types.

Open mouth projection: *See* Reverse-Towne projection.

Oral radiography: Procedures that pertain to producing radiographs of the teeth and/or the oral cavity.

Ossification: The pathological or abnormal conversion of soft tissues into bone.

Osteosclerosis: Abnormal increase in bone density. Appears as in increased radiopacity on a radiograph.

Output: The amount of radiation that an x-ray machine produces, calculated in coulombs per kilogram per second (roentgens per second), measured at the open end of the PID.

Overdevelopment: Leaving the film in the developer solution too long or using developer that is too warm. Overdevelopment results in a dark image.

Overexposure: Exposing the film too long or subjecting the film to an inappropriately increased kVp or mA setting. Overexposure results in a dark image.

Overhang: A restoration that is not contoured to the tooth properly.

Overlapping: Term used to refer to a distortion of the tooth image in which the structures of one tooth are superimposed over the structures of the adjacent tooth. Most often caused by incorrect horizontal angulation of the central beam.

Oxidation: The process during which the chemicals of the developing and fixing solutions combine with oxygen and lose their strength.

Palatoglossal air space: Open space between the tongue and palate. Appears as a radiolucent negative shadow on a panoramic radiograph.

Panoramic radiograph: Generic term pertaining to the radiographic image produced by a panorauic x-ray machine. Images all the teeth and supporting structures of the maxilla and Mardilde on one Film.

Panoramic radiography: Procedure performed with a special-purpose x-ray machine that uses a fixed position of the x-ray source, object, and film to produce a radiograph of the entire dentition and surrounding structures on a single film.

Paralleling technique: Intraoral technique where the film packet is positioned parallel to the long axes of the teeth while the central beam of radiation is directed perpendicularly (at right angles) toward the teeth and the film.

Parenteral exposure: Exposure to blood that results from puncturing the skin barrier.

Particulate radiation (corpuscular radiation): Minute subatomic particles such as protons, electrons, and neutrons; also alpha and beta particles. These particles occupy space; have mass and weight; and, with the exception of neutrons, have an electrical charge.

Pathogen: A disease-causing microorganism.

Patient education: Informing patients about the benefits of oral health and preventive oral hygiene. Providing the patient with necessary information that explains the value of dental radiographs and demonstrates radiation safety measures employed in the practice.

Patient relations: Establishment of the relationship between the patient and the oral healthcare professional.

Pediatric dentistry: Branch of dentistry that specializes in providing comprehensive preventive and therapeutic oral healthcare for children.

Pedodontic film: Any smaller sized film packet used for radiographs of children's teeth.

Penumbra: Partial shadow or fuzzy outline around the image.

Periapical radiograph: Image that shows the entire tooth or teeth and surrounding tissues. Peri means "around" and apical is the root end of the tooth.

Period of injury: Radiation-induced changes that follow the latent period.

Periodontal diseases: Diseases that affects the supporting tissues of the teeth.

Periodontal ligament space: The space between the root of a tooth and the lamina dura where the thin but dense and strong fibrous tissues of the periodontal ligament are located. Radiographically, the periodontal ligament appears as a thin radiolucent line between the lamina dura and the root.

Periodontitis: Inflammation of the periodontium.

Periodontium: Tissues that invest and support the teeth (gingiva and alveolar bone).

Permanent teeth: Teeth that erupt after the primary teeth have been exfoliated (shed). Consists of 32 teeth—8 incisors, 4 canines, 8 premolars, and 12 molars.

Personnel monitoring: The occasional or routine measuring of the amount of radiation to which a person working around radiation has been exposed during a given period of time.

Personnel monitoring device: Device (usually a film badge or thermoluminescent dosimeter [TLD]) worn by a radiation worker to measure the amount of radiation received in a given period of time.

Phleboliths: Calcified masses that are observed as round or oval bodies in the soft tissues of the cheeks.

Phosphors: Fluorescent crystals, calcium tungstate or rare earth, used in the emulsion that coats intensifying screens. Give off light when subjected to radiation.

Photoelectric effect: An attenuation process for x- and gamma radiation in which a photon interacts with an orbital electron of an atom. All of the energy of the photon is absorbed by the displaced electron in the form of kinetic energy.

Photon (x-ray photon): A quantum of energy. Both x-rays and gamma rays are photons.

Photo stimulable phosphors (PSP): Digital imaging sensors that use rare earth phosphor (barium europium fluorohalide) coated plates. When exposed to x-rays, the PSP sensor or plate "stores" the x-ray energy until stimulated by a laser beam to produce a digital image.

PID: *See* Position indicating device.

Pixel: Small, discrete units of digital information that together constitute an image. Pixel is a term shortened from the words "picture" and "element" (pix = plural of picture; el = element).

Point of entry: Spot on the surface of the face toward which the central beam of radiation is directed when aligning the PID for intraoral exposures.

Polychromatic: A term derived from the Greek meaning "having many colors." Used in dental radiography to describe the x-ray beam because it is composed of many different wavelengths.

Port: Opening in the tube head that is covered with a permanent seal of glass, beryllium, or aluminum through which the x-rays exit. The port is opposite the window in the x-ray tube and is the place where the PID attaches to the tube head.

Position indicating device (PID): Also called beam indicating device (BID). An open-ended, cylindrical or rectangular device attached to the tube head at the aperture to direct the useful beam of radiation. PIDs are available in different lengths.

Positive angulation (positive vertical angulation): Angulation achieved by pointing the end of the PID downward from a horizontal plane.

Post and core: Metal restorative material used in an endodontically treated tooth when support for a crown is needed. Appears radiopaque.

Posteroanterior cephalometric radiograph: Extraoral radiograph of the entire skull in the posteroanterior plane. Also called a posterior-anterior projection (PA).

Posteroanterior projection (PA): *See* Posterioanterior cephalometric radiograph.

Potassium alum: One of the components of fixer solution. Shrinks and hardens the gelatin emulsion.

Potassium bromide: Restrains the developing agents from developing the unexposed silver halide crystals.

Pre-disposing factors: Amalgam overhangs, poorly contoured crown margins, and calculus deposits that act as food traps and lead to the build-up of bacterial deposits that cause periodontal disease.

Preservative: One of the chemicals (sodium sulfite) used in both the developer and fixer solutions to slow down the rate of oxidation and prevent spoilage of the solution.

Pressure mark: A black (radiolucent) line that appears on a processed film at the point where a film packet was bent or subjected to excessive pressure.

Primary beam (primary radiation or useful beam): The original undeflected useful beam of radiation that emanates at the focal spot of the x-ray tube and emerges through the aperture of the tube head.

Primary radiation: *See* Primary beam.

Primary teeth: Teeth that fall out or are exfoliated naturally. Consists of 20 teeth—8 incisors, 4 canines, and 8 molars.

Process: Anatomical prominent outgrowth of bone. May be rounded or pointed. Processes of dental importance include alveolar, coronoid, hamular (hamulus), mastoid, and styloid. All appear radiopaque.

Processing: The act of bringing out the latent image and making it permanently visible. Includes the following darkroom procedures: developing, rinsing, fixing, washing, and drying.

Processing tank: Stainless steel receptacle divided into compartments for developer solution, water rinse, and fixer solution. Used to process radiographs.

Protective barrier: Shield of radiation-absorbing material used to protect against radiation exposure.

Proton: A subatomic particle of the atom. The proton is contained in the nucleus and has a positive electrical charge. The proton has mass and weight. The number of protons determines the chemical element.

Proximal caries: Caries found on the proximal surfaces between two adjacent teeth.

Pterygoid plates: Extensions of the sphenoid bone.

Pulp chamber (cavity): Noncalcified tooth tissue containing blood vessels and nerves. Appears radiolucent, as this soft tissue offers only minimal resistance to the passage of x-rays.

Pulp stone: Calcification that appears in the pulp chamber of the teeth, caused by an abnormal disposition of calcium salts. Often described as nodules or denticles. Seen on radiographs as one or more small radiopaque, irregularly shaped, rounded masses within the pulp chamber.

Quality: Term used when describing the intensity of the x-ray beam. Refers to the number of x-rays in the beam.

Quality assurance: The planning, implementation, and evaluation of procedures used to produce high-quality radiographs with maximum diagnostic information while minimizing radiation exposure.

Quality control: A series of tests to assure that the radiographic system is functioning properly and that the radiographs produced are of an acceptable level of quality.

Quantity: Term used when describing the intensity of the x-ray beam. Refers to the penetrating ability of the beam.

Rad: Traditional unit for measuring absorbed dose. 100 rads equals one gray (Gy). One rad equals 0.01 Gy. 1,000 millirads equals 1 rad.

Radiation: The emission and propagation of energy through space or through a material medium in the form of electromagnetic waves, corpuscular emissions such as alpha and beta particles, or rays of mixed and unknown types such as cosmic rays. Most radiations used in dentistry are capable of producing ions directly or indirectly by interaction with matter.

Radiation leakage: Refers to the x-rays that escape out of the tube head at places other than the port.

Radiation worker: Professional who works with or around ionizing radiation or equipment that produces ionizing radiation.

Radiator: A large mass of copper just outside the x-ray tube and connected to the anode terminal. The radiator functions to carry off the excess heat produced in the energy exchange that takes place when the electrons of the cathode stream are converted into about 1% x-rays and 99% heat. The radiator conducts the heat away from the target and cools the tube.

Radicular cyst: A cyst around the apex of a tooth. Generally observed as a small radiolucent circular area that extends away from the apical portions of the root. The sac of the cyst has a distinct wall or capsule that surrounds it and can be distinguished as a faint radiopaque thin line.

Radioactivity: The process whereby certain unstable elements undergo spontaneous disintegration (decay). The process is accompanied by emissions of one or more types of radiation and generally results in the formation of a new isotope.

Radiograph: An image produced on photosensitive film by exposure to x-rays. Developing the film produces a negative image that can be viewed and interpreted.

Radiographer: Professional operating x-ray equipment to make radiographs.

Radiographic contrast: *See* Contrast.

Radiography (roentgenography): The making of radiographs by exposing and processing x-ray film.

Radiology: That branch of medical science that deals with the use of radiant energy in the diagnosis and treatment of disease.

Radiolucent: That portion of the radiograph that is dark. Structures that lack density permit the passage of x-rays with little or no resistance. These structures appear dark on the image.

Radiopaque: That portion of the radiograph that appears light. Dense structures resist the passage of radiation. These structures appear light on the image.

Radioresistant: Refers to a substance or tissue that is not easily injured by ionizing radiation.

Radiosensitive: Refers to a substance or tissue that is relatively susceptible to injury by ionizing radiation.

Rampant caries: Severe, unchecked caries that affect multiple teeth.

Ramus: The ascending portion of each end of the mandible.

Rapid processing: The use of concentrated and/or heated developer to quickly process working films, often with the use of a chairside darkroom.

Rare-earth phosphors: Salt crystals, usually lanthanum (La) and gadolinium (Gd), used to coat intensifying screens. When these absorb x-rays, they fluoresce and emit energy in the form of green light.

Recovery period: Period following exposure to radiation, where some healing can take place.

Rectification: The unidirectional current inside the x-ray tube from the cathode to the anode.

Rectifier: A device within the vacuum tube for converting alternating to direct current.

Recurrent (secondars) caries Caries that occurs under a restoration or around its margins.

Reference film: A radiograph processed under ideal conditions and then used to compare periodically subsequent films. Quality control procedure to monitor processing solution quality.

Rem (roentgen equivalent man): Traditional unit for measuring dose equivalent. Used to compare the biological effects of the various types of radiation. One rem equals 1 rad times a biological effect weighting factor. Since the weighting factor for x- and gamma radiation equals 1, the number of rems is identical to the absorbed dose in rads for these radiations. 100 rem equals one sievert (Sv); one rem equals 0.01 Sv; 1,000 millirems equal 1 rem.

Replenisher: A superconcentrated solution of developer or fixer that is added daily, or as indicated, to the developer or fixer in the processing tank to compensate for loss of volume and loss of strength from oxidation. The act of adding replenisher to the processing solutions is known as replenishment.

Residual cyst: Cyst that remains in the jaw after the tooth that caused it to form is extracted or exfoliated. May remain within the bone, becoming encapsulated with an epithelial lining, or may undergo considerable growth. Appears radiolucent and the lining of the cyst appears as a thin radiopaque line.

Resolution: The discernable separation of closely adjacent image details.

Resorption: Refers to a loss of bone or tooth structure. May originate from natural causes such as the gradual reduction of size of the roots of primary teeth, or may be idiopathic (the result of unknown causes).

Restrainer: Potassium bromide in the developer solution that slows down the action of the elon and hydroquinone and inhibits the tendency of the solution to chemically fog the films.

Retained root: Root remaining after the tooth has been extracted.

Re-take radiographs: Radiographs that have been taken after the first images are deemed undiagnostic.

Retention pin: Metal pin used to support a restoration.

Reticulation: Cracking of the film emulsion caused by a great temperature difference between the developer and the rinse water.

Reverse-Towne radiograph: Extraoral projection used to view the condylar neck of the mandible. Also called open mouth projection.

Rhinoliths: Calcifications within the maxillary sinuses.

Ridge: An extended elevation or crest of bone. On dental radiographs, ridges appear radiopaque.

Rigid cassette: Cardboard panels that are hinged together with a metal clasp that tightly locks. Holds an extraoral film in light-tight conditions for exposure.

Risk: The chance or likelihood of adverse effects or death resulting from exposure to a hazard.

Risk management: Policies and procedures to be followed by the radiographer to reduce the chances that a patient will file legal action against the dentist and oral healthcare team.

Roentgen (R): Traditional unit measurement of exposure to radiation. Measured in air. A simplified definition of the roentgen is the amount of x-radiation or gamma radiation required to ionize 1 cc of air at standard conditions of pressure and temperature (2.083 billion ion pairs).

Roentgen ray: *See* X-ray.

Roentgenograph: *See* Radiograph.

Roller transport system: Moves films through the developer, fixer, water, and drying compartments of an automatic processor. Motor-driven gears or belts propel the roller transport system.

Root canal treatment: *See* Endodontic therapy.

Root surface caries: *See* Cemental caries.

Rotational center: The axis on which the panoramic tube head and the drum rotate. Based on tomographic radiography principles.

Rotational panoramic radiography: Radiographic projection technique that utilizes a narrow beam of x-rays to image a curved layer of tissue.

Rule of isometry: Geometric theorem stating that two triangles with two equal angles and a common side are equal triangles. This theorem is the basis of the bisecting technique.

Safelight: Special filtered light that can be left on in the darkroom while films are processed.

Safelight filter: Removes short wavelengths in the blue-green region of visible light. The longer wavelength red-orange light is allowed to pass through the filter, illuminating the darkroom without fogging the film.

Sanitation: Reducing microorganisms to a level of concentration considered to be safe.

Sarcoma: Malignant tumor of connective tissue origin.

Scatter radiation: Radiation that has been deflected from its path by impact during its passage through matter. This form of secondary radiation is scattered in all directions by the tissues of the patient's head.

Sclerotic bone: A hardening of the bone as a result of inflammation or excessive growth of fibrous tissue and deposition of mineral salts. *See* Condensing osteitis.

Screen film: Extraoral film for use in cassettes with intensifying screens. Emulsion is more sensitive to green, blue, and violet light, emitted when the radiation strikes the phosphors in the intensifying screens than to the x-radiation.

Secondary radiation: Given off by any matter irradiated with x-rays. Created at the instant the primary beam interacts with matter and gives off some of its energy, forming new and less powerful wavelengths. Often referred to as scatter radiation.

Selection criteria: Guidelines developed by an expert panel of healthcare professionals to assist in deciding when, what type, and how many radiographs should be taken.

Selective reduction: Chemical change that takes place within the film emulsion during development. During this change, the non-metallic elements are separated from the silver halide of the exposed crystals, leaving a coating of metallic silver on the film emulsion while the bromide is removed. The process is called selective because the unexposed grains are not reduced.

Self-determination: The legal right of an individual to make choices concerning health care treatment.

Sensor: For use in digital imaging. An electronic or specially coated plate that is sensitive to x-rays. Placed intraorally to capture a radiographic image when exposed to x-rays.

Sepsis: Infection, or the presence of septic matter.

Septum: Thin wall of bone that acts as a partition to separate the nasal cavity or the maxillary sinuses. Appears radiopaque.

Severe caries: A classification of proximal surface caries. Category where caries has penetrated over halfway through the dentin toward the pulp.

Shadow casting: Principle that x-rays cast shadows of images onto the film, producing a radiographic image of the teeth and supporting structures.

Sharp: Any object that can penetrate the skin, such as a needle or scalpel.

Sharpness (*See* Definition): The distinct outlines of structures observed on a radiograph.

Short-scale contrast: High-contrast image. A radiograph that exhibits black and white with few shades. Produced with low kilovoltage.

"Show-Tell-Do": Technique used to orient the patient, especially children to the radiographic procedure. Showing the radiographic equipment—film, film holder, and x-ray machine—to the patient while explaining their use may help to alleviate fear of the unknown and gain patient cooperation.

Sialolith: A salivary calculus or hardened, stonelike mass that forms within the passage of the salivary ducts. If sufficiently large, such masses appear slightly radiopaque on the radiograph.

Sievert (Sv): Systeme Internationale unit for measuring the dose equivalent. The sievert is used to compare the biological effects of various types of radiation. One sievert equals one gray times a biological effect weighting (qualifying) factor. Because the weighting factor for x- and gamma radiation equals 1, the number of sieverts is identical to the absorbed dose in grays for these radiations. One sievert equals 100 rem. *See* Microsievert.

Sigmoid mandibular notch: Notch between the condyle and coronoid process of the mandible.

Silver halide crystals: Compounds of a halogen (either bromine or iodine) with silver. Dental film emulsion is approximately 90 to 99 percent silver bromide and 1 to 10 percent silver iodide. Silver halide crystals are sensitive to radiation. It is the silver halide crystals that, when exposed to x-rays, retain the latent image.

Silver point: Endodontic filling material.

Sinus (maxillary): Large cavity within the body of the maxilla. Appears as a large radiolucency.

Sinus projection: *See* Waters radiograph.

SLOB: Stands for same on lingual, opposite on buccal. Used in localization techniques to determine the facial (buccal) or lingual position of objects. The tube shift method of localization states that if the structure or object in question appears to move in the same direction as the horizontal or vertical shift of the tube, then the structure or object is located on the lingual. Conversely, if the move is in the opposite direction of the shift of the tube, the object is located on the buccal (facial).

Sodium carbonate: Provides required alkalinity of the developer solution to activate developing agents.

Sodium sulfite: Chemical of the developing solution that prevents rapid oxidation of the developing agents.

Sodium thiosulfate: Chemical of the fixer solution that together with the ammonium thiosulfate removes the unexposed and any remaining undeveloped silver halide crystals.

Soft radiation: Longest wavelength of the x-rays. Removed from the polychromatic beam by filtration because soft radiation (Grenz rays) have no value in producing dental radiographs.

Solarized emulsion: Used for duplicating film. Produces a duplicate image that gets lighter the longer the film is exposed to light. Darker images result from shorter exposure times.

Somatic cells: Any body cells except the reproductive cells.

Somatic effect: When radiation affects all body cells except the reproductive cells.

Spatial resolution: Refering to digital imaging. The sharpness of the image is determined by the number and size of pixels and measured in line pairs. When the number of pixels is low, the image appears to have jagged edges and is difficult to see. The greater the spatial resolution, the sharper the image appears.

Speech reading: Method of lip reading used by the hearing impaired.

Sphenoid bone: Cranial bone bordered by the frontal and ethmoid bones.

Split image: Panoramic radiograph with a blank or clear area in the middle of the film. Produced by a panoramic unit with a double-rotation center. The blank middle of the film results when the radiation output is shut off while the unit switches to the second rotation center.

Standard precautions: A practice of care to protect persons from pathogens spread via blood or any other body fluid, excretion, or secretion (except sweat). All-inclusive term that has replaced universal precautions, where the focus was on blood-borne pathogens.

Static electricity: A white-light spark that creates a radiolucent artifact on the film.

Statute of limitations: Time period during which a person may bring a malpractice action against another person.

Step-down transformer (low-voltage transformer): Device consisting of two metal cores and coils so positioned within the circuitry of the tube head to decrease the line voltage to between 3 and 12 volts. Low voltage is required in the cathode to warm up the filament wire.

Step-up transformer (high-voltage transformer): Device consisting of two metal cores and coils positioned within the circuitry of the tube head to increase the potential of the line current to the high kilovoltage required to produce x-radiation.

Step-wedge (penetrometer): A device consisting of increasing increments of an absorbing material. A radiographic exposure made with a step-wedge is used to determine the amount of radiation reaching the film through each of the increments. Measurements of film density may be used to evaluate the intensity and penetrative power of the radiation.

Sterilization: The total destruction of spores and disease-producing microorganisms.

Stochastic effect: When a biological response is based on the probability of occurrence rather than the severity of the change.

Structural shielding: The protection afforded by building materials found in walls, partitions, and cabinetry, present in most buildings where dental radiographs are exposed.

Styloid process: Long, narrow spine that extends downward, from the inferior surface of the temporal bone, just anterior to the mastoid process.

Subject contrast: The difference in density of a radiograph caused by the differing thicknesses of the tissues or objects radiographed.

Submandibular fossa: Irregular depression in the bone near the angle on the lingual of the mandible. Usually observed radiographically below the roots of the molars and extending forward as far as the premolar region. Thin and offering little resistance to the passage of the x-rays, it appears radiolucent.

Submentovertex projection: Extraoral projection showing the base of the skull, the position of the mandibular condyles, and the zygomatic arches. Also called a base projection.

Supernumerary teeth: Extra teeth not normally a part of the dentition. May resemble normal teeth, only smaller with conical crowns, or bear no resemblance to a normal tooth. Often malpositioned or unerupted.

Suture: A line of union of adjacent cranial or facial bones that appears radiolucent on radiographs.

Symphysis: Prominent bone where the right and left sides of the mandible fuse at the midline.

Système Internationale (SI): A metric system of units of that measures radiation quantities. The Système Internationale units are coulombs per kilogram (C/kg), gray (Gy), and sievert (Sv).

Target: Small block of tungsten imbedded in the face of the anode, bombarded by the electrons streaming from the cathode. The focal spot is located on the target.

Target–film distance (source–film distance): Distance between the focal spot on the target and the recording plane of the film.

Target–object distance (source–object distance): Distance between the focal spot on the target and the object being radiographed.

Target–surface distance (source–surface distance): Distance between the focal spot on the target and the skin surface of the patient.

Taurodontia: Teeth characterized by very large pulp chambers and very short roots.

Temporal bone: Cranial bone the makes up the temple, or side of the face. Contains the ear structures, including the auditory meatus.

Temporomandibular disorders (TMD): Currently the accepted term to describe the collection of symptoms and diseases that are generally found involving the temporomandibular joint.

Temporomandibular joint (TMJ): One of two joints connecting the mandible to the temporal bone.

Temporomandibular joint projection: *See* Transcranial radiograph.

Thermionic emission: The release of electrons when a material such as tungsten is heated to incandescence. Electrons are boiled off from the cathode filament in the x-ray tube when electric current is passed through it.

Thermoluminescent dosimeter (TLD): Monitoring device containing certain crystalline compounds (usually lithium fluoride) that store energy when struck by x-rays. When heated, the crystals give off light in proportion to the amount of radiation exposure.

Threshold dose response curve: A graph showing the relationship between the dose of exposure and the response of the tissues, indicating that there is a "threshold" amount of radiation, below which no biological response would be expected.

Thyroid collar: An attached or detachable supplement to the lead apron. Contains 0.25 mm lead or lead-equivalent materials to protect the radiosensitive thyroid gland in the neck region during the exposure of intraoral radiographs.

Timer: A mechanical, electrical, or electronic device that can be set to pre-determine the duration of the interval that current flows through the x-ray machine to produce x-rays.

Time–temperature: Principle of film processing. The length of time the film spends in the developer is based on the temperature of the developer solution. When the temperature is cool, processing time is increased. When the temperature is warm, processing time is decreased. Film manufacturer will usually recommend an ideal temperature and time that will produce quality images.

Tomograph: A radiograph made using the tomography technique.

Tomography: A radiographic technique used to show detailed images of structures located within a predetermined plane of tissue while eliminating or blurring those structures in the planes not selected.

Topographical technique: Occlusal radiography technique that follows the rules of bisecting. The central rays of the x-ray beam are directed through the apices of the teeth perpendicularly toward the bisector to produce an image.

Tori (torus-singular): Outgrowth of bone called exostosis.

Torus mandibularis (lingual torus): Hard, bony protuberance on the lingual surface of the mandible. Usually located above the mylohyoid line near the premolars. Often bilateral.

Torus palatinus: Hard, bony protuberance on the midline of the maxilla.

Total filtration: The combination of inherent and added filtration in an x-ray machine. Many states require a total filtration of 2.5 mm of aluminum equivalent for x-ray machines operating at or above 70 kVp.

Trabecular bone (cancellous bone): The softer spongy bone that makes up the bulk of the inside portion of most bones. The cells of trabecular bone vary in size and density.

Tragus: Small cartilaginous prominence of tissues located near the center and in front of the acoustic meatus (outer ear opening).

Transcranial projection: Extraoral projection used to image the temporomandibular joint (TMJ) in both an open and closed position. Also called a TMJ projection.

Transformer: One of several types of electrical devices capable of increasing or decreasing the voltage of an alternating current by mutual induction between primary and secondary coils or windings on cores of metal. *See* High-voltage transformer and Low-voltage transformer.

Transitional (mixed) dentition: Having both primary and permenent teeth present in the oral cavity. Usually exists between 6 and 12 years of age.

Triangulation: Widening of the periodontal ligament space at the crest of the interproximal bone.

Tube head (tube housing): Protective metal covering that contains the x-ray tube, the high-voltage and low-voltage transformers, and insulating oil. Attached to the flexible extension arm by a yoke. The PID attaches to the tube head at the port.

Tube shift method: Method of localization. *See* Buccal-object rule.

Tube side: Describes the side of an intraoral film packet or extraoral cassette that must face the source of x-rays coming from the tube.

Tubercle: Rounded eminence on a bone.

Tuberosity: Broad eminence on a bone.

Tumor: Swelling or a growth of tissue.

Tungsten (Wolfram): Element with an atomic number of 74. High melting point makes this metal ideal for use as the cathode filament and as the anode target.

Underdevelopment: Not leaving the film in the developer solution long enough or using developer that is too cool or an old, weak solution. Underdevelopment results in a light image.

Underexposure: Not exposing the film long enough or using an inappropriately decreased kVp or mA setting. Underexposure results in a light image.

Universal precautions: A method of infection control in which blood and certain body fluids are treated as if known to be infectious for HIV, HBV, and other bloodborne pathogens. The all-inclusive term standard precautions has replaced universal precautions, where the focus is on bloodborne pathogens.

Useful beam (useful radiation): That part of the primary beam that is permitted to emerge from the tube head and limited by the port, collimator, and lead-lined PID.

Velocity: Property exhibited by electromagnetic radiation. Refers to the speed of the wave as it travels through space. In a vacuum, all electromagnetic radiations travel at the speed of light (186,000 miles/sec or 3×10^8 m/sec).

Verbal communication: Using words to exchange information between two or more persons.

Vertical angulation: The direction of the central beam in an up or down direction achieved by directing the tip of the PID upward or downward. *See* Negative angulation and Positive angulation.

Vertical bone loss (angular bone loss): Occurs in a vertical direction. Alveolar crest is reduced in a manner that creates angular defects.

Vertical bitewing radiograph: Bitewing radiograph placed in the oral cavity with the long dimension of the film packet positioned vertically. Covers an increased area in the vertical dimension, resulting in more information regarding the periodontium being recorded on the film.

Vertical bitewing series: A set of 4 to 7 vertical bitewings. May include both posterior and anterior images.

Vertical placement: *See* Film placement.

Viewbox: Device used to view dental radiographs. Consists of a light source illuminator behind an opaque glass.

Volt: Unit of electromotive force or potential that is sufficient to cause a current of 1 ampere (A) to flow through a resistance of 1 ohm (W).

Voltage: Electrical pressure or force that drives the electric current through the circuit of the x-ray machine. *See* Kilovolt and Kilovolt peak.

Voltmeter: Device for measuring the electromotive force (the difference in potential or voltage) across the x-ray tube.

Waters radiograph: Also called the sinus projection. Similar to the posteroanterior cephalometric radiograph except that the center of interest is focused on the middle third of the face.

Wavelength: In radiography, the length in angstrom units or centimeters of the electromagnetic radiations produced in the x-ray machine. The distance from the crest, or top of one wave to the crest of the next, determines the wavelength—hence its penetration ability.

Weighting factor (qualifying factor): Used to convert absorbed dose to dose equivalent. Takes into consideration the difference in biological effectiveness of various types of radiation (x-, gamma, alpha, beta, etc). Some radiations (such as alpha particles) cause more biological damage than others (such as x-rays). The qualifying factor for dental x-rays is 1; for alpha particles it is 10.

Wet reading: Viewing a radiograph under white light conditions after only two or three minutes of fixation. Used when a diagnosis from the radiograph is needed quickly. Following the wet reading, the film must be returned to the fixer to complete processing.

Working radiograph: A film that is rapidly processed when information is needed quickly. Often used during endodontic procedures. However, short developing and fixing times, combined with minimal washing, result in a substandard radiograph.

X-ray (roentgen ray): Radiant energy of short wavelength that has the power to penetrate substances and to record shadow images on photographic film.

X-ray film: *See* Radiograph and Film packet.

X-ray tube: Electronic tube located in the tube head that generates x-rays.

Yoke: Curved portion of the x-ray machine that is connected to the extension arm. The tube head is suspended within the yoke and can be rotated vertically and horizontally within it.

Zygoma: Cheek bone. Attaches to the zygomatic process of the temporal bone to form the zygomatic arch.

Zygomatic arch: Arch formed by the temporal process of the zygomatic bone and the zygomatic process of the temporal bone. Forms the outer margin of the cheek prominence.

Zygomatic process: Process of the temporal bone that attaches to the zygoma to form the zygomatic arch.

Index

Q

R

T

U

V

W